AF899231

SEX HORMONES

Edited by **Raghvendra K. Dubey**

Sex Hormones
Edited by Raghvendra K. Dubey

Published by InTech
Janeza Trdine 9, 51000 Rijeka, Croatia

Copyright © 2012 InTech
All chapters are distributed under the Creative Commons Attribution 3.0 license, which allows users to download, copy and build upon published articles even for commercial purposes, as long as the author and publisher are properly credited, which ensures maximum dissemination and a wider impact of our publications. After this work has been published by InTech, authors have the right to republish it, in whole or part, in any publication of which they are the author, and to make other personal use of the work. Any republication, referencing or personal use of the work must explicitly identify the original source.

As for readers, this license allows users to download, copy and build upon published chapters even for commercial purposes, as long as the author and publisher are properly credited, which ensures maximum dissemination and a wider impact of our publications.

Notice
Statements and opinions expressed in the chapters are these of the individual contributors and not necessarily those of the editors or publisher. No responsibility is accepted for the accuracy of information contained in the published chapters. The publisher assumes no responsibility for any damage or injury to persons or property arising out of the use of any materials, instructions, methods or ideas contained in the book.

Publishing Process Manager Maja Kisic

Technical Editor Teodora Smiljanic

Cover Designer InTech Design Team

Additional hard copies can be obtained from orders@intechopen.com

Sex Hormones, Edited by Raghvendra K. Dubey
p. cm.
ISBN 978-953-307-856-4

We are IntechOpen, the world's leading publisher of Open Access books

Built by scientists, for scientists

4,000+
Open access books available

116,000+
International authors and editors

120M+
Downloads

151
Countries delivered to

Our authors are among the
Top 1%
most cited scientists

12.2%
Contributors from top 500 universities

CLARIVATE ANALYTICS BOOK CITATION INDEX INDEXED

WEB OF SCIENCE™

Selection of our books indexed in the Book Citation Index
in Web of Science™ Core Collection (BKCI)

Interested in publishing with us?
Contact book.department@intechopen.com

Numbers displayed above are based on latest data collected.
For more information visit www.intechopen.com

For EU product safety concerns:
IN TECH d.o.o., Prolaz Marije Krucifikse Kozulić 3, 51000 Rijeka, Croatia,
info@intechopen.com or visit our website at intechopen.com.

Meet the editor

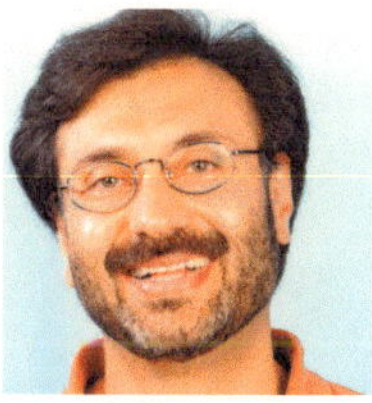

Dr Raghvendra K. Dubey is currently a professor at the Clinic for Reproductive Endocrinology, University Hospital, Zurich. Born in Lucknow, India, he completed his education there, and later obtained his Masters degree in Biochemistry (MSc) from Lucknow University, and went on to earn his PhD from Kanpur University in India. Subsequently, he completed a three year postdoctoral fellowship in Clinical Pharmacology at Vanderbilt University, USA, and later joined the Department of Medicine at West Virginia University as Assistant Professor. After three years, he joined University of Basel as a visiting Professor, and later became Associate Professor at the Department of Medicine in the University of Pittsburgh Medical Center. His current research topic is to study the role of sex hormones in various pathophysiologies, with specific relevance to women's health. He has published more than 100 original peer reviewed papers, several reviews, and book chapters. He is a fellow of the American Heart Association, a member of the American Endocrine Society, and the American Physiological Society. He held a joint associate professorship from 1996 -2010 at the Center for Clinical Pharmacology, Department of Medicine, University of Pittsburgh Medical Center, USA. He has several patents on investigative therapeutic molecules, and he has had competitive research funding for the last two decades. Dr. Dubey's work on estradiol metabolism and the development of 2-methoxyestradiol as a non-carcinogenic therapeutic molecule is ongoing. He has mentored several PhD and Masters students both at ETH Zurich and University of Zurich, Switzerland, and at the University of Pittsburgh, USA.

Contents

Preface

Sex hormones not only regulate reproductive function, but they also play a prominent role in the biology and physiology of several organs/tissues, as well as in the pathophysiology of several diseases. Indeed, accumulating evidence suggests that sex hormones influence different organs and diseases, thereby highlighting the need to assess their roles individually.

During the last two decades, the information on the mechanisms of action of female sex hormones like estradiol have evolved from the conventional nuclear estrogen receptor (ER-alpha) dependent mechanisms to include additional non-nuclear (membrane), non-genomic, and ER-independent (estradiol metabolism driven) mechanisms. This highlights the need to update the current knowledge on sex hormones. Similar to estrogens, the impact of male sex hormones, androgens, and their mechanisms of actions, and association with various disorders, has evolved and needs to be addressed in greater detail. Increasing evidence that exogenous/epigenetic factors can influence sex hormone production and action emphasises the need to understand and update the mechanisms involved.

The current book provides an in-depth and systematic overview of the sex hormones (male and female hormones) and their impact in the biology and pathophysiology of various diseases. Bowling and colleagues provide an overview of the effects of sex hormones on vascular function, Gorazd Drevensek reviews the association with cardiovascular disease, and Leone et al. discuss their role in regulating bacterial infections. Testosterone's impact upon and association with various diseases, and the use of testosterone measurement to diagnose and treat patients is discussed in two chapters on hypogonadism by Andrzej Gomula and Lorna Z. Zaletel, respectively. Additional discussion on this topic is also found in the chapter on urinary tract symptoms, by Sae Chul Kim, and the chapter on osteoporosis by M. Rabijewski and L. Papierska. A unique perspective on sex differences in developmental programming of adult diseases is provided in the chapter by J.S. Gilbert and C.T. Banek. M. Norlin and K. Wikvall go on to lead the readers through the intricate pathways of sex hormone biosynthesis and metabolism. The importance of sex hormones in reproduction is examined in three chapters by S.E. Seeger and U. Kemmerer, by Y.V. Stjernholm, and by I.I. Muderris and Gokalp Oner, respectively. The role of sex hormones in neuromuscular control and physical training is discussed by E.L. Cadore, L.F.M.

Kruel, and Rose Fouladi. Continuing, Stefan Van Dongen and S. Ellen research sex hormones' role in masculinity and sex behavior, and Uner Tan discusses the association of sex hormones with perceptual-verbal and spatial abilities. The impact and importance of sex hormones in sex differentiation is provided in the chapter by I. Negri and M. Pellecchia, and the role of WW domain containing oxidoreductase in regulating hormone action and cancer metastasis is overviewed by W.P. Su and colleagues. Because development of therapeutic estrogens is essential for hormone replacement, the pharmacological aspects of drug development are also reviewed in great detail by C. Wiranidchapong.

The overall aim of this book is to introduce readers to the ever-growing importance of sex hormones in regulating human biology and physiology. The book also discusses the association of sex hormones in various clinical pathologies, as well as their therapeutic importance.

Dr. Raghvendra K. Dubey
Department of Obstetrics & Gynecology,
Clinic for Endocrinology,
University of Zurich Hospital, Zurich,
Switzerland

1

Sex Hormones and Vascular Function

Meaghan Bowling, Suzanne Oparil,
Fadi Hage, Robert Hilgers and Dongqi Xing
University of Alabama at Birmingham
USA

1. Introduction

The relationship between sex hormones and cardiovascular function and disease has long been recognized. As early as the 1950s, researchers concluded that although levels of cholesterol played a major role in the development of cardiovascular disease (CVD), other factors, including gender and hormones, played a role as well. (Anonymous, 1958). Since that time, despite extensive research focusing on the effects of estrogen on vascular function, the relationship remains poorly understood. Furthermore, clinical treatment of postmenopausal women with hormone replacement therapy (HRT) continues to be controversial due to conflicting findings in clinical trials.

Until the 1990s, extensive observational data suggested that HRT was cardioprotective. However, results from the Heart and Estrogen/Progestin Replacement Study (HERS-I and -II) did not confirm a protective effect of HRT on the heart. (Hulley et al 1996; Grady et al 2002). Later, data from the Women's Health Initiative (WHI) reported an increase in coronary heart disease (CHD) risk in women treated with combined estrogen-progestin compared to placebo, while the WHI unopposed-estrogen arm showed no increase in CHD events (Roussow et al, 2002; Anderson et al, 2004). Since release of the WHI, follow-up analyses have shown that the timing of initiation of HRT makes a difference in outcomes. These analyses showed that younger postmenopausal women who initiate therapy at the time of menopause are not at increased risk of CHD events compared to women who initiate therapy at a later age.

In this chapter, we will discuss the pathophysiologic effects of sex hormones on the vasculature, describe both clinical and basic research that has led us to our current understanding, and conclude with future perspectives on avenues of investigation that may lead to innovative treatments for postmenopausal women.

2. Physiology of estrogen actions

2.1 Estrogen metabolism

Estrogen is a steroid hormone that is produced by aromatization of androgen precursors, specifically androstenedione. (Speroff and Fritz, 2005) Estrogens are synthesized primarily in the ovary, with minor contribution from adipose, skin, muscle, and endometrial tissue. In premenopausal women, the primary form of estrogen is 17β-estradiol, often simply referred to as estradiol or E2 (for the two hydroxyl groups located on the basic estrogen ring structure). (Speroff and Fritz, 2005) Estradiol is the form of estrogen used in most pre-clinical studies, and will be abbreviated as 'E2' in this chapter. Clinical studies, particularly studies of HRT, have employed a variety of naturally occurring or synthetic estrogens, which will be identified specifically in the text. Other forms of estrogen include estrone and estriol. Estrone, like estradiol, is produced by aromatization of androstenedione, and is the primary estrogen in postmenopausal women. Estriol is a peripheral metabolite of estrone and estradiol and is not secreted by the ovary. Estriol is the dominant form of estrogen in pregnant women. (Speroff and Fritz, 2005)

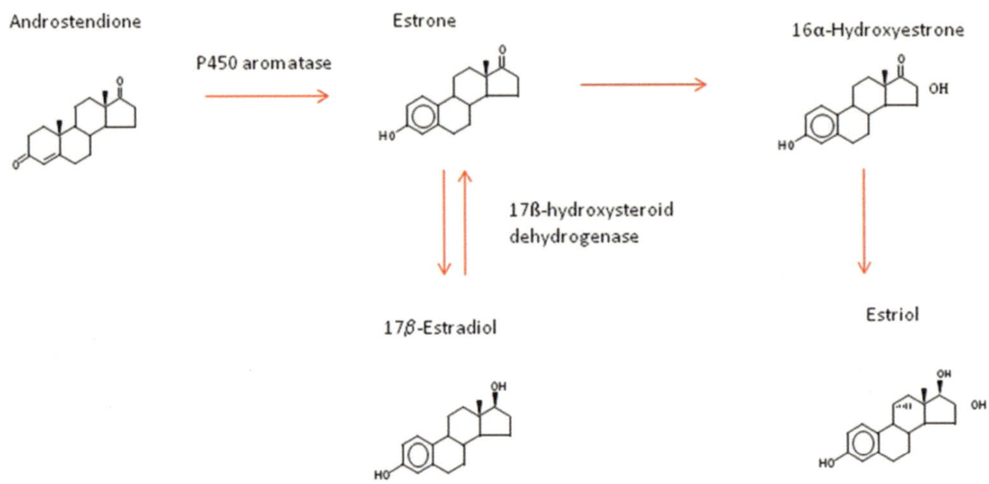

Fig. 1. Estrogen Metabolism (modified from Science Slides Suite © 2010)

The majority of circulating estrogens are bound to carrier proteins, including albumin and sex hormone-binding globulin (SHBG). Albumin binds 30 percent of circulating estrogen and SHBG binds another 69 percent. (Speroff and Fritz, 2005) Only the remaining 1 percent of estrogen that is not protein bound is physiologically active.

2.2 Estrogen receptors

Estrogens act on specific estrogen receptors (ERs) that are differentially expressed in various tissues. There are at least three, and possibly four distinct estrogen receptors. Two of these are the classic ERs: ERα and ER-β. Other ERs include the more recently discovered G protein-coupled receptor (GPER, GPR30, and a putative receptor (ER-X), that has been studied mainly in brain. (Miller et al, 2008)

ERα and ERβ are members of the nuclear steroid hormone receptor superfamily and function as ligand-activated transcription factors. (Speroff and Fritz, 2005) They are expressed in the vasculature and play a role in mediating/modulating responses to vascular injury. Once an estrogen ligand binds to its receptor, the receptor undergoes a conformational change that leads to downstream events in the nucleus, activating or inactivating transcription factors that lead to alterations in gene expression. The conformational plasticity of the ERs is a major reason that estrogen is able to have a variety of agonist/antagonist effects in a given cell or tissue. (Speroff and Fritz, 2005) ERα and ERβ play a pivotal role in vascular remodeling in response to vascular injury.

GPER (GPR30) is an intracellular transmembrane ER that initiates many rapid non-genomic signaling events, including intracellular calcium mobilization and synthesis of phosphatidyl-inositol 3,4,5-triphosphate in the nucleus of multiple cell types. (Revankar et al, 2005). GPER has been indentified in human internal mammary arteries, saphenous veins, and contributes to vasorelaxation in arteries, although this mechanism remains to be fully understood (Haas et al, 2009)

Estrogen acts on various cell types through both genomic and non–genomic mechanisms. Genomic effects occur when estrogen binds to ERs in target tissue cell nuclei, resulting in changes in gene expression. Multiple genes in both the nuclear and mitochondrial genomes are regulated by ERα and ER-β. (O'Lone et al, 2007) In aortic smooth muscle cells and endothelial cells of wild-type ovariectomized mice, E2 treatment resulted in both up- and down-regulation of multiple genes involved in mitochondrial fuction. ERα upregulated four clusters of genes, while ERβ downregulated a different set of mitochondrial genes. E2 also stimulates oxidative phosphorylation and inhibits production of superoxide and other reactive oxygen species in mitochondria. (O'Lone et al, 2007) It is hypothesized that this mechanism decreases the rate of accumulation of mitochondrial DNA mutations over a lifespan, and therefore protects against age-related disease. This notion is relevant to the development of CVD and timing of HRT initiation. (O'Lone et al, 2007)

Estrogen can also trigger non-genomic events by binding to targets other than nuclear receptors, eg., cell membrane ERs. (Kelly and Levin, 2001) Non-genomic effects, such as direct activation of intracellular signaling pathways, can be rapid and do not require changes in gene expression, although the long-term consequences include altered transcription of targeted genes.

3. Physiology of progesterone actions

3.1 Progesterone metabolism and progesterone receptors

Progesterone is a steroid hormone that is synthesized from the precursor pregnenolone (a cholesterol metabolite) by 3β-hydroxysteroid dehydrogenase in the ovaries and adrenal glands. (Figure 2)

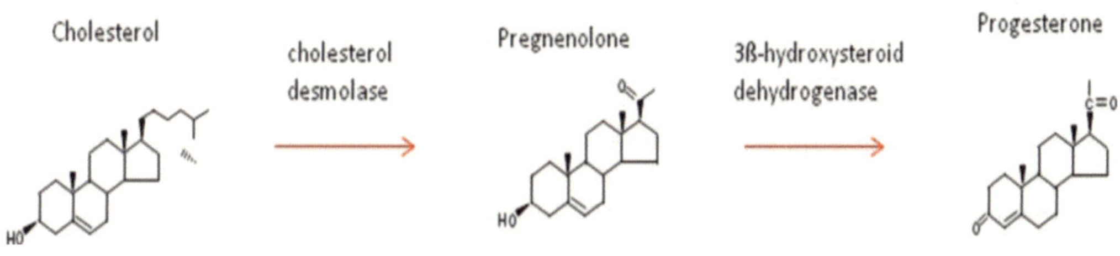

Fig. 2. Progesterone Metabolism ((modified from Science Slides Suite © 2010))

Progesterone acts on two major progesterone receptors (PRs), PR-A and PR-B. (Speroff and Fritz, 2005) While the role of ERs in vascular physiology and pathophysiology is well studied, the literature on PRs is limited and most of what is known about their biological function is derived from studies of reproductive tissues. PR-A and PR-B can form homodimers (AA and BB) or heterodimers (AB) upon binding to a progestin. Downstream effects include protein phosphorylation and modulation of gene transcription. (Speroff and Fritz, 2005) Based on in-vitro studies of endometrium and breast tissue, PR-B is a positive regulator of progesterone-responsive genes, whereas PR-A activation inhibits PR-B activity. Like estrogen, progesterone has both genomic and non-genomic effects, binding both nuclear and cell membrane receptors.

4. Physiologic effects of sex hormones on the vasculature

4.1 Estrogen effects on vascular reactivity

E2 has rapid non-genomic actions on the arterial wall, resulting in vasodilation. Administration of E2 to ovariectomized ewes results in rapid uterine vasodilation, leading to a rise in uterine blood flow within 30 to 45 min (Killam et al, 1973). This rise in uterine blood flow is partially mediated by ER activation and release of nitric oxide (NO), as shown by local infusion of the nonselective ER blocker ICI 182,780 or the NO synthase blocker L-NAME, respectively, into the main uterine artery of nonpregnant ewes (Van Buren et al, 1992) A better understanding of the mechanism(s) by which E2 increases NO production in the vasculature comes from in vitro experiments with cultured endothelial cells. E2 stimulates eNOS activity via an ERα-mediated process in endothelial cells (Chen et al, 1999). ERα and ERβ are present on the endothelial cell membrane and are expressed in a wide range of blood vessels from different vascular beds and species (Andersson et al, 2001). The ERα and eNOS proteins are organized into a functional signaling module in caveolae located on endothelial cell membranes (Chambliss et al, 2000). The role of the ERβ in vasodilation is less clear, but studies from ERβ knockout mice have shown an inhibitory role of ERβ in ERα-mediated NO relaxation (Petterson et al, 2000).
GPER is a seven-transmembrane G protein-coupled ER that has only recently been shown to play a role in the vasculature (Haas et al, 2007). Isoflavones, natural estrogenic compounds (phytoestrogens) found in soy products, e.g. genistein and dadein, and selective ER modulators (SERMs), e.g. tamoxifen and raloxifene, bind to GPER (Filardo et al, 2000). Selective stimulation of GPER by intravenous infusion of the GPER agonist G-1 results in an acute reduction in blood pressure in rats (Haas et al, 2009). G-1 relaxes ex vivo rat and human arteries via an endothelium-dependent and L-NAME-sensitive mechanism (Haas et al, 2009). It is uncertain whether E_2-induced relaxing responses are mediated via GPER or whether crosstalk between ERα/ERβ and GPER exists. Selective GPER antagonists like G-15 (Dennis et al, 2009) might unravel a role for GPER-dependent vasorelaxation upon E2 signaling in the vasculature.
E2 results in vasorelaxation even in the absence of a functional endothelium (Jiang et al. 1991), due primarily to Ca^{2+}-antagonistic effects in smooth muscle cells. E2 inhibits voltage-dependent calcium inward currents on smooth muscle cells, but not on endothelial cells (Shan et al, 1994; Kitazawa et al, 1997). This leads to a reduction in intracellular Ca^{2+} concentration and lower Ca^{2+}-calmodulin-dependent myosin light chain phosphorylation and contraction (Somlyo and Somlyo, 1994). In addition to these Ca^{2+}-antagonistic effects on smooth muscle cells, a variety of endothelium-independent mechanisms have been proposed to account for E_2-induced vasodilation. E2 has been reported to increase cAMP and cGMP levels in the vasculature, thus suggesting a cyclic nucleotide-dependent mechanism of relaxation (Kuehl et al, 1974). For instance, in the porcine coronary artery, E2 causes relaxation via protein kinase G activation and cAMP-dependent opening of large-conductance Ca^{2+}-activated K^+ channels (BK_{Ca}) (Rosenfeld et al, 2000). In human coronary artery smooth muscle cells, E2 has been shown to open BK_{Ca}

channels by stimulating neuronal NOS via a signal pathway involving PI3-kinase and Akt (Han et al, 2007).

In summary, E2 at pharmacological concentrations causes vasorelaxation via a combination of endothelium-dependent, ER-mediated actions and contraction-modulating effects at the level of the smooth muscle cell. The E_2-induced relaxing profile in a specific vascular bed depends on the species, gender, expression patterns and degree of dimerization and crosstalk between the ER subtypes.

4.2 Sex hormone effects on blood pressure

4.2.1 Estrogen effects on blood pressure

Endogenous E_2 lowers BP. Observational studies have demonstrated that BP is lower when E_2 levels peak during the luteal phase than when they are at their nadir during the follicular phase of the menstrual cycle (Dunne et al, 1991; Karpanou et al, 1993; Chapman et al, 1997). Menopause is associated with a significant increase in BP in cross-sectional studies (Staessen et al, 1998). In a prospective study of BP in premenopausal, perimenopausal, and postmenopausal women, an age-independent 4-5 mmHg increase in systolic BP was found in postmenopausal women (Staessen et al, 1997). Further, BP is reduced when endogenous E_2 levels are elevated during pregnancy (Siamopoulos et al, 1996). Data on the BP effects of estrogen replacement therapy (ERT) in menopausal women have been inconsistent, with reports of BP neutral (PEPI Trial Writing Group, 1995), BP lowering (Mercuro et al, 1997; Mercuro et al, 1998; Cagnacci et al, 1999; Seely et al, 1999; Butkevich et al, 2000) and BP elevating effects (Anderson et al, 2004; Wassertheil-Smoller et al, 2000). In the Postmenopausal Estrogen/Progestin interventions (PEPI) trial, which enrolled 875 healthy normotensive early postmenopausal women, assignment to conjugated equine estrogens (CEE), 0.625 mg/d ± a progestin did not impact systolic or diastolic BP when compared with placebo controls (PEPI Trial Writing Group, 1995). In contrast, when transdermal E_2 was administered at physiologic doses to healthy postmenopausal women in two studies that evaluated ambulatory BP, active treatment significantly lowered nocturnal systolic, diastolic and mean BP by 3-7 mmHg compared with placebo (Cagnacci et al, 1999; Seely et al, 1999). The observational study component of the WHI (WHI-OS) collected data on risk factors for CVD, including BP, from 98,705 women aged 50-79 yr, the largest multiethnic, best characterized cohort of postmenopausal women ever studied (Wassertheil-Smoller et al, 2000). WHI-OS found that current HRT use was associated with a 25% greater likelihood of having hypertension compared with past use or no prior use. Further, among 5310 postmenopausal women randomized to CEE (0.625 mg/d) alone compared to a placebo group as part of the randomized controlled trial component of WHI, there was a 1.1-mmHg increase from baseline in systolic BP that persisted throughout the 6.8 yr of follow up (Anderson et al, 2004). There was no difference in diastolic BP between treatment groups.

4.2.2 Progestin effects on blood pressure

Similar to estrogens, the effects of progestins on BP are dependent on the type of progestin. Natural progesterone has been associated with BP lowering or neutral effects. Higher levels of progesterone correlate with lower systolic but not diastolic BP during the second and third trimesters of pregnancy (Kristiansson et al, 2001). In a crossover study of 15 postmenopausal women assigned to placebo or transdermal E_2 ± intravaginal progesterone, addition of progesterone did not affect the nocturnal BP lowering seen with E2 compared with placebo (Seely et al, 1999). Similarly, medroxyprogesterone acetate (MPA) appears to have BP neutral or lowering effects. In a double-blind, crossover study of postmenopausal women assigned to CEE and placebo or increasing doses of MPA, there was a dose-dependent decrease in ambulatory daytime diastolic and mean BPs for women assigned to the progestin compared with placebo (Harvey et al, 2001). In contrast, most studies of synthetic progestins for contraception or hormone therapy have revealed a BP-elevating effect. Oral contraceptives in particular appear to precipitate or accelerate hypertension (Rosenthal et al, 2000).

4.3 Estrogen effects on lipoproteins

E2 also affects serum lipoprotein levels and the interaction of lipoproteins with cellular elements in the vessel wall. E2 has been shown to protect against atherosclerotic lesion formation in multiple animal models. In primate models, E2 results in up to a 66 percent decrease in aortic atherosclerotic plaque size. (Bjarnson et al, 1997) Mouse models have been widely used to study atherosclerosis because of the ability to easily inactivate targeted genes coding for apolipoprotein E (*Apoe*) and the LDL receptor (*Ldlr*) which lead to spontaneous development of atherosclerosis. E2 prevents both initiation and progression of atherosclerotic plaque development in these models. Using subcutaneous implanted E2-releasing pellets to achieve physiologic serum levels, atherosclerotic plaques did not progress beyond the fatty streak stage in apolipoprotein E-deficient mice. (Elhage et al, 1997) Similarly, E2 has been shown to reduce atherosclerotic lesion size in male *Apoe-/-* mice. (Tse et al, 1999) Treatment of minimally-oxidized LDL with E2 leads to decreased cytotoxicity in cultured endothelial cells. (Negre-Salvayre et al, 1993) E2 also inhibits LDL oxidation and decreases formation of cholesterol esters. (Huber et al, 1990)

E2 effects on lipoproteins and atherosclerosis are mediated by both ERα and ERβ. When E2-treated mice that were deficient in ApoE alone were compared to mice that were deficient in both ApoE and ERα, E2 reduced atherosclerotic plaque size in *Apoe-/-* mice by 80%. This effect was not seen in the *Apoe-/- , ERα-/-* mice, indicating that ERα plays a critical role in prevention of aterhosclerosis in this model. (Hodgin et al, 2001)

Clinical studies have shown reductions in serum lipoproteins following oral estrogen replacement therapy. One study randomized women to treatment with CEE (Premarin 0.625 mg) daily versus placebo. (Walsh et al, 1991) The estrogen treatment group had a 15% reduction in serum concentrations of LDL cholesterol and a 16% increase in high density lipoprotein (HDL) cholesterol. Triglyceride levels increased by 24%. These results were consistent across the age spectrum; even women in their 8th decade of life showed similar changes in serum cholesterol levels. Oral estrogens facilitate postprandial clearance of atherogenic lipoproteins and increase serum HDL levels, specifically HDL_2, which may play a major role in reduction of atherogenesis. Oral CEEs appear to increase HDL levels to a greater degree than oral E2. Triglyceride levels are increased with administration of both oral CEE and oral E2, though to a lesser extent by oral E2.

Transdermal E2 formulations also decrease LDL levels, but to a lesser extent than oral preparations. (Stevenson et al 2009) Transdermal estrogens have not been shown to alter postprandial lipoprotein clearance or circulating HDL levels, but may lower triglyceride levels. (Godsland et al, 2001)

4.4 Estrogen effects on C-reactive protein

C-reactive protein (CRP) is an acute phase reactant that has been shown to be both a marker and a mediator of vascular disease. There is an E2-dependent sexual dimorphism in expression of human CRP in experimental models, i.e., the transgenic mouse expressing human CRP (CRPtg) (Szalai et al 1997, 1998, 2002) and in some human populations (Yamada et al, 2001). E2 treatment of male CRPtg can lower baseline CRP levels and removal of E2 can restore its high baseline expression. (Szalai et al, 1998) In postmenopausal women, oral CEE increases baseline CRP levels, but low dose oral or transdermal E2 supplementation does not affect CRP. (Cushman et al, 1999; Vongpatanasin et al, 2003; Lakoski et al, 2005; Mosca et al, 2004) This HRT-induced CRP increase occurs without a significant change in IL-6 or TNF-α, major regulators of CRP under inflammatory conditions, suggesting that the effects of menopausal hormones on CRP do not reflect a generalized inflammatory state. (Vongpatanasin et al, 2003; Mosca et al, 2004) Data from the WHI and the Women's Health Study have demonstrated that CRP predicts CVD risk in post-menopausal women independent of HRT. (Kurtz et al, 2011) HRT use had less predictive value than CRP levels in these studies. Thus, the clinical significance of hormone-related changes in circulating CRP levels remains uncertain.

5. Estrogen effects on inflammation and vascular pathology

5.1 Estrogen modulates pro-inflammatory mediator expression after vascular injury

Inflammation plays a critical role in the pathogenesis of atherosclerosis and subsequent CVD. (Hansson et al, 2005) The process is initiated by activation of endothelial cells due to deposition of lipoproteins, pressure overload, and/or hyperglycemia, leading to increased expression of adhesion molecules (including selectin, vascular cell adhesion molecule 1 [VCAM-1], and intercellular adhesion molecule 1 [ICAM-1]). These molecules cause circulating leukocytes to bind to vascular endothelial cells and release pro-inflammatory cytokines and growth factors. The bound leukocytes then infiltrate the vascular smooth muscle cells layer, leading to a cascade of cytokine secretion, further contributing to the local inflammatory environment within the vessel.

Based on extensive studies using the rat carotid injury model, E2 has been shown to be a negative modulator of injury-induced vascular inflammation and neointima formation. (Bakir et al, 2000; Miller et al, 2004; Xing et al, 2004) There is a sexual dimorphism in the response to vascular injury, with males demonstrating increased neointima formation compared to females. (Chen et al 1996, 1998; Levine et al 1996; Miller et al, 2004) This sexual dimorphism is E2-dependent, based on evidence that physiologic levels of circulating E2 (40-60 pg/ml) decrease neointima formation in both male and female gonadectomized animals. Furthermore, addition of MPA, the progestin used in the Women's Health Initiative, opposes the effects of E2 on injury-induced vascular inflammation and neointima formation. (Levine et al, 1996)

E2 modulates the vascular response to injury by reducing local expression of inflammatory mediators and influx of leukocytes into balloon-injured carotid arteries of ovariectomized rats. (Miller et al, 2004; Xing et al, 2004) In particular, E2 decreases expression of cytokine-induced neutrophil chemoattractant (CINC-2β), a chemoattractant for neutrophils and monocyte chemoattractant protein (MCP-1) in injured arteries. (Xing et al, 2004) This results in significant reductions in influx of these inflammatory leukocyte subtypes, limiting the injury response. (Figure 3)

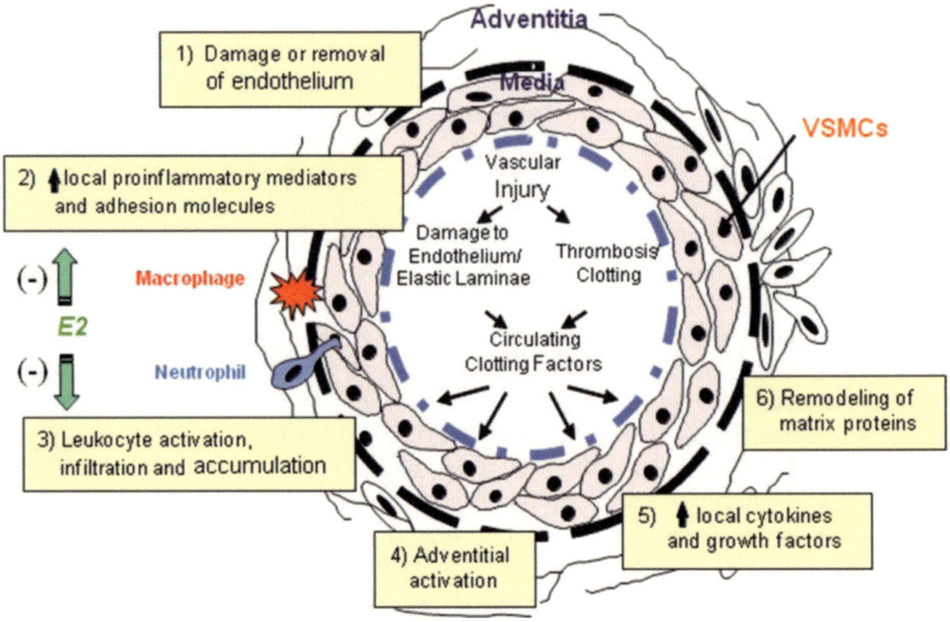

Fig. 3. E2 effects on the early vascular injury response. (*Adapted from Xing et al, 2009*)

5.2 The role of C-reactive protein in E2 modulation of vascular inflammation

E2 also exerts an anti-inflammatory and vasoprotective effect in injured arteries of CRP transgenic (CRPtg) mice. CRPtg mice carry a transgene containing the entire human *CRP* gene and its promoters while the mouse supplies all the required *trans*-acting factors. (Hage et al, 2008) Since in CRPtg mice, human CRP increases several hundred-fold during an acute phase response, analogous to the human condition, this model is convenient for the *in vivo* study of the biologic activities, including vascular effects, of human CRP. Using CRPtg mice, we and others have established that human CRP is a pathogenic mediator of cardiovascular disease. (Danenberg et al, 2003; Paul et al, 2004; Zhang et al, 2010; Nagai et al, 2011; Takahashi et al, 2010)

Using the carotid ligation model of acute vascular injury, we showed that young ovariectomized CRPtg mice develop twofold greater neointima formation than control non transgenic (NTG) mice and that there are extensive deposits of human CRP in the neointima of injured vessels of these animals in the absence of an increase in blood levels of the protein. (Kumar et al, 1997; Hage et al, 2010; Wang et al, 2005; Xing et al, 2008) These findings suggest that local expression of human CRP may exacerbate the adverse remodeling seen after acute arterial injury in the CRPtg model. To test the hypothesis that E2 can inhibit the vascular injury response attributed to human CRP, we treated ovariectomized CRPtg and control NTG mice with E2 prior to carotid ligation and observed that E2-treated CRPtg mice had a significant, ~85%, reduction in neointima formation compared to vehicle-treated CRPtg mice. The E2 effect was directionally similar but somewhat smaller in magnitude in control NTG mice. (Wang et al, 2005) Since the exaggerated vascular injury response in CRPtg mice is mediated by immunoglobulin G Fc receptors (FcγRs) on macrophages, (Xing et al, 2008) and since E2, via its interaction with ERs, can reduce inflammatory cytokine release from activated human macrophages by decreasing expression of the excitatory FcγRs on these cells, (Kramer et al, 2004, 2007) it is plausible that the vasoprotective effects of E2 against CRP-mediated vascular injury response in female mice are regulated by its modulation of macrophage phenotype in order to express less activating receptors (FcγRI and FcγRIII) and more inhibitory receptors (FcγRIIb).

5.3 Estrogen receptors and vascular inflammation

Studies in ERα- and ERβ-deficient mice and in rats treated with pharmacologic antagonists of ERs have provided evidence that both ER subtypes contribute to the vasoprotective effects of E2 in the setting of acute injury. (Mori et al, 2000; Brouchet et al, 2001; Karas et al, 1999; Geraldes et al, 2003; Xing et al, 2007). The ER subtypes contribute to vasoprotection in a cell-specific manner. In porcine endothelial and vascular smooth muscle cells, E2 acts through inhibition of PDGF-BB-induced p38 and p42/44 mitogen-activated protein kinase (MAPK) phosphorylation to stimulate migration and proliferation. (Geraldes et al, 2003) Down-regulation of ERβ, but not ERα, prevented the effects of E2 on smooth muscle cell migration and proliferation. In contrast, in porcine endothelial cells, down-regulation of ERα prevented E2-induced p38 and p42/44 MAPK activation, while down-regulation of ERβ had no effect.

Administration of the ERβ selective agonist DPN has been shown to result in dose-dependednt attenuation of neointima formation induced by injury of the mouse femoral artery. (Krom et al, 2007) The ERα selective agonist PPT prevented neointima formation at low but not high concentrations in this study. In a subsequent study, MPP, an ERα selective antagonist, blocked the inhibitory effect of PPT on neointima formation, but did not block the effects of E2 or DPN. (Harrington et al, 2003) This suggests that E2 acts through a selective ERβ pathway to attenuate neointima formation following restenosis in this mouse model.

The TNF-α-stimulated vascular smooth muscle cell has been used as an in-vitro model of the vascular injury response in order to examine cellular/molecular mechanisms of E2-induced vasoprotection. (Xing et al, 2007) E2 has been shown to attenuate TNF-α induced expression of pro-inflammatory mediators in rat aortic smooth muscle cells through ERβ. (Xing et al, 2007) In this model, DPN reduced TNF-α-induced expression of the neutrophil cytokine CINC-2β in a dose-dependent fashion, while PPT had no effect. The non-selective ER antagonist ICI-182,780 blocked the anti-inflammatory effects of both DPN and E2. Furthermore, both DPN and E2 reduced neutrophil chemotactic activity in TNF-α-treated rat aortic SMCs.

5.4 The role of aging in loss of estrogen-induced vasoprotection

In order to reconcile laboratory findings that E2 provides vascular protection with clinical trial results indicating harmful effects of E2 on the cardiovascular system, studies have been done in models comparing young versus aged animals. Results from one study showed opposing effects of E2 based on age: E2 increased neointima formation in balloon-injured carotid arteries of aged (+75%) versus young (10-12 weeks; -40%) ovariectomized rats. (Miller et al, 2007) The attenuating effect of E2 on inflammatory mediator expression and neutrophil and monocyte infiltration was lost in the injured arteries of aged rats. ERα and ERβ expression was similar in both the young and aged animals. This laboratory evidence was the first of its kind to show that E2 exacerbates the vascular response to injury in aged animals. This seminal finding indicates that the protective effect of E2 is impaired following long periods of hormone deprivation, supporting the timing hypothesis. (Pinna et al, 2008)

The potential role of age-related alterations in ER signaling in these processes remains poorly understood and warrants further study.

6. Reproductive aging, sex hormones, and women's health

Reproductive aging is a function of decreased production of sex hormones by the ovaries. As a woman enters her fifth decade of life, depletion of remaining ovarian follicles occurs. Estrogen production by the ovaries begins to decrease, and women experience progressive loss of menstrual cyclicity. When total depletion of follicles occurs, menses cease, and the woman enters menopause, defined as the absence of menses for a 12-month period. The average age of menopause in the United States is 51 years. (Speroff and Fritz, 2005) Due to increasing lifespan, women can now expect to spend a significant portion of their lives in the postmenopausal state. This prolonged hypoestrogenism may have important consequences for quality of life, as well as various other health parameters, including cardiovascular function, bone health, and cognitive function.

6.1 Age- and sex-specific trends

CHD is rare in premenopausal women, but the incidence of myocardial infarction rises dramatically after menopause. Furthermore, women with premature ovarian failure or early natural menopause (≤ 44 years) have an associated increase in the risk of CVD. (Hu et al, 1999) (Mondul et al 2005) These observations led to the belief that menopause itself is a risk factor for CHD. However, the relationship between menopause, age and CHD is complex and it is not clear that menopause per se is a risk factor for CHD. It is important to recognize that women who develop CHD after menopause have more CHD risk factors (dyslipidemia, family history, hypertension, tobacco use, and diabetes mellitus) compared to postmenopausal women who remain free of disease. Currently available data from randomized controlled trials, e.g., WHI and HERS, do not indicate that HRT is useful in the primary or secondary prevention of CHD. However, a growing body of evidence suggests that initiation of treatment with different HRT preparations in the perimenopausal period may have beneficial effects on the vasculature that may delay the progression of CVD and prevent ischemic events.

6.2 Types and routes of administration of postmenopausal estrogen replacement therapy

ERT is only indicated for the treatment of moderate to severe menopausal symptoms, specifically vasomotor symptoms (eg. hot flushes). Contraindications to ERT include known CHD, breast cancer, a previous venous thromboembolic event or stroke, active liver disease, or high risk for these conditions. ERT should be initiated as close to the time of menopause as possible, typically beginning in the late forties to early fifties. Initiation of therapy beyond age 59 is controversial due to increased risk of CHD events. Most physicians now agree that the benefit of estrogen treatment in healthy, early menopausal women, using the lowest dose and shortest duration of therapy, outweigh the risks of treatment.

Systemic ERT can be given orally or non-orally in the form of transdermal patches and topical creams, gels, and mists. Estrogen can also be given vaginally via tablets, topical formulations and vaginal rings. However, vaginal therapy is only indicated for the treatment of vaginal atrophy and not for systemic/vasomotor symptoms. Assuming that equivalent doses of replacement estrogen are given, the different routes of administration are equivalent in ameliorating menopausal symptoms. Among the oral estrogens, E2 is considered to be the most potent estrogen and estrone is reported to be 50-70% less active. Estriol is the least potent of the three estrogens, with a potency one-tenth that of E2.

While both oral and transdermal estrogens are absorbed systemically, oral estrogens are unique in that they undergo the "first-pass effect" in the liver. Intestinal absorption of estrogens leads to high concentrations of hormone in the portal vein, stimulating hepatic production of thyroxine-binding globulin, corticosteroid-binding globulin, SHBG, triglycerides, HDL, triglycerides, and clotting factors. Transdermal administration of estrogen does not have this effect and there is no resulting increased hepatic production of the above proteins.

Multiple oral estrogen preparations are available, including CEE, E2, esterified estrogen, and conjugated synthetic estrogens. (Table 1)

Estrogen Replacement Therapy					
Drug	**Company**	**Dose**	**Company**	**Drug**	**Dose**
Oral Therapy			*Transdermal Therapy*		
Estradiol			**Estradiol**		
Estrace	Warner Chilcot	0.5, 1, 2 mg	*Patches*		
Gynodiol	Firlding	0.5, 1, 1.5, 2 mg	Alora	Watson	0.025, 0.05, 0.075, 0.1 mg/d
Conjugated equine estrogens			Climara	Berlax	0.025, 0.05, 0.06, 0.075, 0.1 mg/d
Premarin	Wyeth-Ayerst	0.3, 0.45, 0.625, 0.9, 1.25 mg	Esclim	Women First	0.025, 0.0375, 0.05, 0.075, 0.1 mg/d
Esterified Estrogens			Estraderm	Novartis	0.05, 0.1 mg/d
Menest	Monarch	0.3, 0.625, 1.25, 2.5 mg	Vivelle	Novartis	0.025, 0.0375, 0.05, 0.075, 0.1 mg/d
Ogen	Pharmacia	0.75, 1.5, 3 mg	Menostar	Bayer	0.014 mg/d
Ortho-Est	Women First Healthcase	0.5, 1.5, mg	*Gel*		
Conjugated synthetic estrogens			EstroGel	Solvay	0.75 mg/pump
Cenestin	Elan	0.3, 0.45, 0.625, 0.9, 1.25 mg	*Emulsions*		
Enjuvia	Elan	0.625, 1.25 mg	Estrasorb	Novavox	0.025 mg/pouch
Vaginal Therapy			Divigel	Upsher-Smith	0.25, 0.5, 1 mg/pouch
Estradiol			Elestrin	Kenwood	0.52 mg/pump

Rings			*Spray*		
Estring	Pharmacia	0.0075 mg/day	EvaMist	KV pharmaceutical	1.5 mg/spray
Femring	Warner-Chilcott	0.05 mg/day			
Tablet					
Vagifem	Novo Nordisk	0.025 mg/tablet			
Cream					
Estradiol					
Estrace	Warner-Chilcot	0.1 mg/gram			
Conjugated equine estrogen					
Premarin	Wyeth-Ayerst	0.625 mg/gram			

Table 1. Available Estrogen Formulations (*Modified from Martin and Barbieri, 2011*)

CEE is one of the most commonly used preparations and, derived from mare urine, is composed of up to 10 different estrogenic compounds, predominantly the sodium sulfated conjungates of estrone. (Lyman GW 1982) The metabolism of CEE is a complex and still poorly understood process which occurs in the liver. After oral ingestion of CEEs, the compounds are rapidly absorbed by the gastrointestinal tract, then may become conjugated by hepatocytes or excreted in the feces. (Pan CC, 1985) Following oral intake of CEEs, mean serum estrone levels (152 pg/mL) are far higher than estradiol levels (31 pg/mL). (Powers MS et al 1985) However, the estrone component is largely inactive because it is albumin-bound. The clinical response to CEE is hypothesized to be mediated through a mechanism involving conversion of circulating, bound estrone to E2 in the liver. (Barnes RB et al 1987)

E2 is another commonly prescribed oral form of postmenopausal ERT. Native E2 is poorly absorbed; therefore it is manufactured in micronized, sulfated, and esterified forms to improve absorption. (Krantz JC et al 1958) Similar to metabolism of CEE, the majority of E2 is converted to estrone. However, following oral administration of E2, mean circulating levels of estrone (200 pg/mL) and E2 (50 pg/mL) are higher compared to serum levels following ingestion of CEE when equivalent doses are given. (Lobo RA and Cassidenti DL 1992) E2 also induces hepatic production of proteins, but this effect is much less than that of CEEs. (Maschak CA et al 1982).

Esterified estrogens result in serum E2 and estrone levels similar to those seen with CEEs. Synthetic conjugated estrogens are derived from plant sources. They are similar but not identical to CEEs and contain fewer molecular forms of estrogen. (Lobo et al, 2000)

6.3 Types and routes of administration of progesterone replacement therapy

Progesterone is indicated in addition to estrogen as part of a HRT regimen in postmenopausal women with an intact uterus (who have not undergone hysterectomy). Progesterone opposes the effects of estrogen on the endometrial lining and prevents development of endometrial hyperplasia and malignancy which occur in women treated with unopposed estrogen. Both natural and synthetic progestins are available. (Table 2)

Progesterone Formulations			
Generic Name	**Brand Name**	**Company**	**Dose**
Oral Therapy			
Micronized Progesterone	Prometrium	Abbott	100, 200 mg
Medroxyprogesterone Acetate	Provera	Pfizer	2.5, 5, 10 mg
Norethindrone acetate	Aygestin	Teva Pharmaceuticals	2.5, 5, 10 mg
Vaginal Therapy			
Progesterone Cream	Crinone	Columbia Laboratories	90 mg/applicator
Progesterone Gel	Prochieve	Columbia Laboratories	90 mg/applicator
Intrauterine Device (IUD)			
Levonorgestrel IUD	Mirena	Bayer	52 mg/5 yrs
Combination Estrogen-Progesterone Formulations			
Oral Therapy			
CEE/medroxyprogesterone	Prempro	Wyeth	0.3/1.5, 0.45/1.5, 0.625/2.5, 0.625/5 mg
Estradiol/norgestimate	Prefest	Duramed	1/0.9 mg
Estradiol/norethindonr acetate	Activella	Novo Nordisk	1/0.5 mg
Ethinyl estradiol/norethindrone	FemHRT	Warner-Chilcot	5 mcg/1mg
Estradiol/drosperinone	Angeliq	Berlex	1/0.5 mg
Transdermal Patches			
Estradiol/norethindrone	Combi-Patch	Novartis	0.05/0.14, 0.05/0.25 mg
Estradiol/levonorgestrel	Climara Pro	Berlex	0.045/0.015 mg

Table 2. Available Progesterone Preparations. (*Modified from Martin and Barbieri, 2011*)

Micronized progesterone is the major natural progesterone available, and while it has been less well studied than MPA, it appears to be similar in efficacy and is widely prescribed. Synthetic progestins, including MPA, norgestrel, and norethindrone acetate, appear to increase hepatic lipase activity and attenuate the beneficial effects of estrogen on HDL levels (Stevenson 2009), while natural progesterone appears to have no adverse effect on HDL. MPA also opposes the NO-dependent vasodilator effect of E_2, while natural progesterone was found to have no effect. (Williams AK et al 1994)

7. Clinical research in hormone replacement therapy

7.1 Observational studies

The slope of the age-related rise in incidence of CVD in women increases in the post-menopausal period, suggesting that withdrawal of ovarian hormones, particularly E2, has an adverse effect on cardiovascular health. (Lloyd-Jones et al, 2010) This increase is thought to be a consequence of the loss of the multiple protective effects of E2 on the vascular system. Multiple observational studies have suggested that HRT may protect against CVD in postmenopausal women. In a meta-analysis of 16 prospective observational trials, the relative risk of CVD for postmenopausal women who ever used any form of estrogen vs. those who had never used estrogen was 0.70 (95% CI, 0.63-0.77). (Grodstein et al, 1995) The relative risk in current users, calculated from 6 prospective studies, was even more impressive at 0.55 (95% CI, 0.44-0.70). In the Nurses' Health Study, which followed more than 70,000 postmenopausal women for 20 years, the risk for major coronary events was lower among current users of HRT compared with never-users (multi-variate adjusted relative risk, 0.61 [95% CI, 0.52-0.71]). (Grodstein et al, 2000) Buoyed by observational studies suggesting that HRT, including various E2 preparations with or without a progestin (most commonly a synthetic one), reduced CVD risk by ~50%. (Psaty et al, 1994) HRT use increased dramatically during the 2 decades prior to the publication of the WHI. It is estimated that annual hormone therapy prescriptions increased from 58 million in 1995 to 90 million in 1999, representing ~15 million women per year. (Hersh et al, 2004) This rate remained stable until 2002, but after the publication of WHI and other randomized controlled trials that showed no benefit of HRT, fell sharply by 66% in a single year. Many of the studies that prompted the upswing in postmenopausal HRT suffered from the limitations of discordance of the two treatment groups: women who take HRT are on average better educated, have higher incomes and better access to health care and are healthier even before starting therapy. (Barrett-Connor et al, 1989; Matthews et al, 1996) In a meta-analysis that adjusted for socioeconomic status and other risk factors, HRT was not associated with CVD risk reduction. (Humphrey et al, 2002)

7.2 Clinical trials

Publication of the estrogen plus progestin clinical trial component of the Women's Health Initiative (WHI) (Rossouw et al., 2002; Manson et al., 2003) initially sounded a death knell for hormone use in post-menopausal women. This placebo-controlled trial of HRT (CEE 0.625 mg/day plus MPA 2.5 mg/day) in 16,608 post-menopausal women found significant increases in the risk of CHD, stroke, venous thromboembolism and invasive breast cancer in the HRT group. The reductions in colorectal cancer and hip fracture seen with HRT did not balance these increased CVD and cancer risks, and publication of the WHI results stimulated consensus panels to recommend against the use of HRT for chronic disease prevention in post-menopausal women (Mosca et al., 2004). Based on the widely publicized findings of harm in the estrogen plus progestin (E+P) trial of the WHI and a major secondary prevention study that used the same hormone regimen, the Heart and Estrogen/Progestin Replacement Study (HERS) (Hulley et al., 1998; Grady et al., 2002), prescribing of HRT fell drastically. (Hersh et al., 2004) Transdermal hormone preparations were less affected, and transvaginal and low-dose preparations gained somewhat, reflecting caution in the use of the full-dose oral regimens that had been used in WHI and HERS.

Attempts to explain the unanticipated deleterious effects of HRT gave consideration to whether the formulation, dose and route of administration of HRT might play a role (Dubey et al., 2004; Turgeon et al., 2004; Phillips & Langer, 2005). In particular, the progestin MPA was identified as having potential deleterious effects on the vasculature. Pre-clinical studies had shown that MPA negates the vasoprotective and anti-inflammatory effects of E2 in the setting of acute vascular injury (Levine et al., 1996; Oparil et al., 1997; Xing et al., 2004; Miller et al., 2004) and in vitro studies found that MPA signals differently from native progesterone in endothelial cells (Simoncini et al., 2004). The surprising outcomes of the estrogen-alone (EA) component of WHI (WHI SC, 2004) added further evidence that MPA might be a problem and that unopposed estrogen benefits younger post-menopausal women. This trial, which was stopped early, showed no significant effect of unopposed CEE on the primary CHD outcome and a surprising tendency for benefit in the primary safety (invasive breast cancer) outcome.

7.3 The timing hypothesis

The advanced age (63 years in WHI, 67 years in HERS) and long period of hormone deprivation prior to starting HRT may account for deleterious outcomes of hormone treatment in WHI and HERS. Based on a review of pre-clinical studies, as well as observational studies and clinical trials in women, including those with intermediate end-points and CVD outcomes, the "timing hypothesis" was developed (Phillips & Langer, 2005). The timing hypothesis states that the effects of HRT on the vasculature are dependent on the time of initiation of treatment. The timing hypothesis predicts that HRT initiated at the time of or prior to menopause should produce a decrease in CHD over time, while HRT begun years after menopause should produce an increase in CHD events shortly after therapy is begun, followed by later benefit. This hypothesis attributes the complex CHD responses to HRT in human trials to a combination of early erosion/rupture of 'vulnerable' coronary plaque, which is made worse by HRT; long-term reduction in plaque formation, which is improved by HRT; and modulation of the vasoprotective actions of estrogens by systemic progestins.

Indirect support for the timing hypothesis has come from the report of final results from the EA trial in WHI, which included detailed analyses of primary and secondary coronary outcomes and subgroup analyses of participants by age and years since hysterectomy with no menopausal hormone therapy (Hsia J, et al). During the active intervention period, 201 coronary events were confirmed among women assigned to CEE compared with 217 events among women assigned to placebo (HR=0.95%; 95% CI 0.79-1.16). Among women aged 50-59 years at baseline, the HR for the primary outcome (nonfatal myocardial infarction or coronary death) was 0.63 (95% CI 0.36-1.08). In that younger age group, coronary revascularization was less frequent among women assigned to CEE (HR=0.55; 95% CI 0.35-0.86), as were several composite outcomes. Further analyses of the E+P arm of the WHI demonstrated a non-significant trend towards cardioprotection in women who began HRT less than 10 years after menopause (HR = 0.89; 95% CI 0.5-1.5), while women who initiated HRT more than 20 years after menopause had a significantly elevated risk of coronary events (HR = 1.71; 95% CI, 1.1-2.5). (Manson et al, 2003) When the EA and E+P arms from the WHI were combined, a similar trend was seen. (Rossouw et al, 2007)

Another consideration in the relationship between HRT and CVD risk is the duration of HRT. A recent post-hoc analysis of the E+P trial in WHI showed that in women less than 10 years since menopause, HRT resulted in a slightly lower event-free survival rate during the first 5 years of therapy compared to placebo; however, at 6 years, the two curves crossed each other and showed a non-significant trend towards a higher rate of event-free survival in the group using HRT. (Toh et al, 2010) Further analysis of women less than 10 years since menopause in the WHI E+P arm showed an increased risk in the first 2 years of HRT, followed by a decreased risk in the next 2 years, and an overall risk reduction over 8 years.

(Toh et al, 2010). Similar results were seen in the EA arm of the WHI, with a significant decrease in CHD risk after 6 years of CEE alone compared to placebo. (Harman et al, 2011) Among women in the EA arm of the WHI followed up over 10.7 years, there was no difference in CHD risk in those using CEE for a median of 5.9 years compared to placebo at the end of the active treatment period, or overall. (LaCroix et al, 2011) In the post-intervention follow-up period, the annualized rate for CHD in the EA arm was 0.64% compared to 0.67% in the placebo group (HR 0.97, 95% CI, 0.75-1.25). Health outcomes, including CHD, were more favorable for younger women compared to older women (P=0.05 for interaction). These findings support the current clinical recommendations to treat postmenopausal women with HRT for the "shortest possible duration" and may lead to more individualized management.

The WHI was limited by use of only one type of ERT (CEE), by inclusion of women who initiated HRT late after many years of ovarian hormone deprivation, and by exclusion of women who were experiencing menopausal symptoms. Ongoing clinical trials are addressing these deficiencies by examining the timing hypothesis in perimenopausal women. The Kronos Early Estrogen Prevention Study (KEEPS) is a prospective, randomized, double-blind study of 900 healthy perimenopausalwomen aged 45-54 with menopausal symptoms. (Harman et al., 2005) The main hypotheses are 1) HRT initiated early in menopause (before development of atherosclerotic lesions) will prevent progression of atherosclerotic lesions, and 2) both oral CEE and transdermal E2 will be similarly efficacious. Participants were randomized to oral CEE and a placebo patch, oral placebo and a transdermal patch containing E_2, or placebo in both pill and patch. The primary endpoints of KEEPS are carotid intimal medial thickness by ultrasound and the progression of coronary calcium by electron beam tomography, surrogates for CVD. Another ongoing prospective, randomized, controlled trial, the Early versus Late Intervention Trial with Estradiol (ELITE) randomized 643 women who were less than 6 years or more than 10 years since menopause to receive oral E2 versus placebo. (clinicaltrials.gov NCT00114517; Hodis and Mack, 2011) The primary endpoint is rate of change of carotid artery intima-media thickness. These two prospective studies will provide much-needed information regarding the timing hypothesis and use of HRT in reducing CVD risk.

7.4 Oral versus transdermal HRT

To date, few studies have examined the difference in CHD outcomes between postmenopausal women treated with oral versus transdermal therapy. The one existing trial in the literature suggests no difference in CHD outcomes with regard to route. (Clarke SC 2002) This study examined transdermal E2 with or without transdermal norethindrone acetate, and found similar CHD outcomes to the WHI. The literature indicates that dose may be more important than route.

8. Conclusions

Importantly, cellular and molecular studies are urgently needed to elucidate the differential effects of HRT and its components on young, healthy arteries and on older, diseased arteries. Emerging evidence suggests that HRT administered to young healthy women has anti-inflammatory and vasodilator effects that tend to lower blood pressure and slow the progression of atherosclerotic lesions, while the same HRT preparation administered to older women, particularly those with established vascular disease, has a proinflammatory effect, perhaps leading to atherosclerotic plaque instability and neovascularization (Störk et al., 2004; Mendelsohn & Karas, 2005). The mechanisms of these altered vascular responses are not fully understood, but may relate to age-related deterioration in ER expression and signaling. Recent studies of the effects of HRT on blood pressure and vascular function support the age-dependence of the action of HRT on the vasculature. Beneficial effects of HRT appear to be realized only in younger, perimenopausal women in whom hormone response systems remain intact. However, further study of the timing, dose, duration, and route of administration of HRT in postmenopausal women may be informative.

9. References

Anderson, G.L., Limacher, M., Assaf, A.R., Bassford, T., Beresford, S.A., Black, H., Bonds, D., Brunner, R., Brzyski, R., Caan, B., Chlebowski, R., Curb, D., Gass, M., Hays, J., Heiss, G., Hendrix, S., Howard, B.V., Hsia, J., Hubbell, A., Jackson, R., Johnson, K.C., Judd, H., Kotchen, J.M., Kuller, L., LaCroix, A.Z., Lane, D., Langer, R.D., Lasser, N., Lewis, C.E., Manson, J., Margolis, K., Ockene, J., O'Sullivan, M.J., Phillips, L., Prentice, R.L., Ritenbaugh, C., Robbins, J., Rossouw, J.E., Sarto, G., Stefanick, M.L., Van Horn, L., Wactawski-Wende, J., Wallace, R., & Wassertheil-Smoller, S.. Women's Health Initiative Steering Committee. (2004). Effects of conjugated equine estrogen in postmenopausal women with hysterectomy: the Women's Health Initiative randomized controlled trial. *Journal of the American Medical Association*, Vol. 291, No. 14, (April 2004), pp. 1701-1712, ISSN 0098-7484.

Andersson, C., Lydrup, M., Ferno, M., Idvall, I., Gustafson, J. & Nilsson B. (2001). Immunocytochemical demonstration of oestrogen receptor beta in blood vessels of the femal rat. *Journal of Endocrinology*, Vol.169, No. 2, (May 2001), pp. 241-247, ISSN 1479-6805.

Bakir, S., Mori T, Durand J, Chen YF, Thompson JA, & Oparil S. (2000). Estrogen-induced vasoprotection is estrogen-receptor dependent: evidence from the balloon-injured rat carotid artery model. Circulation, Vol.101, No.20, (May 2000), pp. 2342-2344, ISSN: 0009-7322.

Bar, J., Tepper, R., Fuchs, J., Pardo, Y., Goldberger, S., & Ovadia, J. (1993). The effect of estrogen replacement therapy on platelet aggregation and adenosine triphosphate release in postmenopausal women. *Obstetrics & Gynecology*, Vol.81, No.2, (Feb 1993), pp. 261–264, ISSN 1873-233X.

Bar, J., Lahav, J., Hod, M., Ben-Rafael, Z., Weinberger, I., & Brosens, J. (2000). Regulation of platelet aggregation and adenosine triphosphate release in vitro by 17β-estradiol and medroxyprogesterone acetate in postmenopausal women. Journal of Thrombosis and Haemostasis, Vol.84, No.4, (Oct 2000), pp. 695–700, ISSN 0340-6245.

Barnes, R.B., Lobo, R.A. (1987). Pharmacology of Estrogens, In: Menopause: Physiology and Pharmacology, Mishell, D.R., JR, pp. 301-315, Year Book Medical Publishers, Inc., ISBN 0815159145, Chicago, IL.

Barrett-Connor, E., Wingard, D., & Criqui, M. (1989). Postmenopausal estrogen use and heart disease risk factors in the 1980s. Rancho bernardo, calif, revisited. *Journal of the American Medical Association,* Vol. 261, No. 14, (April 1989), pp. 2095-2100, ISSN 0098-7484.

Brouchet, L., Krust, A., Dupont, S., Chambon, P., Bayard, F., & Arnal, J. (2001). Estradiol accelerates reendothelialization in mouse carotid artery through estrogen receptor-alpha but not estrogen receptor-beta. *Circulation*, Vol.103, No.3 (January 2001), pp. 423-428, ISSN 0009-7322.

Butkevich, A., Abraham, C., & Phillips, R.A. (2000). Hormone replacement therapy and 24-hour blood pressure profile of postmenopausal women. *American Journal of Hypertension*, Vol.13, No.9, (September 2000), pp.1039-1041, ISSN 0895-7061.

Cagnacci, A., Rovati, L., Zanni, A., Malmusi, S., Facchinetti, F., & Volpe, A. (1999). Physiological doses of estradiol decrease nocturnal blood pressure in normotensive postmenopausal women. *American Journal of Physiology*, Vol. 276, No.4 Pt 2, (April 1999), pp.H1355-H1360, ISSN 0363-6135.

Chambliss, K.L., Yuhanna, I.S., Mineo, C., Liu, P., German, Z., Sherman, T.S., Mendelsohn, M.E., Anderson, R.G.W., & Shaul, P.W. (2000) Estrogen receptor α and endothelial nitric oxide synthase are organized into a functional signaling module in caveolae. *Circulation Research*, Vol.87, No.11, (November 2000), pp. e44-e52, ISSN: 0009-7330.

Chang, W.C., Nakao, J., Orimo, H., & Murota, S.I. (1980). Stimulation of prostaglandin cyclooxygenase and prostacyclin synthetase activities by estradiol in rat aortic smooth muscle cells. *Biochimica et Biophysica Acta*, Vol.620, No.3 (December 1980), pp. 472-482, ISSN 0006-3002.

Chapman, A.B., Zamudio, S., Woodmansee, W., Merouani, A., Osorio, F., Johnson, A., Moore, L.G., Dahms, T., Coffin, C., Abraham, W.T., Schrier, R.W. Systemic and renal hemodynamic changes in the luteal phase of the menstrual cycle mimic early pregnancy. *American Journal of Physiology*, Vol. 273, No.5 Pt 2, (November 1997), pp.F777-F782, ISSN 0363-6135.

Chen, F.P., Lee, N., Wang, C.H., Cherng W.J., & Soong, Y.K. (1998). Effects of hormone replacement therapy on cardiovascular risk factors in postmenopausal women. *Fertility and Sterility*, Vol.69, No.2, (February 1998), pp. 267–273, ISSN 0015-0282.

Chen, S. J., Li, H., Durand, J., Oparil, S., & Chen, Y.F. (1996). Estrogen reduces myointimal proliferation after balloon injury of rat carotid artery. *Circulation*, Vol.93, No.3, (February 1996), pp. 577-584, ISSN 0009-7322.

Chen, Y.F., & Oparil, S. (1998). Effects of sex steroids in vascular injury, In: Endocrinology of Cardiovascular Function, Levin, E.R., & Nadler, J.L., (Eds), pp.45-49, Kluwer Academic Publishers, ISBN 079238217X, Boston, Massachusetts.

Chen, Z., Yuhanna, I.S., Galcheva-Gargova, Z., Karas, R.H., Mendelsohn, M.E. & Shaul, P.W. (1999). Estrogen receptor α mediates the nongenomic activation of endothelial nitric oxide synthase by estrogen. *The Journal of Clinical Investigation*, Vol.103, No.3, (February 1999), pp. 401-406, ISSN 0021-9738.

Clarke, S.C., Kelleher, J., Lloyd-Jones, H., Slack, M., & Schofield, P.M. (2002). A study of hormone replacement therapy in postmenopausal women with iscaemic heart disease: the Papworth HRT Artherosclerosis Study. *British Journal of Obstetrics and Gynaecology*, Vol.109, No.9, (Sept 2002), pp. 1056-1062, ISSN 0306-5456.

Collins, P. (2001). Vascular effect of hormones. *Maturitas*, Vol.38, No.1, (February 2001), pp. 45-51, ISSN 0378-5122.

Cushman, M., Legault, C., Barrett-Connor, E., Stefanick, M.L., Kessler, C., Judd, H.L., Sakkinen, P.A., & Tracy, R.P. (1999). Effect of postmenopausal hormones on inflammation-sensitive proteins: The postmenopausal estrogen/progestin interventions (pepi) study. *Circulation*, Vol.100, No.7, (August 1999), pp. 717-722, ISSN 0009-7322.

Danenberg, H.D., Szalai, A.J., Swaminathan, R.V., Peng, L., Chen, Z., Seifert, P., Fay, W.P., Simon, D.I., & Edelman, E.R. (2003). Increased thrombosis after arterial injury in human c-reactive protein-transgenic mice. *Circulation*, Vol.108, No.5, (August 2003), pp. 512-515, ISSN 0009-7322.

Darling, G.M., Johns, J.A., McCloud, P.I., & Davis, S.R. (1997). Estrogen and progestin compared with simvastatin for hypercholesterolemia in postmenopausal women. *New England Journal of Medicine*, Vol.337, No.9, (August 1997), pp. 595-601, ISSN 1533-4406.

Demirol, A., Baykal, C., Kiazli, S., & Ayhan A. (2001). Effects of hormone replacement on hemostasis in spontaneous menopause. *Menopause*, Vol.8, No.2, (March 2001), pp. 135-140, ISSN 1530-0374.

Dennis, M.K., Burai, R., Ramesh, C., Petrie, W.K., Alcon, S.N., Nayak, T.K., Bologa, C.G., Leitao, A., Brailoiu, E., Deliu, E., Dun, N.J., Sklar, L.A., Hathaway, H.J., Arterburn, J.B., Oprea, T.I., & Prossnitz, E.R. (2009). In vivo effects of a GPR30 antagonist. *Nature Chemical Biology*, Vol.5, No.6, (June 2009), pp. 421-427, ISSN 1552-4469.

Dubey, R.K., Imthurn, B., Zacharia, L.C., & Jackson, E.K. (2004). Hormone Replacement Therapy and Cardiovascular Disease: What Went Wrong and Where Do We Go From Here? *Hypertension*. Vol.44, No.6, (December 2004), pp. 789-795, ISSN 0194-911X.

Dunne, F.P., Barry, D.G., Ferriss, J.B., Grealy, G., & Murphy, D. (1991). Changes in blood pressure during the normal menstrual cycle. *Clinical Science*, Vol.81, No.4, (October 1991), pp.515-518, ISSN 0143-5221.

Elhage, R. Clamens, S., Reardon-Alulis, C., Getz, G.S., Fievet, C., Maret, A., Arnal J.F., & Bayard, F. (2000). Loss of atheroprotective effect of estradiol in immunodefficient mice. *Endocrinology*, Vol.141, No.1, (January 2000), pp. 462-465.

Faraday, N., Goldschmidt-Clemont, P.J., & Bray, P.F. (1997). Gender differences in platelet GPIIb-IIIa activation. *Journal of Thrombosis and Haemostasis*, Vol.77, No.4, (April 1997), pp. 748-754, ISSN 0340-6245.

Feng, D., Lindpaintner, K., Larson, M.G., Rao, V.S., O'Donnell, C.J., Lipinska, I., Schmitz, C., Sutherland, P.A., Silbershatz, H., D'Agostino, R.B., Muller, J.E., Myers, R.H., Levy, D., & Geoffrey H. Tofler, G.H. (1999). Increased Platelet Aggregability Associated With Platelet *GPIIIa* Pl^{A2} *Polymorphism*: The Framingham Offspring Study. *Arteriosclerosis, Thrombosis, and Vascular Biology*, Vol.19, No.4, (April 1999), pp. 1142-1147, ISSN 1524-4636.

Filardo, E.J., Quinn, J.A., Bland, K.I., & Frackelton, A.R. (2000). Estrogen-induced activation of Erk-1 and Erk-2 requires the G protein-coupled receptor homolog, GPR30, and occurs via trans-activation of the epidermal growth factor receptor through release of HB-EGF. *Molecular Endocrinology*, Vol.14, No.10, (October 2000), pp. 1649-1660, ISSN 1944-9917.

Geraldes, P., Sirois, M.G., & Tanguay, J.F. (2003). Specific contribution of estrogen receptors on mitogen-activated protein kinase pathways and vascular cell activation. *Circulation Research*, Vol.93, No.5, (September 2003), pp. 399-405, ISSN 0009-7330.

Godsland, I.F. (2001). Effects of postmenopausal hormone replacement therapy on lipid, lipoprotein, and apolipoprotein (a) concentrations: analysis of studies published from 1974-2000. *Fertility and Sterility*, Vol.75, No.5, (May 2001), pp. 898-915, ISSN 0015-0282.

Grady, D., Herrington, D., Bittner, V., Blumenthal, R., Davidson, M., Hlatky, M., Hsia, J., Hulley, S., Herd, A., Khan, S., Newby, L.K., Waters, D., Vittinghoff, E., & Wenger, N., for the HERS Research Group. (2002). Cardiovascular Disease Outcomes During 6.8 Years of Hormone Therapy: Heart and Estrogen/Progestin Replacement Study Follow-up (HERS II). *Journal of the American Medical Association*, Vol.288, No.1, (July 2002), pp. 49-57, ISSN 1017-1606.

Grodstein, F. & Stampfer, M. (1995). The epidemiology of coronary heart disease and estrogen replacement in postmenopausal women. *Progress in Cardiovascular Disease*, Vol. 38, No. 3, (November-December 1995), pp. 199-210, ISSN 0033-0620.

Grodstein, F., Stampfer, M., Manson, J., Colditz, G., Willett, W., Rosner, B., Speizer, F., & Hennekens, C. (1996). Postmenopausal estrogen and progestin use and the risk of cardiovascular disease. *The New England Journal of Medicine*, Vol. 335, No. 7, (August 1996), pp. 453-461, ISSN 0028-4793.

Grodstein, F., Manson, J., Colditz, G., Willett, W., Speizer, F., & Stampfer, M. (2000). A prospective, observational study of postmenopausal hormone therapy and primary prevention of cardiovascular disease. *Annals of Internal Medicine*, Vol. 133, No. 12, (December 2000), pp. 933-941, ISSN 1539-3704.

Haas, E., Meyer, M.R., Schurr, U., Bhattacharya, I, Minotti, R., Nguyen, H.H., Heigl, A., Lachat, M., Genoni, M., & Barton, M. (2007). Differential effects of 17beta-estradiol on function and expression of estrogen receptor alpha, estrogen receptor beta, and GPR30 in arteries and veins of patients with atherosclerosis. *Hypertension*, Vol.49, No.6 (June 2007), pp. 1358-1363, ISSN 0194-911X.

Haas, E., Bhattacharya, I., Brailoiu, E., Damjanović, H., Brailoiu, G.C., Gao, X., Mueller-Guerre, L., Marjon, N.A., Gut, A., Minotti, R., Meyer, M.R., Amann, K., Ammann, E., Perez-Dominguez, A., Genoni, M., Clegg, D.J., Dun, N.J., Resta, T.C., Prossnitz, E.R., & Barton, M. (2009). Regulatory role of G protein-coupled estrogen receptor for vascular function and obesity. *Circulation Research*, Vol.104, No.3 (February 2009), pp. 288-291, ISSN 0009-7330.

Hage, F.G., McCrory, M.A., & Szalai, A.J. (2008). C-reactive protein and cardiovascular disease: Lessons learned from studying genetically engineered mice, In: *C-Reactive Protein – New Research*, Nagasawa, S. (Ed), pp.83-116, Nova Publishers, ISBN 978-1-60692-237-8, New York.

Hage, F.G., Oparil, S., Xing, D., Chen, Y.F., McCrory, M.A., & Szalai, A.J. (2010). C-reactive protein-mediated vascular injury requires complement. *Arteriosclerosis, Thrombosis, and Vascular Biology*, Vol.30, No.6, (June 2010), pp. 1189-1195, ISSN 1524-4636.

Haines, C.J., James, A.E., Panesar, N.S., Ngai, T.J., Sahota, D.S., Jones, R.L., Chang, A.M. (1999). The effect of percutaneous oestrediol on atheroma formation in ovariectomized cholesterol-fed rabbits. *Atherosclerosis*, Vol.143, No.2, (April 1999), pp. 369-375, ISSN 0021-9150.

Han, G., Ma, H., Chintala, R., Miyake, K., Fulton, D.J., Barman, S.A., & White, R.E. (2007). Nongenomic, endothelium-independent effects of estrogen on human coronary smooth muscle are mediated by type I (neuronal) NOS and PI3-kinase-Akt signaling. *American Journal of Physiology - Heart and Circulatory Physiology*, Vol.293, No.1, (July 2007), pp. H314-H321, ISSN 1522-1539.

Hansson, G.K. (2005). Inflammation, atherosclerosis, and coronary artery disease. *The New England Journal of Medicine*, Vol.352, No.16, (April 2005), pp. 1685-1695, ISSN 1533-4406.

Harman, S.M., Brinton, E.A., Cedars, M., Lobo, R., Manson, J.E., Merriam, G.R., Miller, V.M., Naftolin, F., & Santoro, N. (2005). KEEPS: The Kronos Early Estrogen Prevention Study. *Climacteric*, Vol.8, No.1 (January 2005), pp. 3–12, ISSN 1473-0804.

Harrington, W.R., Sheng, S., Barnett, D.H., Petz, L.N., Katzenellenbogen, J.A., & Katzenellenbogen, B.S. (2003). Activities of estrogen receptor alpha- and beta-selective ligands at diverse estrogen responsive gene sires mediating transactivation or transrepression. *Molecular and Cellular Endocrinology*, Vol.206, No.1-2, (August 2003), pp. 13-22, ISSN 1944-9917.

Harman, S., Brinton, E., Cedars, M., Lobo, R., Manson, J., Merriam, G., Miller, V., Naftolin, F., & Santoro, N. (2005). KEEPS: The Kronos early estrogen prevention study. Climacteric, Vol. 8, No. 1, (March 2005), pp. 3-12, ISSN 1369-7137.

Harman, S., Vittinghoff, E., Brinton, E., Budoff, M., Cedars, M., Lobo, R., Merriam, G., Miller, V., Naftolin, F., Pal, L., Santoro, N., Taylor, H., & Black, D. (2011). Timing and duration of menopausal hormone treatment may effect cardiovascular outcomes. American Journal of Medicine, Vol. 124, No. 3, (March 2011), pp. 199-205, ISSN 0002-9343.

Harvey, P.J., Molloy, D., Upton, J., & Wing, L.M. (2001). Dose response effect of cyclical medroxyprogesterone on blood pressure in postmenopausal women. *Journal of Human Hypertension*, Vol.15, No.5, (May 2001), pp.313-321, ISSN 0950-9240.

Hersh, A.L., Stefanick, M.L., & Stafford, R.S. (2004). National use of postmenopausal hormone therapy: annual trends and response to recent evidence. *Journal of the American Medical Association*, Vol.291, No.1, (January 2004), pp.47-53, ISSN 1017-1606.

Hodgin, J.B., Krege, J.H., Reddick, R.L., Korach, K.S., Smithies, O., Maeda, N. (2001). Estrogen receptor α is a major mediator of 17β-estradiols atheroprotective effects on lesion size in Apoe(-/-) mice. *The Journal of Clinical Investigation*, Vol.107, No.3, (February 2001), pp. 333-340, ISSN 0021-9738.

Hodis, H & Mack, W. (2011). A "window of opportunity": the reduction of coronary heart disease and total mortality with menopausal therapies is age- and time-dependent. Brain Research, Vol. 1379, pp. 244-252, ISSN 0006-8993.

Hsia, J., Laner, R., Manson, J., Kuller, L., Johnson, K., Crawford, S., Eaton, C., Kostis, J., Caralis, P., & Prentice, R. (2006). Conjugated equine estrogens and coronary heart disease:

Hu, F.B., Grodstein, F., Hennekens, C.H., Colditz, G.A., Johnson, M., Manson, J.E., Rosner, B., & Stampfer, M.J. (1999). Age at natural menopause and risk of cardiovascular disease. *Archives of Internal Medicine*, Vol.159, No.10, (May 1999), pp. 1061-1066, ISSN 1538-3679.

Huber, L.A., Scheffler, E., Poll, T., Ziegler, R., Dresel, H.A. (1990). 17B estradiol inhibits LDL oxidation and cholesterol ester formation in cultured macrophages. *Free Radical Research Communications*, Vol.8, No.3, (n.d. 1990), pp. 167-173, ISSN 8755-0199.

Hulley, S., Grady, D., Bush, T., Furberg, C., Herrington, D., Riggs, B., & Vittinghoff, E. For the Heart and Estrogen/progestin Replacement Study (HERS) Research Group. (1998). Original Contribution Randomized Trial of Estrogen Plus Progestin for Secondary Prevention of Coronary Heart Disease in Postmenopausal Women.

Journal of the American Medical Association, Vol.280, No.7, (August 1998), pp.605-613, ISSN 1017-1606.

Humphrey, L., Chan, B., & Sox, H. (2002). Postmenopausal hormone replacement therapy and the primary prevention of cardiovascular disease. *Annals of Internal Medicine*, Vol. 137, No. 4, (August 2002), pp. 273-284, ISSN 1539-3704.

Iafrati, M.D., Karas, R.H., Aronovitz, M., Kim, S., Sullivan, T.R., Lubahn, D.B., O'Donnell, T.F, Korach, K.S., & Mendelsohn, M.E. (1997). Estrogen inhibits the vascular injury response in estrogen receptor alpha-deficient mice. *Nature Medicine*, Vol.3, No.5, (May 1997), pp. 545-548, ISSN 1078-8956.

Jiang, C., Sarrel, P.M., Lindsay, D.C., Poole-Wilson, P.A., & Collins, P. (1991). Endothelium-independent relaxation of rabbit coronary artery by 17β-oestradiol in vitro. *British Journal of Pharmacology*, Vol.104, No.4, (December 1991), pp. 1033-1037, ISSN 1476-5381.

Karas, R.H., Hodgin, J.B., Kwoun, M., Krege, J.H., Aronovitz, M., Mackey, W., Gustafsson, J.A., Korach, K.S., Smithies, O., & Michael E. Mendelsohn, M.E. (1999). Estrogen inhibits the vascular injury response in estrogen receptor beta-deficient mice. *Proceedings of the National Academy of Sciences*, Vol.96, No.26, (December 1999), pp. 15133-15136, ISSN 1091-6490.

Karpanou, E.A., Vyssoulis, G.P., Georgoudi, D.G., Toutouza, M.G., & Toutouzas, P.K. (1993). Ambulatory blood pressure changes in the menstrual cycle of hypertensive women. Significance of plasma renin activity values. *American Journal of Hypertension*, Vol.6, No.8, (August 1993), pp. 654-659, ISSN 0895-7061.

Kelly, M.J., & Levin, E.R. (2001). Rapid actions of plasma membrane estrogen receptors. *Trends in Endocrinology and Metabolism*, Vol.12, No.4, (May 2001), pp. 152-156, ISSN 1043-2760.

Khetawat, G., Faraday, N., Nealen, M.L., Vijayan, K.V., Bolton, E., Noga, S.J, & Bray, P.F. (2000). Human megocaryocytes and platelets contain the estrogen receptor beta and androgen receptor (AR): testosterone regulates AR expression. *Blood*, Vol.95, No.7 (April 2000), pp. 2289-2296, ISSN 1528-0020.

Killam, A.P., Rosenfeld, C.R., Battaglia, F.C., Makowski, E.L., & Meschia, G. (1973). Effect of estrogens on the uterine blood flow of oophorectomized ewes. *American Journal of Obstetrics & Gynecology*, Vol.115, No.8, (April 1973), pp. 1045-1052, , ISSN 1097-6868.

Kitazawa, T., Hamada, E., Kitazawa, K., & Gaznabi, A.K.M. (1997). Non-genomic mechanism of 17β-oestradiol-induced inhibition of contraction in mammalian vascular smooth muscle. *Journal of Physiology*, Vol.499, No.Pt 2, (March 1997), pp. 497-511, ISSN 1469-7793.

Kramer, P., Kramer, S., & Guan, G. (2004) 17 beta-estradiol regulates cytokine release through modulation of cd16 expression in monocytes and monocyte-derived macrophages. *Arthritis and Rheumatism*, Vol. 50, No. 6, (June 2004), pp. 1967-1975, ISSN 1529-0131.

Kramer, P., Winger, V., & Kramer, S. (2007) 17beta-estradiol utilizes the estrogen receptor to regulate cd16 expression in monocytes. *Molecular and Cellular Endocrinology*, Vol. 279, No. 1-2, (December 2007), pp. 16-25, ISSN 0303-7207.

Krantz, J.C., & Carr, C.J. (1958), The Pharmacologic Principles of Medical Practice, Williams & Wilkins, Baltimore, Maryland.

Kristiansson, P., & Wang, J.X. (2001). Reproductive hormones and blood pressure during pregnancy. *Human Reproduction*, Vol.16, No.1, (January 2001), pp. 13-17, ISSN 0268-1161.

Krom, Y., Pires, N., Jukema, J., de Vries, M., Frants, R., Havekes, L., van Dijk, K., & Quax P. (2007). Inhibition of neointima formation by local delivery of estrogen receptor alpha and beta specific agonists. *Cardiovascular Research*, Vol. 73, No. 1, (January 2006), pp. 217-226, ISSN 008-6363.

Kroon, U.B., Tengborn, L., Rita, H., & Bäckstrom, A.C. (1997). The effects of transdermal oestradiol and oral progestogens on haemostasis variables. *British Journal of Obstetrics and Gynaecology*, Vol.104, No.s16, (November 1997), pp. 32-37.

Kumar, A., Lindner, V. (1997). Remodeling with neointima formation in the mouse carotid artery after cessation of blood flow. *Arteriosclerosis, Thrombosis, and Vascular Biology*, Vol. 17, No. 10, (October 1997), pp. 2238-2244, ISSN 1049-8834.

Kuehl, F.A., Ham, E.A., Zanetti, M.E., Sanford, C.H., Nicol, S.E., & Goldberg, N.D. (1974). Estrogen-related increases in uterine guanosine 3',5'-cyclic monophosphate levels. *Proceedings of the National Academy of Sciences, Vol.*71, No.5 (May 1974), pp. 1866-1870, ISSN 1091-6490.

Kurtz, E., Ridker, P., Rose, L., Cook, N., Everett, B., Buring, J., & Rexrode, K. (2011). Oral postmenopausal hormone therapy, c-reactive protein, and cardiovascular outcomes. *Menopause*, Vol. 18, No. 1, (January 2011), pp. 23-29, ISSN 1072-3714.

LaCroix, A., Chlebowski, R., Manson, J., Aragaki, A., Johnson, K., Martin, L., Margolis, K., Stefanick, M., Brzyski, R., Curb, J., Howard, B., Lewis, C., & Wactawski-Wende, J. (2011). Health outcomes after stopping conjugated equine estrogens among postmenopausal women with prior hysterectomy. *Journal of the American Medical Association*, Vol. 305, No. 13, (April 2011), pp. 1305-1314, ISSN 0098-7484.

Lakoski, S.G., & Herrington, D.M. (2005). Effects of hormone therapy on c-reactive protein and il-6 in postmenopausal women: A review article. *Climacteric*, Vol.8, No.4, (January 2005), pp. 317-326, ISSN 1473-0804.

Lerner, D.J. & Kannal, W.B. (1986). Patterns of coronary heart disease morbidity and mortality in the sexes: A 26-year follow-up of the Framingham population. *American Heart Journal*, Vol.111, No.2 (February 1986), pp.383-90, ISSN 0002-8703.

Levine, R.L., Chen, SJ., Durand, J., Chen YF., & Oparil, S. (1996). Medroxyprogesterone Attenuates Estrogen-Mediated Inhibition of Neointima Formation After Balloon Injury of the Rat Carotid Artery. *Circulation*, Vol.94, No.9, (November 1996), pp. 2221-2227, ISSN 0009-7322.

Lindoff, C., Peterson, F., Lecander, I., Martinsson, G., & Astedt, B. (1996). Transdermal estrogen replacement therapy: Beneficial effects on hemostatic risk factors for cardiovascular disease. *Maturitas*, Vol.24, No.1, (May 1996), pp. 43-50, ISSN 0378-5122.

Lloyd-Jones, D., Adams, R., Brown, T., Carnethon, M., Dai, S., De Simone, G., Ferguson, T., Ford, E., Furie, K., Gillespie, C., Go, A., Greenlund, K., Haase, N., Hailpern, S., Ho, P., Howard, V., Kissela, B., Kittner, S., Lackland, D., Lisabeth, L., Marelli, A., McDermott, M., Meigs, J., Mozaffarian, D., Mussolino, M., Nichol, G., Roger,V., Rosamond, W., Sacco, R., Sorlie, P., Thom, T., Wasserthiel-Smoller, S., Wong, N., & Wylie-Rosett, J. (2010). Heart disease and stroke statistics--2010 update: A report from the american heart association. *Circulation*, Vol. 121, No. 12, (February 2010), pp. e46-e215, ISSN 0009-7322.

Lobo, R.A., & Cassidenti, D.L. (1992). Pharmacokinetics of 17β-estradiol. *Journal of Reproductive Medicine*, Vol.37, No.X, (MO 1992), pp. 77-84, ISSN 0024-7758.

Lobo, R.A., Kelsey, J., & Marcus, R., (Eds). (2000). *Menopause: Biology and Pathobiology*, Academic Press, ISBN 0124537901, New York.

Lyman, G.W., & Johnson, R.N. (1982). Assay for conjugated estrogens in tablets using fused-silica capillary gas chromatography. *Journal of Chromatography*, Vol.234, No.1, (Jan 1982), pp. 234-239, ISSN 0021-9673.

Luster A. (1998) Chemokines- Chemotactic cytokines that mediate inflammation. New *England Journal of Medicine*, Vol. 338, No. 7, (February 1998), pp. 436-445, ISSN 0028-4793.

Manson, J.E., Hsia, J., Johnson, K.C., Rossouw, J.E., Assaf, A., Lasser, N.L., Trevisan, M., Black, H., Heckbert, S.R., Detrano, R., Strickland, O.L., Wong, N.D., Crouse, J.R., Stein, E., & Cushman, M. For the Women's Health Initiative Investigators. (2003). Estrogen plus Progestin and the Risk of Coronary Heart Disease. *The New England Journal of Medicine*, Vol.349, No.6, (August 2003), pp.523-534, ISSN 1533-4406.

Martin, K. & Barbieri, R. (2011). Preparations for postmenopausal hormone therapy, in: *UpToDate.com*, Accessed August 11, 2011, Available from: http://www.uptodate.com/contents/preparations-for-postmenopausal-hormone-therapy?source=search_result&selectedTitle=4%7E150

Mashchak, C.A., Lobo, R.A., Dozono-Takano, R. Eggena, P., Nakamura, R.M., Brenner, P.F., & Mishell, D.R. (1982). Comparison of pharmacodynamic properties of various estrogen formulations. *American Journal of Obstetrics & Gynecology*, Vol.144, No.5, (November 1982), pp. 511-518, ISSN 1097-6868.

Matthews, K., Kuller, L., Wing, R., Meilahn, E., & Plantinga, P. (1996). Prior to use of estrogen replacement therapy, are users healthier than nonusers? *American Journal of Epidemiology*, Vol. 143, No. 10, (May 1996), pp. 971-978, ISSN 0002-9262.

Mendelsohn, M.E., & Karas, R.H. (2005). Molecular and Cellular Basis of Cardiovascular Gender Differences. *Science*, Vol.308, No.5728, (June 2005), pp. 1583-1587, ISSN 1095-9203.

Mercuro, G., Zoncu, S., Pilia, I., Lao, A., Mellis, G.B.,& Cherchi, A. (1997). Effects of acute administration of transdermal estrogen on postmenopausal women with systemic hypertension. *American Journal of Cardiology*, Vol.80, No.5, (September 1997), pp. 652-655, ISSN 0002-9149.

Mercuro, G., Zoncu, S., Piano, D., Pilia, I., Lao, A., Mellis, G.B., & Cherchi, A. (1998). Estradiol-17β reduces blood pressure and restores normal amplitude of the circadian blood pressure rhythm in postmenopausal hypertension. *American Journal of Hypertension*, Vol.11, No.8, (August 1998), pp. 909-913, ISSN 0895-7061.

Miller, A.P., Feng, W., Xing, D., Weathington, N.M., Blalock, J.E., Chen, YF., & Oparil, S. (2004). Estrogen Modulates Inflammatory Mediator Expression and Neutrophil Chemotaxis in Injured Arteries. *Circulation*, Vol.110, No.12, (September 2004), pp. 1664-1669, ISSN 0009-7322.

Miller, A., Xing, D., Feng, W., Fintel, M., Chen, Y., & Oparil, S. (2007). Aged rats lose vasoprotective and anti-inflammatory effects of estrogen in injured arteries. *Menopause*, Vol. 14, No. 2, (March-April 2007), pp. 251-260, ISSN 1072-3714.

Miller, V.M., & Ducklers, S.P. (2008). Vascular actions of estrogens: functional implications. *Pharmacological Reviews*, Vol.60, No.2, (June 2008), pp. 210-241, ISSN 1521-0081.

Mondul, A.M., Rodriguez, C., Jacobs, E.J., & Calle, E.E. (2005). Age at natural menopause and cause-specific mortality. *American Journal of Epidemiology*, Vol.162, No. 11, (December 2005), pp. 1089-1097, ISSN 0002-9262.

Mori, T., Durand, J., Chen, Y., Thompson, J., Bakir, S., & Oparil, S. (2000). Effects of short-term estrogen treatment on the neointimal reponse to balloon injury of rat carotid artery. *American Journal of Cardiology*, Vol. 85, No. 10, (May 2000), pp. 1276-1279, ISSN 0002-9149.

Mosca, L., Appel, L.J., Benjamin, E.J., Berra, K., Chandra-Strobos, N., Fabunmi, R.P., Grady, D., Haan, C.K., Hayes, S.N., Judelson, D.R., Keenan, N.L., McBride, P., Oparil, S., Ouyang, P., Oz, M.C., Mendelsohn, M.E., Pasternak, R.C., Pinn, V.W., Robertson, R.M., Schenck-Gustafsson, K., Sila, C.A., Smith, S.C., Sopko, G., Taylor, A.L., Walsh, B.W., Wenger, N.K., & Williams, C.L. (2004). Evidence-Based Guidelines for Cardiovascular Disease Prevention in Women. *Circulation*, Vol.109, No.5, (February 2004), pp. 672-693, ISSN 0009-7322.

Mosca, L., Banka, C.L., Benjamin, E.J., Berra, K., Bushnell, C., Dolor, R.J., Ganiats, T.G., Gomes, A.S., Gornik, H.L., Gracia, C., Gulati, M., Haan, C.K., Judelson, D.R., Keenan, N., Kelepouris, E., Michos, E.N., Newby, L.K., Oparil, S., Ouyang, P., Oz, M.C., Petitti, D., Pinn, V.W., Redberg, R.F., Scott, R., Sherif, K., Smith, S.C., Sopko, G., Steinhorn, R.H., Stone, N.J., Taubert, K.A., Todd, B.A., Urbina, E., Wenger, N.K., & for the Expert Panel/Writing Group. (2007). Evidence-Based Guidelines for Cardiovascular Disease Prevention in Women: 2007 Update. *Circulation*, Vol.115, No.11, (March 2007), pp. 1481-1501, ISSN: 0009-7322.

Nabulsi, A.A., Folsom, A.R., White, A., Patsch, W., Heiss, G., Wu, K.K., & Szklo, M. for the Atherosclerosis Risk in Communities Study Investigators. (1993). Association of hormone replacement therapy with various cardiovascular risk factos in post menopausal women. *The New England Journal of Medicine*, Vol.328, No.15, (April 1993), pp. 1069-1075, ISSN 1533-4406.

Nagai, T., Anzai, T., Kaneko, H., Mano, Y., Anzai, A., Maekawa, Y., Takahashi, T., Meguro, T., Yoshikawa, T., & Fukuda, K. (2011). C-reactive protein overexpression exacerbates pressure overload-induced cardiac remodeling through enhanced inflammatory response. *Hypertension*. Vol. 57, No. 2, (February 2011), pp. 208-215, ISSN 0194-911X.

Nakano, Y., Oshima, T., Matsuura, H., Kajiyama, G., & and Kambe, M. (1998). Effect of 17β-estradiol on inhibition of platelet aggregation in vitro is mediated by an increase in NO synthesis. *Arteriosclerosis, Thrombosis, and Vascular Biology*, Vol.18, No.6, (June 1998), pp. 961–967, ISSN 1524-4636.

Negre-Salveyre, A., Pieraggi, M.T., Mabile, L., & Salvayre, R. (1993). Protective effects of 17B-estradiol against the cytotoxicity of minimally oxidized LDL to cultured bovine aortic endothelial cells. *Atherosclerosis*, Vol.99, No.2, (March 1993), pp. 209-217, ISSN 0021-9150.

Oparil, S., Levine, R.L., Chen, S.J., Durand, J., & Chen, Y.F. (1997). Sexually Dimorphic Response of the Balloon-Injured Rat Carotid Artery to Hormone Treatment. *Circulation*, Vol.95, No.5, (March 1997), pp.1301-1307, ISSN 0009-7322.

Oparil, S., Chen, S., Chen, Y., Durand, J., Allen, L., & Thompson, J. (1999) Estrogen attenuates the adventitial contribution to neointima formation in injured rat carotid arteries. *Cardiovascular Research,* Vol. 44, No. 3, (December 1999), pp. 608-614, ISSN 0008-6363.

Ottosson, U.B., Johansson, B.G., & von Schoultz, B. (1985). Subfractions of high density lipoprotein cholesterol during estrogen replacement therapy: a comparison between progestogens and natural progesterone. *American Journal of Obstetrics & Gynecology,* Vol.151, No.6, (March 1985), pp. 746-750, ISSN 1097-6868.

Pan, C.C., Woolever, C.A., & Bhavani, B.R. (1985). Transport of equine estrogens: binding of conjugated and uncunjugated equine estrogens with human serum proteins. *Journal of Clinical Endocrinology and Metabolism,* Vol.61, No.3, (September 1985), pp. 499-507, ISSN 1945-7197.

Paul, A., Ko, K., Li, L., Yechoor, V., McCrory, M., Szalai, A., & Chan, L. (2004). C-reactive protein accelerates the progression of atherosclerosis in apolipoprotein e-deficient mice. *Circulation,* Vol. 109, No. 5, (February 2004), pp. 647-655, ISSN 0009-7322.

Pettersson, K., Delaunay, F., & Gustafsson, J.A. (2000). Estrogen receptor beta acts as a dominant regulator of estrogen signaling. *Oncogene,* Vol.19, No.43, (October 2000), pp. 4970-4978, ISSN 1476-5594.

Phillips, L.S., & Langer, R.D. (2005). Postmenopausal hormone therapy: Critical reappraisal and a unified hypothesis. *Fertility and Sterility,* Vol.83, No.3 (March 2005), pp. 558-566, ISSN 0015-0282.

Pinna, C., Cifnarella, A., Sanvito, P., Pelosi, V., & Bolego, C. (2008). Prolonged ovarian hormone deprivation impairs the protective vascular actions of estrogen receptor alpha agonists. *Hypertension,* Vol. 51, No. 4, (April 2010), pp. 1210-1217, ISSN 0194-911X.

Powers, M.S., Schenkel, L, Darley, P.E., Good, W.R., Balestra, J.C., & Place, V.A. (1985). Pharmacokinetics and Pharmodynamics of transdermal dosage froms fo 17ß-estradiol: comparison with conventional oral estrogens used for hormone replacement. *American Journal of Obstetrics & Gynecology,* Vol.152, No.8, (August 1985), pp. 1099-1106, ISSN 1097-6868.

Prossnitz, E.R., & Barton, M. (2009). Signaling, physiological functions and clinical relevance of the G protein-coupled estrogen receptor GPER. *Prostaglandins & Other Lipid Mediators,* Vol.89, No.3-4, (Sept 2009), pp. 89-97, ISSN 1098-8823.

Psaty, B., Heckbert, S., Atkins, D., Lemaitre, R., Koepsell, T., Wahl, P., Siscovick, D., & Wagner, E. (1994). The risk of myocardial infarction associated with the combined use of estrogens and progestins in postmenopausal women. *Archives of Internal Medicine,* Vol. 154, No. 12, (June 1994), pp. 1333-1339, ISSN 1538-3679.

Ranganath, L.R., Christofides, J., & Semple, M.J. (1996). Increase mean platelet volume after estrogen replacement therapy. *Annals of Chemical Biochemistry*, Vol.33, No.Pt 6, (November 1996), pp. 555-560, ISSN 0004-5632.

Revankar, C.M., Cimino, D.F., Sklar, L.A., Arterburn, J.B., & Prossnitz, E.R. (2005). A transmmebrane intracellular estrogen receptor mediates rapid cell signaling. *Science*, Vol.307, No.5715, (March 2005), pp. 1625-1630, ISSN 1095-9203.

Roger, V.L., Go, A.S., Lloyd-Jones, D.M., Adams, R.J., Berry, J.D., Brown, T.D., Carnethon, M.R., Dai, S., de Simone, G., Ford, E.S., Fox, C.S., Fullerton, H.J., Gillespie, C., Greenlund, K.J., Hailpern, S.M., Heit, J.A., Ho, P.M., Howard, V.J., Kissela, B.M., Kittner, S.J., Lackland, D.T., Lichtman, J.H., Lisabeth, L.D., Makuc, D.M., Marcus, G.M., Marelli, A., Matchar, D.B., McDermott, M.M., Meigs, J.B., Moy, C.S., Mozaffarian, D., Mussolino, M.E., Nichol, G., Paynter, N.P., Rosamond, W.D.,

Sorlie, P.D., Stafford, R.S., Turan, T.N., Turner, M.B., Wong, N.D., & Wylie-Rosett, J. (2011). Heart Disease and Stroke Statistics—2011 Update: A Report From the American Heart Association. *Circulation*, Vol.123, No.4, (February 2011), pp. e18-e209, ISSN: 0009-7322.

Rosenfeld, C.R., White, R.E., Roy, T., & Cox, B.E. (2000). Calcium-activated potassium channels and nitric oxide coregulate estrogen-induced vasodilation. *American Journal of Physiology - Heart and Circulatory Physiology*, Vol.279, No.1, (July 2000), pp. H319-H328. ISSN 1522-1539.

Rosenthal, T., &Oparil, S. (2000). Hypertension in women. *Journal of Human Hypertension*, Vol.14, No.10-11 (October-November 2000), pp.691-704, ISSN 0950-9240.

Rossouw, J.E., Garnet L. Anderson, G.L., Prentice, R.L., LaCroix, A.Z., Kooperberg, C., Stefanick, M.L., Jackson, R.D., Beresford, S.A., Howard, B.V., Johnson, K.C., Kotchen, J.M., & Ockene, J. Writing Group for the Women's Health Initiative Investigators. (2002). Risks and Benefits of Estrogen Plus Progestin in Healthy Postmenopausal Women: Principal Results From the Women's Health Initiative Randomized Controlled Trial. *Journal of the American Medical Association*, Vol.288, No.3, (July 2002), pp. 321-333, ISSN 1017-1606.

Rossouw, J., Prentice, R., Manson, J., Wu, L., Barad, D., Barnabei, V., Ko, M., LaCroix, A., Margolis, K., & Stefanick, M. (2007). Postmenopausal hormone therapy and risk of cardiovascular disease by age and years since menopause. *Journal of the American Medical Association*, Vol. 297, No. 13, (April 2007), pp. 1465-1477, ISSN 1538-3598.

Schnoes, K.K., Jaffe, I.Z., Iyer, L., Dabreo, A., Aronovitz, M., Newfell, B., Hansen, U., Rosano, G., & Mendelsohn, M.E. (2008). Rapid recruitment of temporally distinct vascular gene sets by estrogen. *Molecular Endocrinology*, Vol.22, No.11, (November 2008), pp. 2544-2556, ISSN 1944-9917.

Schunkert, H., Danser, A.H., Hense, H.W., Derkx, F.H., Kürzinger, S., & Riegger, G.A. (1997). Effects of estrogen replacement therapy on the renin-angiotensin system in postmenopausal women. Circulation, Vol.95, No.1, (January 1997), pp.39-45, ISSN 0009-7322.

Seely, E.W., Walsh, B.W., Gerhard, M.D., & Williams, G.H. (1999). Estradiol with or without progesterone and ambulatory blood pressure in postmenopausal women. *Hypertension*, Vol.33, No.5, (May 1999), pp. 1190-1194, ISSN 0194-911X.

Shan, J., Resnick, L.M., Liu, Q.Y., Wu, X.C., Barbagallo, M., & Pang, P.K.T. (1994). Vascular effects of 17β-estradiol in male Sprague-Dawley rats. *American Journal of Physiology Heart and Circulatory Physiology*, Vol.266, No.3-Pt 2 (March 1994), pp. H967-H973. ISSN: 0363-6135.

Siamopoulos, K.C., Papanikolaou, S., Elisaf, M., Theodorou, J., Pappas, H., & Papanikolaou, N. (1996). Ambulatory blood pressure monitoring in normotensive pregnant women. *Journal of Human Hypertension*, Vol.10, No.Suppl3 (September 1996), pp.S51-S54, ISSN 0950-9240.

Simoncini, T., Mannella, P., Fornari, L., Caruso, A., Willis, M.Y., Garibaldi, S., Baldacci, C., & Genazzani, A.R. (2004). Differential Signal Transduction of Progesterone and Medroxyprogesterone Acetate in Human Endothelial Cells. *Endocrinology*, Vol.145, No.12 (December 2004), pp. 5745-5756, ISSN 1945-7170.

Somlyo, A.P., & Somlyo, A.V. (1994). Signal transduction and regulation in smooth muscle. *Nature*, Vol.372, No.6503, (November 1994), pp. 231-236, ISSN 1476-4687.

Special Correspondent. (1958). Hormones and atherosclerosis: Meeting in Utah. *British Medical Journal*, Vol.1, No.5078, (May 1958), pp. 1059-1060, ISSN 0959-8138.
Speroff, L. & Fritz, M. (2005). *Clinical Gynecologic Endocrinology and Infertility*. Editor Weinberg, R. Lippincott, Williams, and Wilkins, ISBN 0-7817-4795-3, Philadelphia.
Staessen, J.A., Ginocchio, G., Thijs, L., & Fagard, R. (1997). Conventional and ambulatory blood pressure and menopause in a prospective population study. *Journal of Human Hypertension*, Vol.11, No.8 (August 1997), pp. 507-514, ISSN 0950-9240.
Staessen, J.A., Celis, H., & Fagard, R. (1998). The epidemiology of the association between hypertension and menopause. *Journal of Human Hypertension*, Vol.12, No.9 (September 1998), pp.587-592, ISSN 0950-9240.
Stevenson, L.C. (2009). Type and Route of Estrogen Administration. *Climacteric*, Vol.12, No.s1, (January 2009), pp. 86-90, ISSN 1473-0804.
Störk, S., van der Schouw, Y.T., Grobbee, D.E., & Bots, M.L. (2004). Estrogen, inflammation and cardiovascular risk in women: a critical appraisal. *Trends in Endocrinology and Metabolism*, Vol.15, No.2 (March 2004), pp. 66-72, ISSN 1043-2760.
Szalai, A., Agrawal, A., Greenhough, T., & Volanakis, J.E. (1997) C-reactive protein: structural biology, gene expression, and host defense function. *Immunologic Research*, Vol.16, No. 2, (1997), pp. 127-13, ISSN 0257-277X.
Szalai, A., van Ginkel, F., Dalrymple, S., Murray, R., McGhee, J., & Volanakis, J. (1998) Testosterone and Il-6 requirements for human c-reactive protein gene expression in transgenic mice. *Journal of Immunology*, Vol. 160, No. 11, (June 1998), pp. 5294-5299, ISSN 0022-1767.
Szalai, A, & McCrory, M. (2002). Varied biologic functions of c-reactive protein: Lessons learned from transgenic mice. *Immunologic Research*, Vol. 26, No. 1-3, (2002), pp. 279-287, ISSN 0257-277X.
Takahashi, T., Anzai, T., Kaneko, H., Mano, Y., Anzai, A., Nagai, T., Kohno, T., Maekawa, Y., Yoshikawa, T., Fukuda, K., & Ogawa, S. (2010). Increased c-reactive protein expression exacerbates left ventricular dysfunction and remodeling after myocardial infarction. *American Journal of Physiology - Heart and Circulatory Physiology*, Vol. 299, No. 6, (December 2010), pp. H1795-1804, ISSN 0363-6135.
Tech, H., Quan, A., & Leung, S. (2001). Vascular effects of estrone and DES in porcine coronary arteries. *Menopause*, Vol.16, No.1, (January 2001), pp. 104-109, ISSN 1530-0374.
The Women's Health Initiative Steering Committee. (2004). Effects of Conjugated Equine Estrogen in Postmenopausal Women with Hysterectomy: The Women's Health Initiative Randomized Controlled Trial. *Journal of the American Medical Association*, Vol.291, No.14, (April 2004), pp.1701-1712, ISSN 1017-1606.
The Women's Health Initiative. (2006). Conjugated equine estrogens and coronary heart disease: the Women's Health Initiative. *Archives of Internal Medicine*. Vol. 166, No.3, (February 2006), pp. 357-365, ISSN 1538-3679.
The Writing Group for the PEPI Trial. (1995). Effects of estrogen or estrogen/progestin regimens on heart disease risk factors in postmenopausal women. The Postmenopausal Estrogen/Progestin Interventions (PEPI) Trial. *Journal of the American Medical Association*, Vol.273, No.3, (January 1995), pp. 199-208
Thijs, A., Van Baal, W. A M., Van Der Mooren, M.J., Kenemans, P., Dräger, A.M., Huijgens, P. C., & Stehouwer, C.D.. (2002). Effects of hormone replacement therapy on blood

platelets. *European Journal of Clinical Investigation*, Vol.32, No.8, (August 2002), pp. 613-618, ISSN 1365-2362.

Toh, S., Hernandez-Diaz, S., Logan, R., Rossouw, J., & Hernan, M. (2010). Coronoary heart disease in postmenopausal recipients of estrogen plus progestin therapy: does the increased risk ever disappear? A randomized trial. *Annals of Internal Medicine*, Vol. 152, No. 4, (February 2010), pp. 211-217, ISSN 1539-3704.

Tse, J., Martin-McNaulty, B., Halks-Miller, M., Kauser, K., DelVecchi, V., Vergona, R., Sullivan, M.E., & Rubyani, G.M. (1999).Accelerated atherosclerosis and premature calcified cartilaginous metaplasia in the aorta of diabetic male Apo E knockout mice can be prevented by chronic treatment with 17β-estradiol. *Atherosclerosis*, Vol.144, No.2, (June 1999), pp. 303-313, ISSN 0021-9150.

Turgeon, J.L., McDonnell, D.P., Martin, K.A., & Wise, P.M. (2004). Hormone Therapy: Physiological Complexity Belies Therapeutic Simplicity. *Science*, Vol.304, No.5675, (May 2004), pp. 1269-1273, ISSN 1095-9203.

Van Buren, G.A., Yang, D.S., & Clark, K.E. (1992). Estrogen-induced uterine vasodilatation is antagonized by L-nitroarginine methyl ester, an inhibitor of nitric oxide synthesis. *American Journal of Obstetrics & Gynecology*, Vol.167, No.3, (September 1992), pp. 828-833, ISSN 1097-6868.

Vongpatanasin, W., Tuncel, M., Wang, Z., Arbique, D., Mehrad, B., & Jialal, I. (2003). Differential effects of oral versus transdermal estrogen replacement therapy on c-reactive protein in postmenopausal women. *Journal of the American College of Cardiology*, Vol. 41, No. 8, (April 2003), pp. 1358-1363, ISSN 0735-1097.

Walsh, B.W., Schiff, I., Rosner, B., Greenberg, L., Ravnikar, V., & Sacks, F.M. (1991). Effects of postmenopausal estrogen replacement on the concentrations and metabolism of plasma lipoproteins. *The New England Journal of Medicine*, Vol.325, No.17, (October 1991), pp. 1196-1204, ISSN 1533-4406.

Wang, D., Oparil, S., Chen, Y., McCrory, M., Skibinski, G., Feng, W., & Szalai, A. (2005). Estrogen treatment abrogates neointima formation in human c-reactive protein transgenic mice. *Arteriosclerosis, Thrombosis, and Vascular Biology*. Vol. 25, No. 10, (October 2005), pp. 2094-2099.

Wassertheil-Smoller, S., Anderson, G., Psaty, B.M., Black, H.R., Manson, J., Wong, N., Francis, J., Grimm, R., Kotchen, T., Langer, R., & Lasser N. (2000). Hypertension and its treatment in postmenopausal women: baseline data from the Women's Health Initiative. *Hypertension*, Vol.36, No.5, (November 2000), pp.780-789, ISSN 0194-911X.

Williams, A.K., Honore, E.K., Washburn, S.A., & Clarkson, T.B. (1994). Effects of hormone replacement therapy on reactivity of atherosclerotic coronary arteries in cynomolgus monkeys. *Journal of the American College of Cardiology*, Vol.24, No.7, (December 1994), pp. 1757-1761, ISSN 0735-1097.

Xing, D., Miller, A., Novak, L., Rocha, R., Chen, Y.F., & Oparil, S. (2004). Estradiol and progestins differentially modulate leukocyte infiltration after vascular injury. *Circulation*, Vol.109, No.2, (January 2004), pp.234-241, ISSN 0009-7322.

Xing, D., Feng, W., Miller, A., Weathington, N., Chen, Y., Novak, L., Blalock, E., & Oparil, S. (2007). Estrogen modulates TNF-α-induced inflammation in rat aortic smooth muscles cells through estrogen receptor-ß activation. *American Journal of Physiology - Heart and Circulatory Physiology*, Vol. 292, No. 6, (June 2007), pp. H2607-H2612, ISSN 0363-6135.

Xing, D., Hage, F., Chen, Y., McCrory, M., Feng, W., Skibinski, G., Majid-Hassan, E., Oparil, S., & Szalai, A. (2008). Exaggerated neointima formation in human c-reactive protein transgenic mice is IgG FC receptor type I (fc gamma rI)-dependent. *American Journal of Pathology*, Vol. 172, No. 1, (January 2008), pp. 22-30, ISSN 0002-9440.

Xing D., Nozell, S., Chen, Y.F., Hage, F., Oparil, S. (2009). Estrogen and mechanisms of vascular protection. *Arteriosclerosis, Thrombosis, and Vascular Biology*., Vol.29, No.3 (March 2009), pp. 289-295, ISSN 1524-4636.

Yamada, S., Gotoh, T., Nakashima, Y., Kayaba, K., Ishikawa, S., Nago, N., Nakamura, Y., Itoh, Y., & Kajii, E. (2001). Distribution of serum c-reactive protein and its association with atherosclerotic risk factors in a japanese population : Jichi medical school cohort study. *American Journal Of Epidemiology*, Vol. 153, No. 12, (June 2001), pp. 1183-1190, ISSN 0002-9262.

Yee, D.L., & Bray, P.F. Platelet hyperreactivity: risk factors and the effects of hormones. Adv Stud Med, Vol.4, No.2, (February 2004), pp. 72-78.

Yoshimura, T., Ohshige, A., Maeda, T., Ito, M., & Okamura, H. (1999). Estrogen replacement therapy decreases platelet activating factor acetylhydrolase activity in postmenopausal women. *Maturitas*, Vol.31, No.2, (January 1999), pp. 149-153, ISSN 0378-5122.

Zhang, R., Zhang, Y., Huang, X., Wu, Y., Chung, A., Wu, E., Szalai, A., Wong, B., Lau, C., & Lan, H. (2010). C-reactive protein promotes cardiac fibrosis and inflammation in angiotensin II-induced hypertensive cardiac disease. *Hypertension*, Vol. 55, No. 4, (April 2010), pp. 953-960, ISSN 0194-911X.

Zhu, Y., Bian, Z., Lu, P., Karas, R.H., Bao, L., Cox, D., Hodgin, J., Shaul, P.W., Thoren, P., Smithies, O., Gustafsson, J.A., & Mendelsohn, M.E. (2002). Abnormal vascular function and hypertension in mice deficient in estrogen receptor β. *Science*, Vol.295, No.5554, (January 2002), pp.505-508, ISSN 1095-9203.

2

The Role of Sex Hormones in the Cardiovascular System

Gorazd Drevenšek
University of Ljubljana, Faculty of Medicine,
Institute of Pharmacology and Experimental Toxicology
Slovenia

1. Introduction

In developed countries heart disease is the primary cause of death in men and in women over the age of 60. While premenopausal women have a low incidence of cardiovascular disease as compared to men, the mortality among post-menopausal women rises to the same frequency or even exceeds the rates of men (Adams et al., 1995; Fraser et al., 2000; Gray et al., 2001; Wild & Bartholemew, 1988). This significant gender difference is mostly attributed to the beneficial role of estrogens (Collins et al., 1993; Gray et al., 2001). Many studies have suggested that females have reduced incidence of cardiovascular diseases due to the beneficial effects of estrogen on both the lipid profile and on the vasculature. Lately, many new mechanisms are discovered in cardiovascular diseases and research has been focused on the role of both estrogen and testosterone, as well as some other androgens, but also on the estrogen receptor GPER, which shows an important role in the cardioprotection of both, males and females (Deschamps &Murphy, 2009).

The sex hormones in the cardiovascular system might be viewed at as biomarkers for cardiovascular health status, as well as by itself, as protective agents against myocardial diseases. The estrogens in premenopausal women are modulating health in the regular menstrual cycle. Testosterone is lacking such cycle activity and is probably more expressed in the physically active population. The effects of testosterone are increasing muscle mass induced by higher physical activity, and higher adrenal and hypophysis activity resulting in potential cardiovascular system damage. However, when testosterone or its derivatives are missused, ventricular hypertrophy, diastolic dysfunction and myocardial stiffening appear and the potential risk for infarction increases (Malkin et al., 2010).

The sex hormones, i.e. estrogen, progesterone and androgens and their receptors, ERs, PRs and ARs, have been studied as candidates to mediate sex-specific effects observed in gender related responses of the cardiovascular system and related diseases. Above all estrogen has received major attention, while testosterone is at present studied for its potential beneficial and cardioprotective mechanism of action. However, within several cardiovascular diseases like myocardial infarction, coronary artery disease and other ischemia related diseases, heart failure, ECG gender specific differences, the focus was already turned to the gender related sex hormones differences. These studies presented new approaches and specificities in gender related pathways responses. Recently, most of the approaches of cardiovascular diseases focused on non-genomic action of sex hormones.

1.1 Non-genomic estrogen action

Since estrogens in premenopausal women with regular menstrual cycle are established as a natural protection against cardivoascular diseases, nuclear and non-nuclear mechanisms are evaluated for their mode of action. The non-nuclear modality of estrogens action is for example ascribed to their direct vascular effects, antioxidative activity and a new pathway discovered in the last years shows that the plasma membrane G protein estrogen receptor (GPER1) is involved in cardioprotection of both in females as in males.

1.2 Testosterone and its non-genomic role

For decades, the research reports proposed only cardiotoxic and deleterious effect of testosterone in the cardiovascular system. This was based on epidemiologic human studies, where direct testosterone treatment, especially in supra-physiological androgen abuse, showed an increase in left ventricular mass and hypertrophy, causing myocardial stiffness and diastolic disfunction. Animal studies with castrates showed similar deleterious effects from adrogen receptor antagonist studies. However, later, with the use of better designed studies it was shown that testosterone, in optimal levels, may enable significant and profound cardioprotection expressed in e.g., diminished reperfusion injuries, decreased arrhythmias. It is now obvious that testosterone must posses the comparable non-nuclear activity, at cytoplasmatic level, similar to the non-genomic action of estrogen, through yet unknown mechanism(s).

2. Sex hormones and heart protection

In the cardiovascular tissues the protective effects of estrogen and testosterone are manifested through the instantly responsive arteries of the coronary artery system, which estrogen directly relaxes via the endothelial nitric oxide (NO) mechanism (Dai et al., 2004; Santos et al., 2004; Woodman et al., 2004). It is probable that testosterone relaxes these arteries via a different mechanism, maybe even a non-genomic pathway, which does not involve the nuclear androgen receptors and is independent of the vascular endothelium. This testosterone response is initiated at specific binding sites in the cell membranes of smooth muscles. For example, testosterone directly inhibits voltage-gated calcium channels, with an additional inhibitory action of calcium store-operated calcium channels (Jones et al., 2004; Yildiz et al., 2005). In the myocardium the estrogens reduce the incidence of postischemic ventricular arrhythmias by reducing the accumulation of intracellular Ca^{2+}, protecting mitochondrial structures, inhibiting apoptosis, having antioxidant action and interacting with heat stress proteins, thus protecting the heart from injuries (Fraser et al., 2000; Kim et al., 1998; Knowlton & Sun, 2001; Zhai et al., 2000). Further, both the mitogen activated protein kinase (MAPK) and phosphoinositide-3-kinase (PI3K) are believed to be involved in the regulation of NO synthesis by estrogen (Gray et al., 2001). The acetylcholine-induced and flow-dependent vasodilation are preserved or potentiated by estradiol by increasing the endothelial production of NO and prostacyclin. Estradiol also promotes the endothelial healing and angiogenesis through the activation of estrogen receptor-α, which shows that the protective mechanism in the cardiovascular system is linked to the estrogen activation of ER receptors (Arnal et al., 2010).

In the past the action of androgens on the cardiovascular system has received relatively little attention and authors disagree about possible detrimental or protective effects of testosterone on the heart (Pugh et al., 2000). Later studies showed that cardioprotective effects of testosterone are mediated by a yet not identified androgen-dependent pathway, but only after chronic administration of testosterone (Kuhar at al., 2007; Borst et al., 2010).

2.1 Coronary flow, acute and chronic effects of sex hormones

Direct application as well as estradiol pretreatment increased the coronary flow in isolated female hearts after the onset of reperfusion as well as testosterone pretreated male hearts (which was equally effective to female hearts), showing the vasodilatative effects of sex hormones (Kuhar et al., 2007). The coronary flow was increased after direct application of estradiol, while direct testosterone administration lacked such a vasodilatatory effect (Kuhar et al., 2007). Estradiol is reported to possess a direct artery relaxant action and also a direct effect on myocardium. Similarly, testosterone influenced coronary flow directly and the effects were both beneficial and deleterious (Pugh et al., 2000). Estradiol improved coronary flow of rats directly through the stimulation of NO release from endothelial cells (Dai et al., 2004; Fraser et al., 2000; Santos et al., 2004; Woodman et al., 2004). The vasodilatatory effects of testosterone are mediated by opening the large conductance, calcium-activated potassium channels (Deenadayalu et al., 2001). The short-term administration of testosterone induces a beneficial effect on exercise-induced myocardial ischemia in men with coronary artery disease, which may be related to its direct coronary relaxing effect (Rosano et al., 1999).

In physiological conditions, both estrogens as well as androgens may elicit very rapid effects to keep the homeostasis balanced, without manifesting RNA and protein synthesis (Dechering et al., 2000; Revelli et al., 1998). For example, the plasma membrane estrogen receptor was shown to respond rapidly to estrogen (Peitras & Szego, 1977), while there is no clear evidence yet of a similar effect for androgens.

2.2 Endothelium, estrogen and the heart

The sex hormones in the endothelium were generally believed to have mainly non-genomic effects. The endothelial estrogen receptor-α (ERα) in the endothelium as a whole, is considered one of the most important targets of cardioprotection. The endothelium and, in particular, the endothelial ER-α appear to be a key cellular and molecular targets of the protective actions of estradiol against ischemia/reperfusion (I/R)-induced coronary endothelial dysfunction. The activation of the endothelial estrogen receptor (ER) by estradiol, triggers a protective action on the coronary endothelial structure and function, which, in turn, limits the size of the infarct. This protection may be in part due to reduced cardiac oxidative stress, demonstrated by the decreased production of reactive oxygen species observed during early reperfusion. The signaling mechanisms of cardioprotection are to a great extent dependent on NO, which signals in cardiomyocytes via protein kinases and may possibly protect mitochondria, resulting in decreased cardiomyocyte death. Another indirect effect the reduced neutrophil-mediated cardiomyocyte injury may also play a role as endothelial protection and thus in cardioprotection (Favre et al., 2010).

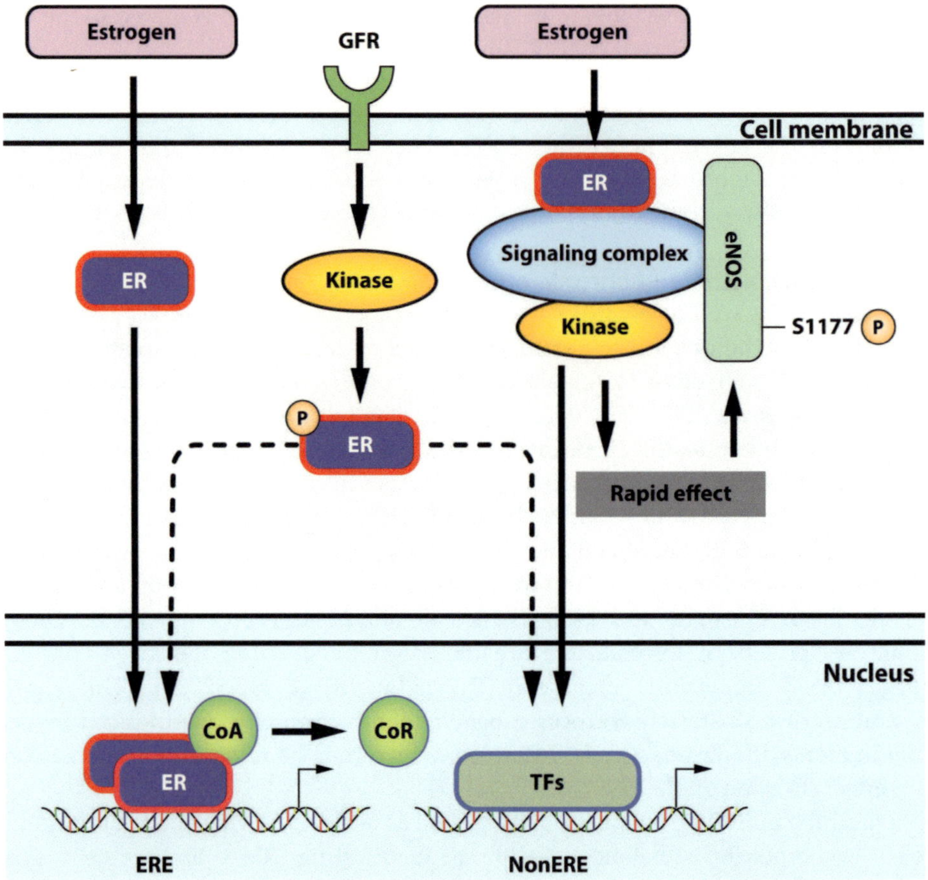

Fig. 1A. Endothelial estrogen-mediated responses. Adopted from Wu et al., (2011).
Left: The first signaling pathway in vascular endothelial cells by estrogen receptor (ER) represent the cytosolic receptors, that are ligand-activated transcription factors, that regulate gene expression. After translocation to the nucleus receptor dimerizes and binds to specific DNA sequences called estrogen response elements (ERE), recruiting coactivator (CoA) proteins, displacing corepressors (CoR) from the DNA, and activating gene expression.
Center: The second signaling pathway are the ERs that can be transcriptionally activated via ligand-independent pathways in which growth factor receptor (GFR) activation leads to activation of specific kinases that directly phosphorylate (circled P) the ER, again leading to altered gene expression, either directly by the ER or via ER interactions with other transcription factors (TFs).
Right: The third signaling pathway is mediated by non-nuclear ERs. In this pathway, estrogen induces a cell membrane–associated ERs to form a signaling complex that results in rapid activation of specific kinases, which in turn phosphorylate and enzymatically activate endothelial nitric oxide synthase (eNOS).

Another important endothelial, cardioprotection factor is the vascular endothelium growth factor (VEGF) and its basic signal molecules (VEGF receptor, Akt, eNOS). ERα knockout mice showed a marked decrease of capillary density, and the absence of receptor β has minimal effect, while the levels of the VEGF receptor, phosphorylated Akt and eNOS in the

ERα knockouts were reduced to half of the values in control group. This leads to the conclusion that VEGF is supposed to act mainly via ERα to regulate VEGF transcription and elements of basic VEGF signaling, which makes it is crucial in the development of microvasculatures in the heart (Jesmin et al., 2010).

2.3 Heart failure

The inability of the heart to supply sufficient cardiac output and blood flow to meet the needs of the body and lungs is defined as a heart failure. The causes of heart failure are myocardial infarction, ischemic heart disease in general, hypertension, valvular heart disease, and cardiomyopathy, with symptoms being shortness of breath, leg swelling,

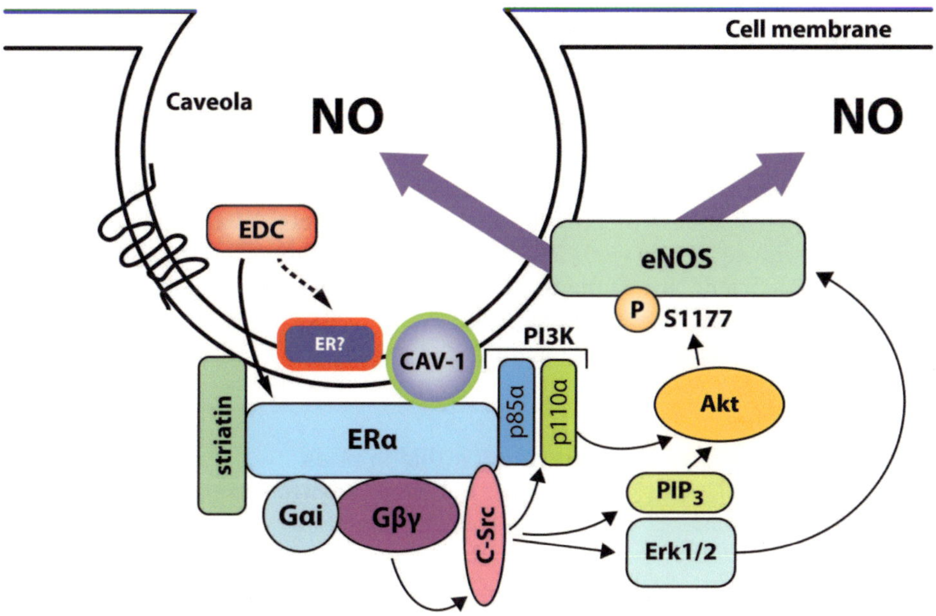

Fig. 1B. Non-nuclear estrogen receptor signaling in vascular endothelial cell caveolae. Adopted from Wu et al., (2011).

The non-nuclear estrogen receptors (ERs) localize to the endothelial cell membrane invaginations called caveolae by direct binding to the caveolar proteins, including the scaffold protein striatin, which is bound to the major caveolar structural protein, caveolin-1 (Cav-1). Upon estrogen binding (EDC), signaling complexes assemble that include the ERs and the G protein $G\alpha_i$, Gβγ and sequentially activate the tyrosine kinase src (C-src), the serine/threonine kinase, phosphoinositide-3 protein kinase (PI3K), consisted of subunits p85a and p110a, that produce phosphatidylinositol (3,4,5)-triphosphate (PIP_3), and the kinase Akt. Akt is serine/threonine protein kinase that plays a key role in multiple cellular processes such as cell proliferation, apoptosis, transcription, cell migration as well as in angiogenesis. Akt then directly phosphorylates endothelial nitric oxide synthase (eNOS) on serine 1,177, leading to its enzymatic activation and the production of nitric oxide (NO). Also, Akt activate extracellular signal-regulated kinases (Erk1/2) or MAP kinases, involved in differentiation of cells, but also in regulation of eNOS. The position of the assembling complex - on the internal or the external side of the cell membrane – remains unclear. This non-nuclear ER dependent pathway confers protection against vascular injury.

exercise intolerance and the overall body becomes congested with fluid. Heart failure is a complex state of progressive multisystem diseases with significant morbidity and mortality and its clinical picture is defined by pathology of the cardiovascular system and is influenced by peripheral cytokine, hormonal, and musculoskeletal dysfunction. The cytokines, catecholamines, and hormones during heart failure have a maladaptive response that leads to a proinflammatory state tipping the metabolic balance toward catabolism. In addition to this procatabolic combination, chronically high levels of catecholamines, angiotensin II, and aldosterone eventually may contribute to testosterone deficiency, which blunts the anabolic compensatory pathways.

Present medical treatments for heart failure have proven to decrease mortality and include treatment with β-adrenergic receptor antagonists, which target adrenergic hyperstimulation of the failing myocardium; angiotensin converting enzyme inhibitors and angiotensin receptor blockers, which attenuate left ventricular remodeling; and aldosterone blockers, which blunt myocardial fibrosis.

Several studies have shown that more than ¼ of men is affected with chronic heart failure are deficient in testosterone. Thus testosterone is directly or indirectly involved in its pathology. Androgen deficient men without heart failure often report similar typical symptoms, such as shortness of breath, fatigue, deterioration of muscle mass, decline in strenght and endurance (Naghi et al., 2011). In male, but not female mice, G protein estrogen receptor GPR30-deficient mice manifested impaired left-ventricular cardiac function, indicating that non-genomic estradiol signalling is important in heart failure. Further, also regulation of vascular tone by GPER1 is indicated to play a role in heart failure (Delbeck et al., 2011).

2.4 Ischemic heart disease and acute myocardial injuries

The protective action of estradiol in cardiac ischemia/reperfusion (I/R) was demonstrated in several animal studies, but most of the cellular targets involved in this protection still need to be defined. Usually, in control animals after cardiac I/R the following are evoked: structural endothelium injuries, including necrosis, associated with altered coronary endothelial NO production. The long-term activation of the endothelial ERα by estradiol protected both the coronary endothelial and myocardial layers and endothelial structures associated with the NO-mediated coronary endothelial response (Favre et al., 2007). However, this was not the case for ovariectomized female mice and male mice, which during I/R showed endothelial dysfunction (Favre et al., 2007). More precisely, the ERα deficiency worsens global I/R-induced alteration in coronary flow and cardiac NO release in male mice and also abolishes the endogenous cardiac protection displayed in intact female mice (Favre et al., 2007).

Genomic pathway for cardioprotection by estrogen receptor (ER) activation is upregulated with chronic ERβ stimulation. This pathway is ligand-activated by transcription factors that, after translocation to the nucleus, bind to DNA sequences and regulate gene expression, resulting in for example modulators of both the NO system and apoptosis processes.

Stimulation of the nuclear G-protein coupled membrane bound estrogen receptor (GPER1) by tyrosine kinase src (C-src) results in activation of matrix metalloproteinase (MMP) leading to the release of epidermal growth factor (EGF) that can transactivate epidermal growth factor receptors (EGFRs). EGFR activation leads to multiple downstream events including activation of kinases within the phosphoinositide-3 protein kinase/ Akt pathways (PI3K/Akt).

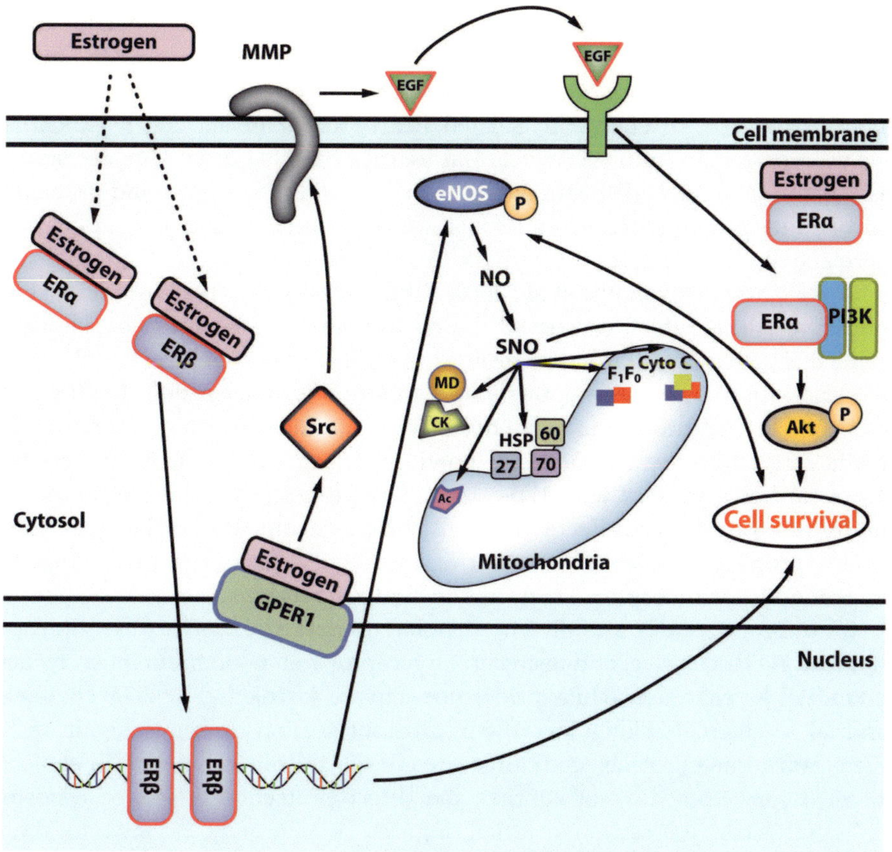

Fig. 2. Cardioprotective signalling pathways induced by estrogen receptor activation. Adopted from Deschamps, Murphy & Sun (2010).
Following after the activation of both PI3K/Akt, nitric oxide (NO) signaling and the chronic activation of ERβ comes a significant increase in S-nitrosylated proteins (SNO) in the mitochondria including F_1F_0-ATPase, aconitase (Ac), cytochrome c oxidase (Cyto C), heat shock proteins (HSP27/60/70), and cytosol like creatine kinase (CK), and malate dehydrogenase (MD). The acute and moreover chronic activation of these pathways leads to enhanced cell survival resulting in cardioprotection.

2.4.1 Amelioration of ischemia and reperfusion induced myocardial injuries

The anti-ischemic effects of sex hormones are considered to protect due to improvement of the coronary flow and due to the reduced incidence of arrhythmias and established cytoprotection during reperfusion. Both estradiol and testosterone in supraphysiological levels significantly decreased ischemia-reperfusion injuries of isolated rat hearts. The reperfusion injuries were reduced both by the direct application of sex hormones, and pretreatment prior to the isolated heart experiment. However, protective effects against ischemia-reperfusion injuries were only observed in the male hearts of animals pretreated with testosterone in a comparable effective way as in estradiol pretreated female hearts. The direct testosterone application was not comparable to the protection by the directly applied estradiol (Kuhar et al., 2007).

Further, in female animals direct administration of estradiol showed protection against cell injuries, and no protection was shown in estradiol pretreatment. In male hearts cytoprotective effects were found only in testosterone pretreated animals, while estradiol lacks direct cytoprotective effects in isolated heart (Kuhar et al., 2007). Amelioration of ischemia and reperfusion induced myocardial injuries has also been demonstrated in some experimental animal models (Delyani et al., 1996). For estradiol a profound protective effect against stroke-like ischemic injuries in female rats was found (Wise et al., 2001), while also the cytoprotective effect of estradiol to hypoxia–reoxygenation induced injuries in cardiac cells has been reported (Jovanovic et al., 2000). Chronic estradiol treatment does show some cardioprotective effects which can be attributed to over expression of heat-shock proteins (HSPs), which is generally regarded as protective against cardiac injury. HSP90 is known to bind the intracellular hormone receptors and therefore it was suggested that the interaction between HSP90, the receptors, and heat-shock factor-1 (HSF-1) was an important element in the activation of HSF-1 by hormones (Knowlton & Sun, 2001). It is known that after treatment of cardiac myocytes with 17β-estradiol or progesterone the HSP90 redistributes. However, testosterone did not effect HSP levels and pretreatment of males with testosterone did not elicit protective effects (Knowlton & Sun, 2001). This is in accordance with the discovery that androgen receptors are absent in cardiac myocytes.

Morover, testosterone acutely and directly depolarizes and oxidizes cardiac mitochondria in a K-dependent, ATP-sensitive, and testosterone receptor-independent manner, by activation of mitochondrial K^+ channels, while it does not activate sarcolemal K^+ ATP channels. Thus, mitochondrial K^+ channels play a key role in cardioprotection during ischemia and via this mechanism testosterone protects cardiomyocytes from ischemic cell death (Er et al., 2004). In contrast, cell injury tests did not confirm the direct protective effects of testosterone in ischemia/reperfusion induced myocardial injuries, which may be due to the limited electrolyte capacity of the mitochondria. To conclude, the action of the sex hormones is attributable not only due to its direct action on coronary arteries, but also due to other non-genomic properties.

The demonstration that estrogen exert a cardioprotective effect in male animals showed, that in vivo supplemental estrogen treatment of male mice reduces the prevalence of cardiac rupture during the acute phase of myocardial infarction (Cao et al., 2011). In other short-term (acute) and long-term (chronic) cardiac function study, myocardial infarction-induced male mice treated with estrogen and female mice treated with testosterone, showed opposing chronic cardiac remodeling and function effects, with favorable (protective) effects exerted by estrogen and detrimental effects exerted by testosterone (Cavasin et al., 2003). During the acute phase of myocardial infarction, however, estrogen appeared to offer no or little protection against acute myocardial infarction-induced cardiac rupture. The castration alone could slightly reduce the prevalence of cardiac rupture in male mice. While a lower prevalence of cardiac rupture was observed in estrogen-treated mice as compared to placebo-treated ones (Cao et al., 2011), no difference was observed in another study (Cavasin et al., 2003).

The observation on the obligatory role of the endothelium for cardiomyocyte protection may appear contradictory to a direct protective action of estradiol on hypoxia/reoxygenation-mediated death of isolated cardiomyocytes. First, the in vitro data used large amounts of immediately administered estradiol and thus with these pharmacological doses, it is possible to elicit direct effects that can not be observed in cardiomyocites. Second, the mechanisms of reperfusion injury to cardiomyocytes in vivo markedly differ from those involved in vitro. The immediate inflammatory response associated with severe oxidative stress appears to be operative in vivo but not in vitro and this phenomenon centrally involves the endothelium as both a target and a trigger of the inflammatory response. Third, another important aspect of reperfusion injury is the no-reflow phenomenon that may worsen I/R injury and that is likely to be reduced by estradiol secondary to endothelial protection (Favre et al., 2010).

2.4.2 Delayed cardioprotection by testosterone

Cardioprotection also can be achieved by preconditioning, a process that can be assesed pharmacologically, by ischemia, or by other stressors. Preconditioning increases the resistance to subsequent longer stress. Among the most important benefits are reduction of reperfusion injuries, diminished arrhythmia, prevention of myocardial stunning and post-ischemic contractile dysfunction, marked limitation and decrease of infarct size, and reduction of endothelial injury (Geršak & Drevenšek, 2002). The receptors involved in preconditioning are mainly coupled to protein kinase C. In mice with removed testicles, the immediate cardioprotection of ischemic preconditioning is abolished, thus testosterone is needed for the acute cardioprotection of preconditioning. In the absence of testosterone, the preconditioning with metabolic inhibition in vitro or k-opioid agonist in vivo, failed to establish delayed cardioprotection against ischemic insult in ventricular myocytes or isolated perfused male rat hearts, respectively (Liu et al., 2006). This was the first evidence that testosterone at physiological concentrations is needed for the delayed cardioprotection of preconditioning.

3. Atherogenesis, sex hormones and gender differences

Estrogen is known to relax arteries directly via endothelial NO and thus exert potential antiatherogenic effects (Dai et al., 2004; Santos et al., 2004; Woodman et al., 2004). Also, estradiol prevents early atheroma through endothelial-mediated mechanisms (Arnal et al., 2010). Androgens on the other hand, have been associated with possible proatherogenic effects and an increased cardiovascular risk by adversely affecting the plasma lipid and lipoprotein profile, increasing the risk of thrombosis and cardiac hypertrophy (Adams et al., 1995). On the contrary, short-term administration of testosterone causes vasodilatation in a range of species including humans (Costarella et al., 1996; Crews & Khalil, 1999; Honda et al., 1999; Perusquia et al., 1996; Yue et al., 1995). However these beneficial early on atherogenesis effects of testosterone were not explained by changes in lipid levels. Besides, estradiol administration to orchidectomized males attenuated lesion formation to the same extent as testosterone administration. These results indicate that testosterone attenuates early atherogenesis and that this is most likely be caused by being converted to estrogens by the enzyme aromatase expressed in the vessel wall (Nathan et al., 2000). The latest study in an androgen receptor knockout mice on apolipoprotein E-deficient basis, showed acceleration of atherosclerosis, while testosterone treatment reduced this atherosclerosis. In conclusion, the male mice showed testosterone atheroprotection which has both androgen receptor-dependent and androgen receptor-independent components (Bourghardt et al., 2010).

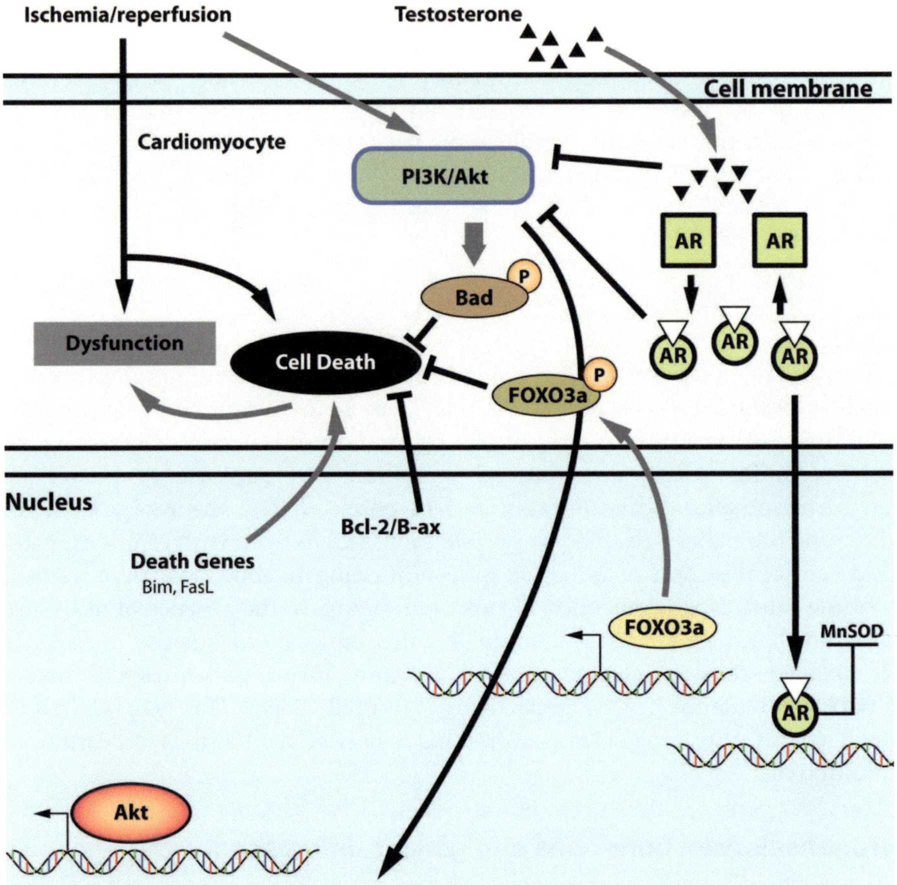

Fig. 3. Acute ischemia/reperfusion induced testosterone signalling pathways in cardiomyocites during androgen receptor activation. Adopted from Huang et al. (2010). The activation by myocardial Akt in PI3K/Akt downstream signaling after activation of androgen receptor (AR) due to ischemia reperfusion causes increased release of cell death signals (Bad, Bcl-2, FOXO3a) and decrease apoptotic mediator FasL. The Akt protein at normal sex hormone status is more active in female then in male hearts and thus in this pathway testosterone is a negative factor in cardioprotection processes.
The genomic actions of the AR activation consist out of changes in gene expression involved in cardiac protection/injury, like modulators of the superoxide dismutase (MnSOD) system, apoptotic and death genes. Besides, testosterone in acute ischemia down-regulates FOXO3a, a trigger protein for apoptosis, and decreases antiapoptotic activator targets as Bim and FasL that are probably post-translational products with little or no influence on acute ischemia/reperfusion injuries. Overall, genomic pathway probably leads to testosterone induced cardioprotection.

4. Arrhythmias

The ventricular arrhythmias, mostly being the malignant ones of all arrhythmias, show important gender differences. Torsades de pointes, a ventricular tachyarrhythmia that can lead to ventricular fibrilation, is associated with long QT syndrome and is more common in females than in males. The long QT syndrome can be inherited as congenital mutations of the ion channels that carry the cardiac action potential or acquired as a result of drugs that block these cardiac ion currents. The higher male incidence of the Brugada syndrome is associated with the early phase of ventricular repolarization, that is larger in the right ventricular epicardium of males than in females, resulting in a characteristic ST elevation in males. The early repolarization syndrome is characterized by a prominent J wave and by elevation of the ST-segment in the left precordial leads; it is most commonly seen in young males (Ezaki et al., 2010).

The evaluation of arrhythmias during ischemic-reperfusion induced injuries using high doses of hormones, showed that cardioprotection with testosterone is established only after pretreatment (Kuhar et al., 2007), but no protective effect was detected when testosterone was applied directly to the isolated animal hearts. Animals pretreated with testosterone as well as with estradiol showed high level of cardioprotection against post-ischemic injuries. Most of the beneficial effects shown in post-ischemic hearts were expressed as improved coronary flow, decreased release of lactate dehydrogenase rate and shorter lasting arrhythmias (Kuhar et al., 2007). The increased coronary flow in the hearts of pretreated animals of both sexes with estradiol and testosterone may be the result of induced NO production. The diminished arrhythmias in chronically treated hearts in rats of both sexes could be the consequence of both, vasodilatation and the direct cardioprotective effects of the hormones. The reduced lactate dehydrogenase release rate in the estradiol pretreated group showed more complex activity; cardioprotection might be induced also due to HSP activation with estradiol.

During reperfusion in the hearts of the animals pretreated with both testosterone and estradiol, all types of arrhythmias were reduced compared to the directly treated groups (Kuhar et al., 2007). The heart arrest was most severely decreased followed by, decreasing intensities in ventricular fibrilation, and ventricular premature complexes (Kuhar et al., 2007). The protective effect of sex hormones against the appearance of arrhythmias, fibrillation and ventricular tachycardia, was proposed by some other studies (Kim et al., 1998; Zhai et al., 2000).

4.1 Electrocardiogram, QTc and ST

The QT interval in the electrocardiogram (ECG) is defined as the interval from the onset of the QRS complex to the end of the T wave (Figure 4), it is the sum of ventricular myocardial action potential duration and the ventricular repolarization. The ST segment of the ECG represents the duration of ventricular repolarization only, with -J, -M, and –E segment representing the right and left ventricles and are measured by the ECG leads V2 and V5 respectively. The sex hormones, like estrogens, progesterones and androgens, can modulate a variety of ionic currents and are reported to influence the duration of the ECG (James et al., 2007).

4.1.1 Molecular basis for QTc differences

The QTc represents the rate-corrected QT interval that is calculated using the method of Fridericia (QTc=QT/RR1/3, Schwartz et al., 2011). On molecular level, the duration of the QT interval is the net effect of the activity of multiple ion-channels and transporters. The combined activity of two delayed rectifier currents I_{Kr} (rapid delayed rectifier potassium channel) and I_{Ks} (slow delayed potassium channel) account for the majority of phase 3 repolarization of the ventricles. Several mutations in genes regulating these channels are responsible for the more common forms of inherited long QT syndromes. But also acquired conditions such as cardiac disease, electrolyte derangements (e.g. hypokalemia, hypocalcemia), and renal insufficiency (Genovesi et al., 2008), and iatrogenic causes, as cardiac as well as non-cardiac drugs are known to prolong the QT interval (Roden, 2004). Moreover, I_{ks}, but not I_{kr}, is highly influenced by β-adrenergic stimulation and blockade.

4.1.2 Gender related QTc differences

In men left ventricular mass is greater than in women (Hayward et al., 2001) and besides, the hearts from a small number of young and middle-aged non-diseased women showed reduced expression of a variety of K^+ channel subunits (HERG, mink, Kir2.3, Kv1.4, Kir6.2, KchIP2, SUR2) as compared to male hearts (Gaborit et al., 2010). In general, the QT interval durations of men are generally shorter than of women. The androgen receptors expressed in the heart muscle cells might play an important role in gender-dependent heart function differences, in particular the electrical activity of the left ventriculum. The QT interval at birth is comparable between genders (Stramba-Badiale et al., 1995) and up to 10 years of age, then at puberty it shortens by some 20 msec in young males (Pham & Rosen, 2002). The normal upper limit for QTc in men is 440 msec (Schwartz et al., 2011) and the shorter the QT interval the more it protects men from developing malignant ventricular arrhythmias such as Torsade de pointes (Abi-Gerges et al., 2004). Women which have a faster heart rate and thus a shorter QT interval show a higher incidence of Torsade de pointes. So the QT differences can be attributed to gender.

In women, repolarization lasts longer and proceeds slower compared with men and, indeed, surface ECG reveals longer QT interval and lower T-wave amplitude in adult women of all ages as compared with men (Bidoggia et al., 2000a). Also, the method of Fridericia to correct the QT intervals for heart rate (QTc) showed longer QTc intervals in women (about 1%) compared with men (Kadish et al., 2004; Schwartz et al., 2011). Moreover, the gender difference in QT interval is larger at long cardiac cycle lengths (Genovesi et al., 2007). The gender-related differences in QTc interval and T-wave amplitude are not present at birth (Stramba-Badiale et al., 1995) and during childhood, but appear during the teenage years (Pham & Rosen, 2002; Surawicz & Parikh, 2002), and decrease at older ages suggesting that this gender related QT difference of cardiac repolarization can be attributed to the life cycle: first an increase followed by a decrease of the sex hormones. The average sex differences in QTc intervals range from 10–15 ms (approximately 2-6 %). Besides, the longitudinal assessment of QT interval is independent of the menstrual cycle of women (Burke et al., 1996; Surawicz & Parikh, 2002), whereas in men the QT intervals shorten by some 20 msec at puberty (Surawicz & Parikh, 2002), and in both men and women testosterone levels directly shorten the QT interval independently of the heart rate (Schwartz et al., 2011), with differences in men of about 4% between high and low testosterone levels (Charbit et al., 2009; Pecori Giraldi et al., 2010). Further, these differences were larger than expected in older men and women during decreased hormonal status, where for women, testosterone decreased QT and QTc intervals but were longer in comparison with men (Schwartz et al., 2011). Moreover, a direct shortening of QT intervals by testosterone in older men and older women or hypogonadal status is known to exist independent of heart rate changes

(Schwartz et al., 2011). Male hypogonadism is associated with an increased prevalence of prolonged QT interval, over 2.5%, as compared to the control and the healthy population (Schwartz et al., 1993), and hence, a higher risk for fatal ventricular arrhythmias. The QTc interval in the hypogonadal state is prolonged and by hormone replacement therapy normalized (Pecori Giraldi et al., 2010). This evidence led to the conclusion that testosterone is the main determinant of gender-related differences in the ventricular refractory periods (James et al., 2007), and several experimental studies support this hypothesis.

In vitro and data on animals showed that sex hormones increased the QTc intervals in females, or conversely, decreased the QTc intervals in males (Fülöp et al., 2006). Women with excess androgen secretion present shorter and faster repolarization (Bidoggia et al., 2000b). In orchiectomized rabbits testosterone administration shortens the QT interval and drug-induced QT prolongation (Liu et al., 2002).

4.1.3 Gender related ST differences

Gender differences in the ST segment are known for healthy subjects and the ST level is elevated in young males compared to females (Ezaki et al., 2010). Also females showed longer JT intervals than males. These differences of ventricular repolarization are not observed in early childhood, but they become apparent after puberty (Ezaki et al., 2010), suggesting an important role of sex hormones. After puberty the leads that represent the right and left ventricles show that the J point amplitude is higher and besides that the ST segment and angle is steeper in males.

Brugada syndrome has higher incidence in young males than in females and causes sudden death by ventricular fibrillation: in the early phase of the ventricular repolarization of males, the transient outward potassium current I_{to} is stronger and contributes more largely to the repolarisation of the right ventricular epicardium. In the early repolarization syndrome an important elevation of the J wave and ST-segment is detected in males (Ezaki et al., 2010).

In pre-pubescent subjects of age 5–12 years, there is no significant gender differences in the ST levels. In males, the ST levels from both leads increase significantly after puberty and reach a maximum after 20 to 29 years of age and decrease during the 3rd decade of life (Nankin & Calkins, 1986). While for females, with increasing age there was a reduction in lead V5 only and irrespective of female age, from lead V2 the ST levels remained low and almost constant. For both sexes, all 3 ST segments were significantly higher in lead V2, which shows a more potent left ventricle. After puberty, the ST levels from both leads V2 and V5 were significantly higher in males than in females, suggesting that the effect of sex hormones on ST levels might be smaller in females than in males (Ezaki et al., 2010). In males, androgen-deprivation therapy significantly lowered all 3 ST segments and they closely resembled the ST segments of age-matched control females (Ezaki et al., 2010). Further, the J point amplitude was significantly lower in males with secondary hypogonadism and in castrated males.

These significant age- and gender differences in the ST segment suggest that sex hormones modulate the early phase of ventricular repolarization (Ezaki et al., 2010). For example, in healthy adults, estrogen prolongs the repolarization (ST segment), while testosterone shortens it (James et al., 2007). Sex differences in the ST segment elevation showed an important role for the male hormone testosterone. Since the plasma testosterone concentration increases around puberty, reaches peaks at 20–30 years of age, and decreases gradually due to the physiologic effects of aging in both males and females, the ST segment fluctuation with age is correlated to the level of testosterone. In contrast, the female sex hormone, which also increases around puberty, has little effect on the ST levels because it does not change the ST segment in pubescent females (Ezaki et al., 2010).

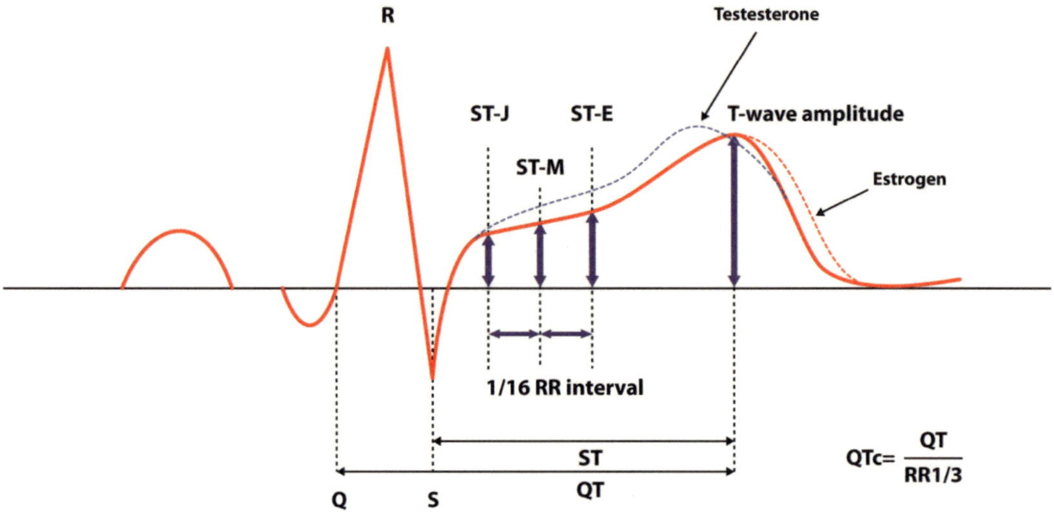

Fig. 4. Electrocardiogram of the heart
ST-J: The J point level at the end of the QRS complex with respect to the baseline. The middle or **ST-M** level is the level at 1/16th of the preceding RR interval of the following ST segment. **ST-E**: The level at 2/16th of the preceding RR interval of the following ST segment. T-wave amplitude is defined as the absolute distance from the baseline from the S point to the apex of the T-wave. In men the level of repolarizarion (ST) is elevated in all 3 segments and the duration is shortened (blue hatched line), while testosterone deprivation therapy in men decreases the elevation of these segments. The duration of the repolarization (ST) is prolonged by estrogens (red hatched line). The method of Fridericia for calculating the rate-corrected QT interval: QTc=QT/RR1/3 is described in text. Adopted from Ezaki et al. (2010) and James et al. (2007).

5. Sex hormone receptors and their role in the cardiovascular system

Androgen receptors are expressed both in the atria and the ventricles, while estrogen receptors are more pronounced in atrial myocytes (Lizotte et al., 2009). Anti-androgen drugs inhibit the androgen receptors of cardiac ventricular myocytes and decrease the hormonal modulation of ventricular repolarization (Ezaki et al., 2010). The actions of estrogen are mediated through (1) receptor-α and -β, (2) an unknown cytosolic membrane receptor and (3) another membrane based GPER1. ERα directly modulates transcription of target genes through two activation functions, AF1 and AF2. ERα demonstrates to have a prominent role in vascular biology, i.e., an AF1-deficient ERα isoform can be physiologically expressed in the endothelium and appears sufficient to mediate most of the vasculoprotective actions of estradiol (Arnal et al., 2010). Pretreatment of cardiac myocytes with estradiol protects against cell death during ischemia and decreases the extent of cell death (Wise et al., 2001). Testosterone is known to act via nuclear receptors and regulate protein synthesis (Reid et al., 2003), and experimental data also indicates a non-genomic pathway of testosterone action on the cardiovascular system, i.e. direct testosterone mediated vasodilatation (English et al., 2002).

5.1 Estrogen receptors

At present, there are three known estrogen receptors. The two »classical« nuclear estrogen receptors, ERα and ERβ, are ligand-activated nuclear transcription factors that bind regulatory response elements in the promoters of genes (Carroll & Brown, 2006). The third estrogen receptor, GPER1 or GPER (previously GPR30) was identified as an orphan 7-transmembrane G protein-coupled receptor (GPCR) with low homology to other known GPCRs (Carmeci et al., 1997; Kvingedal & Smeland, 1997; O'Dowd et al., 1998; Takada et al., 1997).

Although the distinction between the modes of cellular activation, rapid signaling versus transcription, there exists extensive overlap between these artificially defined categories. Classical estrogen receptors are traditionally thought of as regulators of transcription, however, there is extensive evidence of their ability to mediate rapid signaling events (Moriarty et al., 2006). In addition, rapid signaling events, whether initiated by nuclear steroid receptors, growth factor receptors or GPCRs, result in the modification of transcriptional activity of conventional transcription factors (Ma & Pei, 2007). Thus the cellular effects of estrogen will depend on the specific receptors expressed and the integration of their stimulatory and inhibitory signaling pathways.

5.1.1 ERα

In cardiomyocytes ERα is distributed in the cytosolic, nuclear and membrane compartments (Lizotte et al., 2009), in T-tubular membranes (Ropero et al., 2006) and in the caveolae (Chung et al., 2009), which suggests that the ERα is localized in these complexes as an estrogen non-genomic rapid signaling, and its cytosolic and nuclear distribution suggest a genomic signaling. Moreover, ERα is more densely expressed in ventricular tissue as compared to the atrium, having higher densities in men than in women (Lizotte et al., 2009).

Estradiol induces the translocation of ERα to the PI3K regulatory domain and results in endothelial NOS (eNOS) activation (Simoncini et al., 2000). In an in vivo rabbit ischemia/reperfusion (I/R) model, acute treatment with estradiol significantly decreases the infarct size in female hearts after ischemia (Booth et al., 2005), suggesting that activation of ERα is required for the acute cardioprotective effects of estrogen. Also an in vivo study with ovariectomized female rats found that acute estrogen-mediated cardioprotection, following I/R, is mimicked by pretreatment with an ERα agonist and unaffected by ERβ antagonist pretreatment (Jeanes et al., 2008). In a model of ERα knockout mice cardioprotection in the ischemia model was blocked in female animals (Zhai et al., 2000). Subchronical estradiol pretreated female rats showed cardioprotection comparable, but lower, than the protection of directly applied estradiol (Kuhar et al., 2007). In conclusion, the importance of ERα in cardioprotection is confirmed in many models, despite being controversial and more protection is dedicated to direct estrogen effects.

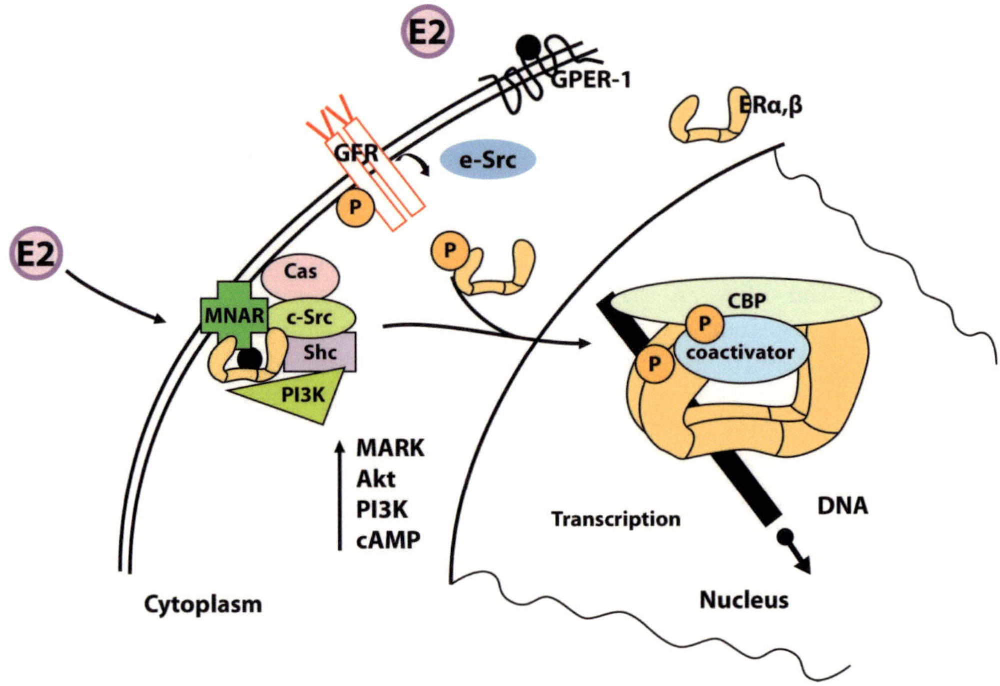

Fig. 5. Overview of genomic and non-genomic action of estrogen receptors
Estradiol stimulates cytoplasmic as well as nuclear signaling. Estradiol (E2) binds to the estrogen receptors (ERα, ERβ), stabilizes ER dimers, and stimulates direct interaction with growth factor receptors (GFR), association with proto-oncogenic tyrosine kinase Src (c-Src) and adaptor molecules: modulator of non-genomic activity of the estrogen receptor (MNAR), apoptotic protein (Shc), cellular apoptosis susceptibility protein, an exportin (Cas), and stimulation of common cytoplasmic signaling pathways via phosphoinositide-3 protein kinase (PI3K). ER can also initiate gene transcription in the absence of estradiol via phosphorylation (circled P) and activation of receptors and coactivators (cAMP-response element-binding protein - CBP), by growth factor signaling cascades, or by a ligand-stimulated mechanism. Testosterone stimulates, probably similarly to estrogens, both cytoplasmic and nuclear androgen receptors. Adopted from Fox et al. (2009) and Huang et al. (2010) and Wu et al. (2011).

5.1.2 ERβ

ERβ is predominantly localized in the nucleus and cytosol of adult murine cardiomyocytes (Lizotte et al., 2009), and has been reported to be localized in the mitochondria (Yang et al., 2004). Being primarily found in the sarcolemma, the possible ERβ-mediated effects will depend mostly on gene transcription. ERβ is evenly distributed in the heart (Lizotte et al., 2009), with females showing a higher density than males. Direct application of a specific ERβ agonist showed no antiischemic effects (Booth et al., 2005) thus suggesting that acute activation of ERβ is lacking cardioprotection.

Most studies have found that female ERβ knockout mice had more I/R injury than control (Wang et al., 2008). However, the knockouts showed increased damage, i.e., decreased gene expression of fatty acids and nitric oxide (NO) production (Gabel et al., 2005), and further reduced activation of the PI3K/Akt proteins (Wang et al., 2009). In ovariectomized female mice long-term treatment with ERβ agonists has been shown to be cardioprotective and reduce I/R injury. The gene profiling of this experimental model showed that a number of protective genes were upregulated, i.e., encoding the NO biosynthesis and the anti-apoptotic proteins. Through activation of ERβ, estrogen plays a cardioprotective role against I/R injury (Nikolic et al., 2007). Other reported that estrogen-mediated cardioprotection following I/R is unaffected by an ERβ antagonist and is activated by ERα agonists (Jeanes et al., 2008). The chronic treatment with estradiol and/or ERβ activation leads to activation of protein-S nitrosylation and cardioprotection, which could be blocked by NOS inhibition (Lin et al., 2009), suggesting that chronic estrogen exposure protects the hearts largely via activation of ERβ and NO signaling.

5.2 GPER receptors

The G protein-coupled estrogen receptor (GPR30 or now GPER-1) was initially identified as an orphan G-protein coupled receptor (GPCR), and were traditionally recognized as mediating rapid changes in the levels of second messengers and to regulate various pathways of kinases (Luttrell, 2006). Then estrogen was identified as an endogenous ligand, and estradiol binding to GPER1 was found to result in Gbg activation of Src and resulting in the matrix metalloproteinase (MMP) cleavage of heparan-bound epidermal growth factor (EGF). Subsequently, the activated EGF receptor results in acute PI3K and ERK activation (Filardo et al., 2000). Thus, as a transmembrane estrogen receptor, GPER1 activation may mediate rapid cell signaling (Prossnitz et al., 2008). GPER1 is expressed in both the ventricles and the atria of the human heart, although more in ventricles than in atria, and besides, in the atrioventricular sinus and aorta. It is absent in the atrioventricular node and in the heart apex (Lizotte et al., 2009).

5.2.1 GPER1 and ischemia

GPER1 appears to be present in all tissues where ischemic injuries takes place. Under hypoxic conditions the up-regulation of GPER1 in estrogen receptor-negative HL-1 cardiomyocytes is activated by HIF-1-responsive elements located within the promoter region of GPER1 (Recchia et al., 2011), and required for this cardiomyocyte pathway is the ROS-induced activation of EGFR/ERK signaling. Thus the adaptive cell responses to hypoxia induced by estrogen are most likely GPER mediated (Recchia et al., 2011). In Langendoff perfused male and female rat hearts, the acute activation of GPER1 by its specific agonist G-1 reduced the myocardial infarct size and improved the functional recovery of contractility when compared to control (Deschamps & Murphy, 2009). Besides, less myocardial inflammation was found, indicated by decreased levels of tumor necrosis factor α (TNF-α), interleukin 1β (IL-1β), and IL-6 (Wang et al., 2006). Also increased phosphorylation of both Akt and ERK were found, which could be reversed by the use of the PI3K/Akt inhibitor (Filardo et al., 2000). Moreover, the mitochondria permeability transition pore opening was inhibited through the activation of the extracellular signal regulated kinase (ERK) pathway (Bopassa et al., 2010). Further, administration of G1 prior to global ischemia also improved the cardiac contractility function, while the improvements were abolished both by co-administration of GPER1 specific antibodies, or an inhibitor of the PI3K pathway (Deschamps & Murphy, 2009). Further, the acute administration of G-1 causes the activation of the ERK pathway, inducing phosphorylation of eNOS (Filice et al., 2009).

In ovariectomized rats, G-1 was able to prevent an elevation in systolic blood pressure that occurs due to estrogen depletion, and in a GPER1 deficient mouse model, female mice develop a significant increase in mean arterial blood pressure (Mårtensson et al., 2009).

5.2.2 GPER1 and other pathways

Under hypoxic conditions the GPER1 may also mediate additional effects that are separate from those of both genomic and nongenomic classic ERs signaling. From isolated female mouse hearts with knockout mutations for ERα or ERβ, the role for both of these receptors in mediating the protective effects of estrogen through GPER1 against I/R injury was established (Wang et al., 2009; Weil et al., 2010). The upregulation of protein kinase A and the following inhibition of apoptosis was contributed to GPER1 and not to the ER. The acute administration of estradiol in the isolated rat heart was protective against acute I/R injury, and both ERα and/or ERβ may mediate these effects. ERβ mediates the upregulation of extracellular receptor kinase (ERK)-signaling and the antiapoptotic PI3K/Akt pathways and ERα mediates the downregulation of proapoptotic c-Jun N-terminal kinase (JNK) pathways. The GPER1 activation provides cardioprotection by decreasing inflammation, including activation of proinflammatory cellular pathways, upregulation of protective mitogen activated kinase (p38 MAPK) and/or JNK pathways (Weil et al., 2010), in addition to decreasing cellular apoptosis, and to promote survival.

5.2.3 GPER mediates cardioprotection

These results show that the G protein estrogen receptor GPER1 plays an important role in mediating the acute cardioprotective effects of estrogen against global ischemia/reperfusion. They can be upregulated by ischemia and mediate protection through adaptation to low oxygen and reactive oxygen species generation conditions and may contribute to progression of disease in the metabolic function, impulse cell proliferation and improve the contractility of myocites (Patel et al., 2010; Recchia et al., 2011). It is suggested that these mechanisms of protection by GPER1 activation are mediated through the EGF receptor/extracellular signal regulated kinase (ERK) and the PI3K/AKT, and eNOS signaling pathways (Filardo et al., 2000; Filice et al., 2009).

Just like ERα and ERβ the membrane estrogen receptor GPER1 is involved in estradiol induced cardiac activity. The cardiotropic effects induced by estrogen include the ERK, PI3K and PKA transduction cascades. A potential functional interactivity between GPER1, ERα and ERβ, might exert their combined cardioprotection, and involves all of the ERK, PI3K, PKA pathways and converge downstream on the eNOS transduction pathway, suggesting that NO production plays a central role in the response of male heart to estrogen stimulation (Filice et al., 2009).

5.3 Androgens

5.3.1 Angiogenesis

The androgen receptors have independent of their genomic function, which changes gene transcription, a second mode of action, in which cytoplasmic androgen binding to androgen receptors causes rapid changes in cell function, such as changes in ion transport. The most potent natural androgen is dihydrotestosterone (DHT), that in contrary to testosterone, cannot be aromatised to estradiol and thus no secondary estrogen receptor mediated effects can be produced. Endothelial cells exposed to DHT produce a dose-dependent increase in

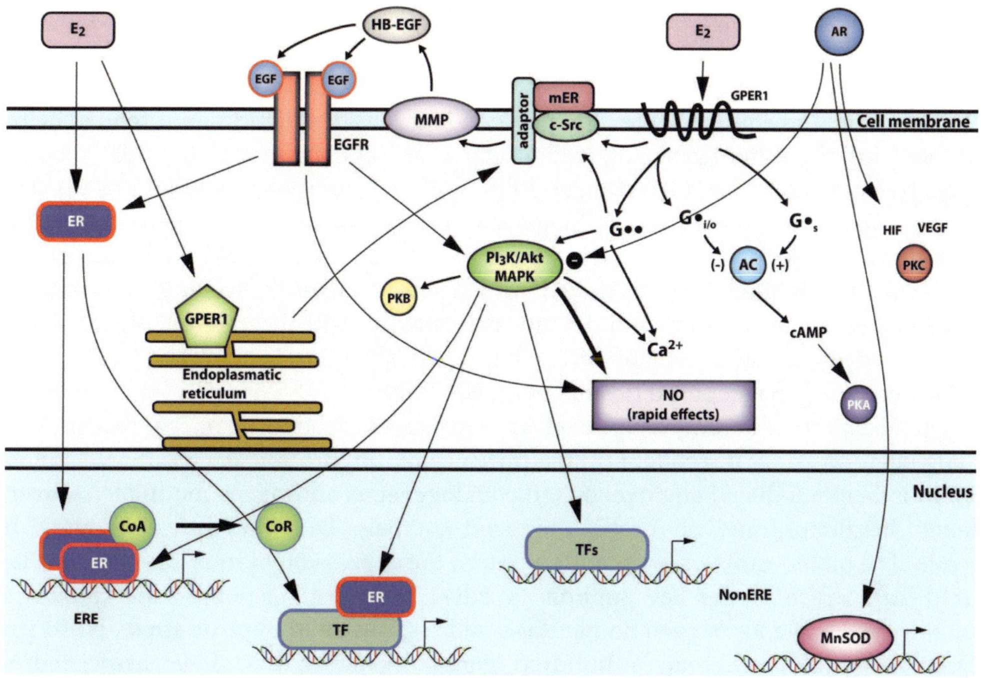

Fig. 6. Signaling pathways activated by estrogens and androgens. Adopted from Meyer et al. (2009) and Nilsson et al. (2011).

Specific cellular actions of estradiol (E2) are activated through both genomic and non-genomic transduction pathways. In the primary genomic pathway (left), activated estrogen receptors (ER) influence the nuclear transcription as well as rapid signaling by nitric oxide (NO) and phosphoinositide-3 protein kinase (PI3K) / Akt activation. In the secondary (center) non-genomic pathway, stimulation of membrane bound G protein-coupled estrogen receptor (GPER1) activates G proteins, which trigger multiple effectors. Both pathways activate $G\alpha_{i/o}$ proteins and activate adenylate cyclase (AC) to either, positively or negatively regulate the cAMP level and the subsequent cAMP-dependent protein kinase (PKA) activity. Also, the stimulation of $G\alpha_{i/o}$ leads to activation of PI3K and subsequent Akt/PKB protein kinase (Akt/PKB). Activation of c-Src protein kinase, forming the complex with adaptor protein, activaties matrix metalloproteinase (MMP), that liberate heparin-bound epidermal growth factor (HB-EGF) and activates the EGF receptor (EGFR). The EGFR activation leads to multiple downstream events including activation of mitogen activated protein kinases (MAPK) and PI3 kinases (PI3K), which increase expression of transcription factors (TFs). Besides, the GPER1 stimulation also leads to elevation of intracellular Ca^{2+} through unknown mechanisms that involve either primary signaling through G proteins or secondary signaling through EGFR transactivation. Moreover, the estrogen stimulation can lead to the expression of target genes whose promoters do not contain steroid response elements (nonEREs). The combined effects of these signaling and transcriptional events often lead to cell cycle progression and cell proliferation.

The androgen receptors (AR, right) are known to activate hypoxia induced factors (HIF), vascular endothelium growth factor (VEGF) and effects resulting in activation of protein kinase C (PKC), and besides AR activation leads to deactivation of PI3K, thus leading also to diminished cardioprotection, and direct effects on calcium metabolism is also described.

the production of vascular endothelial growth factor (VEGF), a key angiogenic growth factor and show increased messenger RNA expression of VEGF receptors 1 and 2 (Flt-1 and KDR respectively, Sieveking et al., 2010). This suggests that the proangiogenic effects of DHT in male endothelial cells are VEGF dependent. Besides, it is known that KDR is the main mediator of the mitogenic/angiogenic action of VEGF in endothelial cells, while Flt-1 is a negative regulator of VEGF action and Flt-1 mRNA is indeed expressed less upon DHT exposure. This upregulated anti-VEGF action, and also the activated inhibitor of phosphoinositol 3-kinase (PI3K), a key enzyme in the PI3K– AKT pathway of VEGF signaling, both inhibited DHT-mediated tubulogenesis genes (Sieveking et al., 2010). In comparison, estrogen receptor α and β are both involved in the cerebral VEGF/Akt/NO pathway in angiogenesis in female mice, while VEGF signaling is disrupted in the hearts of mice lacking estrogen receptor α (Jesmin et al., 2010a, b).

Also, orchidectomy markedly decreased in vivo vascularization in males, and in females this angiogenesis is not dependent on the presence of dihydrotestosterone (Sieveking et al., 2010). In ischemia induced angiogenesis, the endogeneous androgens modulate recovery in ischemic hindlimbs, and in orchidectomized animals DHT enhances recovery from ischemia. The orchidectomy significantly reduced the expression of hypoxia-inducible factor 1α (HIF-1α), which is the key subunit to HIF-1, a critical, genome-wide transcription regulator responsible for oxygen homeostasis and responsive to hypoxic stress. HIF-1 drives the expression of more than a hundred genes, including the genes associated with angiogenesis (e.g., VEGF and its receptors). In conclusion, the endogenous androgens play an important role in the coordination of ischemia-mediated angiogenesis by the regulation of key angiogenesis-related genes (Sieveking et al., 2010).

5.3.2 Vascular tone

The castration of animals causes reduced arterial pressure and reduced responses to angiotensin II (Song et al., 2010). In the castrated animals, treatment with testosterone restored the response to angiotensin II. It is concluded that long term effects of testosterone is pressor-related to angiotensin II responses. Treatment of the castrates with a protein kinase C (PKC) inhibitor attenuated the differences in arterial pressure to angiotensin II. Also, mRNA expression of PKCδ and PKCε are attenuated by castration, but are restored by testosterone. The expression of protein kinase C (CPI-17) and phospho-CPI-17 was decreased in the castrated group, whereas drug replacement of testosterone in castrated rats reversed this effect (Song et al., 2010). These findings suggest that in genetically hypertensive rats the PKC/CPI-17 pathway may contribute to androgenic potentiation of the pressor and renal vascular responses of angiotensin II (Song et al., 2010).

6. Pathway basis of sex hormones action in cardiovascular system

The estrogen binding to GPER1 activates downstream PI3K, MAPK, and NOS along a similar path as the non-genomic signaling of the classic ERs-mediated signaling. However, the GPER1 also may mediate additional effects that are separate from those of both genomic and non-genomic signaling mediated by the classic ERs. For example, it seems that GPER1 and not ERα is responsible for the upregulation of protein kinase A and the inhibition of apoptosis.

6.1 NO and protein S-nitrosylation

Most of the present cardioprotective effects are dedicated to the NO-related mechanisms that play a role in the regulation of cardiovascular function. Beside the activation of cyclic guanosine monophosphate (cGMP)-dependent pathway, NO also regulates cell function through protein S-nitrosylation. This is a reversible redox-sensitive posttranslational protein modification, which involves the attachment of a NO moiety to the nucleophilic protein sulfhydryl, resulting in S-nitrosothiol (SNO) formation. It is very likely that the protein S-nitrosylation plays an important role in cardioprotection (Sun & Murphy, 2010).

Estrogen-induced protein S-nitrosylation has been shown to be involved in a murine model of I/R resulting in a cardioprotection (Lin et al., 2009). During the Langendorff model of I/R, hearts of ovariectomized female mice pretreated with estradiol and/or ERβ-selective agonists, showed increased post-ischemic recovery. This protection was blocked by a NOS inhibitor (Lin et al., 2009), suggesting that increased NO signaling contributes to the cardioprotection. These chonic estradiol or ERβ agonist exposed hearts showed increased S-nitrosylated proteins and this protein S-nitrosylation could be abolished by pretreating hearts with the NOS inhibitor (Lin et al., 2009). These data suggest that chronic estrogen treatment and activation of ERβ would indeed lead to increased NO/SNO signaling, playing an essential role in cardioprotection.

Many of the S-nitrosylated proteins found in ERβ-selective agonist-treated hearts (Lin et al., 2009) have also been shown to be increased in preconditioned hearts (Sun et al., 2007), including the mitochondrial F_1F_0-ATPase, aconitase, malate dehydrogenase, creatine kinase, cytochrome c oxidase and heat shock proteins (HSP 27, 60, and 70). The protein S-nitrosylation might also elicit cardioprotective effects by regulating intracellular Ca^{2+} handling, apoptosis, and post-infarct myocardial remodeling (Sun & Murphy, 2010).

Estradiol, the naturally occuring major form of estrogen, increases protein S-nitrosylation levels in cultured endothelial cells and besides in intact endotheliums where, the estradiol was shown to act through ERα, activates eNOS and generates NO which leads to S-nitrosylation (Sun & Murphy, 2010). The S-nitrosylation also mediates the inhibitory effects of estradiol on endothelial ICAM-1 expression by angiotensin II (Chakrabarti et al., 2010). It is a post-translational protein modification induced by both, endogenous NO, generated by NOS in endothelium, and exogenous NO in a variety of cells. Over 100 different cellular proteins have been shown to be S-nitrosylated in processes that reduce the generation of harmful free radicals on one hand, and activate the free radical scavengers on the other (Chakrabarti et al., 2010). Both processes contributing to a reduction in oxidative stress, but also reducing pro-inflamatory signaling, processes which are crucial in I/R injury protection (Chakrabarti et al., 2010).

6.2 PI3K/Akt pathway and its activation by sex hormones

The Akt pathway is considered as one of the most important molecular kinase that mediates cardioprotection during ischemia reperfusion (Wang et al., 2009). Female hearts have higher level of Akt activity and thus, compared to male hearts, have better protection against I/R injuries and better heart recovery. Indeed, male hearts showed lower Akt activity and worse I/R recovery. In ovariectomized rat hearts the Akt activity is reduced, the recovery decreased (Huang et al., 2010), and supposedly the occurance of apoptosis during the myocardial infarction is one of the potential reasons.

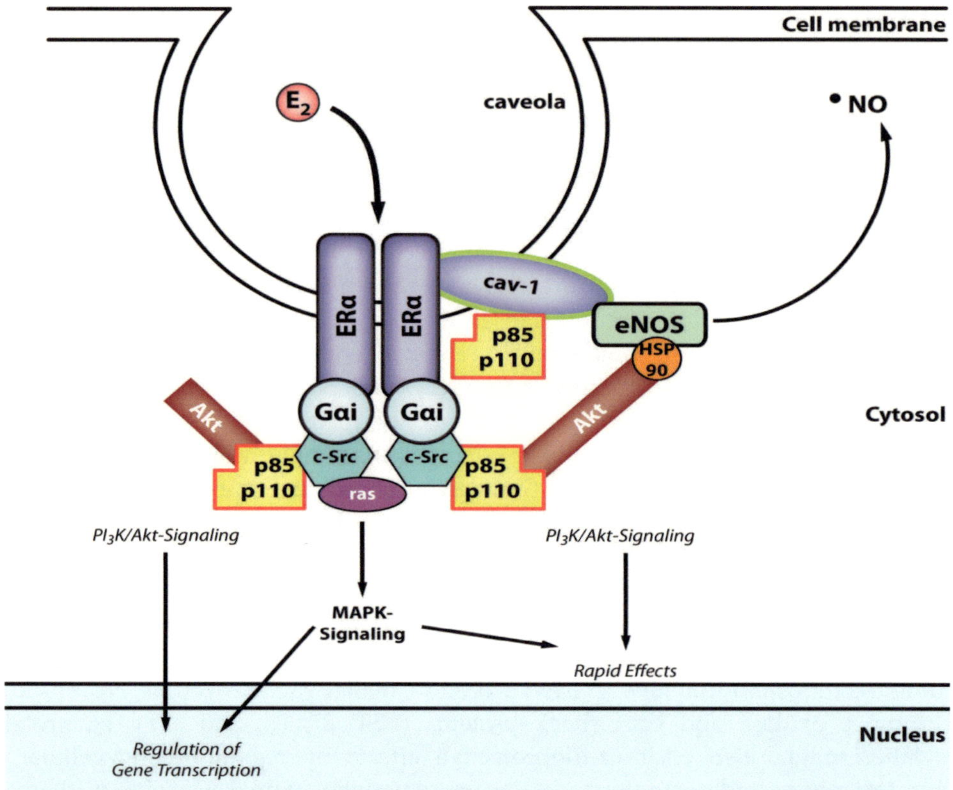

Fig. 7. Integrative model of putative mechanism of non-genomic estrogen signaling. Modified from Meyer et al. (2009) and Moriarty et al. (2006).
Caveolae, invaginations of the endothelial plasma membrane, are centers for signaling processing, providing localization for the molecules involved. Here, estradiol (E2) binds to the estrogen receptor α (ERα) and the "modulator of non-genomic activity of the ER" (MNAR) promotes complex formation with ERα, c-Src, and p85, the regulatory subunit of phosphoinositide-3 protein kinase (PI3K; with subunits p85 and p110), facilitating activation of the PI3K/Akt-signaling. Alternatively, c-Src activates the monomeric GTPase p21ras (ras), which is capable of directly recruiting downstream the mitogen activated protein kinases (MAPK) pathway. Essential for the activation of c-Src is the direct interaction of the G protein $G\alpha_i$ with ERα. Once activated, both PI3K/Akt- and MAPK-pathways can modulate gene transcription, and besides in endothelial cells, alternatively, the activation of PI3K/Akt-signaling leads to the phosphorylation of endothelial nitric oxide synthase (eNOS) protein, which is localized to caveolae through interaction with caveolin-1 (cav-1), a protein that also targets ERα. The molecular chaperone heat shock protein 90 (Hsp90) enhances the PI3K/Akt-eNOS interaction. Once eNOS is activated, the release of nitric oxide (NO) induces rapid cellular effects.

The ablation of ERβ significantly decreased postischemic functional recovery in female, but not in male hearts (Wang et al., 2009), and besides, a reduced activation of PI3K/Akt was noted in the female ERβ knockout hearts. Since, females show higher densities in cardiac ERβ expression in women than in men, the activation of the PI3K/Akt signaling cascade plays a crucial role in the cardioprotection against I/R injury through an acute gender-dependent ER-mediated and gender-independent GPER1 signaling.

6.2.1 Estrogen

At present, PI3K seems to be the most important activation pathway in the cardioprotection of sex hormones. This pathway involves further Akt and NOS activation. Both in vivo and in vitro studies show that acute estradiol treatment reduces cardiomyocyte apoptosis and elicits cardioprotection via ERα activation and PI3K/Akt signaling (Patten et al., 2004). In endothelial cells a direct protein-protein interaction between ligand-activated ERα and the regulatory subunit p85 of PI3K through a nongenomic mechanism is suggested (Simoncini et al., 2000), by which estradiol rapidly activates eNOS via the activation of PI3K/Akt.

6.2.2 Testosterone

Decreased testosterone in castrated animals showed increased myocardial Akt activation (Huang et al., 2010), so some researchers suggested its negative role in I/R induced injuries and others confirmed increased Akt activity. In isolated rat hearts, testosterone used in acute ischemia reperfusion caused gender differences in myocardial Akt activation and its dowstream signaling molecules (p-Bad, Bcl-2, p-FOXO3a). Bad and Bcl are triggers for apoptosis and once these levels increase, apoptosis is suppressed. FOXO, another downstream target of Akt pathway, enables cell survival by inducing death genes. Also, the use of the testosterone antagonist flutamide or castration of the animals prior to the experiment showed an increase in myocardial Akt pathway and increased all three markers (p-Bad, Bcl-2, p-FOXO3a) in the male hearts. Moreover, the effect of castration in the activation of the Akt pathway can be reversed by some agonists, but not by dihydrotestosterone (Huang et al., 2010).

6.3 Matrix metalloproteinase in ischemia

The degradation of the extracellular matrix by metalloproteinases (MMPs) is involved in post-myocardial infarction processes of healing and remodeling. Knockout mice targeting the MMP-9 gene (the primary MMP protein functioning in post-myocardial infarction cardiac remodeling) were reported to have a reduced prevalence of cardiac rupture and attenuated left ventricular remodeling compared to control mice. Also a temporal change in the expression of MMP-9 and MMP-2 after myocardial infarction has been found (Tao et al., 2004). With estrogen treatment a significant reduction in MMP-9 expression was exerted regardless of castration status, and no reduction was observed in the MMP-2 protein. The decreased activity of matrix MMP-9 by estrogen induced cardioprotection in males after acute myocardial infarction was accompanied with increased Akt-Bcl-2 anti-apoptotic signaling (Cao et al., 2011).

6.4 Apoptosis in cardiac ischemia-reperfusion

Apoptosis of cardiomyocytes in infarct zones can be determined by the anti-apoptotic protein marker Bcl-2. Estrogen treated mice showed higher amounts of Bcl-2 expression during myocardial infarction as compared to control mice (Cao et al., 2011). This study has established a pivotal role for the Akt gene in estrogen-induced inhibition of apoptosis. However, which of the ER isoforms (α or β) play a role is uncertain.

To established the protective effects of estrogen on hypoxia-induced apoptosis cells with minimal ERα expression were used (Cao et al., 2011), and it was revealed that 17β-estradiol protects against apoptosis induced by H_2O_2-induced oxidative stress through the glutathione/glutaredoxin-dependent redox regulation of the Akt protein. After estrogen treatment, the activity of the pro-apoptotic Akt (P-Akt) began to decrease, while the expression of the anti-apoptotic Bcl-2 began to increase. Cell-cycle analyses indicated that hypoxia-induced apoptosis was efficiently inhibited through supplemental of 17β-estradiol, which shows that ERβ is at least partly involved in the estrogen-mediated cardioprotection (Cao et al., 2011).

6.5 Gonadotrophin releasing hormone as a new target in the heart

Among the other potential hormones acting in the heart, gonadotrophin releasing hormone is the potential cardiac marker, responsible for the release of luteinizing hormone and follicle-stimulating hormone from the anterior pituitary, that is synthesized and released from neurons in the hypothalamus. Treatment may be associated with an increased risk of cardiac dysfunction that is attributed to the accompanying androgen deprivation. Gonadotrophin releasing hormone by itself may be a major contributor to the cardiac pathology. The chronically administered agonists may prolong QT interval in men and in women and reduce cardiac index, and decreased blood pressure. The potential pathway of activation is the PKA pathway and not the PKC pathway, that leads to gonadotrophin releasing hormone-mediated increased contractility. The PKA-mediated pathway has targets for phosphorylation, promotes cardiomyocyte contractile function, including the L-type Ca^{2+} channel on the sarcolemma and components of the contractile apparatus. Besides, PKA also phosphorylates the ryanodine receptor and Ca^{2+} release channels in the cardiomyocytes, which in turn regulates channel opening and leads to increased sensitivity to Ca^{2+}-induced activation. Higher doses of gonadotrophin releasing hormone elevated resting intracellular Ca^{2+} and may be a reflection of increased sarcoplasmic reticulum Ca^{2+} release and cardiac contractility (Dong et al., 2011).

6.6 Other potential mechanism of sex hormones mediated protection

Some other potential mechanisms may contribute to the cardioprotective effects of sex hormones. For example, it has been reported that estrogen exerts cardioprotective effects by modulating the cardiac expression of tumor necrosis factor-α (TNFα) and its receptor (Xu et al., 2006). Additionally, nitric oxide synthase (NOS) has also been shown to mediate estrogen-induced cardioprotection (Lin et al., 2009). Therefore, the entire mechanism may be far beyond our current knowledge. Also, understanding the exact functional relationship between estrogen and androgen in the cardiovascular system should be the goal of future research.

7. Conclusion

Many studies of the last years focused not only on estrogen, but also on testosterone for a role in cardiovascular diseases. Importantly, as a new approach of non-nuclear modulation of cardioprotection the estrogen receptor GPER1 was mentioned.

The actions of estrogen are mediated by estrogen receptors -α and -β, by two cytosolic receptors and another, membrane bound receptor GPER1. In the cardiovascular system the

ERα demonstrates to have a more prominent role compared to ERβ, which might be gender-related. ERα is widely distributed in cardiomyocytes (Lizotte et al., 2009), thus indicating its important role, and its membrane position suggests important estrogen non-genomic rapid signaling, while its cytosolic and nuclear distribution suggest genomic signaling. Among the rapid signalling effects, estradiol induces the translocation of ERα to the PI3K regulatory domain and shows NOS (eNOS) activation in endothelium (Simoncini et al., 2000) as one of the most important effector product. Also, GPER1 activation results in matrix metalloproteinase cleavage of heparin-bound epidermal growth factor, that is able to activate the EGF receptor, that subsequently results in acute PI3K and ERK activation (Filardo et al., 2000). Besides, being a transmembrane estrogen receptor, GPER1 activation mediates rapid cell signaling too (Prossnitz et al., 2008). GPER1 deactivation of the PI3K pathway was confirmed by abolishing the agonist-mediated protective effect, suggesting that the more important mechanism of protection by GPER1 activation is through the PI3K/AKT pathway. The activation of the PI3K pathway by GPER1-mediated transactivation of the EGF receptor (Filardo et al., 2000), leads not only to activation of PI3K but also to activation of ERK. Also, HIF- 1 in hypoxic conditions activates the up-regulation of GPER1 in cardiomyocytes and ROS-induced activation of EGFR/ERK signaling is required for this pathway. Hypoxia-induced expression of GPER1 may be included among the mechanisms involved in the anti-apoptotic effects elicited by estrogens. Blocking the PI3K activation resulted in reduced phosphorylation of Akt and in reduced recovery and larger infarct sizes compared to agonist-treated hearts. The acute activation of the estrogen receptor GPER1 is gender-independent cardioprotective (Deschamps & Murphy, 2009).

Androgenes, mostly testosterone, have been known up till now for their deleterious effects in cardiovascular system, and are supposed to potentiate ischemic/reperfusion injuries; but those effects are present only in acute heart injuries. Rapid androgen receptor activation, analogous to estrogen receptor cytosolic activation, probably enable yet unknown cardioprotective pathways, which are expressed as diminished ischemic effects, and decreased arrhythmias. Most of such protective effects, beyond their nuclear cardioprotection pathway, are proposed to be mainly long-term activated. Also, endothelial cells exposed to dihydrotestosterone, produced a dose-dependent increase in the production of a key angiogenic growth factor - vascular endothelial growth factor, and further increased the expression of VEGF receptors Flt-1 and KDR. VEGF receptor KDR is the main mediator of the mitogenic/angiogenic action of VEGF in endothelial cells, and VEGF receptor Flt-1 is a negative regulator of VEGF action, so dihydrotestosterone plays a proangiogenic role for VEGF signaling. Anti-VEGF action inhibits tubulogenesis, and also the inhibitor of phosphoinositol 3-kinase (PI3K), a key enzyme in the PI3K–AKT pathway of VEGF signaling, inhibited dihydrotestosterone-mediated tubulogenesis.

The main pathways for cardioprotection are known to be PI3K-mediated. Estradiol induces the translocation of ERα to the PI3K regulatory domain and results in endothelial NOS (eNOS) activation (Simoncini et al., 2000). ERβ activation leads to protein S-nitrosylation and thus cardioprotection, which could be blocked by NOS inhibition, suggesting that chronic estrogen exposure protects hearts largely via activation of ERβ and NO signaling (Lin et al., 2009). The role for the Akt gene in estrogen-induced inhibition of apoptosis is probably a crucial step. However, which ER isoform plays the major role, ERα or ERβ, and whether gender-dependent, is uncertain. In short, ERα and GPER1 might be more important in acute protection, and ERβ in more long term, estrogen chronically exposed conditions.

Cardioprotective effects induced by estrogen involved ERK, PI3K and PKA transduction cascades. In endothelial cells, ERα activation culminates in two major signal transduction events, one is the ERK pathway, and a second is increased PI3K/Akt activity. In both pathways, the final event involves a rapid NO production by eNOS. A potential functional interactivity between GPER1, ERα and ERβ leads to cardioprotective action, responsible for estrogen involvement in ERK, PI3K, PKA and eNOS. Gender-independent GPER1 activation of eNOS plays a central role in the response to estrogen stimulation (Filice et al., 2009). Testosterone on the other hand, is known to act via PKC; PKC inhibition attenuates the differences in arterial pressure to Ang II. Also, expression of PKCδ and PKCε are attenuated by castration, but are restored by testosterone. Undoubtly, testosterone cardioprotection is the focus of present studies and search for its protective pathways, independent from nuclear action.

Of course, some clinical findings predicts even more potential clinical protection by sex hormones, by yet unknown mechanisms. A review analysis of physiologic responses to critical illnesses and injury as well as their relative rates of survival and recovery, proposed estrogen to have protective effects in numerous conditions ranging from global ischemic insults and massive systemic inflammatory responses to devastating focal injury and apoptosis in vital organs. Furthermore, the authors suggested even exogenous infusion of estrogen, not only as a direct therapeutic agent, that can benefit in some instances, but proposed estrogen administration for synergism with other resuscitative interventions (Wigginton et al., 2010).

8. Acknowledgement

This manuscript was proofread by Dr. Cécil J.W. Meulenberg. Figures were prepared by Mr. Jura Štok. Publication was made possible by Grant J3-0024 »Pharmacological protection against ischemic-reperfusion injuries in brain and cardiovascular tissues« from the Slovenian Research Agency. The author declare no conflicts of interest.

9. References

Abi-Gerges, N., Philp, K., Pollard, C., Wakefield, I., Hammond, T.G. & Valentin, J.P. (2004). Sex differences in ventricular repolarization: from cardiac electrophysiology to torsades de pointes. *Fundamental and Clinical Pharmacology*, Vol. 18, No. 2, pp. 139–151.

Adams, M.R., Williams, J.K. & Kaplan, J.R. (1995). Effects of androgens on coronary atheroslcerosis and atherosclerosis-related impairment of vascular responsiveness. *Arteriosclerosis, Thrombosis, and Vascular Biology,* Vol.15, No. 5, pp. 562–570.

Arnal, J.F., Fontaine, C., Billon-Galés, A., Favre, J., Laurell, H., Lenfant, F. & Gourdy, P. (2010). Estrogen receptors and endothelium. *Arteriosclerosis, Thrombosis, and Vascular Biology,* Vol. 30, No. 8, pp. 1506-1512.

Bidoggia, H., Maciel, J.P., Capalozza, N., Mosca, S., Blaksley, E.J., Valverde, E., Bertran, G., Arini, P., Biagetti, M.O. & Quinteiro, R.A. (2000a). Sex differences on the electrocardiographic pattern of cardiac repolarization: possible role of testosterone. *American Heart Journal,* Vol. 140, No. 4, pp. 678-683.

Bidoggia, H., Maciel, J.P., Capalozza, N., Mosca, S., Blaksley, E.J., Valverde, E., Bertran, G., Arini, P., Biagetti, M.O. & Quinteiro, R.A. (2000b). Sex-dependent electrocardiographic pattern of cardiac repolarization. *American Heart Journal*, Vol. 140, No. 3, pp. 430-436.

Booth, E.A., Obeid, N.R. & Lucchesi, B.R. (2005). Activation of estrogen receptor-alpha protects the in vivo rabbit heart from ischemia-reperfusion injury. *American Journal of Physiology. Heart and Circulatory Physiology*, Vol. 289, No. 5, pp. 2039-2047.

Bopassa, J.C., Eghbali, M., Toro, L. & Stefani, E. (2010). A novel estrogen receptor GPER inhibits mitochondria permeability transition pore opening and protects the heart against ischemia-reperfusion injury. *American Journal of Physiology. Heart and Circulatory Physiology*, Vol. 298, No. 1, pp. 16-23.

Borst, S.E., Quindry, J.C., Yarrow, J.F., Conover, C.F. & Powers, S.K. (2010). Testosterone administration induces protection against global myocardial ischemia. *Hormone and Metabolic Research*, Vol. 42, No. 2, pp. 122-129.

Bourghardt, J., Wilhelmson, A.S., Alexanderson, C., De Gendt, K., Verhoeven, G., Krettek, A., Ohlsson, C. & Tivesten, A. (2010). Androgen receptor-dependent and independent atheroprotection by testosterone in male mice. *Endocrinology*, Vol. 151, No. 11, pp. 5428-5437.

Burke, J.H., Goldberger, J.J., Ehlert, F.A., Kruse, J.T., Parker, M.A. & Kadish, A.H. (1996). Gender differences in heart rate before and after autonomic blockade: evidence against an intrinsic gender effect. *American Journal of Medicine*, Vol. 100, No. 5, pp. 537-543.

Cao, J., Zhu, T., Lu, L., Geng, L., Wang, L., Zhang, Q., Yang, K., Wang, H. & Shen, W. (2011). Estrogen induces cardioprotection in male C57BL/6J mice after acute myocardial infarction via decreased activity of matrix metalloproteinase-9 and increased Akt-Bcl-2 anti-apoptotic signaling. *International Journal of Molecular Medicine*, Vol. 28, No. 2, pp. 231-237.

Carmeci, C., Thompson, D.A., Ring, H.Z., Francke, U. & Weigel, R.J. (1997). Identification of a gene (GPR30) with homology to the G-protein-coupled receptor superfamily associated with estrogen receptor expression in breast cancer. *Genomics*, Vol. 45, No. 3, pp. 607-617.

Carroll JS, Brown M. (2006). Estrogen receptor target gene: an evolving concept. Mol Endocrinol. 2006 Aug;20(8):1707-14.

Cavasin, M.A., Sankey, S.S., Yu, A.L., Menon, S & Yang, X.P. (2003). Estrogen and testosterone have opposing effects on chronic cardiac remodeling and function in mice with myocardial infarction. *American journal of physiology. Heart and Circulatory Physiology*, Vol. 284, No. 5, pp. 1560-1569.

Chakrabarti, S., Lekontseva, O., Peters, A. & Davidge, S.T. (2010). 17beta-Estradiol induces protein S-nitrosylation in the endothelium. *Cardiovascular Research*, Vol. 85, No. 4, pp. 796-805.

Charbit, B., Christin-Maître, S., Démolis, J.L., Soustre, E., Young, J. & Funck-Brentano, C. (2009). Effects of testosterone on ventricular repolarization in hypogonadic men. *American Journal of Cardiology*, Vol. 103, No. 6, pp. 887-890.

Chung, T.H., Wang, S.M., Liang, J.Y., Yang, S.H. & Wu, J.C. (2009). The interaction of estrogen receptor alpha and caveolin-3 regulates connexin43 phosphorylation in metabolic inhibition-treated rat cardiomyocytes. *International Journal of Biochemistry and Cell Biology*. Vol. 41, No. 11, pp. 2323-2333.

Collins, P., Rosano, G.M., Jiang, C., Lindsay, D., Sarrel, P.M. & Poole-Wilson, P.A. (1993). Cardiovascular protection by oestrogen—a calcium antagonist effect? *Lancet*, Vol. 341, No. 8855, pp. 1264–1265.

Costarella, C.E., Stallone, J.N., Rutecki, G.K. & Whittier, F.C. (1996). Testosterone causes direct relaxation of rat thoracic aorta. *Journal of Pharmacology and Experimental Therapeutics*, Vol. 277, No. 1, pp. 34–39.

Crews, J.K. & Khalil, R.A. (1999). Gender-specific inhibition of Ca^{2+} entry mechanisms of arterial vasoconstriction by sex hormones. *Clinical and Experimental Pharmacology and Physiology*, Vol. 26, No. 9, pp. 707–715.

Dai, Z., Zhu, H.Q., Jiang, D.J., Jiang, J.L., Deng, H.W. & Li, Y.J. (2004). 17beta estradiol preserves endothelial function by reduction of the endogenous nitric oxide synthase inhibitor level. *International Journal of Cardiology*, Vol. 96, No. 2, pp. 223–227.

Dechering, K., Boersma, C. & Mosselman, S. (2000). Estrogen receptors α and beta: two receptors of a kind? *Current Medicinal Chemistry*, Vol. 7, No. 5, pp. 561–576.

Delbeck, M., Golz, S., Vonk, R., Janssen, W., Hucho, T., Isensee, J., Schäfer, S. & Otto, C. (2011). Impaired left-ventricular cardiac function in male GPR30-deficient mice. *Molecular Medicine Reports*, Vol. 4, No. 1, pp- 37-40.

Deschamps, A.M. & Murphy, E. (2009). Activation of a novel estrogen receptor, GPER, is cardioprotective in male and female rats. *American Journal of Physiology. Heart and Circulatory Physiology*. Vol. 297, No. 5 pp. 1806-1813.

Deschamps, A.M., Murphy, E. & Sun, J. (2010). Estrogen receptor activation and cardioprotection in ischemia reperfusion injury. *Trends in Cardiovascular Medicine*, Vol. 20, No. 3, pp. 73-78.

Delyani, J.A., Murohara, T., Nossuli, T.O. & Lefer, A.M. (1996). Protection from myocardial reperfusion injury by acute administration of 17 beta-estradiol. *Journal of Molecular and Cellular Cardiology*, Vol. 28, No. 5, pp. 1001–1008.

Deenadayalu, V.P., White, R.E., Stallone, Y.N., Gao, X. & Garcia, A.Y. (2001). Testosterone relaxes coronary arteries by opening the large conductance, calcium activated potassium channel. *American Journal of Physiology. Heart and Circulatory Physiology*, Vol. 281, No.4, pp. 1720–1727.

Dong, M., Niklewski, P.J. & Wang, H.S. (2011). Ionic mechanisms of cellular electrical and mechanical abnormalities in Brugada syndrome. *American Journal of Physiology. Heart and Circulatory Physiology*, Vol. 300, No. 1, pp. 279-287.

Dong F, Skinner DC, Wu TJ, Ren J. The heart: a novel gonadotrophin-releasing hormone target. J Neuroendocrinol. 2011 May;23(5):456-63.

English, K.M., Jones, R.D., Jones, T.H., Morice, A.H. & Channer, K.S. (2002). Testosterone acts as a coronary vasodilator by a calcium antagonistic action. *Journal of Endocrinological Investigation*, Vol. 25, No. 5, pp. 455–458.

Er, F., Michels, G., Gassanov, N., Rivero, F. & Hoppe, U.C. (2004). Testosterone induces cytoprotection by activating ATP-sensitive K channels in the cardiac mitochondrial inner membrane. *Circulation*, Vol. 110, No. 19, pp. 3100–3107.

Ezaki, K., Nakagawa, M., Taniguchi, Y., Nagano, Y., Teshima, Y., Yufu, K., Takahashi, N., Nomura, T., Satoh, F., Mimata, H. & Saikawa, T. (2010). Gender differences in the ST segment: effect of androgen-deprivation therapy and possible role of testosterone. *Circulation Journal*, Vol. 74, No. 11, pp. 2448-2454.

Favre, J., Musette, P., Douin-Echinard, V., Laude, K., Henry, J.P., Arnal, J.F., Thuillez, C. & Richard, V. (2007). Toll-like receptors 2-deficient mice are protected against postischemic coronary endothelial dysfunction. *Arteriosclerosis, Thrombosis, and Vascular Biology*, Vol. 27, No. 5, pp. 1064 -1071.

Favre, J., Gao, J., Henry, J.P., Remy-Jouet, I., Fourquaux, I., Billon-Gales, A., Thuillez, C., Arnal, J.F., Lenfant, F. & Richard, V. (2010). Endothelial estrogen receptor α plays an essential role in the coronary and myocardial protective effects of estradiol in ischemia/reperfusion. *Arteriosclerosis, Thrombosis, and Vascular Biology*, Vol. 30, No. 12, pp. 2562-2567.

Filice, E., Recchia, A.G., Pellegrino, D., Angelone, T., Maggiolini, M. & Cerra, M.C. (2009). A new membrane G protein-coupled receptor (GPR30) is involved in the cardiac effects of 17beta-estradiol in the male rat. *Journal of Physiology and Pharmacology*, Vol. 60, No. 4, pp. 3-10.

Filardo, E.J., Quinn, J.A., Bland, K.I. & Frackelton, A.R. Jr. (2000). Estrogen-induced activation of Erk-1 and Erk-2 requires the G protein-coupled receptor homolog, GPR30, and occurs via trans-activation of the epidermal growth factor receptor through release of HB-EGF. *Molecular Endocrinology*, Vol. 14, No. 10, pp. 1649-1660.

Fox, E.M., Andrade, J. & Shupnik, M.A. (2009). Novel actions of estrogen to promote proliferation: integration of cytoplasmic and nuclear pathways. *Steroids*, Vol. 74, No. 7, pp. 622-627.

Fraser, H., Davidge, S.T. & Clanachan, A.S. (2000). Activation of Ca^{2+}-independent nitric oxide synthase by 17beta-estradiol in post-ischemic rat heart. *Cardiovascular Research*, Vol. 46, No. 1, pp. 111–118.

Fülöp L, Bányász T, Szabó G, Tóth IB, Bíró T, Lôrincz I, Balogh A, Petô K, Mikó I, Nánási PP. (2006). Effects of sex hormones on ECG parameters and expression of cardiac ion channels in dogs. Acta Physiol (Oxf). Nov-Dec;188(3-4):163-71.

Gabel, S.A., Walker, V.R., London, R.E., Steenbergen, C., Korach, K.S. & Murphy, E. (2005). Estrogen receptor beta mediates gender differences in ischemia/reperfusion injury. *Journal of Molecular and Cellular Cardiology*, Vol. 38, No. 2, pp. 289-297.

Gaborit, N., Varro, A., Le Bouter, S., Szuts, V., Escande, D. & Nattel, S. (2010). Gender-related differences in ion-channel and transporter subunit expression in non-diseased human hearts. *Journal of Molecular and Cellular Cardiology*, Vol. 49, No. 4, pp. 639–646.

Genovesi, S., Zaccaria, D., Rossi, E., Valsecchi, M.G., Stella, A. & Stramba-Badiale, M. (2007). Effects of exercise training on heart rate and QT interval in healthy young individuals: are there gender differences? *Europace*, Vol. 9, No. 1, 55-60.

Genovesi, S., Dossi, C., Viganò, M.R., Galbiati, E., Prolo, F., Stella, A. & Stramba-Badiale, M. (2008). Electrolyte concentration during haemodialysis and QT interval prolongation in uraemic patients. *Europace*, Vol. 10, No. 6, pp. 771-777.

Geršak, B. & Drevenšek, G. (2002). Combining coronary revascularization and valvular surgery on a beating heart: an analysis. *Heart surgery forum*, 2002, Vol. 5, No. 1, pp. 1-4.

Gray, G.A., Sharif, I., Webb, D.J. & Seckl, J.R. (2001). Oestrogen and the cardiovascular system: the good, the bad and the puzzling. *Trends in Pharmacological Sciences*, Vol. 22, No. 3, pp. 152–156.

Honda, H., Unemoto, T. & Kogo, H. (1999). Different mechanisms for testosterone-induced relaxation of aorta between normotensive and spontaneously hypertensive rats. *Hypertension*, Vol. 34, No. 6, pp. 1232–1236.

Hayward, C.S., Webb, C.M. & Collins, P. (2001). Effect of sex hormones on cardiac mass. *Lancet*, Vol. 357, No. 9265, pp. 1354–1356.

Huang, C., Gu, H., Zhang, W., Herrmann, J.L. & Wang, M. (2010). Testosterone-down-regulated Akt pathway during cardiac ischemia/reperfusion: a mechanism involving BAD, Bcl-2 and FOXO3a. *Journal of Surgical Research*, Vol. 164, No. 1, pp. 1-11.

James, A., Choisy, S. & Hancox, J. (2007). Recent advances in understanding sex difference in cardiac repolarization. *Progress in Biophysics and Molecular Biology*, Vol. 94, No. 2, pp. 265–319.

Jeanes, H.L., Tabor, C., Black, D., Ederveen, A. & Gray, G.A. (2008). Oestrogen-mediated cardioprotection following ischaemia and reperfusion is mimicked by an oestrogen receptor (ER)alpha agonist and unaffected by an ER beta antagonist. *Journal of Endocrinology*, Vol. 197, No. 3, pp. 493-501.

Jesmin, S., Mowa, C.N., Sultana, S.N., Shimojo, N., Togashi, H., Iwashima, Y., Kato, N., Sato, A., Sakuma, I., Hiroe, M., Hattori, Y., Yamaguchi, N. & Kobayashi, H. (2010). VEGF signaling is disrupted in the hearts of mice lacking estrogen receptor alpha. *European Journal of Pharmacology*, Vol. 641, No. 2-3, pp. 168-178.

Jesmin, S., Mowa, C.N., Sultana, S.N., Mia, S., Islam, R., Zaedi, S., Sakuma, I., Hattori, Y., Hiroe, M. & Yamaguchi, N. (2010). Estrogen receptor alpha and beta are both involved in the cerebral VEGF/Akt/NO pathway and cerebral angiogenesis in female mice. *Biomedical Research*, Vol. 31, No. 6, pp. 337-346.

Jones, R.D., English, K.M., Jones, T.H. & Channer, K.S. (2004). Testosterone induced coronary vasodilatation occurs via a non-genomic mechanism: evidence of a direct calcium antagonism action. *Clinical Science (London)*, Vol. 107, No. 2, pp. 149–158.

Jovanovic, S., Jovanovic, A., Shen, W.K. & Terzic, A. (2000). Low concentrations of 17b-estradiol protect single cardiac cells against metabolic stress-induced Ca^{2+} loading. *Journal of the American College of Cardiology*, Vol. 36, No. 3, pp. 948–952.

Kadish, A.H., Greenland, P., Limacher, M.C., Frishman, W.H., Daugherty, S.A. & Schwartz, J.B. (2004). Estrogen and progestin use and the QT interval in postmenopausal women. *Annals of noninvasive electrocardiology*, Vol.9, No. 4, pp. 366-374.

Kim, Y.D., Farhat, M.Y.,Myers, A.K., Kouretas, P., DeGroot, K.W., Pacquing, A., Ramwell, P.W., Suyderhoud, J.P. & Lees, D.E. (1998). 17-Beta estradiol regulation of myocardial glutathione and its role in protection against myocardial stunning in dogs. *Journal of Cardiovascular Pharmacology*, Vol. 32, No. 3, pp. 457–465.

Knowlton, A.A. & Sun, L. (2001). Heat-shock factor-1, steroid hormones, and regulation of heat-shock protein expression in the heart. *American Journal of Physiology. Heart and Circulatory Physiology*. Vol. 280, No. 1, pp. 455–464.

Kvingedal, A.M. & Smeland, E.B. (1997). A novel putative G-protein-coupled receptor expressed in lung, heart and lymphoid tissue. *FEBS Letters*, Vol. 407, No. 1, pp. 59-62.

Kuhar, P., Lunder, M. & Drevenšek, G. (2007). The role of gender and sex hormones in ischemic-reperfusion injury in isolated rat hearts. *European Journal of Pharmacology*, Vol. 561, No. 1-3, pp. 151-159.

Lin, J., Steenbergen, C., Murphy, E. & Sun, J. (2009). Estrogen receptor-beta activation results in S-nitrosylation of proteins involved in cardioprotection. *Circulation*, Vol. 120, No. 3, pp. 245-54.

Liu, X.K., Katchman, A., Whitfield, B.H., Wan, G., Janowski, E.M., Woosley, R.L. & Ebert, S.N. (2002). In vivo androgen treatment shortens the QT interval and increases the densities of inward and delayed rectifier potassium currents in orchiectomized male rabbits. *Cardiovascular Research*, Vol. 57, No. 1, pp. 28-36.

Liu. J., Tsang, S. & Wong, T.M. (2006). Testosterone is required for delayed cardioprotection and enhanced heat shock protein 70 expression induced by preconditioning. *Endocrinology*, Vol. 147, No. 10, pp. 4569-4577.

Lizotte, E., Grandy, S.A., Tremblay, A., Allen, B.G. & Fiset, C. (2009). Expression, distribution and regulation of sex steroid hormone receptors in mouse heart. *Cellular Physiology and Biochemistry: International Journal of Experimental Cellular Physiology, Biochemistry, and Pharmacology*, Vol. 23, No. 1-3, pp. 75-86.

Luttrell, L.M. (2006). Transmembrane signaling by G protein-coupled receptors. *Methods in Molecular Biology*, Vol. 332, pp, 3-49.

Ma. L. & Pei, G. (2007). Beta-arrestin signaling and regulation of transcription. *Journal of Cell Science*, Vol. 120, No. 2, pp. 213-218.

Malkin CJ, Channer KS & Jones TH. (2010). Testosterone and heart failure. *Current Opinion in Endocrinology, diabetes, and obesity*, Vol. 17, No. 3, pp. 262-268.

Mårtensson, U.E., Salehi, S.A., Windahl, S., Gomez, M.F., Swärd, K., Daszkiewicz-Nilsson, J., Wendt, A., Andersson, N., Hellstrand, P., Grände, P.O., Owman, C., Rosen, C.J., Adamo, M.L., Lundquist, I., Rorsman, P., Nilsson, B.O., Ohlsson, C., Olde, B. & Leeb-Lundberg, L.M. (2009). Deletion of the G protein-coupled receptor 30 impairs glucose tolerance, reduces bone growth, increases blood pressure, and eliminates estradiol-stimulated insulin release in female mice. *Endocrinology*, Vol. 150, No. 2, pp. 687-698.

Meyer, M.R., Haas, E., Prossnitz, E.R. & Barton, M. (2009). Non-genomic regulation of vascular cell function and growth by estrogen. *Molecular and Cellular Endocrinology*, Vol. 308, No. 1-2, pp. 9-16.

Moriarty, K., Kim, K.H. & Bender, J.R. (2006). Minireview: estrogen receptor-mediated rapid signaling. *Endocrinology*, Vol. 147, No. 12, pp. 5557-5563

Naghi, J.J., Philip, K.J., DiLibero, D., Willix, R. & Schwarz, E.R. (2011). Testosterone therapy: treatment of metabolic disturbances in heart failure. *Journal of Cardiovascular Pharmacology and Therapeutics*, 16, No. 1, pp. 14-23.

Nankin HR, Calkins JH. (1986). Decreased bioavailable testosterone in aging normal and impotent men. J Clin Endocrinol Metab, 63: 1418 - 1420.

Nathan, L., Shi, W., Dinh, H., Mukherjee, T.K., Wang, X., Lusis, A.J. & Chaudhuri, G. (2001). Testosterone inhibits early atherogenesis by conversion to estradiol: critical role of aromatase. *Proceedings of the National Academy of Sciences of the United States of America*, Vol. 98, No. 6, pp. 3589-3593.

Nikolic, I., Liu, D., Bell, J.A., Collins, J., Steenbergen, C. & Murphy, E. (2007). Treatment with an estrogen receptor-beta-selective agonist is cardioprotective. *Journal of Molecular and Cellular Cardiology*, Vol. 42, No. 4, pp. 769-780.

Nilsson, B.O., Olde, B. & Leeb-Lundberg, L.F. (2011). G protein-coupled oestrogen receptor 1 (GPER1)/GPR30: a new player in cardiovascular and metabolic oestrogenic signalling. *British Journal of Pharmacolology*, Vol. 163, No. 6, pp. 1131-1139.

O'Dowd, B.F., Nguyen, T., Jung, B.P., Marchese, A., Cheng, R., Heng, H.H., Kolakowski, LF. Jr., Lynch, K.R. & George, S.R. (1998). Cloning and chromosomal mapping of four putative novel human G-protein-coupled receptor genes. *Gene*, Vol. 187, No. 1, pp. 75-81.

Patel, V.H., Chen, J., Ramanjaneya, M., Karteris, E., Zachariades, E., Thomas, P., Been, M. & Randeva, H.S. (2010). G-protein coupled estrogen receptor 1 expression in rat and human heart: Protective role during ischaemic stress. *International Journal of Molecular Medicine*, Vol. 26, No. 2, pp. 193-199.

Patten, R.D., Pourati, I., Aronovitz, M.J., Baur, J., Celestin, F., Chen, X., Michael, A., Haq, S., Nuedling, S., Grohe, C., Force, T., Mendelsohn, M.E. & Karas, R.H. (2004). 17β-estradiol reduces cardiomyocyte apoptosis in vivo and in vitro via activation of phospho-inositide-3 kinase/Akt signaling. *Circulation Research*, Vol. 95, No. 7, pp. 692-699.

Pecori Giraldi, F., Toja, P.M., Filippini, B., Michailidis, J., Scacchi, M., Stramba Badiale, M. & Cavagnini, F. (2010). Increased prevalence of prolonged QT interval in males with primary or secondary hypogonadism: a pilot study. *International Journal of Andrology*, Vol. 33, No. 1, pp. 132-138.

Perusquia, M., Hernandez, R., Morales, M.A., Campos, M.G. & Villalon, C.M. (1996). Role of endothelium in the vasodilating effect of progestins and androgens on the rat thoracic aorta. *General Pharmacology*, Vol. 27, No.1, pp. 181–185.

Peitras, R.J. & Szego, C.M. (1977). Specific binding sites for oestrogen at the outer surfaces of isolated endometrial cells. *Nature*, Vol. 265, No. 5589, pp. 69–72.

Pham, T.V. & Rosen, M.R. (2002). Sex, hormones, and repolarization. *Cardiovascular Research*, Vol. 53, No. 3, pp. 740–751.

Prossnitz, E.R., Arterburn, J.B., Smith, H.O., Oprea, T.I., Sklar, L.A., & Hathaway, H.J. (2008). Estrogen signaling through the transmembrane G protein-coupled receptor GPR30. *Annual Review of Physiology*, Vol. 70, pp. 165-190.

Pugh, P.J., English, K.M., Jones, T.H. & Channer, K.S. (2000). Testosterone: a natural tonic for the heart? *Quarterly Journal of Medicine*, Vol. 93, No. 10, pp. 689–694.

Recchia, A.G., De Francesco, E.M., Vivacqua, A., Sisci, D., Panno, M.L., Andò, S. & Maggiolini, M. (2011). The G protein-coupled receptor 30 is up-regulated by hypoxia-inducible factor-1alpha (HIF-1alpha) in breast cancer cells and cardiomyocytes. *Journal of Biological Chemistry*, Vol. 286, No. 12, pp. 10773-10782.

Reid, J., Betney, R., Watt, K. & McEwan, I.J. (2003). The androgen receptor transactivation domain: the interplay between protein conformation and protein–protein interactions. *Biochemical Society transactions*, Vol. 31, No. 5, pp. 1042–1046.

Revelli, A., Massobrio, M. & Tesarik, J. (1998). Nongenomic actions of steroid hormones in reproductive tissues. *Endocrine Reviews*, Vol. 19, No.1, pp. 3–17.

Roden, D.M. (2004). Drug-induced prolongation of the QT interval. *New England Journal of Medicine*, Vol. 350, No. 10, pp. 1013-1022.

Ropero, A.B., Eghbali, M., Minosyan, T.Y., Tang, G., Toro, L. & Stefani, E. (2006). Heart estrogen receptor alpha: distinct membrane and nuclear distribution patterns and regulation by estrogen. Journal of Molecular and Cellular Cardiology. Vol. 41, No. 3, pp. 496-510.

Rosano, G.M., Leonardo, F., Pagnotta, P., Pelliccia, F., Panina, G., Cerquetani, E., DellaMonica, P.L., Bonfigli, B., Volpe, M. & Chierchia, S.L. (1999). Acute anti-ischemic effect of testosterone in men with coronary artery disease. *Circulation*, Vol. 99, No. 13, pp. 1666–1670.

Santos, R.L., Abreu, G.R., Bissoli, N.S. & Moyses, M.R. (2004). Endothelial mediators of 17 beta-estradiol-induced coronary vasodilation in the isolated rat heart. *Brazilian Journal of Medical and Biological Research*, Vol.37, No. 4, pp. 569–575.

Schwartz PJ, Moss AJ, Vincent GM, Crampton RS. Diagnostic criteria for the long QT syndrome. An update. Circulation. 1993 Aug;88(2):782-4

Schwartz, J.B., Volterrani, M., Caminiti, G., Marazzi, G., Fini, M., Rosano, G.M. & Iellamo F. (2011). Effects of testosterone on the Q-T Interval in older men and older women with chronic heart failure. *International Journal of Andrology*, 2011 May 25. doi: 10.1111/j.1365-2605.2011.01163.

Sieveking, D.P., Lim, P., Chow, R.W., Dunn, L.L., Bao, S., McGrath, K.C., Heather, A.K., Handelsman, D.J., Celermajer, D.S. & Ng, M.K. (2010). A sex-specific role for androgens in angiogenesis. *Journal of Experimental Medicine*, Vol. 207, No. 2, pp. 345-352.

Simoncini, T., Hafezi-Moghadam, A., Brazil, D.P., Ley, K., Chin, W.W. & Liao, J.K. (2000). Interaction of oestrogen receptor with the regulatory subunit of phosphatidylinositol-3-OH kinase. *Nature*, Vol. 407, No. 6803, pp. 538-541.

Song, J., Eyster, K.M., Kost, C.K. Jr., Kjellsen, B. & Martin, D.S. (2010). Involvement of protein kinase C-CPI-17 in androgen modulation of angiotensin II-renal vasoconstriction. *Cardiovascular Research*, Vol. 85, No. 3, pp. 614-621.

Stramba-Badiale, M., Spagnolo, D., Bosi, G. & Schwartz, P.J. (1995). Are gender differences in QTc present at birth? *American Journal of Cardiology*, Vol. 75, No. 17, pp. 1277–1278.

Sun, J., Morgan, M., Shen, R.F., Steenbergen, C. & Murphy, E. (2007). Preconditioning results in S-nitrosylation of proteins involved in regulation of mitochondrial energetics and calcium transport. *Circulation Research*, Vol. 101, No. 11, pp. 1155-1163.

Sun, J. & Murphy, E. (2010). Protein S-nitrosylation and cardioprotection. *Circulation Research*, Vol. 106, No. 2, pp. 285-96.

Surawicz, B. & Parikh, S.R. (2002). Prevalence of male and female patterns of early ventricular repolarization in the normal ECG of males and females from childhood to old age. *Journal of the American College of Cardiology*, Vol. 40, No. 10, pp. 1870-1876.

Takada Y, Kato C, Kondo S, Korenaga R, Ando J. (1997). Cloning of cDNAs encoding G protein-coupled receptor expressed in human endothelial cells exposed to fluid shear stress. Biochem Biophys Res Commun. Nov 26;240(3):737-41.

Tao, Z.Y., Cavasin, M.A., Yang, F., Liu, Y.H. & Yang, X.P. (2004). Temporal changes in matrix metalloproteinase expression and inflammatory response associated with cardiac rupture after myocardial infarction in mice. *Life Sciences*, Vol. 74, No. 12, pp. 1561-1572.

Wang, M., Crisostomo, P.R., Markel, T., Wang, Y., Lillemoe, K.D. & Meldrum, D.R. (2008). Estrogen receptor beta mediates acute myocardial protection following ischemia. *Surgery*, Vol. 144, No. 2, pp. 233-238.

Wang, M., Wang, Y., Weil, B., Abarbanell, A., Herrmann, J., Tan, J., Kelly, M. & Meldrum, D.R. (2009). Estrogen receptor beta mediates increased activation of PI3K/Akt signaling and improved myocardial function in female hearts following acute ischemia. *American Journal of Physiology. Regulatory, Integrative and Comparative Physiology*, Vol. 296, No. 4, pp. 972-978.

Weil, B.R., Manukyan, M.C., Herrmann, J.L., Wang, Y., Abarbanell, A.M., Poynter, J.A. & Meldrum, D.R. (2010). Signaling via GPR30 protects the myocardium from ischemia/reperfusion injury. *Surgery*, Vol. 148, No. 2, pp. 436-443.

Wigginton, J.G., Pepe, P.E. & Idris, A.H. (2010). Rationale for routine and immediate administration of intravenous estrogen for all critically ill and injured patients. Critical Care Medicine, Vol. 38, No. 10, pp. 620-629.

Wild, R.A. & Bartholemew, M.J. (1988). The influence of body weight on lipoprotein lipids in patients with polycystic ovary syndrome. *American Journal of Obstetrics and Gynecology*, Vol. 159, No. 2, pp. 423–427.

Wise, P.M., Dubal, D.B., Wilson, M.E., Rau, S.W., Böttner, M. & Rosewell, K.L. (2001). Estradiol is a protective factor in the adult and aging brain: understanding of mechanism derived from in vivo and in vitro studies. *Brain research. Brain Research Reviews*, Vol. 37, No. 1-3, pp. 313–391.

Woodman, O.L., Missen, M.A. & Boujaoude, M. (2004). Daidzein and 17beta estradiol enhance nitric oxide synthase activity associated with an increase in calmodulin and a decrease in caveolin-1. *Journal of Cardiovascular Pharmacology*, Vol. 44, No. 2, pp. 155–163.

Wu, Q., Chambliss, K., Umetani, M., Mineo, C. & Shaul, P.W. (2011). Non-nuclear estrogen receptor signaling in the endothelium. *Journal of Biological Chemistry*, Vol. 286, No. 17, pp. 14737-14743.

Xu, Y., Arenas, I.A., Armstrong, S.J., Plahta, W.C., Xu, H. & Davidge, S.T. (2006). Estrogen improves cardiac recovery after ischemia/reperfusion by decreasing tumor necrosis factor-alpha. *Cardiovascular Research*, Vol. 69, No. 4, pp. 836-844.

Yildiz, O., Seyrek, M., Gul, H., Un, I., Yildirim, V., Ozal, E., Uzun, M. & Bolu, E. (2005). Testosterone relaxes human internal mammary artery in vitro. *Journal of Cardiovascular Pharmacology*, Vol. 45, No. 6, pp. 580–585.

Yang, S.H., Liu, R., Perez, E.J., Wen, Y., Stevens, S.M. Jr., Valencia, T., Brun-Zinkernagel, A.M., Prokai, L., Will, Y., Dykens, J., Koulen, P. & Simpkins, J.W. (2004). Mitochondrial localization of estrogen receptor beta. *Proceedings of the National Academy of Sciences of the United States of America*, Vol. 101, No. 12, pp. 4130-4135.

Yue, P., Chatterjee, K., Beale, C., Poole-Wilson, P.A. & Collins, P. (1995). Testosterone relaxes rabbit coronary arteries and aorta. *Circulation*, Vol. 91, No. 4, pp. 1154–1160.

Zhai, P., Eurell, T.E., Cotthaus, R., Jeffery, E.H., Bahr, J.M. & Gross, D.R., 2000. Effect of estrogen on global myocardial ischemia–reperfusion injury in female rats. *American Journal of Physiology. Heart and Circulatory Physiology*, Vol. 279, No. 6, pp. 2766–2775.

3

Serum Free Testosterone and Estradiol Levels in Perceptual-Verbal and Spatial Abilities; Differences in Sex and Hand Preference

Üner Tan
Çukurova University, Medical School, Department of Physiology, Adana, Turkey

1. Introduction

Cognitive sex differences have been demonstrated in humans: men usually outperform women on spatial ability (Linn & Peterson, 1985; Gladue et al., 1990; Mann et al., 1990; Gouchie & Kimura, 1991; Gladue & Bailey, 1995; Halpern & Tan, 2001; Tan et al., 2003a, b; Herlitz & Lovén, 2009); women outperform men on verbal tasks (Hyde & Linn, 1988; Mann et al., 1990; Halpern & Tan, 2001; Tan et al., 2003a, 2003b; Herlitz & Lovén, 2009). The sex hormones were thought to be responsible for the observed sex differences in cognitive abilities, but the available scientific literature does not provide any generally acceptable conclusion on this topic. For instance, testosterone has been reported to be beneficial for visuospatial ability in men (Hier & Crowly, 1982; Gordon & Lee, 1986; Christiansen & Knussmann, 1987; Tan, 1990a, b; Tan & Akgun, 1992; Christiansen, 1993; Janowsky et al., 1994; Van Goozen et al., 1994; Van Goozen et al., 1995; Tan & Tan, 1998; Barrett-Connor et al., 1999a; Silverman et al., 1999; Aleman et al., 2001; Kutlu et al., 2001; Kenny et al., 2002; Yaffe et al., 2002; Azurmendi et al., 2005), and women (Shute et al., 1983; Resnick et al., 1986; McKeever, 1987; Gouchie & Kimura, 1991; Van Goozen et al., 1995; Moffat & Hampson, 1996; Barrett-Connor et al., 1999b; Celec et al., 2002; Ostatnikova, et al., 2002). On the other hand, testosterone has also been reported as having no benefit for spatial ability in either men or women (Shute et al., 1983; Gouchie & Kimura, 1991; Moffat & Hampson, 1996; Van Goozen et al., 1995). Contrarily, some authors did not accept any significant association between testosterone and spatial cognition (McKeever et al., 1987; Kampen & Sherwin, 1996; Herlitz & Lovén, 2009). An inverse U-shaped relation between testosterone and spatial cognition was also reported, that is, the optimal performance was found in moderately high levels of testosterone (Shute et al., 1983; Gouchie & Kimura, 1991; Moffat & Hampson, 1996; Alexander et al., 1998; Neave, et al., 1999). With regard to handedness, significant relationships have been found between testosterone and spatial ability in right-handers, but not in left-handers (Moffat & Hampson, 1996).

Verbal abilities have also been studied in relation to sex-hormone concentrations in men and women. Some authors could not demonstrate any significant association between testosterone and verbal tasks (Gordon & Lee, 1986; Gouchie & Kimura, 1991; Neave, et al., 1999; Herlitz & Lovén, 2009), but others reported beneficial effects of testosterone on verbal ability (Cherrier, 1999; Alexander et al., 1998), but detrimental influence of androgen levels pn the vocabulary ability in girls (Azurmendi et al., 2005) . In female-to-male transsexuals, verbal skills have been shown to dramatically decline within three months following high doses of testosterone (Van Goozen et al., 1995). In contrast, high estrogen levels have been reported to be advantageous for verbal skills in women, and vary according to their ovarian cycle (Kimura, 1996; Halpern & Tan, 2001).

Cattell`s Culture Fair Intelligence Test measuring the sex-neutral IQ (Tan et al., 1993; Tan & Tan, 1998; Halpern & Tan, 2001) shows menstrual cycle fluctuations, being lower during the pre-ovulatory and post-ovulatory phases; in fact, an inverse U-shaped relation has been found between serum estradiol concentration and Cattell IQ in women (see Halpern & Tan, 2001). Despite the sex-neutrality of this IQ test, a direct relation has been found between Cattell IQ and total serum testosterone level in left-handed men (Tan et al., 1993). An inverse U-shaped relation has also been demonstrated between the total serum testosterone level and Cattell IQ in men and women (Tan & Tan, 1998). Students successful in exams for university entrance have also been shown to have higher total testosterone than those unsuccessful in university exams (Kutlu et al., 2001). On the other hand, matrices taken from the Kaufman Brief Intelligence Test, measuring the fluid intelligence similar to the Cattell's Culture Fair Intelligence Test, showed negative correlation with serum testosterone levels in 5-year-old children (Azurmendi et al., 2005).

Tan et al. (2003a) recently reported that an observed sex difference in visuo-spatial ability was not a real sex difference but merely depended upon the body size, because with covariates of height, weight, and vital capacity, sex differences in mental rotation completely disappeared. Under a combined co-variation of height, weight, and testosterone, the sex difference in mental rotation ability reversed, women scoring better than men (Tan et al., 2003b). In perceptual-verbal ability studies (Finding As test), with covariates of estradiol and progesterone, the sex difference also disappeared, suggesting the prominent role of these sex hormones in different verbal abilities of men and women with related differences in height and weight associated with *nature vs nuture* (Tan et al., 2003b). In accord, the height and weight are correlated with brain size, which is also correlated with IQ ($r = .40$) (Rushton, 1992, 1997; Raz et al., 1993; Tan et al., 1999; McDaniel, 2005). These results suggest that the body size should also be considered as a co-variate in studies of sex-related differences in cognitive abilities.

Under light of the above mentioned controversial results about the relations of sex hormones, testosterone and estrogens, on the verbal and non-verbal, visuo-spatial abilities, the aim of the present work was to evaluate the relations of the serum free testosterone and estradiol levels to the verbal, and non-verbal, visuo-spatial ability scores in right- and left-handed men and women. Although there are numerous reports on this subject with numerous controversial results, the present work will be the first, in the scientific literature, taking only the participants within the similar range of body size in male and female young adults, following the interrelationships among the body size, intelligence, and sex hormones. Controlling the body size could help to obtain a more reliable, homogenous sample of men and women within the same age range.

2. Methods

Participants in the study were 52 male and 24 female university students. All volunteers were between 18 and 20 years old, and willing to participate in this study since they wanted to know their IQs and sex-hormone levels. They were healthy and did not exhibit neurological signs and symptoms. Their cognitive functions were measured using three tests: "Finding As Test", "Mental Rotation Test," and "Cattell's Culture Fair Intelligence Test.

2.1 Finding As test

To measure the perceptual-verbal ability, the Finding As test from the ETS kit of Factor-Referenced Cognitive Tests (Ekstrom et al., 1976), classified as "feminine," was administered to the subjects. The test-retest correlation has been reported to be r = .87 for this test (Ekstrom et al., 1976). This test is usually used to assess the perceptual speed, and favors women, with very large effect size (Jensen, 1998 and e.g., Kimura & Hampson, 1994; Halpern & Tan, 2001; Tan et al., 2003b).

In each column of 40 words, the respondents were required to identify the five words containing the letter "a." In the Turkish version of this test (see Halpern & Tan, 2001), the subjects were asked to read the words in several columns as fast as possible, and cross out the letter "a" whenever it appears in the word list. This is a timed test of two minutes was allowed to read one page out of three pages, which the subjects should examine consequently. After completing the test, the number of the correctly chosen words was determined for each subject.

2.2 Mental Rotation Test (MRT)

To study mental rotation functions and the ability to solve spatial problems, the "Mental Rotation Test" (MRT) was used. This test was originally developed by Vandenberg and Kuse (1978), based on a design by Shepard and Metzler (1971). This test is a timed, group-administered paper-and-pencil test comprising problems in which participants are required to say whether pairs of two- or three-dimensional drawings of cubes from different angles and perspectives were the same or mirror images of each other. There were 25 problems, giving a maximum possible score of 25.

2.3 Cattell nonverbal intelligence test (Test of "g": Culture Fair)

The Cattell's Culture Fair Intelligence Test was originally designed to be a general measure of inborn intelligence without utilizing verbal material (Cattell, 1973, 1987). We applied the Institute for Personality and Ability (IPAT) Culture Fair Intelligence Test, Scale 3A, Form A to university students. The test primarily measures fluid intelligence, with part-whole relations, similarities, causal and spatial relations, inductive reasoning, inferential relations, including series, classification, matrices, and topology. There were 13 items on Subset 1 (3 min), 14 items in Subset 2 (4 min), 13 items in Subset 3 (3 min), and 10 items in Subset 4 (4 min). Raw scores were converted to normalized scores expressed by age group, and scoring was performed by using score key overlays with the response forms. Factor analysis showed validity in the 1970s and 1980s when the general ability factor was correlated with the concepts featured in the subtests (see Cattell, 1987). The spatial ability seems to be the most important factor with some loading on verbal and numerical abilities.

2.4 Hormone tests

Following the tests for cognitive abilities, blood was taken from the cubital vein the same day, and stored in the deep freeze for later analysis of hormone concentrations. The serum free testosterone and estradiol concentrations were measured using a radioimmunoassay technique (Diagnostic Product Corporation, USA), which is commercially available. Because testosterone shows diurnal and circadian variations (Kimura & Hampson, 1994; Moffat & Hampson, 1996), all the tests were completed and blood samples were taken before noon in the spring semester (May).

3. Results

3.1 Sex hormone levels

The mean testosterone levels were found to be 7.56±2.7 ng/dL and 5.2±3.7 ng/dL for the right-handed men (N = 33) and left-handed men (N = 19), respectively. The difference between these means was statistically significant: $t = 2.67$, $df = 50$, $p = .01$.

There was no significant difference between the mean estradiol levels of the right-handed (28.26±15.04 pg/mL)) and left-handed (29.16±14.93 pg/mL) male subjects, $t = 0.21$, $df = 50$, $P > .80$. The number of the left-handed females was not statistically suitable to make any comparison with right-handed women.

3.2 Mental rotation ability

Test	N	Mean	Minimum	Maximum	25%-75%
Mental rotation					
RH males	29	10.55±3.40	5.00	20.00	8.00-13.25
RH females	24	8.17±3.12	3.00	16.00	5.50-10.00
LH males	19	8.16±3.18	2.00	8.00	6.00-10.75
Cattell					
RH men	25	115.8±6.6	104	128	108-120
RH women	18	117.9±8.3	106	133	114-124
As					
RH men	25	37.9±5.4	27	47	33-42
RH women	20	40.7±.9	23	59	35-46

Table 1. Mental rotation, Cattell IQ and Finding As Test results

3.3 Sex hormones

3.3.1 Right-handers

Figure 1 illustrates the relation between serum testosterone and estradiol levels (abscissa) and mental rotation ability (ordinate) in the right-handed men (A, B) and women (C, D). In right-handed men, the relation between serum testosterone level and the number of correct answers on the mental rotation test could be best described by a quadratic equation (Figure 1A), i.e., the lowest mental rotation scores were at both ends of the inverted U-shaped curve. This quadratic relation was statistically significant: $r = .61$, $F(1, 24) = 7.7$, $p < .001$. In right-handed women, there was a direct relation between serum testosterone level and mental rotation scores, $r = .61$, $F(1, 22) = 13.2$, $p < .001$ (Figure 1C).

The serum estradiol level directly correlated with mental rotation test scores in the right-handed men (Figure 1B); the relation was statistically significant, $r = .61$, $F(1, 24) = 13.9$, $p < .001$. Similar to testosterone versus mental rotation in right-handed men, there was a quadratic relation (inverse U) between serum estradiol level and mental rotation ability in right-handed women, $r = .57$, $F(1, 22) = 5.3$, $p < .05$ (Figure 1D).

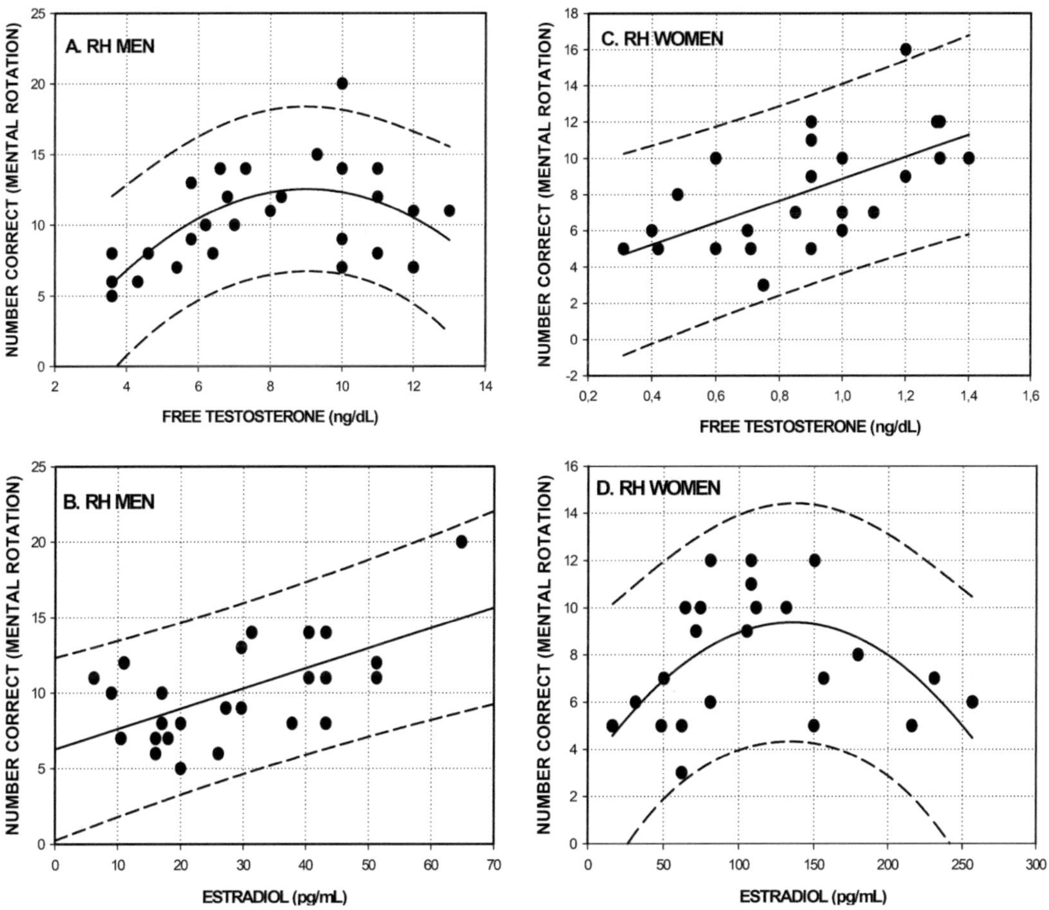

Fig. 1. Relations of serum testosterone and estradiol concentrations (abscissa) to mental rotation test scores (ordinate) in right-handed men (A, B) and women (C, D).

3.3.2 Left-handers

The scattergrams in Figure 2 illustrate the variations in mental rotation scores (ordinate) with various serum testosterone (left) and estradiol (right) levels in left-handed subjects. Since there were only a few left-handed females (N = 6), all left-handers were analyzed together (Figure 2), and the results were essentially similar to the right-handed male subjects. The relation of mental rotation ability versus testosterone could best be described by a quadratric equation, $r = .49$, $F(1, 17) = 5.5$, $P < .05$, with a slight decrease in mental rotation ability towards the higher testosterone levels. The relation of mental rotation to estradiol was best described by a direct correlation, $r = .68$, $F(1, 17) = 14.3$, $p < .001$.

3.4 Cattell`s culture fair intelligence test

There was no significant sex difference in Cattell IQ, $F(1, 161) = 0.31$, $p > .55$. Since there were only a few left-handed subjects who took the Cattell IQ test, only the right-handers will be analyzed in this section. Figure 3 illustrates the relation between the serum testosterone and estradiol levels (abscissa) to Cattell IQ (ordinate) in the right-handed male

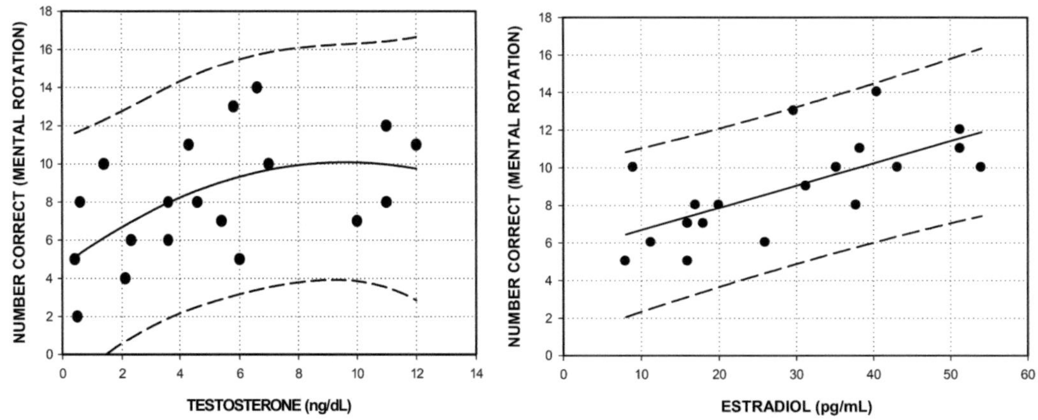

Fig. 2. Relations of mental rotation test scores (ordinate) to serum testosterone (left) and estradiol (right) levels in left-handed subjects.

(A, B) and female (C, D) subjects. In males, there was no significant correlation between testosterone and IQ (Figure 3A; r = .00; N = 25). The relation between estradiol and IQ could best be described by a quadratic (inverse U shaped) function (Figure 3B). This relation was found to be statistically significant (r = .47, F = 7.2, p < .05).

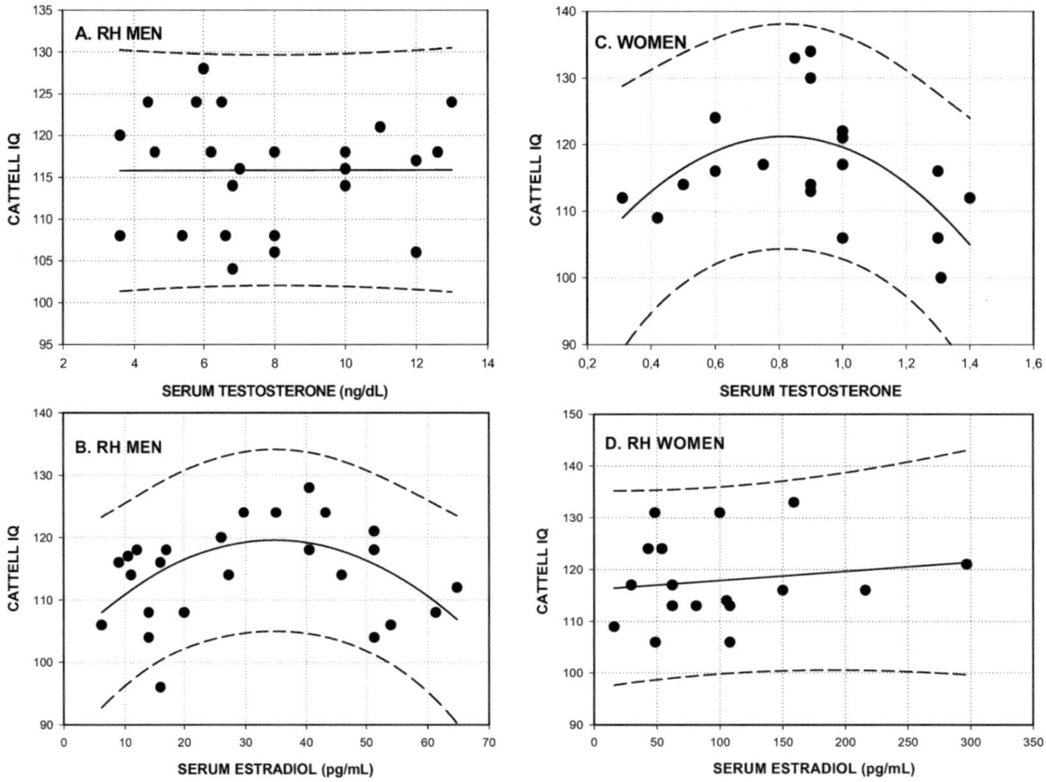

Fig. 3. Relations of serum testosterone and estradiol levels (abscissa) to Cattell IQ (ordinate) in male (left) and female (right) right-handed subjects.

An opposite picture was found for the female subjects. Namely, there was a quadratic, inverse U-shaped relation between testosterone and IQ (Figure 3C; $N = 16$, $r = .55$, $F = 7.3$, $p < .05$), and there was no significant correlation between estradiol and Cattell IQ (Figure 3D; $N = 16$, $r = .15$, $F = 0.4$, $p > .55$).

3.5 Perceptual-verbal ability ("Finding As Test")

3.5.1 Right-handers

Figure 4 illustrates the relation between the number of correct answers on the "Finding As Test" (ordinate) to the serum testosterone and estradiol levels (abscissa) in right-handed male (A, B) and female (C, D) subjects.

There was an inverse relation between the serum free testosterone levels and the number of correct answers, and this was best described by a quadratic relation, $r = .73$, $F = 12.9$, $p < .001$ (see Figure 4A). The serum estradiol level exhibited an inverse U-shaped (quadratic) relation to the perceptual-verbal ability ($N = 25$, $F = 19.3$, $p < .001$). In right-handed female subjects, the serum testosterone level significantly correlated with the numbers of correct answers on the test (see Figure 4C; $r = .53$, $F = 7.1$, $p < .05$). The relation between serum estradiol level and the number of correct answers was inverse U-shaped (Figure 4D; $r = .57$, $F = 9.0$, $p < .01$).

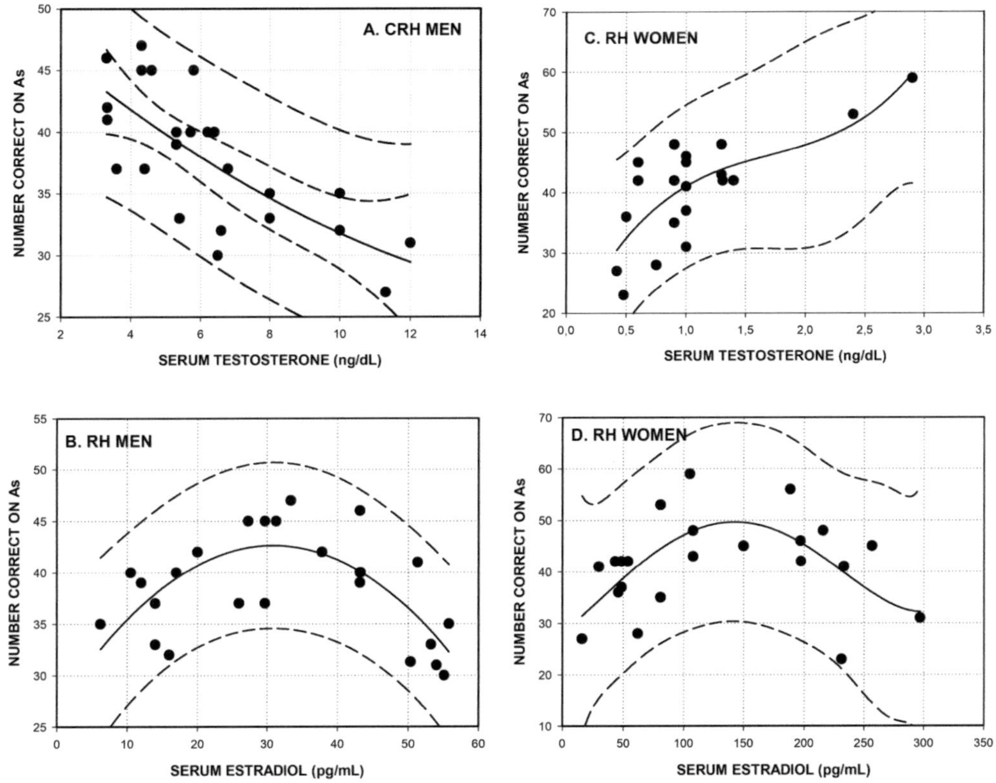

Fig. 4. Relations of number correct on As (ordinate, perceptual-verbal ability) to serum testorterone and estradiol levels (abscissa) in right-handed male (left) and female (right) subjects.

3.5.2 Left-handers

Since there were so few left-handed females, only the male left-handers were analyzed. Figure 5 illustrates the relation between the serum free testosterone and estradiol levels and the number of correct answers on the "Finding As Test". There were positive correlations between the number of correct answers and the serum testosterone and estradiol levels in these subjects. The correlation between the number of correct answers and serum free testosterone level was best described by a quadratic equation: $r = .62$, $F(2, 15) = 12.1$, $p = .001$; the serum estradiol level was positively linearly correlated by the equation: $r = .88$, $F(1, 12) = 20.0$, $p < .001$.

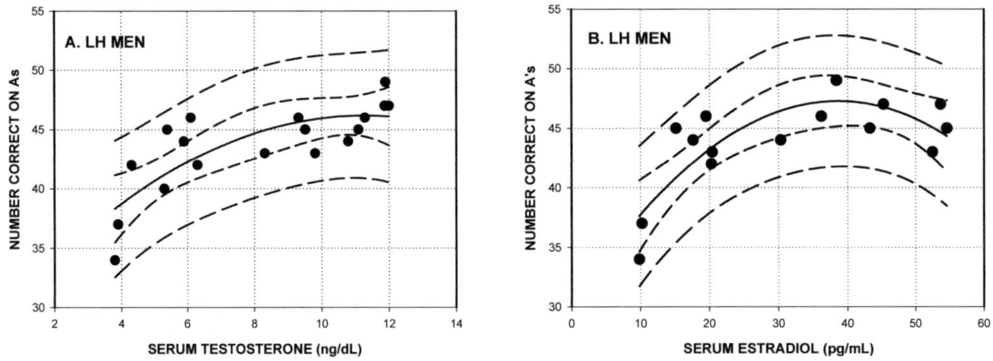

Fig. 5. Relations between perceptual-verbal ability (ordinate: number correct on A`s test) and serum free testosterone (A) and estradiol (B) levels in left-handed male subjects.

4. Discussion

4.1 Mental rotation ability

The results suggest that testosterone may be beneficial for mental rotation ability in women (see Figure 1C). Moffat and Hampson (1996) also found a positive correlation between visuospatial performance and salivary testosterone level in right-handed females, but there was no significant correlation in left-handed females. The sample size for the left-handed women was not large enough in the present work to make any statistical inferences.

The beneficial effects of testosterone on spatial ability has also been experimentally verified in humans and animals. Aleman et al (2004) found that a single testosterone administration improved mental rotation ability in young women; Roof and Havens (1992) found in rats that males outperformed females in the Morris water maze (spatial ability), and females given testosterone performed better than females without testosterone.

In right- and left-handed men, the mental rotation ability increased with testosterone for a large testosterone spectrum, but tended to decrease with very high testosterone levels, which was especially visible in right-handers (see Figures 1A and 2). In contrast to women, there are inconsistencies in the scientific literature with regard to testosterone effects on spatial ability in men. Some authors found a direct correlation, while others found an inverse relation, or an inverse U-shaped relation. The present work suggests relatively high testosterone levels would be advantageous, but very low and very high testosterone levels would be disadvantageous for the mental rotation ability in right- and left-handed men.

The present results favor the hypothesis that serum free testosterone is beneficial for visuospatial ability for a large part of the testosterone spectrum regardless of hand preference. Consistent with a curvilinear relation, Beech (2001) found that moderate baldness reflecting high levels of blood dihydrotestosterone is related to better performance in the mental rotation test in males. Supporting the dominant beneficial effect of testosterone on spatial ability in men, Christiansen and Knussman (1987) found a positive linear correlation between testosterone (salivary and serum) and spatial performance. There are many other examples supporting beneficial testosterone effects on spatial ability, such as in female-male transsexuals (Van Goozen et al., 1994), older men (Janowsky et al., 1994, 2000), and hypogonadal men (Alexander et al., 1998). According to Silverman et al. (1999), mental rotation scores are positively correlated with mean testosterone levels, but not with changes in testosterone. Gonadectomized male rodents have been shown to exhibit reduced cognitive performance (object recognition, radial arm maze, testosterone-maze, inhibitory avoidance), which could be reversed by testosterone-replacement (Frye et al., 2003). There are also inconsistent reports of low salivary testosterone levels being advantageous and high salivary testosterone levels being disadvantageous for visuospatial ability (Gouchie & Kimura, 1991; Moffat & Hampson, 1996). There are also studies showing null relations (e.g., McKeever et al., 1987; McKeever & Deyo, 1990).

The possible reasons for these inconsistencies may be diverse sample characteristics such as differences in educational levels (see Kutlu et al., 2001), hand preferences, and different measurement techniques(e.g., salivary versus serum testosterone levels), which, however, may not be related to inconsistent results , according to Silverman et al. (1999). On the other hand, differences in body size may also play a role in inconsistent results (Tan et al., 2003a, 2003b). The results of the present work suggest that serum free testosterone may be beneficial for the mental rotation ability in men and women, except that when levels of testosterone are too high in men there is a detrimental effect on mental rotation ability.

The relation of estradiol to mental rotation ability exhibited an inverse U-shaped relation to serum estradiol levels in right-handed women (Figure 1D), similar to that found in right-handed men as shown in Figure 1A. On the other hand, estradiol positively linearly correlated with mental rotation in right- and left-handed men (see Figures 1B and 2), like testosterone in right-handed women (Figure 1C). Inconsistent with these results, Wolf and Kirschbaum (2002) could not find a significant relation between endogenous estradiol levels and mental rotation in older men and women, suggesting no beneficial effects of estradiol in older people. There are, however, studies suggesting that high estradiol levels may be disadvantageous for spatial ability, consistent with the present results. For instance, in elderly women high estrogen levels showed negative relations to visuospatial functions (Drake et al., 2000; Barrett-Connor & Goodman-Gruen, 1999); performances on spatial tasks are hindered in the midluteal phase of the menstrual cycle as well as during pregnancy (Hampson, 1990; Hampson & Kimura, 1988; Maki et al., 2002; Silverman & Phillips, 1993). The inverse U-shaped variation of mental rotation ability is best seen during the menstrual cycle, parallel with the endogenous estradiol concentrations (see Figure 6 in Halpern & Tan, 2001). The above mentioned studies suggesting disadvantageous effects of high estradiol (E2) levels on spatial cognition in women support the present results. There are, however, advantageous effects of estradiol in relatively moderate concentrations; very low E concentrations were associated with low mental rotation scores (see Figure 1D).Beneficial effects of estrogen replacement therapy have frequently been reported, especially in post-menopausal women and in women with Alzheimer's disease (see Yaffe, Lui et al., 2000), so an optimal estradiol level would be most beneficial, but too much estradiol would be harmful for the spatial ability in women. The same was true for men in relation to serum testosterone levels, as seen Figure 1A.

These two relations partly support Nyborg's (1983) optimal gonadal hormone theory, which argues that there is an inverted U-shaped relationship between brain estrogen and spatial ability, with males tending more than females to occupy the peak of the curve. Nyborg assumed, however, that testosterone does not affect the brain directly, but exerts its effects by aromatization to estrogen in the brain.

There was a positive correlation between serum estradiol level and mental rotation ability in the right-handed male subjects (see Figure 1B) and this suggests that estradiol is beneficial for the mental rotation ability in men. The free testosterone level was also found to be beneficial for this ability for a large spectrum of testosterone levels. Consequently, the positive relation of serum estradiol level to mental rotation ability is to be expected, since testosterone is a circulating pro-hormone, which, through aromatization, is converted to E2, the principal ligand for estrogen receptors (see Simpson, et al., 2002). The male estradiol should be very important, since men maintain a high circulating level of the active precursor testosterone, which is available for conversion to estradiol (estradiol, or active estrogen) throughout life in extragonadal sites.

The activating effects of testosterone and estradiol on the mental rotation ability was also observed in left-handed male subjects (see Figure 2), in contrast to the results of Moffat and Hampson (1996), who could not find any relation of testosterone to spatial ability either in left-handed males or in left-handed females.

Jordan et al. (2002) have reported that women and men exhibited activations in different cortical areas during mental rotation even when performances were similar. This suggests the sex-related differences in the relations between sex hormones and mental rotation ability may be accounted for by different cerebral origins of the visuospatial abilities.

4.2 Cattell's culture fair intelligence test

There is no significant sex difference in Cattell IQ (see also Tan et al., 2003 a, b). Despite that, there were some significant relations between sex hormones and IQs. The results did not support the notion that there is no relation between testosterone and performance on some cognitive abilities at which men are not usually better (Gouchie & Kimura, 1991). The fluid intelligence, as measured by Cattell's Culture Fair Intelligence Test, has frequently been reported to be related to serum total testosterone levels in men and women (Tan, 1990 a, b; Tan & Akgun, 1992; Tan et al., 1993).

Athough Cattell's Culture Fair Intelligence Test also measures the visuospatial ability, which is similar to mental rotation ability, the relations between testosterone and estradiol to Cattell IQs were quite different from those for the mental rotation test (see Figure 3). So, different visuospatial tests may produce different results. Here again, the correlations exhibited sex-dependent results: there was no significant relation between testosterone and IQ in males, and no significant relation between estradiol and IQ in females. testosterone in women and estradiol in men exhibited curvilinear correlations with Cattell IQ. These results suggest the possible effects of testosterone and estradiol on Cattell IQ may reflect the independent, direct effects of these sex hormones on nonverbal intelligence. The differential sex-related correlations may be due to the sex-related cortical activation patterns as for the mental rotation task (see Jordan et al., 2002).

The results are good examples for the optimal hormone levels for the highest cognitive abilities. Halpern and Tan (2001) showed fluctuations in Cattell IQ with menstrual cycle, and found an inverse U-shaped relation between serum estradiol level and Cattell IQ using a larger sample size. Using the total serum testosterone level, Tan and Tan (1998) reported there were curvilinear correlations (close to inverse U) between testosterone and Cattell IQ, especially in young women. The present results showed the relations of serum free testosterone vs Cattell IQ in men, and serum estradiol vs Cattel IQ in women were insignificant, but the relations of testosterone to Cattell IQ in women, and estradiol to Cattell IQ in men showed inverse-U shaped relations (see Figure 3). So, only optimal estradiol concentrations in men and optimal testosterone concentrations in women are beneficial for this visuospatial ability.

4.3 Perceptual-verbal ability ("Finding As Test")

The finding As test is a perceptual-verbal test, usually yielding higher scores for females than males (e.g., Kimura & Hampson, 1994; Halpern & Tan, 2001). In the current study this test also exhibited sex-related differential correlations with testosterone and estradiol (see Figure 4). In left-handed male subjects, testosterone and estradiol levels showed positive correlations with the score on the test, but the relations were different in right-handers. The results were inconsistent with Gouchie and Kimura (1991) who reported that sex hormones may not influence mental ability tests that favor women or do not typically show a sex difference. Interestingly, Tan et al. (2003a) have reported the sex difference on the Finding As Test increased using testosterone as covariate; but disappeared with covariates of estradiol and progesterone, suggesting the remarkable dependence of this test on hormonal milieu.

Serum free testosterone level was inversely related to perceptual-verbal ability in right-handed men: increasing testosterone levels seemed to be detrimental (Figure 4A). Van Goozen et al. (1994) have also found that verbal fluency deteriorated after testosterone levels were increased into the physiological range for men. Alexander et al. (1998) could not find any significant association between testosterone and perceptual speed in this test in eugonadal and hypogonadal men.

In women, there was a positive relation between testosterone and perceptual-verbal ability: the score on the test increased with serum free testosterone levels (Figure 4C). In support, Drake et al. (2000) reported that higher testosterone levels were associated with superior verbal fluency in older women. A positive correlation was also found between testosterone and verbal memory in healthy elderly women (Wolf & Kirschbaum, 2002). It was argued that high levels of male sex steroids may impair performance on tests in which women outperform men (see Almeida, 1999; Wolf et al., 2000). In the present work, women outperformed men in the Finding As Test, but, despite that, testosterone was not detrimental; rather it seemed to be beneficial for this ability.

Interestingly, there was an inverse U-shaped relation between estradiol and the Finding As Test score in right-handed males and females. This means there is an optimum estradiol level for this perceptual-verbal ability, as also shown for the pre-ovulatory phase of the menstrual cycle, where serum estradiol level first increases and then decreases towards the ovulation (see Figure 5 in Halpern & Tan, 2001). So, advantageous and disadvantageous effects of estradiol are both recorded in the scientific literature.

The serum testosterone and estradiol levels were found to be positively correlated with the perceptual-verbal ability in the left-handed male subjects (Figure 5). There is no report from the current literature to compare the present results on this topic. The results suggest opposite relations of serum testosterone and estradiol levels to the perceptual-verbal ability in right- and left-handers, accentuating the importance of cerebral laterality in sex-hormone relations to cognitive abilities.

The scientific literature abounds with examples of hormonal effects on various abilities. For example, estrogen was found to have a possible positive effects on oral reading in post-menopausal women (Shaywitz et al., 2003), but an association between estrogen level and verbal memory has not been generally supported (see Green et al., 2000). Wolf & Kirschbaum, (2002) have indeed shown that in older women higher estradiol levels were associated with better verbal memory (paired associates). Anti-androgen therapy in combination with estrogen treatment was shown to have no enhancing effect on verbal fluency in adult men (Slabbekoorn et al., 1999). Women were shown to have enhanced verbal articulation during the pre-ovulatory phase of the menstrual cycle when only estrogren levels were high (Hampson, 1990).Manipulations of sex hormone levels appeared to be unrelated to verbal skills and perceptual speed in transsexuals (Slabbekoorn et al., 1999), while in menopausal women estrogen replacement therapy have been shown to improve cognition, especially verbal memory (Wolf, 2003). Serum free and bioavailable estradiol may have beneficial effects for cognitive decline in older women (Yaffe, Haan et al., 2000), but this benefit may be obtained with a low dose of estrogen (Tierney, 2000).

5. Conclusions and perspectives

Since the most prominent sex difference in mental rotation ability—being better in men than women— reversed under covariation of bodily measures such as height and weight, to be better in women than men, and similar changes were observed in other cognitive tests, the sex differences in perceptual-verbal and spatial abilities were re-studied in the present work, which recruited men and women with similar height and weight and with known right- or left-hand preference.

The mental rotation ability predominantly increased with serum free-testosterone levels in right- and left-handed men and women, but there were detrimental effects of very large testosterone concentrations in the same individuals. The serum estradiol concentrations showed a direct relationship to mental rotation test scores in right- and left-handed men, but an inverse U-shaped relation in right-handed women. The relation of perceptual-verbal ability *vs* testosterone exhibited a different pattern: in right-handers the correlation was negative, while in left-handers it was positive. This suggests an optimum estradiol level could be beneficial for this ability in men and women.

The sex-neutral Cattell IQ did not show any significant relationship either to the serum testosterone level in right-handed men or to the estradiol level in right-handed women. Optimal testosterone and estradiol levels (not too high and not too low) were needed for the highest Cattell IQs in right-handed men and women, but if levels of these hormones were too high or too low this was detrimental for the sex-neutral fluid intelligence.

The results of the present work suggest that the sex-related differences in cognitive abilities may depend upon the hand preference and the cognitive tests used to measure the cognitive abilities. Sex-hormones may exert beneficial or detrimental effects on the cognitive abilities, depending upon their serum concentrations and cerebral laterality differences. The results also suggest that bodily measures, hand preference, and sex as basic variables should be considered in basic research and clinical evaluations, as well as in future treatment for cognitive impairments and related cognitive disorders such as dementia in men and women. The results may also be enlightening for future research on the physiological mechanisms of cognitive abilities.

6. Acknowledgments

This study was partly supported by the Turkish Academy of Sciences.

7. References

Aleman, A, de Vries, W.R. & Koppeschaar H.P., et al. (2001). Relationship between circulating levels of sex hormones and insulin-like growth factor-1 and fluid intelligence in older men. *Experimental Aging Research,* Vol.27, No.3, pp. 283-91.

Aleman, A., Bronk, E., Kessels, R.P.C., Koppeschaar, H.P.F., & van Honk, J. (2004). A single administration of testosterone improves visuospatial ability in young women. *Psychoneuroendocrinology,* Vol.29, No.5, pp. 612-617.

Alexander, G. M., Swerdloff, R. S., Wang, C., Davidson, T., et al. (1998). Androgen-behavior correlations in hypogonadal men. II. Cognitive abilities. *Hormones and Behavior,* Vol.33, pp. 85-94.

Almeida, O. P. (1999). Sex playing with the mind. Effects of oestrogen and testosterone on mood and cognition. *Arquivos de neuro-psiquiatria,* Vol.57, No.3A, pp. 701-706.

Azurmendi, A., Braza, F., Sorozabal, A., et al. (2005). Cognitive abilities, androgen levels, and body mass index in 5-year-old children. *Hormones and Behavior,* Vol. 48, pp. 187-195.

Barrett-Connor, E., & Goodman-Gruen, D. (1999a). Cognitive function and endogenous sex hormones in older women. *Journal of American Geriatric Society,* Vol. 47, No. 11, pp. 1289-1293.

Barrett-Connor, E. & Goodman-Gruen, B. (1999b). Endogenous sex hormoınes and cognitive function in older men. *Journal of Clinical Endocrinology and Metabolism,* Vol. 84, No. 10, pp. 3681-3685.

Beech, J.R. (2001). A curvilinear relationship between hair loss and mental rotation and neuroticism: a possible influence of sustained dihydrotestosterone production. *Personality & Individual Differences,* Vol.31, pp. 185-192.

Cattell, R. B. (1973). Manual for the Cattell culture fair intelligence test. Champaign, IL: Institute for Personality and Ability Testing.

Cattell, R. B. (1987). Intelligence: its structure, growth and action. Advances in Psychology. (Vol. 35) Amsterdam, The Netherlands: Elsevier Science

Celec, P., Ostatnikova, D., Putz, Z. & Kudela, M. (2002). The circalunar cycle of salivary testosterone and the visual-spatial performance. *Bratislavské Lékarske Listy,* Vol. 103, No.2, pp. 59-69.

Cherrier, M. M. (1999). Androgens, aging, behavior and cognition: complex interactions and novel areas of inquiry. *New Zealand Journal of Psychology,* Vol.28, pp. 4-9.

Cherrier, M.M., Asthana, S., Plymate, S., Baker, L., Matsumoto, A.M., Peskind, E., Raskind, M.A., Brodkin, K., Bremmer, W., Petrova, A., Latendresse, S., & Craft, S. (2001). Testosterone supplementation improves spatial and verbal memory in healthy older men. *Neurology,* Volo.57, pp. 80-88.

Christiansen, K. (1993). Sex-hormone-related variations of cognitive perfomance in !Kung San hunter-gatherers of Namibia. *Neuropsychobiology,* Vol.27, pp. 97-107.

Christiansen, K. & Knussman, R. (1987). Sex hormones and cognitive functioning in men. *Neuropsychobiology,* Vol.18, pp. 27-36.

Drake, E.B., Henderson, V.W., Stanczyk, F.Z., et al. (2000). Associations between circulating sex steroid hormones and cognition in normal elderly women. *Neurology,* Vol. 54, No. 3, pp. 599-603.

Ekstrom, R.B., French, J. W., Harman, H., & Derman, D. (1976). Kit of factor-referenced Cognitive tests (rev. ed.). Princeton, NJ: Eduactional Testing Service.

Frye, C. A., Petralia, S. M., Rhodes, M. E. & Stein, B. (2003). Fluoxetine may influence lordosis of rats through effects on midbrain 3 alpha,5 alpha-THP concentrations. *Annual of New York Academy of Sciences,* Vol. 1007, pp. 37-41.

Gladue, B.A., Beatty, W.W., Larson, J. & Staton, R.D. (1990). Sexual orientation and spatial ability in men and women. *Psychobiology,* Vol. 18, pp. 101-108.

Gladue, B.A. & Bailey, J.M. (1995). Aggressiveness, competitiveness, and human sexual orientation. *Psychoneuroendocrinology,* Vol. 20, pp. 475-485.

Gordon, H.W. & Lee, P.L. (1986). A relationship between gonadotropins and visuospatial function. *Neuropsychologia,* Vol. 24, pp. 563-576.

Gouchie, C. & Kimura, D. (1991). The relationship between testosterone levels and cognitive ability patterns. *Psychoneuroendocrinology,* Vol. 16, pp. 323-334.

Green, H.J., Pakenham, K.I. & Gardiner, R.A. (2000). Effects of luteinizing releasing hormone analogs on cognititon in women and men. *Psychology, Health and Medicine,* Vol. 5, pp. 407-418.

Halpern, D. F., & Tan, U. (2001). Stereotypes and steroids using a psychobiosocial model to understand cognitive sex differences. *Brain and Cognition,* Vol. 45, pp. 392–414.

Hampson, E. (1990). Estrogen-related variations in human spatial and articulatory-motor skills. *Psychoneuroendocrinology,* Vol. 15, pp. 97-111.

Hampson, E., & Kimura, D. (1988). Reciprocal effects of hormonal fluctuations on human motor and perceptual-spatial skills. *Behavioral Neuroscience,* Vol. 102, pp. 456-459.

Herlitz, A. & Lovén, J. (2009). Sex differences in cognitive functions. *Acta Physiologica Sinica,* Vol. 41, No. 11, pp. 1081-1090.

Hier, D.B. & Crowley, W.F. (1982). Spatial ability in androgen-deficient men. *New England Journal of Medicine,* Vol. 306, pp. 1202-1205.

Hyde, J.S. & Lin, M.C. (1988). Gender differences in verbalability. A meta-analysis. *Psychological Bulletin,* Vol. 104, pp. 53-69.

Janowsky, J.S., Oviatt, S.K. & Orwoll, E.S. (1994). Testosterone influencs spatial cognition in older men. *Behavioral Neuroscience,* Vol. 108, No. 2, pp. 325-332.

Janowsky, J.S., Cahvez, B. & Orwoll, E. (2000). Sex steroids modify working memory. *Journal of Cognitive Neuroscience,* Vol. 12, pp. 407-414.

Jensen, A.R. (1998). The G factor: the science of mental ability. Westport, CT: Praeger.

Jordan, K., Wuestenberg, T., Heinze, H.-J., Peters, M. & Jancke, L. (2002). Women and men exhibit different cortical activation patterns during mental rotation tasks. *Neuropsychologia,* Vol. 40, pp. 2397-2408.

Kampen, D.L. & Sherwin, B.B. (1996). Estradiol is related to visual memory in healthy young men. *Behavioral Neuroscience,* Vol. 110, No. 3, pp. 613-617.

Kenny, A.M., Bellantonio, S., Gruman, C.A., Acosta, R.D. & Prestwood, K.M. (2002). Effects of transdermal testosterone on cognitive function and health perception in older men with low bioavailable testosterone levels. *Journal of Gerontology A,* Vol. 57, No. 5, pp. M321-325.

Kimura, D. (1996). Sex, sexual orientation and sex hormones influence human cognitive function. *Current Opinion in Neurobiology,* Vol. 6, pp. 259-263.

Kimura, D., and Hampson, E. (1994). Cognitive pattern in men and women is influenced by fluctuations in sex hormones. *Current Directions in Psychological Science,* Vol. 3, *pp.* 57–61.

Kutlu, N., Ekerbicer, N., Ari, Z., Uyanik, B.S., Zeren, T., & Tan, U. (2001). Testosterone and nonverbal intelligence in right-handed men with successful and unsuccessful educational levels. *International Journal of Neuroscience,* Vol. 111, No. 1-2, pp. 1-9.

Linn, M.C. & Petersen, A.C. (1985). Emergence and characterization of sex differences in spatial ability. *Child Development,* Vol. 56, pp. 1479-1498.

Maki, P.M., Rich, J.B., & Rosenbaum, R.S. (2002). Implicit memory varies across the menstrual cycle: estrogen effects in young women. *Neuropsychologia*, Vol. 40, pp. 518-529.

Mann, V.A., Sasanuma, S., Sakuma, N. & Masaki, S. (1990). Sex differences in cognitive abilities: a cross-cultural perspective. *Neuropsychologia,* Vol. 28, N. 10, pp. 1063-1077.

McDaniel, M.A. (2005). Big-brained people are smarter: a meta-analysis of the relationship between in vivo brain volume and intelligence. *Intelligence,* Vol. 33, pp. 337-346.

McKeever, S. (1987). Mental health nursing. Working together. *Nurse Times,* Vol. 83, No. 2, pp. 58-59.

McKeever, W.F., Rich, D.A., Deyo, R.A. & Conner, R.L. (1987). Androgens and spatial ability: failure to find a relationship between testosterone and ability measures. *Bulletin of the Psychonomic Society,* Vol. 25, pp. 438-440.

McKeever, W.F. & Deyo, R.A. (1990). Testosterone, dihydrotestosterone, and spatial task performance of males. *Bulletin of the Psychonomic Society,* Vol. 28, pp. 305-308.

Moffat, S. D., & Hampson, E. (1996). A curvilinear relationship between testosterone and spatial cognition in humans: Possible influence on hand preference. *Psychoneuroendocrinology,* Vol. 21, pp. 323-337.

Neave, N., Menaged, M & Weightman, D.R. (1999). Sex differences in cognition: the role of testosterone and sexual orientation. *Brain and Cognition,* Vol. 41, No. 3, pp. 245-262.

Nyborg, H. (1983). Spatial ability in men and women: review and new theory. *Advances in Behaviour Rsesearch and Therapy,* Vol. 5, pp. 89-140.

Ostatnikova, D., Putz, Z., Celec, P. & Hodosy, J. (2002). May testosterone levels and their fluctuations influence cognititve performance in humans?. *Scripta Medica,* Vol. 75, No. 5, pp. 245-254.

Raz, N., Torres, I.J., Spencer, W.D. et al. (1993). Neuroanatomical correlates of age-sensitive and age-invariant cognitive abilities. *Intelligence,* Vol. 17, pp. 407-422.

Resnick, S.M., Berenbaum, S.A., Gottesman, I.I. & Bouchard, T. (1986). Early hormonal influences on cognitive functioning in congenital adrenal hyperplasia. *Developmental Psychology,* Vol. 22, pp. 191-198.

Roof, R.L. & Havens, M.D. (1992). Testosterone improves maze performance and induces development of a male hippocampus in females. *Brain Research,* Vol. 572, No. 1-2), pp. 310-313.

Rushton, J.P. (1992). Cranial capacity related to sex, rank, and race in a stratified random sample of 6325 US military personnel. *Intelligence,* Vol. 16, pp. 401-413.

Rushton, J.P. (1997). *Race, evolution, and behavior.* New Bruswick (USA) and London (UK): Transaction Publishers.

Shaywitz, S.E., Naftolin, F., Zelterman, D., et al. (2003). Better oral reading and short-term memory in midlife, postmenopausal women taking estrogen. *Menopause,* Vol. 10, No. 5, pp. 420-426.

Shephard, R. N., & Metzler, J. (1971). Mental rotation of three-dimensional objects. *Science,* Vol. 17, pp. 701-703.

Shute, V.J., Pellegrino, J.W., Hubert, L. & Reynolds, R.W. (1983). The relationship between androgen levels and human spatial abilities. *Bulletin of the Psychonomic Society,* Vol. 21, pp. 465-468.

Silverman, I., Phillips, K. (1993). Effects of estrogen changes during the menstrual cycle on spatial performance. *Ethology and Sociobiology,* Vol. 14, pp. 257-270.

Silverman, I., Kastuk, D., Choi, J. & Phillips, K. (1999). Testosterone levels and spatial ability in men. *Psychoneuroendocrinology,* Vol. 24, No. 8, pp. 813-822.

Simpson, E.R., Clyne, C. & Rubin, G. et al. (2002). "Aromatase—abrief overview". *Annual Review of Physiology,* Vol. 64, pp. 93-127.

Slabbekoorn, D., van Goozen, S.H.M., Megens, J., Gppren, L.J.G., & Cohen-Kettenis, P. T. (1999). Activating effects of cross-sex hormones on cognitive functioning: a study of short-term and long-term hormone effects in transsexuals. *Psychoneuroendocrinology*, 24, 423-447.

Tan, U. (1990a). Testosterone and nonverbal intelligence in right-handed men and women. *International Journal of Neuroscience,* Vol. 54, pp. 277-282.

Tan, U. (1990b). Relationship of testosterone and nonverbal intelligence to hand preference and hand skill in right-handed young adults. *International Journal of Neuroscience,* Vol. 54, pp. 283-290.

Tan, U. & Akgun, A. (1992). There is a direct relationship between nonverbal intelligence and serum testosterone level in young men. *International Journal of Neuroscience,* Vol. 64, pp. 213-216.

Tan, U. & Tan, M. (1998). Curvelinear correlations between total testosterone levels and fluid intelligence in men and women. *International Journal of Neuroscience*, Vol. 95, pp. 77-83.

Tan, U., Akgun, A. & Telatar, M. (1993). Relationships among nonverbal intelligence, hand speed, and serum testosterone level in left-handed male subjects. *International Journal of Neuroscience,* Vol. 71, pp. 21-28.

Tan, U. Tan, M., Polat, P., et al. (1999). Magnetic resonance imaging brainsize/IQ relations in Turkish university students. *Intelligence,* Vol. 27, No. 1, pp. 83-92.

Tan, U. Okuyan, M., Bayraktar, T. & Akgun, A. (2003a). Covariation of sex differences in mental rotation with body size. *Perceptual and Motor Skills, Vol.* 96, pp. 137-144.

Tan, U. Okuyan, M., Bayraktar, T. & Akgun, A. (2003b). Sex difference in verbal and spatial ability reconsidered in relation to body size, lung volume, and sex hormones. *Perceptual and Motor Skills,* Vool. 96, pp. 1347-1360.

Tierney, M.C. (2000). Oestradiol concentrations in prediction of cognitive decline in women. The Lancet, Vol. 356, pp. 694-695.

Vandenberg, S. G. & Kuse, A. R. (1978). Mental rotations, a group test of three-dimensional spatial visualization. *Perceptual and Motor Skills,* Vol. 47, pp. 599-604.

Van Goozen, S.H.M., Cohen-Kettenis, P.T., Gooren, L.J.G. et al. (1994). Activating effects of androgens on cognitive performance: causal evidence in a group of female-to-male transsexuals. *Neuropsychologia,* Vol. 32, No. 10, pp. 1153-1157.

Van Goozen, S.H.M., Cohen-Kettenis, P.T., Gooren, L.J.G. et al. (1995). Gender differences in behavior: activating effects of cross-sex hormones. *Psychoneuroendocrinology,* Vol. 20, No. 4, pp. 343-363.

Wolf, O.T., Preut, R., Hellhammer, D.H. et al., (2000). Testosterone and cognition in elderly men: a single testosterone injection blocks the practice effect in verbal fluency, but has no effecton spatial or verbal memory. *Biological Psychiatry,* Vol. 47, No. 1, pp. 650-654.

Wolf, O.T. (2003). Cogntive functions and sex steroids. *Annales d' endocrinologie*, Vol. 64, pp. 158-161.

Wolf, O.T. & Kirschbaum, C. (2002). Endogenous estradiol and testosterone levels are associated with cognitive performance in older women and men. *Hormone and Behavior,* Vol. 41, No. 3, pp. 259-266.

Yaffe, K., Lui, L-Y., Grady, D. , et al. (2000). Cognitive decline in women in relation to non-protein-bound oestradiol concentrations. *Lancet*, Vol. 356, pp. 708-712.

Yaffe, K., Haan, M., Byers, A., Tangen, C., & Kuller, L. (2000). Estrogen use, APOE, and cognitive decline. Evidence of gene-environment interaction. *Neurology*, Vol. 54, pp. 1949-1953.

Yaffe, K., Lui, L.Y., Zmuda, J. & Cauley, J. (2002). Sex hormones and cognitive function in older men. *Journal of American Geriatry Society,* Vol. 50, No. 4, pp. 707-712.

4

Sex Hormones and Infertility

Iptisam Ipek Muderris and Gokalp Oner
Erciyes University / Department of Obstetric and Gynecology
Turkey

1. Introduction

The normal physiology of the female reproductive system involves a hypothalamus that secretes gonadotropin-releasing hormone (GnRH)in a pulsatile manner, a pituitary gland that can be stimulated by the hypothalamus to regularly secrete both luteinizing hormone (LH) and follicle-stimulating hormone (FSH), an ovary that has both methodical enzymatic system and steroidogenesis for producing the sex hormones such as estrogen and progesteron, and a functional uterus that can be responded by these hormones.
Sex hormones play a crucial role in reproductive biology as well as in general physiology. The most important aim of sex hormones is to design the cycle and to produce an optimal environment for pregnancy according to form ovarian physiology including follicular growth, ovulation, and corpus luteum formation and endometrial response including proliferative and secretuar phase for implantation. Among the various functions, sex hormones influence pregnancy, cardiovascular function, bone metabolism, and an individual's sense of general well-being. The action of sex hormones is mediated via extracellular signals to the nucleus to affect a physiologic response.

2. Gonadotropin-releasing hormone (GnRH)

Gonadotropin-releasing hormone (GnRH) is a decapeptide pulsatile produced by neurons with cell bodies primarily in the arcuate nucleus of the hypothalamus (1). Embryologically, these neurons originate from the olfactory area and then migrate to their adult locations (2). These GnRH-secreting neurons project axons that terminate on the portal vessels at the median eminence where GnRH is secreted for delivery to the anterior pituitary. The continual pulsatile secretion of GnRH is necessary because its short half-life is only 2–4 minutes as a result of rapid proteolytic cleavage.
GnRH stimulates the production, secretion and storage of FSH and LH from anterior hypophysis. (3). It is also an unique releasing hormone for the regulation of the simultaneous secretion of two hormones in human body (4). GnRH performs this special affect according to its pulsatile secretion. In the follicular phase, its secretion is characterized by frequent, small-amplitude pulses, however during the luteal phase, there is a progressive lengthening of the interval between pulses with higher amplitude (5).
GnRH is primarily involved in endocrine regulation of gonadotropin secretion from the pituitary. However, the regulation of GnRH secretion is various (Table 1). The pulsatile secretion of GnRH is directly affected by catecholaminergic system including the activator of

Inhibitors of GnRH secretion	Activators of GnRH secretion
Dopamine	Norepinephrin
Gonadotrophins (negative feedback)	Catecholamins
Endogenous opioids	Neuropeptide Y
Estradiol	Acetylcholine
Progesterone	VIP
CRH	Naloxone
Melatonin	
Serotonin	
GABA	

Table 1. The control of GnRH secretion

norepinephrine and the inhibitor of dopamin. This system is basically regulated by endogenous opioids (6).
These opioids are three groups;

1. Endorphins
2. Enkephalins
3. Dynorphins

Endogenous opioids, inhibit the gonadotropin secretion to swage the GnRH secretion from hypothalamus.
Sex steroids affect GnRH by increasing the secretion of the endogenous opioids in the central nervous system (7).
Although estrogen stimulates the secretion of endogenous opioids, estrogen plus progesterone increase this effect. Clinically, increased endogenous opioids may cause hypothalamic amenorrhea.

3. GnRH analogs

3.1 GnRH agonists (leuprolide, goserelin, nafarelin, buserelin)

GnRH agonists are modifications of the native molecule to either increase receptor affinity or decrease degradation (8). The pulsatile usage of GnRH agonists that resemble endogenous GnRH leads to increase the secretion of FSH and LH. However the constant GnRH usage leads to suppression of gonadotropin secretion by the downregulation of its receptor. An initial release of gonadotropins is followed by a profound suppression of secretion. The initial release of gonadotropins represents the secretion of pituitary stores in response to receptor binding and activation. With continued activation of the gonadotroph GnRH receptor, however, there is a downregulation effect and a decrease in the concentration of GnRH receptors. As a result, gonadotropin secretion decreases and sex steroid production falls to castrate levels (9).
The most commonly used regimen for superovulation in ART is called the long, or luteal, downregulation protocol. In this protocol, GnRH agonist is started in the luteal phase (day 21) of the previous cycle, which minimizes its flare effect and prevents the follicular recruitment that is thought to begin in the luteal phase. The couple undergoing treatment is advised to abstain from intercourse during the cycle before the start of COH; however, concomitant use of GnRH agonist in the presence of an unsuspected pregnancy has not been reported to be associated with increased spontaneous abortion, congenital abnormalities, or pregnancy

complications. Most importantly, clinical pregnancy rates and live birth rates per retrieval were significantly higher using the long protocol. The benefits including higher pregnancy rates and lower OHSS rates of using the long protocol for administration of GnRH agonists greatly outweigh its disadvantages, which include daily administration, increased requirement for gonadotropins, and an overall increase in the cost of medication (10, 11).

3.2 GnRH antagonists (cetrorelix, ganirelix)

GnRH antagonists produce a competitive blockage of GnRH receptors, preventing stimulation by endogenous GnRH and causing an immediate fall in gonadotropin and sex steroid secretion. The clinical effect is generally observed within 24 to 72 hours. Moreover, antagonists may not show flare-up affect comparing with GnRH agonists. GnRH antagonists are also used in ART for the prevention of premature ovulation and displays similar efficacy comparing GnRH agonist (long protocol) (12). However, there were significantly fewer pregnancies with the GnRH antagonist protocol. A significant reduction in the incidence of severe OHSS and the number of gonadotropin injections were observed in the antagonist regimen compared with the long GnRH-agonist protocol.
When we searched the Cochrane Library and ACOG Commitee on Practice Bulletins.;
Clinically usage of GnRH analogs listed below;

- Endometriosis
- Hormon dependent neoplasia such as endometrium cancer, breast cancer.
- Myomas of uterus
- Precocious puberty
- Dysfunctional uterine bleeding
- Ovarian hyperandrogenism
- Premenstrual syndrome
- ART for control of premature ovulation

Side effects of GnRH analogs listed below;

- Hypoestrogenic state
- Vasomotor symptoms
- Vaginal dryness
- Mood changes
- Loss of bone mineral density

Usage of these agents is generally limited to 6 months because of the adverse effects as listed above. The most important side effect is osteoporosis. Many side effects can be minimized by providing add-back therapy in addition to the agents.The addition of 2.5 mg of norethindrone or 0.625 mg of conjugated estrogens with 5 mg/d of medroxyprogesterone acetate seems to relieve these side effects of GnRH analogs. The addition of 5 mg daily of norethindrone acetate alone or in conjunction with low-dose conjugated equine estrogen seems to eliminate the loss of bone mineral density effectively as well (13).

4. Gonadotropins

The gonadotropins FSH and LH are produced by the anterior pituitary gonadotroph cells and are responsible for ovarian follicular stimulation. Structurally, there is great similarity between FSH and LH. They are both glycoproteins that share identical α subunits and differ only in the structure of their β subunits, which confer receptor specificity (14). The synthesis

of the β subunits is the rate-regulating step in gonadotropin biosynthesis (Lalloz MRA, et al. GnRH desensitization preferentially inhibits expression of the LH β-subunit gene in vivo. Endocrinology 1988;122:1689–1694.). Thyroid-stimulating hormone and placental human chorionic gonadotropin (hCG) also share identical α subunits with the gonadotropins. The structural similarity between FSH, LH, TSH and hCG defines as the α subunits identical and the β subunits differ.
The gonadotropins were metabolized in liver and kidney then excreted by the way of urine. The half life of LH, FSH and hCG is 20 minute, 3-4 hours and 24-36 hours, respectively.

4.1 FSH

Receptors of FSH are found on granulosa cells.
FSH plays role in; granulosa cell proliferation in follicules and estrogen production
- the production of FSH and LH receptors on granulosa cells
- the activation of aromatase and 3 beta-hydroxysteroid dehydogenase
- enzymes
- the stimulation of follicules and prevention of apoptosis of them

In the beginning of follicular development, there is no LH receptor on granulosa cells, however, during the 11-12nd days of cycle, FSH stimulates the production of LH receptors on granulosa cells.

4.2 LH

Receptors of LH are found on theca cells.
LH plays role in; internal thecal cell proliferation in follicules and androgen production
- luteinization and the production of progesterone when LH receptors found on
- granulosa cells during the 11-12nd days of cycle
- providing of ovulation
- the completion of I. myosis (the transformation of primary oocyte to
- secondary oocyte)

Although FSH plays an important role for the early maturation of follicules, FSH and LH are responsible together for the maturation of follicules before the ovulation.

5. Inhibin

Inhibin secretes from granulosa cells, sertoli cells, placenta and the basophilic cells of hypophysis. In the cycle, Inhibin selectively inhibits the secretion of FSH. There are two forms; Inhibin A and Inhibin B. The affect of Inhibin B mostly shows on follicular phase, but the affect of Inhibin A mostly shows on luteal phase of cycle. During luteofollicular transition of cycle FSH increase by decreasing of Inhibin A levels. Inhibin also stimulates LH activity and IGF secretion from granulosa and theca cells to increase androgen production.

6. Activin

Activin secretes from granulosa cells and the basophilic cells of hypophysis. In the cycle, Activin selectively activates the secretion of FSH. Therefore, it activates all affects of FSH on granulosa cells. Activin also inhibits LH activity, androgen production from theca cells and progesterone production from granulosa cells. Additionally, activin inhibits the secretion of IGF from ovary and the secretion of prolactin, ACTH, and GH from hypophysis. These affects of activin is inhibited by inhibin and follistatin. Follistatin that secretes from granulosa cells and the basophilic cells of hypophysis inhibits FSH activity by binding activin.

6.1 IGF

IGF secretes from granulosa cells and theca cells. Its affect is similar to GH.

IGF plays role in; the stimulation of LH activity on theca cells to increase androgen production

- the production of FSH and LH receptors on granulosa cells
- the activation of aromatase enzyme
- the proliferation of granulosa cells
- the improvement of progesterone synthesis

All of IGF binds insulin like growth factor binding protein (IGF-BP) in the circulation. FSH and insulin inhibit the synthesis of IGF-BP, so efficacy of IGF may increase by increasing free IGF.

Epidermal growth factor (EGF) that is an important inhibitor of FSH in the ovary is another growth factor.

7. Steroid hormones in reproduction

Sex steroid hormones are synthesized in the gonads, adrenal gland, and placenta. Cholesterol is the primary building block in steroidogenesis, and all steroid-producing tissues except the placenta are capable of synthesizing cholesterol from the 2-carbon precursor, acetate. Steroid hormone production, which involves at least 17 enzymes, primarily occurs in the abundant smooth endoplasmic reticulum found in steroidogenic cells.

Steroids are metabolized mainly in the liver and to a lesser extent in the kidney and intestinal mucosa. Accordingly, administration of certain pharmacologic steroid hormones may be contraindicated in those with active liver disease. Sex steroids are divided into three groups based on the number of carbon atoms that they contain. Each carbon in this structure is assigned a number identifier, and each ring is assigned a letter. The 21-carbon series includes progestins as well as glucocorticoids and mineralocorticoids. Androgens contain 19 carbons, whereas estrogens have 18. However the ovary is deficient in 21-hydroxylase and 11 -hydroxylase and therefore is unable to produce corticosteroids. Most important steroidogenic enzymes are listed in Table 2. Steroidogenesis is summarized in Figure 1.

Enzyme Cellular	Location	Reactions
P450scc	Mitochondria	Cholesterol side chain cleavage
P450c11	Mitochondria	11-Hydroxylase 18-Hydroxylase 19-Methyloxidase
P450c17	Endoplasmic reticulum	17-Hydroxylase 17, 20-Lyase
P450c21	Endoplasmic reticulum	21-Hydroxylase
P450arom	Endoplasmic reticulum	Aromatase

Table 2. Steroidogenic enzymes

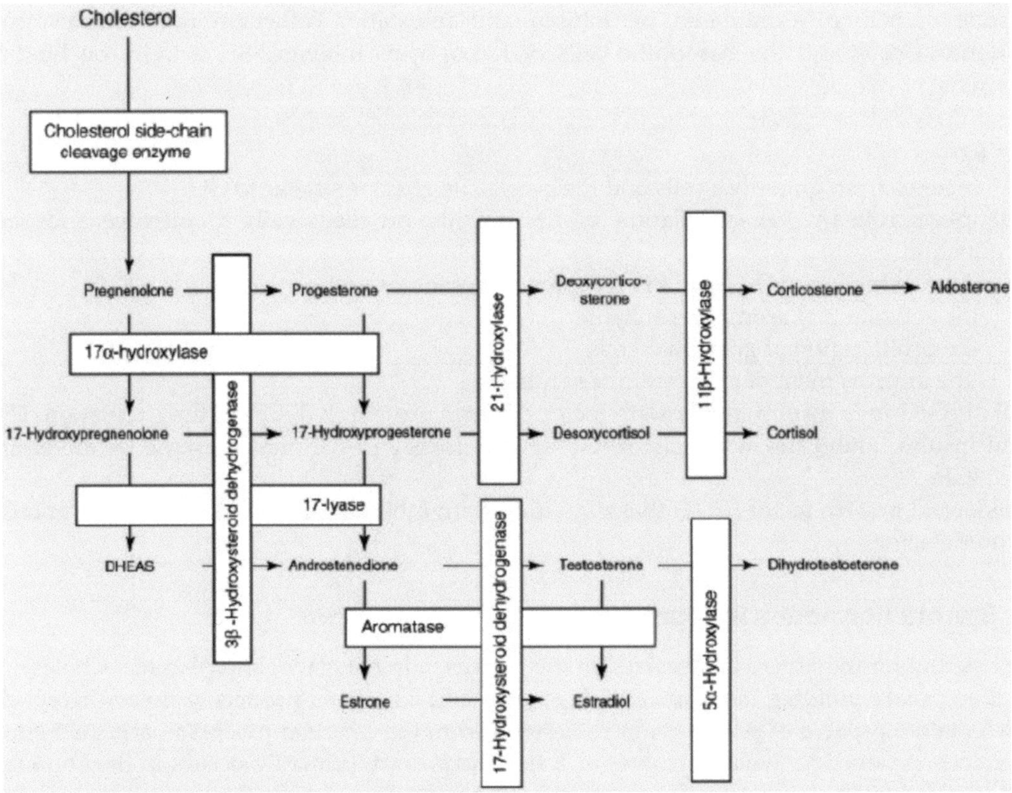

Fig. 1. The steps of the steroidogenesis pathway

Most steroids in the peripheral circulation are bound to carrier proteins, either specific proteins such as sex-hormone binding globulin (SHBG) or corticosteroid-binding globulin, or to nonspecific proteins such as albumin. Only 1 to 2 percent of androgens and estrogens are unbound or free. Tablo 3 shows the steroid transformations. Levels of SHBG are increased by hyperthyroidism, pregnancy, and estrogen administration. In contrast, androgens, progestins, GH, insulin, and corticoids decrease SHBG levels.

8. Estrogens

Steroids with 18 C classified as;

Estron (E1): Poor estrogenic affect, basically peripheric estrogen are the properties. It is dominant estrogen in prepubertal and postmenopausal periods.

Estradiol (E2): The most potent estrogen is mainly produced in the reproductive age.

Estratriol (E3): The least potent estrogen is mainly produced in pregnancy and synthesized by maternal and fetal units together. Therefore, E3 is an indicator to show the normal fetoplacental unit.

Estetrol (E4): There is not estrogenic affect. It is synthesized from fetal liver and increases in term.

Estrogens are produces by the aromatization of androstenedione and testosterone in ovary and the peripheral aromatization of androstenedione in skin, fat tissue, muscle and endometrium (Figure 2). There is a two-cell theory of ovarian steroidogenesis. The two-cell theory of ovarian steroidogenesis explains that estrogen biosynthesis requires the combined action of two gonadotropins (LH and FSH) on two cell types (theca and granulosa cells) (15). Until the late antral stage of follicular development, LH-receptor expression is limited to the thecal compartment and FSH-receptor expression is limited to the granulosa cells. Theca cells express all of the genes needed to produce androstenedione. This includes high levels of CYP17 gene expression, whose enzyme product catalyzes 17-hydroxylationation the rate-limiting step in the conversion of progesterones to androgens (16). This enzyme is absent in the granulosa cells, so they are incapable of producing the precursor needed to produce estrogens by themselves. Granulosa cells therefore rely on the theca cells as their primary source for estrogen precursors. In response to LH stimulation, theca cells synthesize the androgens, androstenedione and testosterone. These androgens are secreted into the extracellular fluid and diffuse across the basement membrane to the granulosa cells to provide precursors for estrogen production. In contrast to theca cells, granulosa cells express high levels of aromatase activity in response to FSH stimulation. Thus, these cells efficiently convert androgens to estrogens, primarily the potent estrogen, estradiol. In sum, ovarian steroidogenesis is dependent on the effects of LH and FSH acting independently on the theca cells and granulosa cells, respectively.

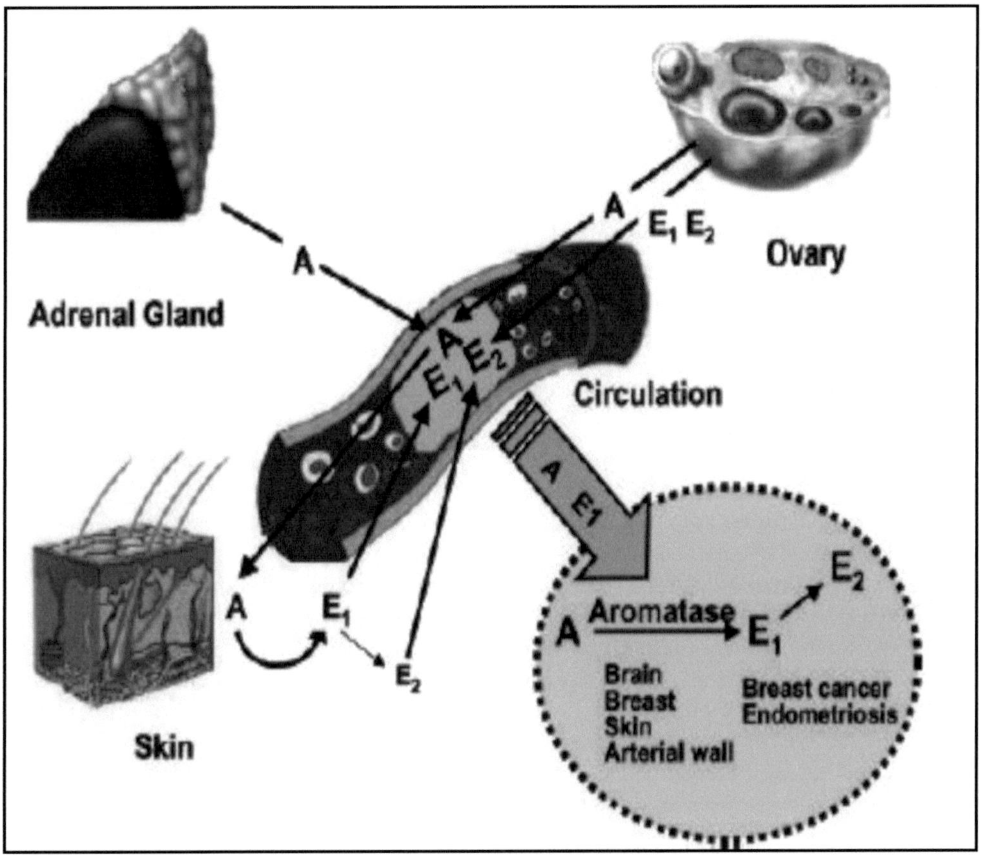

Fig. 2. Estrogen biosynthesis

Estrogen is metabolized in liver and excreted to bile.

The effects of estrogen on;
Genitourinary system:

- Stimulation of urethral epithelial proliferation
- Stimulation of vaginal epithelial proliferation and superficial cells of epithelium may become dominant in vagina.
- Decreases the vaginal pH (3.8-4.5)
- Increases the cervical mucus and elasticity and decreases the cervical viscosity (Spinn-Barkeit)
- Increases the crystallization of NaCl in cervical mucus and may cause ferning image.
- Increase cervical mucus pH
- Proliferation of endometrial stroma and glands
- Production of endometrial progesterone receptor
- Increase the gap junctions, connexion proteins, and oxytocin sensitivity of smooth muscles in uterus. Therefore, estrogen increases the uterin contractility.
- Increase the ciliary activity and motility in fallopian tubes
- Facilitate follicular stimulation
- Inhibits FSH (negative feed-back effect)
- Positive feed-back on LH before the ovulation
- Inhibits GnRH (Increase central opioids)

Breast

- Development of ductus

Seconder sex characters

- Development of axillary and pubic hairs in puberty (pubarche)
- Development of breast in puberty (thelarche)

Bone

- Increase the osteoblastic activity in bone and bone mineral density

Skin

- Increase vascularity and collagen

Liver

- Increase SHBG synthesis
- Increase transcortin synthesis
- Increase angiotensinogen
- Increase coagulation factors as Factor II, VII, VIII, IX, and X
- Decrease antithrombin production
- Increase triglycerides, total cholesterol, and HDL
- Decrease LDL
- Increase concentration of bile acids and the development of cholelithiasis

Estrogens exert a variety of effects on growth and development of different tissues. The effects of estrogens are mediated via estrogen receptors (ER), intracellular proteins that function as ligand-activated transcription factors and belong to the nuclear receptor superfamily. Two mammalian ERs have been identified, denoted ERα and ERβ. The structure of both receptors is similar and consists of six domains named A through F from the N- to C-terminus, encoded by 8 to 9 exons. Genes that are regulated by activated ERs include early gene responses such as c-myc, c-fos, and d-jun, as well as genes encoding for growth factors such as insulin growth factor (IGF-1 and IGF-2), epidermal growth factor (EGF), transforming growth factor-α, and colony-stimulating factor (CSF-1).

In addition to the described genomic effects of estrogens, there is growing evidence for nongenomic effects of estrogens on intracellular signal transduction pathways. These effects include, for example, rapid activation of the adenylate cyclase, which results in cyclic adenosine monophosphate (cAMP)-dependent activation of protein kinase A (PKA). Estrogens can also stimulate the mitogen-activated protein kinase (MAPK) pathways and rapidly activate the Erk1/Erk2 proteins (17).

	Free	Albumin	SHBG	Transcortin
Estrogen	% 1	% 30	% 69	-
Testosterone	% 1-2	% 20-32	% 66-78	-
DHEA	% 4	% 88	% 8	-
Androstenedione	% 7	% 85	% 8	-
DHT	% 1	% 71	% 28	-
Progesterone	% 2	% 80	% 1>	% 18
Cortisol	% 10	% 15	-	% 75

Table 3. Steroid transformations

The combined production of estradiol and inhibin B by the dominant follicle results in the decline of follicular phase FSH levels, and at least in part, may be responsible for the failure of other follicles to reach preovulatory status during any one cycle. This model predicts that follicles that lack adequate FSH receptor and granulosa cell number will remain primarily androgenic and will therefore become atretic. In support of this model, an increased androgen:estrogen ratio is found in the follicular fluid of atretic follicles and a number of studies have demonstrated that high estrogen levels prevent apoptosis. IGF also has apoptosis-suppressing activity, and is produced by granulosa cells. This action of IGF-I is suppressed by certain IGF-binding proteins that are present in the follicular fluid of atretic follicles. The action of FSH to prevent atresia may therefore result, in part, from its ability to stimulate IGF-I synthesis and suppress the synthesis of the IGF-binding proteins.

Clinically, there are some selective estrogen receptor modulators (SERM) such as clomiphene citrate (CC), tamoxifen, and raloxifen (Table 4).

	Breast	Genital	Kemik	Lipid
Clomiphene citrate	+	_	+	+
Tamoxifen,	_	+	+	+
Raloxifen	_	_	+	+

Table 4. The effects of selective estrogen receptor modulators on some tissues

CC is the initial treatment for most anovulatory infertile women. Chemically similar to tamoxifen, CC is a nonsteroidal triphenylethylene derivative that demonstrates both estrogen agonist and antagonist properties. Antagonist properties predominate except at very low estrogen levels. As a result, negative feedback that is normally produced by estrogen in the hypothalamus is reduced. Gonadotropin-releasing hormone (GnRH) secretion is improved and stimulates pituitary gonadotropin release. The resulting increase in follicle-stimulating hormone (FSH), in turn, drives ovarian follicular activity.

The SERM tamoxifen is an estrogen antagonist in the breast that is used in the treatment of estrogen-receptor positive breast cancer. Tamoxifen (20 mg) also has been approved for the prevention of breast cancer in high-risk women, resulting in an approximately 50% reduction in the risk of disease (18).
Raloxifene is a SERM that has been approved for both the prevention and treatment of osteoporosis. Raloxifene exercises estrogen-like actions on bone and lipids without stimulating the breast or endometrium. Raloxifene also may reduce the risk of breast cancer. Postmenopausal women receiving raloxifene as part of a large osteoporosis treatment trial experienced a 76% reduction in the risk of invasive breast cancer compared with placebo-treated women (19).

Androgens	Potence	Ovary	Adrenal	Peripheral
DHEA	_	% 25	% 50	% 25
DHEAS	5	_	% 100	_
Androstenedione	10	% 50	% 50	_
Testosterone	100	% 25	% 25	% 50
DHT	300	_	_	% 100

Table 5. Androgen biosynthesis

9. Progesterone

Progesterone is the 21 C steroid that secretes mainly from corpus luteum and placenta. It minimally secretes from the cortex of adrenal gland. Although its level is 1 ng/mL in preovulatuary phase, it is 3-15 ng/mL in luteal phase. Also, progesterone has a thermogenic affect.
The effects of progesterone on;
Genitourinary system:

- Intermediate cells of epithelium may become dominant in vagina.
- Increases the vaginal pH (> 4.5)
- Increases the cervical viscosity and decreases the cervical mucus and elasticity
- Decreases cervical mucus pH
- Antiproliferative and antimitotic effects on endometrial stroma and glands
- Secretuar changes on endometrium for implantation
- Decraeses the gap junctions, connexion proteins, and oxytocin sensitivity of smooth muscles in uterus. Therefore, progesterone decreases the uterin contractility
- Decrease the ciliary activity and motility in fallopian tubes
- Antiestrogenic activity according to the decrease in estrogen receptor and the increase in transformation of E2 to E1 (stimulates 17 OHSD enzyme)
- Inhibits LH (negative feed-back effect)
- Positive feed-back on FSH before the ovulation
- Inhibits GnRH (Increase central opioids)

Breast

- Development of alveols and lobules

Bone
- Antiresorptive effects on bone and increase bone mineral density

Liver
- Decrease SHBG synthesis

Most progesterone actions on the female reproductive tract are mediated through nuclear hormone receptors. Progesterone enters cells by diffusion and in responsive tissues becomes associated with progesterone receptors (Conneely OM, et al: Reproductive functions of progesterone receptors. Recent Prog Horm Res 57:339, 2002). There are multiple isoforms of the human progesterone receptor. The best understood isoforms are the progesterone receptor type A (PR-A) and B (PR-B). Both arise from a single gene, are members of the steroid receptor superfamily of transcription factors, and regulate transcription of target genes. These receptors have unique actions. When PR-A and PR-B receptors are co-expressed, it appears that PR-A can inhibit PR-B gene regulation. The inhibitory effect of PR-A may extend to actions on other steroid receptors, including estrogen receptors.

10. Androgens

The ovary produces primarily androstenedione and dehydroepiandrosterone (DHEA) with small amounts of testosterone. Although the adrenal cortex primarily produces mineralocorticoids and glucocorticoids, it also contributes to approximately one-half of the daily production of androstenedione, DHEA, and essentially all of the sulfated form of DHEA (DHEAS). Twenty-five percent of circulating testosterone is secreted by the ovary, 25 percent is secreted by the adrenal gland, and the remaining 50 percent is produced by peripheral conversion of androstenedione to testosterone (Figure 3).

11. Anti-Müllerian hormone (AMH)

AMH has been identified as a dimeric glycoprotein and a member of the transforming growth factor beta (TGFb) family of growth and differentiation factors. The pool of primordial follicles in the ovary is related to the number of growing antral follicles. Antral follicles are responsive to gonadotrophin stimulation and the measure of ovarian reserve can be defined as the total number of follicles, which can be stimulated to grow under maximal stimulation. Classically, age, FSH levels in the early follicular phase, antral follicle count and inhibin B have been used as markers of ovarian reserve. More recently, AMH, have been used by various groups to assess the ovarian reserve (20).

AMH is initially expressed in ovarian granulosa cells of primary follicles, maximal expression occurs in pre-antral and small antral follicles. Antral follicles measuring <6 mm express the greatest amount of AMH, and that expression declines as antral follicles increase in size. AMH is not expressed by atretic follicles and during FSH dependent final stages of follicular growth. AMH inhibits initial primordial follicles recruitment and decreases the sensitivity of preantral and small antral follicles to FSH. Serum AMH concentrations decline with increasing age and constitute a sensitive marker for ovarian aging. Recently, AMH is used as pretreatment assessment of ovarian reserve.

Basal serum levels of AMH may more accurately reflect the total developing follicular cohort and consequently potential ovarian response to FSH in cycles of ART. AMH, antral follicle count, inhibin B, FSH and ovarian volume have been demonstrated to reflect ovarian reserve.

12. Infertility

Infertility is defined as 1 year of unprotected intercourse without pregnancy. This condition may be further classified as primary infertility, in which no previous pregnancies have occurred, and secondary infertility, in which a prior pregnancy, although not necessarily a live birth, has occurred. Infertility affects about 10% to 15% of reproductive age couples. (21). Various factors may be responsible for the inability to achieve a successful pregnancy. Ovulatory, anatomic, immunologic, or hormonal factors on the woman's side and abnormalities of the semen parameters on the man's side are the most common (Table 6). After a thorough work-up, treatment can be planned that aims to correct the problem identified or, in the case of unexplained infertility, tries to improve all steps of the reproductive process.

	Prevalence of the etiologies of infertility (%)
Male factor	25–40
Female factor	40–55
- Ovulatory dysfunction	30–40
- Tubal or periotoneal factor	30–40
- Unexplained infertility	10–15
- Miscellaneous causes	10–15
Both male and female factors	10
Unexplained infertility	10

Table 6. Causes of Infertility

13. Evaluation of infertility

The most important tests for evaluation of infertility are to assess the ovarian function.

13.1 Ovarian function

Ovarian function can be evaluated by various methods. Regular menstrual cycles are a sign of ovulation in 95% of the cycles. Because the ovaries also "age," however, the regularity of the cycles alone is not enough to characterize ovarian function. The number of follicles in the ovaries decreases from birth. As a result, from the age of 30 onward a slow decline in fertility occurs. This decline parallels the reduction in the number and quality of the follicles and oocytes. The first sign of reduced ovarian activity is the shortening of the follicular phase, which reduces the length of the ovulatory cycle. The decrease in the number of follicles is followed by hormonal changes. Inhibin B is produced by the small antral follicles, and as their number declines, the ovarian output of inhibin B decreases. This is paralleled by a rise in FSH level.

For the everyday practice, there are several tests to assess ovarian reserve. Measurement of the early follicular phase FSH and estradiol levels to determine the FSH/estradiol ratio; measurement of inhibin B or anti-Müllerian hormone levels; or the early follicular phase antral follicle count are options (Table 7). Dynamic tests evaluate the ovaries during clomiphene citrate (CC) challenge or during gonadotropin-releasing hormone agonist (GnRHa) or gonadotropin stimulation.

Test	Normal Value	Abnormal Value
Cycle Day 3 FSH	< 10-15 mIU/mL	> 10-15 mIU/mL
Cycle Day 3 estradiol	< 80 pg/mL	> 80 pg/mL
Inhibin B	> 45 pg/mL	< 45 pg/mL
Anti-Müllerian hormone	> 2.7 ng/mL associated with improved oocyte quality as reflected in a higher implantation rate and trend toward better clinical pregnancy rate[56]	Low levels
Clomiphene citrate challenge test	FSH < 26 mIU/mL on Day 10	FSH > 26 mIU/mL on Day 10
Gonadotropin stimulation test	Estradiol level elevation and subsequent decrease	No elevation of estradiol level
Antral follicle count on ultrasound	> 3-4	< 3-4
Ovarian volume on ultrasound	> 3 mL	< 3 mL

*Note: Different infertility centers use different tests. Cut-off values may differ from center to center on the basis of their experience and results.

Table 7. Cut-off Values* for the Most Commonly Used Ovarian Reserve Tests

On the one hand, the results of these tests will help with designing treatment (to choose the appropriate treatment, stimulation protocol, and gonadotropin dose), and on the other hand they will be useful for counseling the couple. It is very important that a couple undergoing any form of assisted reproduction has realistic expectations (22).

In addition to these tests, it is useful to perform an ultrasound midcycle to assess the ovary and uterus and to document ovulation. Midcycle ultrasound will document follicle growth and allow us to look at the endometrial lining (eg, thickness and type). Ovulation can be documented in several ways. The easiest is to measure a midluteal phase progesterone level. Changes in the basal body temperature, urinary LH kits, luteal phase endometrial biopsy, and serial ultrasounds are alternatives for assessing ovulation.

When the cycles are irregular, other hormonal measurements -- such as testosterone, dehydroepiandrosterone sulfate (DHEAS), 17-OH progesterone, cortisol, prolactin -- as well as thyroid function tests and dynamic evaluation of pituitary function may be necessary for the infertility work-up. If the results of any of these tests are considered abnormal, conducting imaging studies (eg, MRI, CT, thyroid scan) may be the appropriate step.

13.2 Ovulation induction, controlled ovarian hyperstimulation

Ovulation induction has a role in the management of patients with anovulation/oligo-ovulation or regular cycles. In the case of oligo-ovulation, the goal is to restore mono-ovulatory cycles.

Various drugs can be used to restore ovulation. Selective estrogen receptor modulators (eg, CC, tamoxifen) are usually administered first. CC is the agent for which most experience has accumulated. It is administered from Day 3 or 5 of the cycle for 5 days. The starting dose is 50 mg, but if needed the dose can be increased by 50 mg daily during subsequent stimulation. Usually, a daily dose > 150 mg is not recommended, as higher doses compromise endometrial development, and pregnancy rates are very low. Ovulation rates are high (80%)

with CC, but cumulative pregnancy rates are only around 40%. The difference between the high ovulation rates and relatively low pregnancy rates is most likely due to the antiestrogenic effects of CC on the periphery, most prominently at the level of the endometrium. If pregnancy does not occur after a maximum of 6 cycles, other options need to be explored (23).
CC stimulation can be combined with ovulation induction with human chorionic gonadotropin (hCG), especially when a spontaneous LH surge cannot be documented. The multifetal gestation rate is about 10% with CC use. CC has relatively few side effects, with gastrointestinal symptoms, visual changes, and hot flashes being more common.
Aromatase inhibitors (eg, letrozole, anastrozole) have been explored recently. Aromatase is an enzyme that regulates the androgen-estrogen conversion. Aromatase inhibitors work by reducing estradiol level and therefore increasing pituitary gonadotropin output (resulting in decreased estradiol negative feedback). Their use is seldom associated with multifollicular development. Pregnancy rates are about 15% to 20 % per cycle. No adverse perinatal outcome following aromatase inhibitor use has yet been reported in the published, peer-reviewed literature, although the authors of a study presented during the American Society for Reproductive Medicine meeting in 2005 reported a higher rate of congenital anomalies with 5 mg anastrozole (24, 25, 26). Notably, letrozole has warned clinicians against prescribing drugs for ovulation induction on the basis of reports of birth defects and spontaneous miscarriages in its safety database (27). Letrozole is not approved for ovulation induction.
Insulin-sensitizing agents have been successfully used to treat infertile patients with PCOS. Metformin (1500 to 2000 mg daily) has been used most widely. With metformin, ovulation can be documented in about 50% to 60% of cases. Metformin can also be combined with CC in CC-resistant cases. Lower miscarriage rates and fewer cases of gestational diabetes have been reported with metformin use. Metformin is a category B drug; no serious adverse effects have been reported with use during pregnancy. Gastrointestinal side effects are often reported upon initiation of treatment. It is a good approach to start with a lower daily dose and slowly increase it to the therapeutic range. Metformin should not be used in women with liver or renal disease. It takes at least 2 to 3 months for insulin sensitizers to take full effect (28, 29, 30, 31, 32).
Gonadotropins can be administered when oral preparations are ineffective or do not lead to pregnancy after repeated attempts. Gonadotropins can be used alone or in combination with oral preparations and are usually started on Day 3 of the cycle at an initial dose of 75 to 150 IU. Cycle monitoring (ultrasound ± estradiol measurement) begins after 5 days of stimulation. When gonadotropins are combined with oral preparations, the pill is initiated first (usually on Day 3) and the injections are administered starting 2 days later. Injections are usually administered on every other day. These protocols can be adjusted depending on the response. Although pregnancy rates are higher following gonadotropin stimulation, the risks for multiple gestations and ovarian hyperstimulation syndrome (OHSS) are increased as well.
Ovulation induction cycles can be completed in different ways. Urinary LH kits can be used to predict ovulation and to time intercourse or insemination. Alternatively, when the lead follicle is around 18 to 20 mm in diameter, human chorionic gonadotropin (hCG) can be administered to induce ovulation. When hCG is used, intercourse or insemination is scheduled 36 to 40 hrs after the injection.

14. Intrauterine Insemination

Intrauterine insemination (IUI) further improves the chances of pregnancy. IUI is more effective than intracervical or intravaginal insemination. Its use is especially indicated when mild male factor or cervical factor infertility is diagnosed. A wide range of pregnancy rates have been reported after insemination (5% to 20% per cycle). Pregnancy rates are higher when gonadotropin stimulation is used in conjunction with IUI. Pregnancy rates are affected by the age of the female partner, semen parameters, tubal status, the presence of endometriosis, and the order of the treatment cycle. The pregnancy and multiple gestation rates are highest with the first treatment cycle. Some even recommend performing the first IUI in a natural unstimulated cycle to avoid multiple gestations and only to proceed with stimulation if the first attempt fails. Usually IUI should not be repeated more than 3 or 4 times. Two exceptions are when donor sperm is used and when the patient has oligo-ovulation; in these cases, a significant number of further pregnancies have been reported in a 5th or 6th cycle. The decision should be made individually, and the availability of IVF obviously influences the decision (33, 34).

15. In vitro fertilization, intracytoplasmic sperm injection

The first baby conceived after IVF treatment was born in 1978. Since then, the field has undergone enormous development, and IVF is now routinely used in the management of various forms of infertility. Initially, it was used for the treatment of tubal factor infertility, but today it is used to help patients with male factor infertility, unexplained infertility, genetic problems, and those who fail in vivo treatments.

Early on, IVF was carried out during the patients' natural cycle. Later, CC was added to the protocol to increase efficacy. These cycles were characterized by relatively high cancellation rates as a result of premature ovulation and low pregnancy rates. With the advent of GnRH agonists, antagonists, and different types of gonadotropins, new stimulation protocols have been developed. Cycles with these protocols, by contrast, are characterized by very low cancellation rates, a higher number of oocytes, better-quality embryos, and significantly higher implantation and pregnancy rates.

A typical IVF cycle is made up of 3 parts: stimulation, egg retrieval, and embryo transfer. Stimulation usually consists of pretreatment and stimulation. Pretreatment with oral contraceptive pills or a GnRH agonist allows flexible cycle scheduling and a more simultaneous follicle growth. In the various stimulation protocols, GnRH agonist or antagonist can be given to prevent premature LH surges. The GnRH agonist can be initiated in the luteal phase of the preceding cycle (long protocol) or with the onset of menstruation together with gonadotropins (short, ultrashort protocols). The GnRH agonist initially depletes the pituitary gonadotropin stores ("flare up" effect) before it prevents further FSH and LH release (usually after 7 to 12 days). This initial flare effect is used with the short protocols.

A GnRH antagonist has a different mechanism of action. It competes with GnRH for its pituitary receptors. Upon administration it immediately prevents FSH and LH release. In GnRH antagonist cycles, the antagonist is administered either on Day 6 of stimulation (fixed protocol) or when the lead follicle reaches 14 mm in diameter (flexible protocol).

There are 5 or 6 different stimulation protocols in use by IVF centers. Subtle differences in the management of the pretreatment phase or in the type and dose of gonadotropins do exist between IVF clinics. Several patient characteristics are considered before one decides about the protocol to be used. Typically, age, results of the ovarian reserve testing, and response to previous stimulation help with the decision about the appropriate stimulation protocol (35).

Cycle monitoring (ultrasound and estradiol measurements) usually starts after 5 days of stimulation. When at least 2 follicles reach 17 to 18 mm in diameter, the final steps of oocyte maturation are induced by 5000 to 10,000 IU hCG. In those cycles during which GnRH agonist downregulation is not applied, the final maturation of the oocytes can be induced with GnRH agonist as well. This method is associated with a lower incidence of OHSS. Oocyte retrieval is scheduled 35 to 36 hours after the final injection.

Oocyte retrieval is an ultrasound-guided vaginal procedure that is performed under intravenous sedation. Oocytes are collected in culture medium and are processed for fertilization. Human tubular fluid was used as an example to design culture medium. Currently, several companies produce culture medium. Use of sequential media tries to satisfy the changing needs of the developing embryo.

Fertilization may occur spontaneously when the sperm number, motility and morphology are within the normal range or can be done using intracytoplasmic sperm injection (ICSI). ICSI is used when the sperm parameters are suboptimal or when fertilization was poor in a previous cycle. During ICSI, the immobilized sperm is transferred through the zona pellucida with a fine glass needle to allow fertilization to take place (36).

The day after the retrieval, the oocytes are checked for signs of fertilization (presence of 2 pronuclei) and are cultured for an additional 2 to 4 days. Transfer usually takes place on Day 3 or 5 after the retrieval. Embryos are assessed on the basis of blastomere number and morphology. Usually 2 or 3 good-quality embryos are transferred. The decision is influenced by the order of the cycle, the patient's age, the number and quality of the embryos, the couple's wishes, and by regulations in those countries where the number of embryos to be transferred is limited. Surplus good-quality embryos can be frozen and stored for later use. To reduce the number of multiple gestations, there is tendency toward transferring fewer embryos. In some countries, the transfer of only a single embryo is allowed. Although pregnancy rates per transfer are lower, following the transfer of 1 fresh and 1 cryopreserved embryo, the cumulative pregnancy rates are comparable to rates following the transfer of 2 embryos. Multiple pregnancies occur significantly less often. An efficient cryopreservation program needs to be in place, however, before one can comfortably offer elective single embryo transfer (37).

This patient has oligo-anovulation; therefore, the assessment of her hormonal status is important. Most commonly, irregular ovarian activity has an endocrine etiology including thyroid disease, hyperprolactinemia, androgen excess, PCOS, premature ovarian failure. Transvaginal ultrasound will assess the morphology of the ovaries (ie, whether they are polycystic or not), myometrium, and endometrium. Serial ultrasound will document follicle growth and allows us to look at the changes in the endometrial lining (eg, thickness and type). Once the etiology of the irregular cycles is known, the appropriate treatment can be planned.

Women with PCOS are at increased for impaired glucose tolerance (and diabetes), dylipidemia, and hypertension. Therefore, the baseline evaluation of these metabolic markers should be part of the work-up for this patient.

Weight loss (life-style modification), CC, or insulin sensitizers could be recommended. At least half of women with PCOS are obese. Obesity is associated with insulin resistance that will further compromise ovarian activity. Weight loss and regular exercise are integral parts of their treatment. Weight loss is associated not only with improved ovarian function but also with lower risk for metabolic complications. CC and insulin sensitizers have both been shown to be effective for ovulation induction among women with oligo-ovulation.

Adding an insulin sensitizer such as metformin would be the next step. A daily dose > 150 mg of CC is not recommended, as higher doses compromise endometrial development, and pregnancy rates are very low. Insulin-sensitizing agents have been successfully used to treat infertile patients with PCOS. Metformin (1500-2000 mg daily) has been used most widely. With metformin, ovulation can be documented in about 50% to 60% of the cases. Metformin can be combined with CC in CC-resistant cases. Lower miscarriage rates and fewer cases of

gestational diabetes have been reported with metformin use. Metformin is a category B drug; no adverse effects have been reported with use during pregnancy. Once follicle growth is achieved, adding hCG can help the timing (intercourse or insemination). Without a mature follicle, however, hCG alone does not work.
The patient's husband has a low sperm count. Therefore, IUI could improve this couple's chances for conception. IVF/ICSI would be recommended if IUI was not successful after 3 to 6 attempts.

16. References

[1] Plant TM, et al. The arcuate nucleus and the control of the gonadotropin and prolactin secretion in the female rhesus monkey. Endocrinology 1978;102:52–62.

[2] Schwanzel-Fukuda M, et al. Origin of luteinizing hormone releasing hormone neurons. Nature 1989;338:161–164.

[3] Blackwell RE. Concomitant release of FSH and LH induced by native and synthetic LRF. Am J Physiol 1973;224:170–175.

[4] Knobil E. Neuroendocrine control of the menstrual cycle. Recent Prog Horm Res 1980;36:53–88.

[5] Filicori M, et al. Characterization of the physiological pattern of episodic gonadotropin secretion throughout the human menstrual cycle. J Clin Endocrinol Metab 1986;62: 1136–1144.

[6] Howlett TA, et al. Endogenous opioid peptide and hypothalamo-pituitary function. Annu Rev Physiol 1986;48:527–536.

[7] Reid Rl, et al. Effects of exogenous β-endorphin on pituitary hormone secretion and its disappearance rate in normal human subjects. J Clin Endocrinol Metab 1981;52:1179–1184.

[8] Karten MJ, et al. Gonadotropin-releasing hormone analog design. Structure function studies towards the development of agonists and antagonists: rationale and perspective. Endocr Rev 1986;7:44–66.

[9] Conn PM, Crowley WF Jr. Gonadotropin-releasing hormone and its analogs. Annu Rev Med 1994;45:391–405.

[10] Ron-El R, et al. Gonadotropins and combined gonadotropin- releasing hormone agonist gonadotropins protocols in a randomized prospective study. Fertil Steril 1991;55:574–578.

[11] San Roman GA, et al. A prospective randomized comparison of luteal phase versus concurrent follicular phase initiation of gonadotropin-releasing hormone agonist for in vitro fertilization. Fertil Steril 1992;58:744–749.

[12] Al-Inany H, et al. Gonadotrophin-releasing hormone antagonists for assisted conception. Cochrane Database Syst Rev 2001;CD001750.

[13] Surrey ES, et al. Prolonged GnRH agonist and add-back therapy for symptomatic endometriosis: Long term follow-up. Obstet Gynecol 2002; 99: 709.

[14] Vaitukaitis JL, et al. Gonadotropins and their subunits: basic and clinical studies. Recent Prog Horm Res 1976;32:289–331.

[15] Peters H, Joint A: The Ovary: A Correlation of Structure and Function in Mammals. Berkeley, University of California Press, 1980.

[16] Sasano H, et al. Immunolocalization of aromatase, 17 alpha-hydroxylase and side-chain-cleavage cytochromes P-450 in the human ovary. J Reprod Fertil 85:163, 1989.

[17] Speroff L, et al: Neuroendocrinology. In Clinical Gynecologic Endocrinology and Infertility, 7th ed. Baltimore, Lippincott Williams & Wilkins, 2005.

[18] Fisher B, et al. Tamoxifen for prevention of breast cancer: report of the national surgical adjuvant breast and bowel project P-1 study. J Natl Cancer Inst 1998;90:1371–1388.

[19] Cummings S, et al. The effect of raloxifene on risk of breast cancer in postmenopausal women: results from the MORE randomized trial. JAMA 1999;281:2189–2197.

[20] Jayaprakasan K, et al. A prospective, comparative analysis of anti-Mullerian hormone, inhibin-B, and three-dimensional ultrasound determinants of ovarian reserve in the prediction of poor response to controlled ovarian stimulation. Fertil Steril 2010; 93: 855-864.

[21] National Center for Health Statistics. Infertility. Available at: http://www.cdc.gov/nchs/fastats/fertile.htm. 2005.

[22] Hillier SG Gonadotropic control of ovarian follicular growth and development Mol Cell Endocrinol. 2001; 179: 39-46.

[23] Hopps CV, et al. The diagnosis and treatment of the azoospermic patient in the age of intracytoplasmic sperm injection. Urol Clin North Am. 2002; 29: 895-911.

[24] Adashi EY. Clomiphene citrate-initiated ovulation. A clinical update. Semin Reprod Endocrinol. 1986; 4: 255-275.

[25] Mitwally MF, et al. Use of an aromatase inhibitor for induction of ovulation in patients with an inadequate response to clomiphene citrate. Fertil Steril. 2001; 75: 305-309.

[26] Healy S, et al. Effects of letrozole on superovulation with gonadotropins in women undergoing intrauterine insemination. Fertil Steril. 2003; 80: 1325-1329.

[27] Biljan MM, et al. The outcome of 150 babies following treatment with letrozole or letrozole and gonadotropins. ASRM/CFAS Annual Meeting; October 15-19, 2005.

[28] Novartis warns doctors on off-label Femara use. Reuters Health. November 30, 2005. Available at: http://www.medscape.com/viewarticle/518136. 2005.

[29] The Rotterdam ESHRE/ASRM-sponsored PCOS consensus workshop group Revised 2003 consensus on diagnostic criteria and long-term health risks related to polycystic ovarian syndrome (PCOS). Hum Reprod. 2003; 19: 41-47.

[30] Costello MF, et al. A systematic review of the reproductive system effects of metformin in patients with polycystic ovary syndrome. Fertil Steril. 2003; 79: 1-13.

[31] Glueck CJ, et al Metformin therapy throughout pregnancy reduces the development of gestational diabetes in women with polycystic ovary syndrome. Fertil Steril. 2002; 77: 520-525.

[32] Glueck CJ, et al. Continuing metformin throughout pregnancy in women with polycystic ovary syndrome appears to safely reduce first-trimester abortion: a pilot study. Fertil Steril. 2001; 75: 46-52.

[33] Nestler JE, et al. Strategies for the use of insulin-sensitizing drugs to treat infertility in women with polycystic ovary syndrome. Fertil Steril. 2002; 77: 209-215.

[34] Hughes EG The effectiveness of ovulation induction and intrauterine insemination in the treatment of persistent infertility: a meta-analysis. Hum Reprod. 1997; 12: 1865-1872.

[35] Dickey R, et al. Effect of diagnosis, age, sperm quality, and number of preovulatory follicles on the outcome of multiple cycles of clomiphene-citrate intrauterine insemination. Fertil Steril. 2002; 78: 1088-1095.

[36] Arslan M, et al. Controlled ovarian hyperstimulation protocols for in vitro fertilization: two decades of experience after the birth of Elizabeth Carr. Fertil Steril. 2005; 84: 555-569.

[37] Palermo GD, et al. Pregnancies after intracytoplasmic injection of single spermatozoon into an oocyte. Lancet. 1992; 340: 17-18.

5

Progesterone in Human Pregnancy and Parturition

Ylva Vladic Stjernholm
Department of Woman and Child Health, Karolinska University Hospital and Institute, Stockholm, Sweden

1. Introduction

1.1 Progesterone synthesis

Progesterone was independently discovered by different research groups (Butenandt & Westphal 1934, Allen 1935). Allen and collaborators discovered progesterone in 1933, and were the first to determine the molecular weight and partial molecular structure. The name *progesterone* derives from progestational steroidal ketone *(Allen 1935)*.

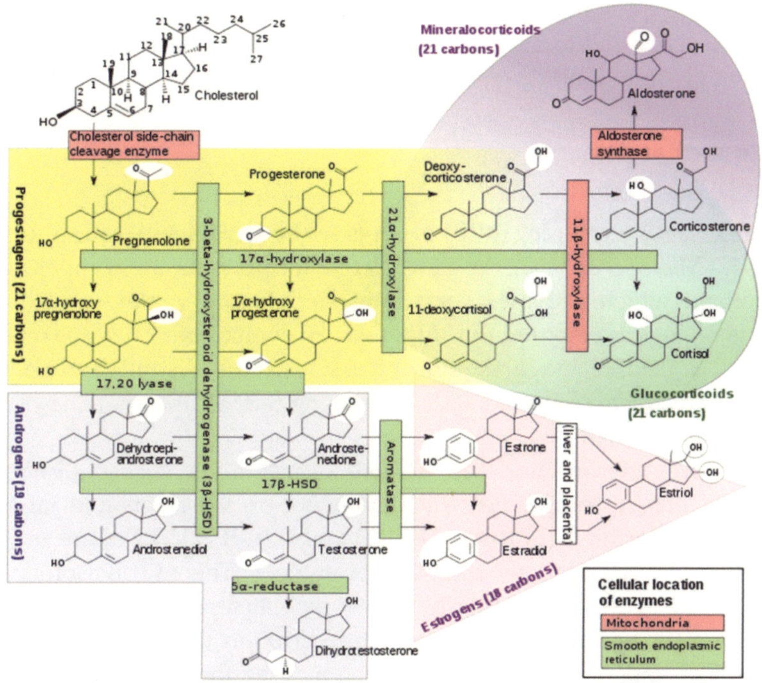

Fig. 1. Steroid hormone synthesis. The precursor cholesterol from the maternal circulation is converted to 21 carbon (C21) progestagens. Progestagens can be converted to C21 glucocorticoids, or to C19 androgens. Androgens serve as precursors for C18 estrogens. Source: Wikipedia.

Progesterone belongs to the C21 group of progestagens and is the evolutionary most conserved of the reproductive steroid hormones. The synthesis of progesterone from its precursor cholesterol in the maternal circulation requires only two enzymatic steps to form pregnenolone, which is readily transformed to progesterone. The main source of progesterone in humans is the corpus luteum in the ovary. After conception, the corpus luteum is supported by the secretion of human chorionic gonadotropin (hCG) from the conceptus, and produces progesterone until approximately the 10th gestational week. After a transition period by 7-10 gestational weeks the placenta becomes the major progesterone source, using circulating cholesterol as a substrate, after which maternal serum levels of progesterone increase markedly. Progesterone in serum is to 95-99% bound to corticosteroid binding globulin (CBG) almost as tightly as glucocorticoids *(Speroff et al 1994).*

Progesterone accompanies and modulates estrogen action. Whereas progesterone is synthesized in the placenta, neither the placenta nor the fetal adrenal glands are capable of producing sufficient quantities of precursors for estrogen synthesis. This observation led to the coining of the unique endocrine system "the maternal-fetal-placental unit" (*Diczfalucy 1969*). In early pregnancy, the maternal circulation provides androgen precursors for estrogen synthesis. By 20 gestational weeks the majority of androgen precursors, predominantly dehydroepiandrosterone sulphate (DHEAS), are derived from the fetal adrenals. The fetal compartment is extremely efficient in sulphate conjugation of steroid hormones, protecting the fetus from high steroid concentrations. About 30% of circulating estrogens are loosely bound to albumin, whereas the major amount is tightly bound to sex hormone binding globulin (SHBG) *(Speroff et al 1994).*

2. Mechanisms of action

2.1 Genomic effects

The nuclear progesterone receptor (nPR) belongs to the steroid supergroup of transcription factor proteins (*O´Malley et al 1990*). All steroid receptor proteins are composed of a variable N-terminal domain which activates gene transcription and protein-protein interactions, determining the biological response of the steroid, an evolutionary highly conserved DNA-binding domain, a flexible hinge region and a C-terminal ligand-binding domain. The classic genomic mechanism of steroid action involving mRNA and protein synthesis is slow, occurring over hours to days.

The nPR binds to progesterone, and with a much less affinity to cortisol *(Sanborn et al 1976).* The biological response to progesterone is dependent on the levels and ratios of the nPR isoforms. The nPR isoforms A (nPR-A) (94 kDa) and nPR-B (116 kDa) are transcribed from the same gene, being activated by different promoters. The nPR-B isoform contains an additional 164 amino acids at the N-terminal and activates progesterone responsive genes. The nPR-A isoform is a weaker activator of transcription than nPR-B and can act as an inhibitor of nPR-B and other steroid receptors such as the nuclear estrogen (nER) and nuclear glucocorticoid (nGR) receptors *(Vegeto et al 1993, Pieber et al 2001).* A third nPR-C isoform has been identified in human myometrium *(Condon et al 2006).* nPR-C lacks a large segment of the N-terminal and a major part of the DNA-binding domain, and therefore cannot bind to DNA.

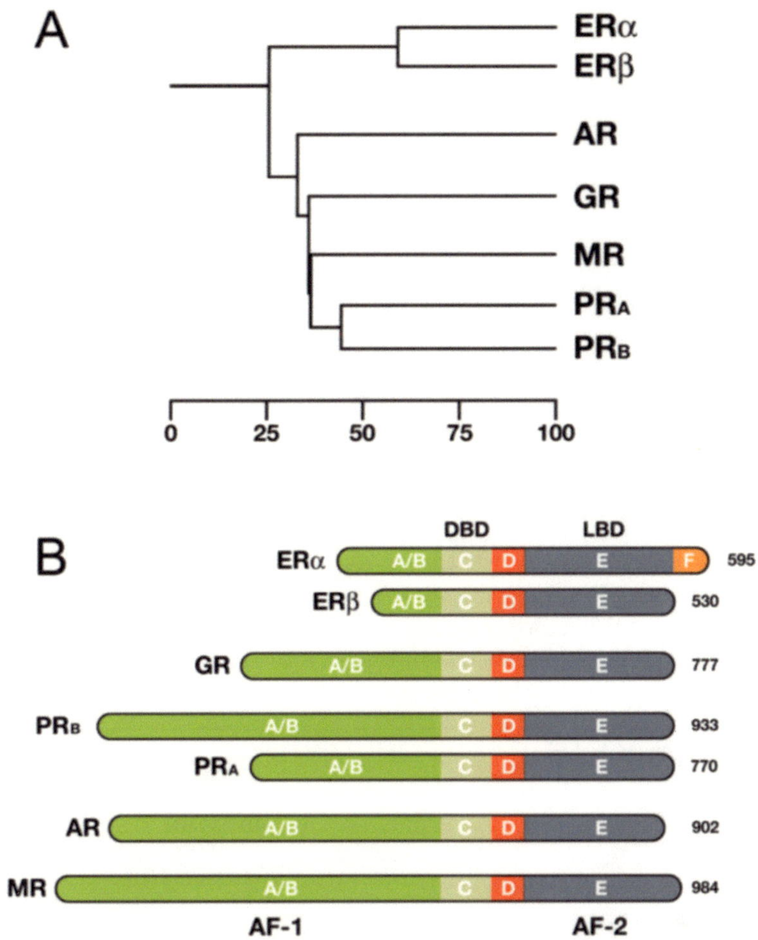

Fig. 2. The steroid hormone receptor family. A. Phylogenetic tree of the steroid hormone receptors showing the evolutionary interrelationships between the receptors . B. Sequence homologies of intracellular steroid hormone receptor proteins showing the N-terminal domain (A/B), the DNA-binding domain (DBD, C), the hinge region (D) and the C-terminal ligand binding domain (LBD, E). The human estrogen receptor subtypes (ERα and ERβ), glucocorticoid receptor (GR), progesterone receptor isoforms (PRA and PRB), androgen receptor (AR), and mineralocorticoid receptor (MR) are described. The estrogen receptor α is unique in that it contains an additional C-terminal F domain. Numbers represent the amino acid sequency of the receptors. In Griekspoor A, et al. Nuclear Receptor Signaling (2007) 5, e003.

2.2 Non-genomic effects

Steroid hormones have been shown to initiate rapid actions, which cannot be explained by the slow genomic mechanisms. Such rapid actions occur within seconds through the activation of intracellular signaling pathways resulting in alterations in ion fluxes and intracellular free calcium concentrations *(Blackmore et al 1991)*, and within minutes through the activation of other second messengers, such as cyclic nucleotides and extracellular-regulated kinase (ERK) 1 and 2 (*Filardo et al 2000*). Recently, three new putative membrane progesterone receptors (mPRs), mPRα, mPRβ, and mPRγ were identified in humans (*Zhu et al 2003*).

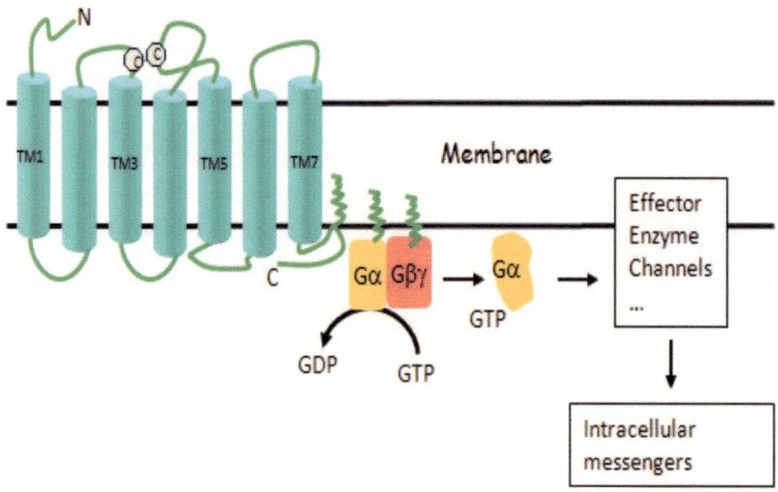

Fig. 3. G (guanine nucleotide-binding) protein-coupled transmembrane (TM) receptors communicate signals from hormones and other signaling factors to intracellular messengers. They consist of the Gα and the tightly associated Gβ,γ subunits. Here guanosine-triphosphate (GTP) is hydrolyzed by Gα subunit to guanosine-diphosphate (GDP). Source: CellMosaic, Worcester, MA, US.

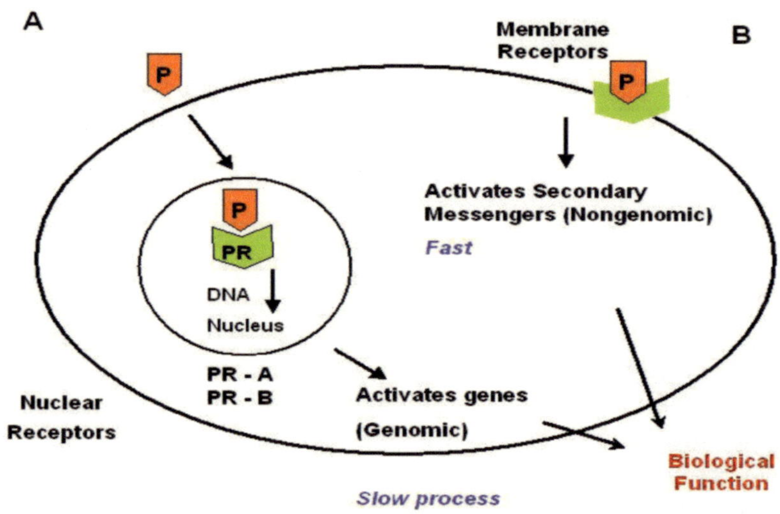

Fig. 4. Nuclear and transmembrane-bound progesterone receptors mediating genomic and non-genomic effects. Progesterone (P) activates A. Genomic pathways through nuclear receptor proteins (PR-A, PR-B) resulting in gene activation (slow process) and/or B. Non-genomic pathways via membrane-bound receptors, which activate secondary messengers (fast process).

3. Systemic effects

Serum levels of progesterone increase progressively during human pregnancy and remain high until delivery of the placenta *(Csapo et al 1973, Speroff et al 1994, Stjernholm et al 1997).* In other species, such as rodents and rabbits, which depend on an active corpus luteum for progesterone synthesis throughout pregnancy, labor is initiated by prostaglandin $F_2\alpha$ (PG–$F_2\alpha$) from the endometrium, activating prostaglandin F (FP)-receptors in the corpus luteum leading to luteolysis *(Sugimoto et al 1997).* These observations led to the concept of a "functional progesterone withdrawal" at parturition in humans *(Hertelendy & Zakar 2004).*

3.1 The placenta

Placental concentrations of progesterone reach 1-10 μM (*Stites & Siiteri 1983, Miyaura & Iwata 2002),* whereas serum concentrations reach 100-500 nM until term pregnancy before labor *(Stjernholm et al 1997; Miyaura & Iwata 2002).*

3.2 The vascular system

Increased levels of prostacyclin (PGI_2) are considered to be a factor behind the physiological angiotensin resistance observed in normal pregnancy *(Friedman 1988).* A progesterone induced mechanism behind this refractoriness to angiotensin has been suggested *(Everett et al 1978, Rupnow et al 2002).* Nitric oxide (NO) and protein kinase C (PKC) pathways are involved in the regulation of vascular tone during pregnancy *(Kublickiene et al 1997, Chang et al 2008).*

3.3 The respiratory system

The pulmonary function is not impaired by pregnancy, but the tidal volume, minute ventilator volume and minute oxygen uptake increase with advancing gestation. This pregnancy-induced respiratory alkalosis is partially compensated for by increased renal excretion of bicarbonate. As a consequence, maternal arterial pH is increased to 7.46. The increased respiratory effort and decrease in PCO_2 has been related to progesterone and to a lesser degree to estrogen *(Wolfe et al 1998, Jensen et al 2005).*

4. The uterus

4.1 The decidua at implantation

Successful maintenance of pregnancy depends on maternal tolerance of the fetal semi-allograft *(Szekeres-Bartho 2002).* Progesterone, cortisol and prolactin have strong immunomodulatory effects leading to immunotolerance during pregnancy (*Stites & Siiteri 1983, Speroff et al 1994).* The human decidua is adjacent to the myometrium, the fetal trophoblasts of the placenta and to the fetal membranes. Natural killer (NK) cells is the predominant immune cell in the decidua before implantation and in early pregnancy, constituting 70% of decidual immune cells, followed by macrophages constituting about 10%of total decidual cells, dendritic cells (DC) and T lymphocytes. The local endocrine environment regulates the recruitment of monocytes into the uterus, and the subsequent differentiation of monocytes into macrophages with specific phenotypes promoting immunotolerance or inflammation (*Stout et al 2004*). Colony-stimulating factor (CSF)-1, macrophage migration inhibitory factor (MIF), monocyte chemoattractant protein (MCP)-1 and regulated on activation, normal T cell expressed, and secreted (RANTES) have been suggested as factors involved in the recruitment and modulation of decidual macrophages, and are synthesized by decidual stromal cells, NK-cells and trophoblasts at the maternal-fetal interface (*Wood et al, 1997; Lockwood et al 2006*). Resident decidual macrophages appear to express immunosuppressive actions that favor the maintenance of pregnancy. In contrast, monocytes/macrophages migrating into the lower uterine segment prior to parturition are involved in the inflammatory process associated with cervical ripening and labor initiation *(Nagamatsu et al 2010)*. A switch in decidual type 1 (Th1) to type 2 (Th2) T cell dominance in the fetal-placental interface has been suggested to play a crucial role in the establishment of pregnancy (*Wegmann et al 1993*). Human Th1 T-cells are the main effectors of host defence and Th1-type cytokines produce proinflammmtory responses. The Th-1 response involves interferon (IFN)-γ, interleukin-2 (IL-2), tumor necrosis factor (TNF)-α, and the generation of cell-mediated immunity. On the contrary, human Th2 T cells inhibit macrophage functions. A Th2 response involves IL-4, IL-5, anti-inflammatory IL-10, IL-10, IL-13, and the stimulation of humoral immunity *(Abbas et al 1996, Weiner et al 2001)*.

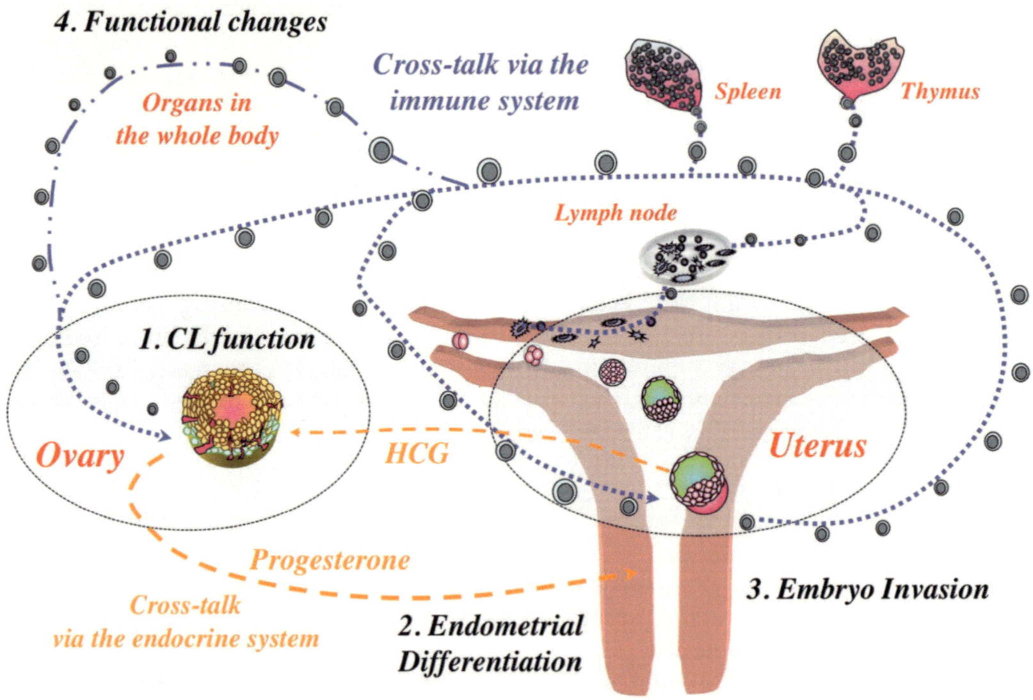

Fig. 5. Endocrine and immune cross-talk in the fetal-maternal interface at implantation. CL= corpus luteum, HCG= human chorionic gonadotropin. In Fujiwara H. Molecular Human Reproduction (2009) 15, 335–343.

Progesterone at concentrations higher than in serum but comparable to those in the maternal-fetal interface induces differentiation of T cells along the Th2 pathway (*Stites & Siiteri 1983; Piccinni et al 1995, Miyaura & Iwata 2002*). Glucocorticoids and 1,25-dihydroxy Vitamin D increase IL-4 (*Rook et al 1994*), whereas dihydrotestosterone decreases IL-4 and IL-5 production (*Vacca et al 1990*).

The progesterone induced protective immune environment in the decidua during early pregnancy includes production of the immunomodulatory progesterone-induced blocking factor (PIBF) protein by decidual cells *(Szekeres-Bartho et al 1985, Piccinni et al 1995).* The presence of nPRs in immune cells has been debated. nPRs in the thymus are necessary for progesterone induced involution of the thymus during pregnancy (*Tibbetts et al 1999).* Most studies have showed an absence of nPRs in lymphocytes from nonpregnant women *(Szekeres-Bartho et al 1990, Mansour et al 1994, Bamberger et al 1999).* Recently, transcripts for mPRα and mPRβ but not mPRγ, were detected in human peripheral blood leukocytes and T lymphocytes. Progesterone activated an inhibitory G-protein (Gi), suggesting that mPRs are coupled to Gi. These results suggest a potential novel mechanism for progesterone's immunoregulatory function through activation of mPRs (*Dosiou et al 2008*).
The establishment of human pregnancy is associated with an adequate synthesis of leukemia inhibitory factor (LIF), and macrophage colony-stimulating factor (M-CSF) producing T-cells. Progesterone at concentrations comparable to those in the maternal-fetal interface induces LIF and M-CSF (*Piccinni 2010*).

4.2 The myometrium

The corpus uteri is a muscular organ with about 70% smooth muscle cells surrounded by extracellular matrix (Danforth 1954). Progesterone is holding the uterine myometrium in a quiescent state, "a progesterone block", during pregnancy by suppressing the propagation of electrical activity between the excitable myocyte membranes (*Csapo 1956, Csapo et al 1973*). The genomic and nongenomic pathways co-operate to maintain myometrial relaxation. At parturition, a functional progesterone withdrawal occurs by increased expression of the nPR-A and/or nPR-C to nPR-B ratios and changes in nPR co-regulator levels which result in repression of the nPR-B transcriptional activity. The diminished progesterone influence leads to an estrogen dominance *(Mesiano et al 2002).* Prostaglandins have been shown to induce an increased nPR-A/nPR-B ratio through the protein kinase C (PKC) pathway in human myometrial cells *(Madsen et al 2004).* Proinflammatory IL-1β up-regulates nPR-C in human myometrial cells, leading to diminished activation of nPR-B *(Condon et al 2006).* The increased expression of specific membrane-associated PRs (mPRs) at parturition augments contractility by decreasing intracellular cyclic adenosine monophosphate (cAMP) and altering intracellular Ca_{2+} levels. *(Pieber et al 2001, Mesiano et al 2002, Madsen et al 2004, Mesiano 2007).*

5. The cervix uteri

The cervix uteri is up to 85% composed by connective tissue, which is dominated by collagen fibers. Fibroblasts, smooth muscle cells, T and B lymphocytes, leukocytes and Langerhans cells are scattered within the tissue (Danforth & Evanston 1954, Schwalm & Dubrauszky 1966, White et al 1997). Cervical remodeling is a prerequisite for cervical effacement and dilatation prior to labor and is characterized by increased levels of vascular adhesion molecules (VCAM), diapedesis and activation of neutrophils, monocytes/macrophages, T lymphocytes, mast cells, eosinophils, the release of proinflammatory cytokines such as IL-1β and the strong chemotactor IL-8, and increased tissue concentrations of metalloproteinase enzymes (MMPs) (*Junquiera et al 1980, Liggins 1981, Uldbjerg et al 1983, Bokström et al 1997, Sennström et al 2000, Stygar et al 2002, Winkler et al 2003*). At parturition, a functional progesterone withdrawal occurs in the cervix uteri with decreased total nPR and an increased nPR-A/nPR-B ratio

(Stjernholm et al 1997, Vladic Stjernholm et al 2004). These endocrine and inflammatory events are followed by an up to 30-50% decreased collagen concentration, and an altered proteoglycan composition with a decreased density of the small proteoglycan decorin and an increased density of the large proteoglycan Versican. These events result in dispersed collagen fibrils clinically recognized as cervical effacement and dilatation (*Uldbjerg et al 1983, Ekman et al 1986, Norman et al 1993, Stjernholm et al 1997).* Evidence suggest that progesterone effects on the cervix uteri are even more pronounced than its effects on the myometrium (*Romero 2007*).

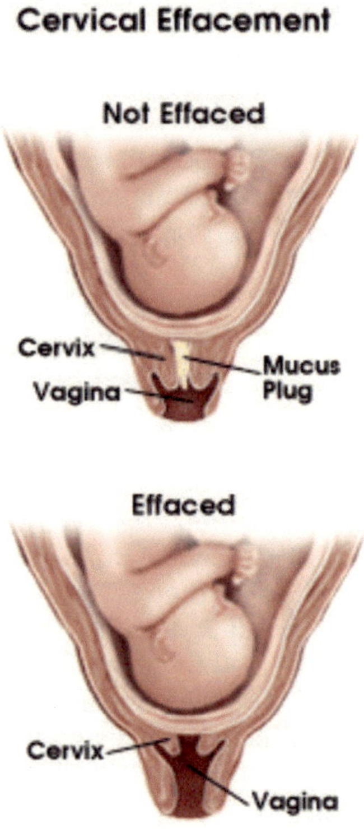

Fig. 6. Cervical effacement and dilatation before labor onset.

6. Parturition

6.1 Animal studies

Classical experiments in sheep demonstrated that parturition in this species is initiated by activation of the fetal hypothalamic pituitary adrenal (HPA) axis leading to increased fetal cortisol secretion and induction of placental P450 enzymes (17α-hydroxylase and 17-20-lyase activities), which favor the conversion of C21 to C18 steroids *(Liggins 1974, Anderson et al 1975).*

6.2 Human parturition

Progesterone is the main progestational hormone in humans, whereas the HPA axis has a modulatory function *(Hertelendy & Zakar 2004).* Prostaglandins (PGs) from the E and F series are considered to be the main promoters of cervical ripening and myometrial contractility, and the influence of PG-E_2 in promotion of cervical maturation and uterine vasodilatation has been

suggested as the primary functions of PGs in human parturition *(Hertelendy & Zakar 2004)*. Human decidual macrophages synthetize PGs (*Norwitz 1991*). Mechanical stretch of the lower uterine segment, proinflammatory cytokines such as IL-1β and the peptide hormone oxytocin induce PG synthesis *(Molnar et al 1999, Allport et al 2001, Leguizamon et al 2001)*.
Successful treatment with PG-E_2 for cervical priming before labor induction, allowing for resulting in cervical effacement and dilatation allowing for parturition was associated with diminished cervical progesterone and androgen receptor concentrations *(Vladic Stjernholm, 2009)*.

7. The puerperium

After delivery of the placenta, serum concentrations of estrogen and progesterone decrease within hours, and the puerperuim (*puer*: infant, *pario*: give birth) is a hypoestrogenic and hypoprogestagenic state. The high progesterone level during pregnancy inhibits lactation. The fall in progesterone levels after delivery is one factor that stimulates milk production *(Tucker 1979)*.

8. Progestin and progesterone treatment

Natural progesterone and synthetic progestins do both exert a progestogenic effect, defined as the decidualizing effect on estrogen-primed rabbit endometium *(Elton 1966, Schindler et al 2003)*.

8.1 Progestins and progesterone for preventing miscarriage

In clinical practice, progestin treatment was practised since the 1950s as luteal phase support to prevent miscarriage during the first trimester of pregnancy. The amount of data from well-controlled clinical trials is limited. Further studies are required to establish the optimal treatment situation as well as type and dose of progestin *(LeVine et al 1964, Daya & Gunby 2004)*.

8.2 Progestins and progesterone for preventing premature birth

Since the 1960s studies on treatment with synthetic progestins for preventing premature childbirth have reported beneficial effects. Human pregnancy lasts 40 gestational weeks and birth between 22 and 37 weeks is defined as premature (*WHO 1977*). The highly active progesterone ester 17α-hydroxyprogestrone caproate has a long duration allowing for

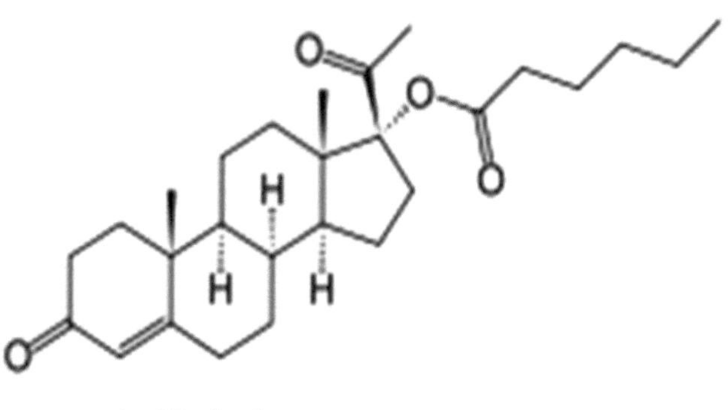

Fig. 7. The synthetic progestin 17α-hydroxyprogesterone caproate.

intramuscular administration 1-3 times weekly. It has been administered to risk groups with previous recurrent abortions or previous premature births and to patients with premature contractions and short cervices *(Johnsson et al 1976, Meis et al 2003, Dodd et al 2006)*. Natural progesterone has been administered as of vaginal gel to such risk groups and in situations with premature contractions and short cervices *(daFonseca et al 2003, deFranco et al 2007, O´Brien et al 2007)*. Reduced incidence of premature birth before 32, 34 and 37 gestational weeks and improved neonatal outcome were reported *(Brent 2005)*. Further studies are required to establish the optimal dose and type of agent as well as long term effects on the newborn.

9. Summary

Progesterone is the evolutionary most conserved of the reproductive steroid hormones. It is the main progestational hormone in humans, and its strong immunomodulatory effects are important for the physiological immunotolerance at implantation. After a transition period by 7-10 gestational weeks the placenta becomes the major progesterone source. Placental concentrations of progesterone reach 1-10 μM and serum concentrations 100-500 nM until term pregnancy. Progesterone exerts its effects through genomic nuclear receptor mediated and non-genomic transmembrane receptor mediated processes, keeping the myometrium in a quiescent state and stabilizing the cervix uteri during pregnancy. A functional progesterone withdrawal occurs at human parturition with a diminished total receptor density and altered isoform ratios. In clinical practice, progestin treatment has been given as luteal phase support to prevent miscarriage during the first trimester of pregnancy. Treatment with synthetic progestins and natural progesterone has been shown to reduce the incidence of premature birth. Further studies are required to establish the optimal dose and type of agent as well as long term effects on the newborn.

10. Acknowledgements

I thank the editor for inviting me to present this work and Dr Tomislav Vladic for critical comments.

11. References

Abbas AK, Murphy KM & Sher A (1996) Functional diversity of helper T lymphocytes. Nature 383:787–793.

Allen WM (1935) The isolation of crystalline progestin. Science 82 (2118): 89–93.

Allport VC, Pieber D, Slater R, Newton JO, White PR & Bennett PR (2001) Human labour is associated with nuclear factor-kappaB activity which mediates cyclo-oxygenase-2 expression and is involved with the "functional progesterone withdrawal". Mol Hum Reprod 7:581-586.

Anderson AB, Flint AP & Turnbull AC (1975) Mechanisms of action of glucocorticoids in induction of ovine parturition: effects on placental steroid metabolism. J Endocrinol 66:61-70.

Bamberger CM, Else T, Bamberger AM, Beil FU & Schulte HM (1999) Dissociative glucocorticoid activity of medroxyprogesterone acetate in normal human lymphocytes. J Clin Endocrin Metab 84:4055–4061.

Blackmore PF, Neulen J, Lattanzio F & Beebe SJ (1991) Cell surface-binding sites for progesterone mediated calcium-uptake in human sperm. J Biol Chem 266:18655–18659.

Bokström H, Brännström H, Alexandersson M & Norström A (1997) Leukocyte subpopulations in cervical stroma at early and late pregnancy. Hum Reprod 12:586-590.

Brent RL (2005) Nongenital malformations following exposure to progestational drugs. The last chapter of an erroneous allegation. Birth Defects Res 73: 906-918.

Butenandt A & Westphal U (1934) Zur Isolierung und Charakterisierung des Corpusluteum-Hormons. Berichte Deutsche Chemische Gesellschaft 67:1440–1442.

Chang K & Zhang L (2008) Steroid hormones and uterine vascular adaptation to pregnancy. Reprod Sci 15: 336–348.

Condon JC, Jeyasuria P, Faust JM & Mendelson CM (2004) Surfactant protein secreted by the maturing mouse fetal lung acts as a hormone that signals the initiation of parturition. Proc Natl Acad Sci USA 101:4978–4983.

Csapo AI (1956) A progesterone block. Am J Anat 98:273-291.

Csapo AI, Pulkkinen MO & Wiest WG (1973) Effects of lutectomy and progesterone replacement therapy in early pregnant patients. Am J Obstet Gynecol 115:759-765.

Danforth DN & Evanston MD. The distribution and functional activity of the cervical musculature (1954) Am J Obstet Gynecol 68:1261-1271

Daya S & Gunby J (2004) Luteal phase support in assisted reproduction cycles (review). Cochrane Database Syst Rev 2:CD004830. Update in: Cochrane Database Syst Rev 2008; (3):CD004830.

da Fonseca EB, Bittar RE, Mario HB & Zugaib M (2003) Prophylactic administration of progesterone by vaginal suppository to reduce the incidence of spontaneous preterm birth in women at increased risk: a randomised placebo controlled double blind study. Am J Obstet Gynecol 188:419-24.

deFranco EA, O´Brien JM, Adair CD,Lewis DF, Hall DR, et al (2007) Vaginal progesterone is associated with a decrease in risk for early preterm birth and improved neonatal outcome in women with a short cervix: a secondary analysis from a randomized, double-blind, placebo-controlled trial. Ultrasound Obstet Gynecol 30:697-705.

Diczfalucy E (1969) Steroid metabolism in the human feto-placental unit. Acta Endocrinol 61:649-664.

Dodd JM, Flenady V & Cincotta R (2006) Prenatal administration of progesterone for preventing preterm birth (Review). Cochrane Database Syst Rev CD004947.

Dosiou C, Hamilton AE, Pang Y, Overgaard MT, Tulac S, Dong J, et al (2008) Expression of membrane progesterone receptors on human T lymphocytes and Jurkat cells and activation of G-proteins by progesterone. J Endocrinol 196:67–77.

Ekman G, Malmström A, Uldbjerg N & Ulmsten U (1986) Cervical collagen. An important regulator of cervical function in term labor. Obstet Gynecol 67:663-666.

Elton RL (1966) The decidual cell responses in rabbits. Acta Endocrinol (Copenh) 51:543-550.

Everett RB, Worley RJ, MacDonald PC & Gant NF (1987) Modification in vascular responsiveness to angiotensin II in pregnant women by intravenously infused 5α-dihydroprogesterone. Am J Obstet Gynecol 131:352.

Filardo EJ, Quinn JA, Bland KI & Frackelton AR (2000) Estrogen-induced activation of ERK-1 and ERK-2 requires the G protein-coupled receptor homolog, GPR30, and occurs via trans-activation of the epidermal growth factor receptor through release of HB-EGF. Mol Endocrinol 14:1649–1660.

Fonseca EB, Celik E, Parra M, Singh M & Nicolaides KH (2007) Progesterone and the risk of preterm birth among women with a short cervix. New England J Med 357 (5): 462–469.

Friedman SA (1988) Preeclampsia: A review of the role of prostaglandins. Obstet Gynecol 71:122-137.

Hertelendy F & Zakar T (2004) Prostaglandins, the myometrium and the cervix. Prostagl, Leukot Essen Fatty Acids 70:207-222.

Jensen D, Wolfe LA, Slatkovska L, Webb KA, Davies GA & O'Donnell D (2005) Effects of human pregnancy on the ventilatory chemoreflex response to carbon dioxide . Am J Physiol Regul Integr Comp Physiol 288:1369-75.

Johnson JW, Austin KL, Jones GS, Davis GH % King TM (1975) Efficacy of 17α– hydroxyprogestrone caproate in the prevention of premature labour. New Engl J Med 293:675-680.

Junquiera LCU, Zugaib M, Montes G, Toledo O, Krisztan R & Shigihara K (1980) Morphologic and histological evidence for the occurrence of collagenolysis and for the role of leukocytes during cervical dilatation. Am J Obstet Gynecol 138:273-281.

Kublickiene KR, Nisell H, Poston L, Krüger K & Lindblom B (2000) Modulation of vascular tone by nitric oxide and endothelin 1 in myometrial resistance arteries from pregnant women at term. Am J Obstet Gynecol 182:87-93.

Leguizamon G, Smith J, Younis H, Nelson DM & Sadovsky Y (2001) Enhancement of amniotic cyclooxygenase type 2 activity in women with preterm delivery associated with twins or polyhydramnios. Am J Obstet Gynecol 184:117-122.

LeVine L (1964) Habitual abortion. A controlled clinical study of progestational therapy. West J Surg Gynecol 72: 30.

Liggins GC (1974) Parturition in the sheep and the human. Basic Life Sci 4:423-443.

Liggins GC (1981) Cervical ripening as an inflammatory reaction. In The Cervix in pregnancy and labour. Eds: Ellwood DA, Anderson ABM, Edinburg, Scotland, UK. Churchill Livingstone pp 1-9.

Lockwood CJ, Matta P, Krikun G, Koopman LA, Masch R, Toti P, et al (2006) Regulation of monocyte chemoattractant protein-1 expression by tumor necrosis factor-α and interleukin-1β in first trimester human decidual cells: implication for preeclampsia. Am J Pathol 168:445-452.

Madsen G, Zakar T, Ku CY, Sanborn BM, Smith R & Mesiano S (2004) Prostaglandins differentially modulate progesterone receptor A and -B expression in human myometrial cells: evidence for prostaglandin-induced functional progesterone withdrawal. J Clin Endocrinol 89:1010-13.

Mansour I, Reznikoff-Etievant MF & Netter A (1994) No evidence for the expression of the progesterone receptor on peripheral blood lymphocytes during pregnancy. Hum Reprod 9:1546–1549.

Mastorakos G & Ilias I (2000) Maternal hypothalamic-pituitary-adrenal axis in pregnancy and the postpartum period. Ann NY Acad Sci 900:95-106.

Meis P, Klebanoff M, Thom E, Dornbrowski MP, Sibai B, Moawad AF, et al (2003) Prevention of recurrent preterm delivery by 17 alpha-hydroxyprogesterone caproate. New England J Med 348:2379-2385.

Mesiano S, Chan EC, Fitter JT, Kwek K, Yeo G & Smith R (2002) Progesterone withdrawal and estrogen activation in human parturition are coordinated by progesterone receptor A expression in the myometrium. J Clin Endocrinol Metab 87:2924-2930.

Mesiano S (2007) Myometrial progesterone responsiveness. Semin Reprod Med 25:5-13.

Miyaura H & Iwata M (2002) Direct and indirect inhibition of Th1 development by progesterone and glucocorticoids. J Immunol 168: 1087-1094.

Molnar M, Rigo J Jr, Romero R & Hertelendy F (1999) Oxytocin activates mitogen-activated protein kinase and up-regulates cyclooxygenase-2 and prostaglandin production in human myometrial cells. Am J Obstet Gynecol 181:42-49.

Mulac-Jericevic B & Conneely OM (2004) Reproductive tissue selective actions of progesterone receptors. Reproduction 128:139-146.

Norman M, Ekman G & Malmström A (1993) Changed proteoglycan metabolism in human cervix immediately after spontaneous vaginal delivery. Obstet Gynecol 81; 217-223.

Norman AW, Mizwicki MT & Norman DP (2004) Steroid-hormone rapid actions, membrane receptors and a conformational ensemble model. Nature Rev 3: 27–41.

Norwitz ER, Starkey P, Lopez Bernal A & Turnbull A (1991) Identification by flow cytometry of the prostaglandin-producing cells of term human decidua. J Endocrinol 131:327-334.

O´Brien JM, Adair CD, Lewis DF, Hall DR, deFranco EA, Fusey P, et al (2007) Progesterone vaginal gel for the reduction of recurrent preterm birth: primary results from a randomised, double blind, placebo-controlled trial. Ultrasound Obstet Gynecol 30: 687-696.

O´Malley B (1990) The steroid receptor superfamily. More excitement predicted for the future. Mol Endocrinol 4:363-369.

Piccinni MP, Giudizi MG, Biagiotti R, Beloni L, Giannarini L, Sampognaro S, et al (1995) Progesterone favours the development of human T helper cells producing Th2-type cytokines and promotes both IL-4 production and membrane CD30 expression in established Th1 cell clones. J Immunol 155:128-133.

Piccinni MP (2010) T cell tolerance towards the fetal allograft. J Reprod Immunol 85:71-75. Review.

Pieber D, Allport VC, Hills F, Johnson M, Bennett PR (2001) Interaction between progesterone receptor isoforms in myometrial cells in human labor. Mol Hum Reprod 7:875-879.

Romero R, Scoccia B, Mazor M, Wu YK & Benaviste R (1988) Evidence for a local change in the progesterone/estrogen ratio in human parturition at term. Am J Obstet Gynecol 159:657-660.

Romero R (2007) Prevention of spontaneous preterm birth: the role of sonographic cervical length in identifying patients who may benefit from progesterone treatment. Ultrasound Obstet Gynecol 30 :675–686.

Rook GA, Hernandez-Pando R & Lightman SL (1994) Hormones, peripherally activated prohormones and regulation of the Th1/Th2 balance. Immunol Today 13:301-303.

Rupnow HL, Phernetton TM, Modrick ML, Wiltbank MC, Bird IM & Magness RR (2002) Endothelial vasodilator production by uterine and systemic arteries. VIII. Estrogen and progesterone effects on cPLA2, COX-1, and PGIS protein expression. Biol Reprod 66:468-474.

Sanborn BM, Held B & Kuo HS (1976) Hormonal action in human cervix - II Specific progestogen binding proteins in humans. J Ster Biochem 7:665-672.

Schindler AE, Campagnoli C, Druckmann R, Huber J, Pasqualini JR, Schweppe KW & Thijssen JH (2003) Classification and pharmacology of progestins. Maturitas Suppl 1: S7–S16.

Schwalm H & Dubrauszky V. The structure of the musculature of the human uterus muscles and connective tissue (1966) Am J Obstet Gynecol 94:391-404.

Sennström M, Ekman G, Westergren-Thorsson G, Malmström A, Byström B, Endresen U et al (2000) Human cervical ripening, an inflammatory process mediated by cytokines. Mol Hum Reprod 6:375-381.

Speroff L, Glass & Kase N, eds (1994) Clinical gynecologic endocrinology and infertility (5th Edition) Williams and Wilkins, USA.

Stites DP & Siiteri PK (1983) Steroids as immunosuppressants in pregnancy. Immunol Rev 75:117-138.

Stjernholm Y, Sahlin L, Malmström A, Barchan K, Eriksson HA & Ekman G (1997) Potential roles for gonadal steroids and insulin-like growth factor I during final cervical ripening. Obstet Gynecol 90:375-380.

Stout RD & Suttles J (2004) Functional plasticity of macrophages: reversible adaptation to changing microenvironments. J Leukoc Biol 76:509-513.

Stygar D, Wang H, Vladic Stjernholm Y, Ekman G, Eriksson HA & Sahlin L (2002) Increased levels of matrix metalloproteinases 2 and 9 in the ripening process of the human cervix. Mol Hum Reprod 67:889-894.

Sugimoto Y, Yamasaki A, Segi E, Tsuboi K, Aze Y, Nishimura T, et al (1997) Failure of parturition in mice lacking the prostaglandin F receptor. Science 277:681-683.

Szekeres-Bartho J, Kilar F, Falkay G, Csrnus V, Torok A & Pacsa AS (1985) Progesterone-treated lymphocytes of healthy pregnant women release a factor inhibiting cytotoxicity and prostaglandin synthesis. Am J Reprod Immunol Microbiol 9:15-19.

Szekeres-Bartho J, Szekeres G, Debre P, Autran B & Chaouat G (1990) Reactivity of lymphocytes to a progesterone receptor-specific monoclonal antibody. Cell Immunol 125:273–283.

Szekeres-Bartho J (2002) Immunological relationship between the mother and the fetus. Int Rev Immunol 21:471-495.

Tibbetts TA, de Mayo F, Rich S, Conneely OM & O´Malley B (1999) Progesterone receptors in the thymus are required for for thymic involution during pregnancy and for normal fertility. Proc Natl Acad Sci USA 96:12021-6.

Tucker HA (1979) Endocrinology of lactation. Semin Perinatol 3: 199-223.

Uldbjerg N, Ekman G, Malmström A, Olsson K & Ulmsten U (1983) Ripening of the human uterine cervix is related to changes in collagen, glycosaminoglycans and collagenolytic activity. Am J Obstet Gynecol 147:662-666.

Vacca A, Martinotti S, Screpanti I, Maroder M, Felli MP, Farina AR, et al (1990) Transcriptional regulation of the interleukin 2 gene by glucocorticoid hormones. J Biol Chem 265: 8075-8080.

Vegeto E, Shahbaz MM, Wen DX, Goldman ME, O'Malley BW & McDonnell DP (1993) Human progesterone receptor A form is a cell- and promoter specific repressor of human progesterone receptor B function. Endocrinology 7:1244-1255.

Wegmann TG, Lin L, Guilbert L & Mosmann TR (1993) Bidirectional cytokine interactions in the maternal-fetal relationship: is successful pregnancy a Th2 phenomenon? Immunol Today 14:353-356.

Weiner LH (2001) Induction and mechanism of action of transforming growth factor beta secreting Th3 regulatory cells. Immunol Rev 182:207-214.

White HD, Yeaman G, Givan A & Wira C. Mucosal immunity of the female reproductive tract: cytotoxic T lymphocyte function in the cervix and vagina of premenopausal and postmenopausal women (1997) Am J Reprod Immunol 37:30-38.

WHO (1977) recommended definitions, terminology and format for statistical tables related to the perinatal period and use of a new certificate for cause of perinatal deaths. Modifications recommended by FIGO as amended October 14, 1976. Acta Obstet Gynecol Scand 56(3):247-253.

Winkler M, Kemp B, Fischer DC, Ruck P & Rath W (2003) Expression of adhesion molecules in the lower uterine segment during term and preterm parturition. Microsc Res Tech 1:430-444.

Vladic Stjernholm Y, Wang H, Stygar D, Ekman G & Sahlin L (2004) Differential regulation of the progesterone receptor A and B in the human uterine cervix. Gynecol Endocrinol 18:41-46.

Vladic Stjernholm Y, Vladic T, Blesson CS, Ekman-Ordeberg G & Sahlin L (2009) Prostaglandin treatment is associated with a withdrawal of progesterone and androgen at the receptor level in the uterine cervix. Reprod Biol Endocrinol 7:116.

Wolfe LA, Kemp JG, Heenan AP, Preston RJ & Ohtake PJ (1998) Acid-base regulation and control of ventilation in human pregnancy. Can J Physiol Pharmacol 76: 815–827.

Wood GW, Hausmann E & Choudhuri R (1997) Relative role of CSF-1, MCP-1/JE, and RANTES in macrophage recruitment during successful pregnancy. Mol Reprod Dev 46:62-70.

Zhu Y, Bond J & Thomas P (2003) Identification, classification, and partial characterization of genes in humans and other vertebrates homologous to a fish membrane progestin receptor. Proc Natl Acad Sci USA 100:2237–2242.

6

Late - Onset Hypogonadism - New Point of View

Andrzej Gomuła*
The Andropause Institute, Warsaw, Poland

1. Introduction

Long-term testosterone deficiency related to age may adversely affect health, anatomy and physiology of man. The implementation of testosterone boost therapy only at the time, when for many years, as the result of testosterone deficiency, irreversible anatomical changes have occurred, is clearly too late. Age-related progressive decrease in testosterone serum concentration levels causes anatomical and functional abnormalities. It is the cause of lipid disorders; it excarberates type-2 diabetes, it is also the common cause of cardiovascular diseases. It contributes to other health problems such as atherosclerosis, hypertension, osteoporosis and obesity and it manifests itself by decreased libido and potency. There is also a strong relationship between age-related decrease in testosterone and Parkinson's disease and Alzheimer's disease. Benign prostatic hyperplasia (BPH) and carcinoma of the prostate are closely associated with testosterone deficiency and comedo-carcinoma — the most malignant form of prostate cancer — is directly proportional to the decrease in serum testosterone. A good therapy for increasing testosterone serum levels can reverse the problems associated with aging such as type-2 diabetes, sexual dysfunction, osteoporosis, hyper-lipidemia and ischemic heart disease. It can even reverse symptoms of Parkinson's disease. Using synthetic testosterone is often recommended in the treatment of testosterone deficiency. Unfortunately, synthetic testosterone can cause side effects such as infertility and a long-term use of testosterone may also lead to irreversible testicular atrophy. Therefore, patients receiving long-term testosterone therapy are all dependent on adequate doses of synthetic testosterone until the end of their lives. Meanwhile, intramuscular administration of hCG to stimulate the endogenous testosterone synthesis, has been known since the 1950s. The induction of endogenous testosterone production by hCG has been effective in all age groups while being safe at the same time. In this paper, the author presents problems caused by testosterone deficiency and outlines the possibility of the treatment, which increases the induction of testosterone endosynthesis by hCG. It has not yet been determined how to diagnose testosterone deficiency. The age-related serum testosterone concentration reference range has not been established yet either. The paper presents the first attempt to establish international standards for testosterone serum concentration levels in different age groups.

2. Late-onset hypogonadism

Late-onset hypogonadism (LOH) is a testosterone deficiency syndrome resulting in the aging process. LOH leads to metabolic disorders and functional or anatomical abnormalities. It is

* Corresponding Author

now beyond dispute that, as testosterone deficit increases with age, it adversely affects the function of multiple organ systems. Therefore the implementation of appropriate strategies to increase testosterone levels only when as a result of testosterone deficiency irreversible anatomical changes have occurred, is clearly too late, which operates to the detriment of men.
Recent studies suggest that there are large numbers of men in the community whose testosterone deficiency is neither being diagnosed nor treated (Trinick et al., 2011).
Testosterone exerts influence on multiple life processes such as blood cell production, bone formation, lipid metabolism, protein metabolism, carbohydrate metabolism, liver function, and spermiogenesis (Gooren, 2000). This can affect the structure and function of many organs in human body. They include skin, hair, muscle, brain and bones. It also has a significant effect on fertility and sexual behaviour. Testosterone plays a very important role in a man's life. At the mitochondrial level of each single cell it is the catalyst for protein synthesis. It has an effect on the brain's function, and thus determines the physical and sexual condition. It increases libido and improves sexual potency. It stimulates the immune system and affects multiple metabolic processes. It reduces body fat accumulation. It can affect muscle mass and strength. It increases bone mass and accelerates wound healing. Testosterone is responsible for our memory processes. Computer memory circuits are manufactured using metal arranged on silicon. In the process of human memory, proteins are involved. The testosterone that catalyzes the synthesis of various proteins is also a catalyst for storage protein synthesis. Protein synthesis becomes less efficient with age, proteins formed are unstable. Their decay means that an old man remembers what was years ago and cannot remember what just happened. In the literature, there have been isolated reports about the role of testosterone in the aetiology of Alzheimer's disease (Hogervorst, 2004).
Testosterone also aids in immune system protein synthesis, which protects us against infection. Hormone intake in pregnant women during the first trimester of pregnancy significantly affects hormone balance in young men. Although hormone therapy allows the woman to keep her pregnancy from failing, it is also essential for organogenesis, and in particular for the reproductive organs of male foetuses. According to the definition in Standards of Endocrinology, "Testosterone deficit disorder manifests itself in a decrease in libido and potency, in constant fatigue, in deterioration of mood and in sleep quality, in nervousness, in hot flushes, in low testosterone, and in elevated serum gonadotropin concentrations" (Zgliczyński & Zgliczyński, 2002). However, according to the definition provided by ISSAM, the International Society of Andrology (ISA) and the European Association of Urology (EAU), it is "a clinical and biochemical syndrome associated with advancing age, characterized by typical symptoms and a deficiency in serum testosterone levels. It can cause a significant deterioration in over-all quality of life and adversely affect the function of many different organs and systems" (Nieschlag, et al., 2005). It is now beyond dispute that, as testosterone deficit increases with age, it adversely affects the function of multiple organ systems. Previously adopted minimum standard testosterone levels, at which there has been best evidence for treatment, are far too low. The implementation of the therapy to boost testosterone levels at the time when for many years, as a result of testosterone deficiency, irreversible anatomical changes have occurred, is clearly too late, which operates to the detriment of men (Gomuła & Rabijewski, 2010). According to Tenover, if we consider the norm based on the level of total testosterone, in a group of 55-year-old men, 20% of them will be hypogonadal; and in the same group of men, when we adopt a standard based on the level of bio-available testosterone, hypogonadism will be diagnosed in half of them (Tenover, 1997). Cross-sectional studies have shown that, since

this is associated with a simultaneous increase of SHBG levels, bioavailable testosterone may decline more significantly than apparent total testosterone (Snyder, 2001, Vermeulen, 2001). Only the testosterone circulating in the body which is not bound to SHBG is biologically active in the target organs. Therefore the measurement of bioavailable testosterone levels more accurately reflects a patient's clinical status than the measurement of total testosterone levels. The study of 810 men aged 24-90 years showed a strong correlation between age and a decrease in bioavailable testosterone level and in estradiol level (r =- 0.52). It was still strong when other variables were taken into account such as alcohol intake, BMI, smoking, caffeine intake, and diabetes (Ferrini & Barrett-Connor, 1998). Also significant but weaker (r=- 0.13) correlations were found between age and total testosterone and estradiol levels. Both the decreased testosterone production and its increased conversion can explain a reduction in total testosterone levels, while age-related increase in sex hormone binding capacity can cause reduced biologically available testosterone production. The correlation between age and the level of bioavailable and of total estradiol in men has not been studied previously. Bioavailable estradiol levels might decrease due to a decline in levels of testosterone, which is the main substrate for male estradiol production. It also contributes to an increase of SHBG with age. In one of the largest studies, which involved 2,623 men aged 65 and over, enjoying good health, levels of free and bioavailable testosterone and estradiol levels correlated with each other (Orwoll, et al. 2006). Higher age, higher BMI, and worse health status were associated with slightly lower total testosterone levels. The concentration of SHBG rose with age. The decrease in testosterone levels fell approximately 10% for 10 years. Many old men still had testosterone levels established for young men. However, it is unknown which level of testosterone is sufficient for an elderly person and for that person's specific tissues (i.e. muscles, bones, and nervous system). The number of androgen binding sites in the hippocampus and the number of the layers of the skin tissues that cover the penis increase with age (Hijazi & Cunningham, 2005). Testosterone production peaks at age 20 and then begins a gradual decline, usually giving rise to the first symptoms after the age of 50. In a group of men aged 80, the level of free testosterone is half of what they had when they were younger (Vermeulen, et al., 1996).

2.1 Hypogonadism – Primary, secondary, LOH

Classic categorization of hypogonadism differentiates its primary and secondary types. In the case of primary hypogonadism, testicles are unable to synthesize estosterone, while in case of secondary hypogonadism low testosterone is caused by pituitary insufficiency. Until present from the pathophysiology point of view, LOH has been regarded as a mixed type of hypogonadism conditioned by the changes undergoing both in gonads (component of primary hypogonadism) and on the level of central controllers of testicular functions; hypothalamus and pituitary (components of secondary hypogonadism). Hypothalamus and pituitary regulate, on the basis of feedback, functions of Leydig cells in testicles. Gonadotrophin-releasing hormone is a trophin hypothalamus hormone relative to the Leydig cells. Its effect on pituitary results in the synthesis of luteinizing hormone (LH) and folicule stimulating hormone (FSH) in gonadotrophin cells. Gonadotrophin LH stimulates the synthesis of testosterone through the Leydig cells in testicle. With age, pulsating secretion of LH becomes disturbed. Pulses become more scarce (decreased frequency), of lower amplitude and their duration extends. The result is an increase of LH concentration with age. If LH concentration increases with age, thus pituitary insufficiency, i.e. secondary hypogonadism, does not exist and testicles retain their capability of high endosynthesis of testosterone, hence in case of LOH features of primary or of secondary hypogonadism are non-existent. It has been acknowledged that testicle stimulation with hCG does not cause any substantial, sufficient increase of endosynthesis of testosterone. And here lies the fundamental error – the statement that hCG does not result in any substantial increase of testosterone endosynthesis is untrue!!! Therapy based on hCG allows doubling the concentration of testosterone, which in over 90% of those treated enables restoring a normal hormone condition. I base my statement on over a 10-year long observation of 1200 patients I treated with hCG to induce endosynthesis of testosterone.

Secretion of GnRH is distorted as well. Hypothalamus response to change of LH pulse nature and to lowered secretion of androgens is incommensurate. The phenomenon is referred to as dysregulation of hypothalamus pulse generator. The reasons for alternations of pulsating secretion of GnRH and LH are unclear, however of importance are genetic factors and backward changes in gonadotrophin cells and in reflective microcirculation on hypothalamus and pituitary axis (Snyder, et al., 2000). Ferrini, Wang, Hakim et al. have established that changes in functioning of hypothalamus and pituitary may not be the major cause of gonads dysfunctions in men (Ferrini, et al., 2001). They have found evidence for a substantial increase of hypothalamus and pituitary apoptosis, two changes clarifying development of hypogonadism at old age. Until now it was believed that together with hypothalamus and pituitary dysfunction gonadal backward changes played an important role in etiopathogenesis of gonads. The process of decreasing testosterone synthesis starts approximately at the age of 35-40 years and is of extreme individual variability. Changes within testicles are noted for progressive decrease of the number of Leydig cells and deterioration of Sertoli cells functions and as a result decrease of secretion of inhibin, impaired micro-circulation and blood-supply of testicle cells and backward changes within perivascular parenchyma (Deslypere & Vermulen, 1984, Snyder, 2001). From the analysis of own material it is considered that to-date views on TDS aetiology are unfounded. As it has been demonstrated in the material consisting of 908 men treated with induction of endosynthesis, it is possible with every age group, but it decreas in terms of physiology with age. Nevertheless, the capability of efficient endosynthesis is retained until advanced years, which contradicts views of atrophy of Leydig cells functions. From a clinical point of view, LOH resembles pathology of incorrect LH bioactivity described in men of 47XY karyotype who after adolescence undergo hypogonadism with decrease of testosterone and increase of LH concentration. These patients demonstrate correct gonads response to LH stimulation. It has been acknowledged that in these cases LH bioactivity is decreased, while immunoreactivity is normal. It results from glutamine changing into arginine in position 54 of beta chains.

Currently, it is not possible to define explicitly the aetiologic factor of LOH leading to testosterone shortfall. Testosterone shortfall results in metabolic syndrome causing disorders of many bodily functions such as memory disorders, difficulties with falling asleep, excessive nervousness, deterioration of ability to associate and concentrate, heat waves, depression tendencies, vertigo and headache, fall of strength and muscle bulk, as well as numerous cardiovascular system complaints. Testosterone concentration drop leads to lipid disorders and diabetes type 2.

2.2 Andropause, ADAM, PADAM, LOH, TDS

The concept of "male menopause" has been known since 1960s (Wang, et al., 1996) yet until today it has not been unambiguously defined. The names of the clinical state caused by testosterone shortfall have changed many times over decades which explicitly proves lack of firm facts based on indisputable ground. Names of andropause, sarcopenia, viropause were followed by andropause, (Morley & Perry, 2003) which stayed in medicine for good. Many learned societies with the term of andropause in the centre were established around the world. However the term of andropause is erroneous by definition. Such a phenomenon as pause, break in production of testosterone with men does not exist. Since a pause is a stage of an activity as discontinuation and a pause (a break) is followed by return to the activity from before the pause. At the end of previous century notions of *Androgen Deficiency in Aging Male* or *Androgen Deficiency in Adult Male* /ADAM/ (Carruthers, 2004) came to being. It must be emphasized that an adult man is aged between 20-25 years, while an aging man according to *International Society for the Study of the Aging Male* (ISSAM) is a gentleman above 60-65 (Carruthers, 2004). This is where the dilemma arises, does the testosterone shortfall issue concern exclusively elder men or younger, adult men? Testosterone shortfall has earned yet another name— PADAM (*partial androgen deficiency in aging male*), which defines the testosterone shortfall in a not sufficiently explicit manner. The concept lacks specification of boarder testosterone concentration and thus the value according to which a shortfall can be recognized. Therefore the term PADAM should not be used at all. What does partial shortfall mean? No accounting system recognizes partial deficit, it either exists or does not. Can a woman be partially pregnant? Another term was established; secondary or late onset hypogonadism but it still did not represent the core of the problem (Morales, et al., 2006). As clinical symptoms of androgen shortfall manifest themselves already at the break of forth and fifth decade (Mosby, 1998) (35–45 years), i.e. in the first half of life, can it be said that hypogonadism appears late? The latest name of the disease, which so far has not been explicitly defined, is *testosterone deficiency syndrome /TDS /* (Morales, et al., 2006) – currently a fashionable term. Yet science and fashion follow totally different criteria. What counts in fashion is a one-season success, while in science exact, indisputable facts forming a solid basis for many years should be essecial. In the meantime, testosterone shortfall, an unfavourable phenomenon leading to various metabolic disorders or issue pathologies, has not been named a disease until now.

2.3 Late - onset hypogonadism and age related testosterone levels

Many studies have now demonstrated that as men age, their serum testosterone concentrations fall at an average rate of 0.8%-1% per year (Feldman, et al., 2002, Kaufmann & Vermeulen, 2005). Concurrently, free and bioavailable testosterone levels fall by 2% per year (Kaufmann & Vermeulen, 2005). Obesity, alcohol abuse, diabetes, hypertension, heart disease, cancer and ulcers have intensified the negative impact (Harman, et al., 2001).

Therefore, and also due to an increase in the concentrations of carrier proteins, significantly decreased testosterone levels characterise approximately 8% of men of 40-60 and 20% men of 60-80 (Kaufmann & Vermeulen, 2005). The question arises: how to measure the decrease in testosterone levels during the life of a man? By the hormonal status of young people today? The hormonal status of their fathers? What was the hormonal status of their grandparents in their youth, since testosterone levels in men over age 70 often reach the upper range of the standard? And another question: what was the testosterone level of a 30-year-old man, whose level now, at 70, is more than 35 nmol/L?

Standard testosterone levels vary in different analytical laboratories. In American research laboratories alone, the lower limit of normal testosterone level ranges from 4.5 to 15.6 nmol/L - 350% difference (Lazarou, et al., 2006)

The effects of an objectively measurable drop in testosterone levels may also vary. Researchers wonder if it would be most appropriate to establish separate ranges of normal testosterone levels for the young and for the old (Lunenfeld & Gooren, 2002). It is also unknown whether the plasma testosterone threshold values vary with age. There is preliminary evidence that the threshold value necessary for the proper functioning and for the proper effects of testosterone also increases with age (Schiavi, et al., 1993). Bancroft hypothesizes that the threshold required for the behavioral effects of testosterone increases with age (Bancroft, 1989). Although many older men have testosterone levels within the normal range, their levels may not be sufficient for normal sexual functioning. Probably organ sensitivity to androgens is not the same for the young and for the old. Schiavi reported that nocturnal erections are androgen-dependent and are disrupted in healthy elderly men who do not meet the criteria for hypogonadism, which seems to confirm Bancroft's hypothesis (Bancroft, 1989, Schiavi, et al. (1993). Based on the analysis of the material provided by 1267 men of 20-89, together with the material provided by 908 men under treatment, standard levels of testosterone have been age-determined (Gomuła & Rabijewski, 2010). Among the respondents between 20-29, the average level of testosterone was 21.99 nmol/L; among the respondents between 30-39 – 21.91 nmol/L among the respondents between 40-49 – 19.18 nmol / L; among the respondents between 40-49 - 19.18 nmol/L; among the respondents between 50-59 – 17.74 nmol/L; among the respondents between 60-69 – 15.94 nmol/L among the respondents between 70-79 – 17.66 nmol/:L and among the respondents between 80-89 – 16.65 nmol/l. The standard testosterone levels in individual age groups (minimum and maximum, average level, standard deviations and medians) are shown in Table 1.

Age/min-max, median,average,SD	**n, Testosterone in nmol/L**	**Age/min-max, median,average,SD**	**n, Testosterone in nmol/L**
20–29 years	n = 78	**60–69 years**	n = 281
Min., max.	4.64; 49.10	Min., max.	2; 40.40
Average (SD)	21.99 (9.33)	Average (SD)	15.94 (6.68)
Median (25%, 75%)	19.75 (15.40; 26.20)	Median (25%, 75%)	15 (11.30; 19.70)
30–39 years	n = 102	**70–79 years**	n = 213
Min., max.	8.90; 46.80	Min., max.	2.71; 45.60
Average (SD)	21.91 (8.18)	Average (SD)	17.66 (7.87)
Median (25%, 75%)	21.70 (15.80; 25.20)	Median (25%, 75%)	16.10 (12.70; 21.30)
40–49 years	n = 176	**80–89 years**	n = 50
Min., max.	3.40; 47.20	Min., max.	3.70; 38.80
Average (SD)	19.18 (8.92)	Average (SD)	16.65 (7.55)
Median (25%, 75%)	17 (12.6; 24.30)	Median (25%, 75%)	15.75 (12; 20.60)
50–59 years	n = 367		
Min., max.	3.10; 53.50		
Average (SD)	17.74 (8.01)		
Median (25%, 75%)	16.20 (12.10; 21.70)		

n - number of patients in the age group , SD - standard deviation

Table 1. Testosterone levels of 1267 men in different age groups

The evaluation of 1267 men aged 20-89 years has found that the average testosterone level in all age groups is higher than 12 nmol/L - what is shown in Fig. 1.

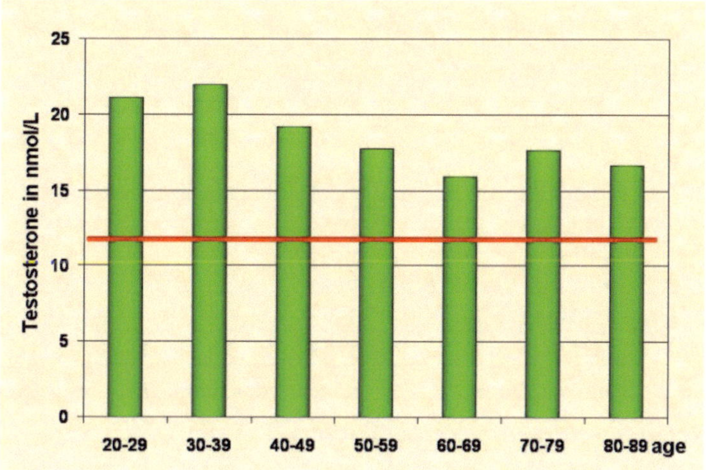

Fig. 1. The average testosterone levels of 1267 men in different age groups. The horizontal line on the graph represents an accepted lower limit of normal testosterone level 12 nmol/L /according to the International Society for the Study of the Aging Male/ (Lunenfeld, B. Et al., 2005, Nieschlag, et al., 2005). If we assume that the standard testosterone level is higher than 12 nmol/L, in the age group 20-29 years testosterone deficit has been found in 11.5% of those examined. In the age group 30-39 years the deficit has been found in 5.9% of those examined. In the age group 40-49 years - in 21% of those examined; in the age group 50-59 years - in 24% of those examined; in the age group 60-69 years - in 27.8%; in the age group 70-79 years - in 20.6%; and in the age group 80-89 years - in 24% of those examined. Testosterone deficiency (serum testosterone concentrations below 12 nmol/L) in different age groups is shown in Table 2.

Age	N pts	%
20–29	9/78	11.5%
30–39	6/102	5.9%
40–49	37/176	21%
50–59	88/367	24%
60–69	78/281	27.8%
70–79	44/213	20.6%
80–89	12/50	24%

Table 2. Testosterone deficiency in different age groups.

On the basis of the TDI ratio, testosterone deficiency has been found in 49.55% of those in the study group. The smaller number of patients who had TDI determined is due to the absence of the ratio of LH for 48 out of 1267 patients. Summary of parameters to provide a basic index of the Andropause status for 1219 patients is shown in Table 3.

Parameter n = 1219 pts
T (ng/mL)
Min., max. = 0.58; 15.41 Average (SD)= 5.22 (2.33) Median (25%, 75%) = 4.78 (3.59; 6.48)
LH (IU/L)
Min., max. = 0.2; 47 Average (SD) = 5.8 (4.6) Median (25%, 75%) = 4.8 (3.3; 6.7)
T/LH
Min., max. = 0.02; 41.76 Average (SD) = 1.36 (1.67) Median (25%, 75%) = 1 (0.63; 1.61)
TDI < 1 = 604/1219 (49.55%)

T – testosterone; LH – luteinizing hormone; SD – standard deviation; TDI – testosterone deficit index.

Table 3. Average serum testosterone concentrations , LH and TDI

The findings in Table 4 show, on the basis of the TDI ratio, an increased incidence of testosterone deficiency with age.

Age	TDI < 1
20–29	21/78 (28%)
30–39	29/101 (28.7%)
40–49	56/165 (33.9%)
50–59	160/355 (45.1%)
60–69	174/271 (64.2%)
70–79	124/197 (62.9%)
80–89	38/47 (80.85%)

Table 4. Testosterone deficiency in different age groups for 1219 male respondents, calculated on the basis of TDI.

Two methods of assessing testosterone deficiency have been compared, based on global standards and on TDI. Figures 2 and 3 show the material discussed above under analysis. In the group of 1267 patients, there were only 274 males with serum testosterone concentrations levels below 12 nmol/L, which amounts to 21.62% of those examined, whereas, in accordance with TDI standards, 604 out of 1219 men had testosterone deficiency, which amounts to 49.55% of those examined. The observed difference between the groups is statistically significant.

If we put on the two graphs (Figure 2 and Figure 3) the lines connecting testosterone level in young men when they have the highest testosterone level (i.e., 30-39 year olds), it turns out that the testosterone deficit estimation results in accordance with the standardised testosterone-below-12-nmol/l approach are different from those in accordance with TDI standards. As shown in Figure 2, in accordance with the most rigorous standards of serum testosterone concentration, men aged 60-70 years have been diagnosed with testosterone

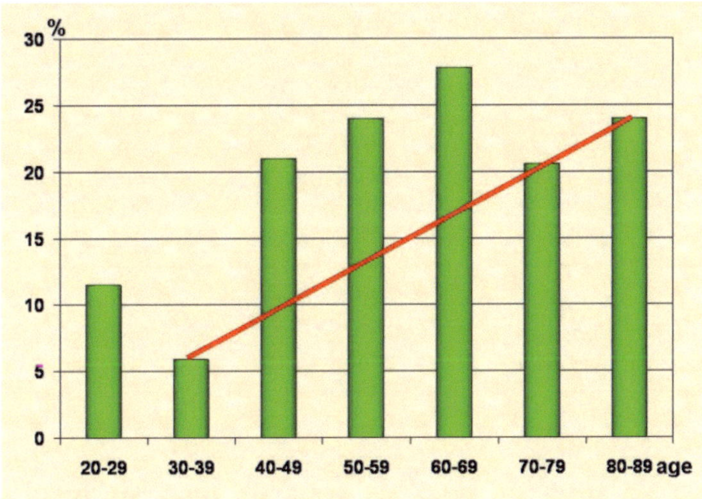

Fig. 2. Testosterone levels below 12 nmol/L in relation to age.

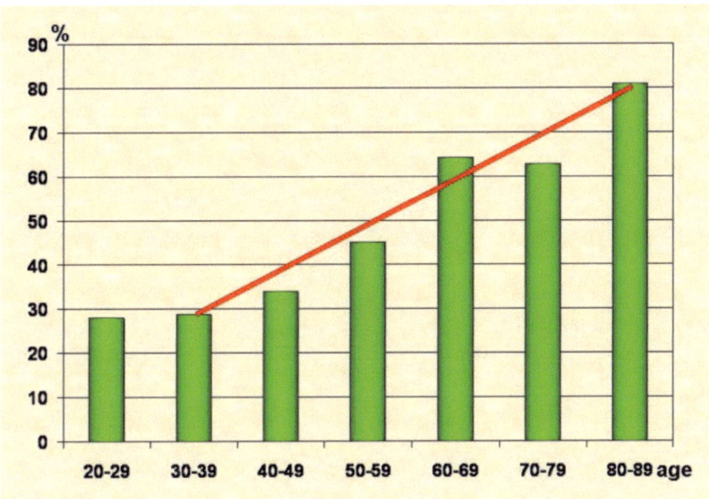

Fig. 3. TDI (Testosterone Deficit Index) in relation to age.

deficiency, while testosterone deficiency levels have clearly been lower in the age group 70-79 years and in the age group 80-89 years. An assessment in accordance with the testosterone-concentrations-below-12-nmol/L parameter exhibits significant deviations. It shows that, as men age, testosterone deficiency does not increase in a linear fashion. However, Figure 3 shows that the analysis of the same material on the basis of the testosterone deficiency index (TDI) demonstrates that, as men age, testosterone deficiency increases in a linear fashion. The study proves the effectiveness of the testosterone deficiency index (TDI) in assessing the degree of testosterone deficiency. On the basis of the TDI results and/or on the basis of a patient's clinical status, 903 of those examined were involved in testosterone endosynthesis induction treatment with human chorionic gonadotropin /hCG/ (Gould, 1951, Gomula, 2001, Gomula, 2002). Testosterone levels in response to hCG treatment are shown in Table 5, and graphically in Figure 4.

Age	T-0 nmol/L	T-1 nmol/L	Change	p
20-29	n=44	n=44	n=44	
Min., max. Average (SD) Median (25%, 75%)	6.2, 49.1 21.13 (9.7) 19.7 (14.05, 24.55)	20.30, 89.10 44.03 (13.45) 44.05 (34.70, 51.15)	1.5, 42.2 22.9 (10.9) 23.55 (14.35, 30.9)	<0.001
30–39	n = 63	n = 63	n = 63	
Min., max. Average (SD) Median (25%, 75%)	8.9; 46,8 21.78 (8.31) 21.7 (15.9; 24)	20.50; 96.20 49.62 (16.12) 46.80 (37.60; 60.40)	3.9; 63.6 27.8 (13.5) 28.9 (16.6; 35.7)	
40–49	n = 131	n = 131	n = 131	
Min., max. Average (SD) Median (25%, 75%)	6.3; 46.6 18.5 (8.47) 16.5 (12.3; 23.6)	11.40; 78.20 41.72 (14.36) 39.60 (31.60; 50.50)	2.1; 58.5 23.2 (12.09) 23.13 (13.8; 32.6)	< 0.001
50–59	n = 277	n = 277	n = 277	
Min., max. Average (SD) Median (25%, 75%)	3.1; 46.4 17.14 (7.72) 15.7 (11.9; 20.5)	10.30; 78.30 39.23 (12.63) 38.50 (29.80; 46.20)	4.9; 62.6 22.08 (11.7) 20.1 (13.7; 29.6)	< 0.001
60–69	n = 205	n = 205	n = 205	
Min., max. Average (SD) Median (25%, 75%)	2.71; 40.4 15.59 (6.45) 14.4 (10.8; 19.1)	7.50; 82.30 34.48 (13.32) 32.30 (24.70; 41.90)	4.3, 69.2 18.9 (11,.9) 16.8 (10.6; 25)	< 0.001
70–79	n = 154	n = 154	n = 154	
Min., max. Average (SD) Median (25%, 75%)	2.71; 45.6 17.09 (7.5) 15.15 (12.5; 19.9)	6.80; 89 34.08 (14.83) 32 (23.50; 42.70)	7.2; 59 16.99 (13.32) 15.6 (6.3; 24.2)	< 0.001
80–89	n = 29	n = 29	n = 29	
Min., max. Average (SD) Median (25%, 75%)	3.7; 27.8 14.39 (5.43) 14.8 (12; 17.6)	11,50; 48,50 27.10 (10.36) 24.50 (18.80; 35.40)	4.9; 29.6 12.72 (9.86) 12.4 (5.4; 19)	< 0.001

Table 5. Testosterone concentration before (T-0) and during hCG treatment (T-1) in different age groups.

Using Student's t-test or the Wilcoxon rank-sum test, it has been examined whether the testosterone concentration change is significantly different from 0. Statistically significant results have been achieved both for the whole group and when broken down by age group.

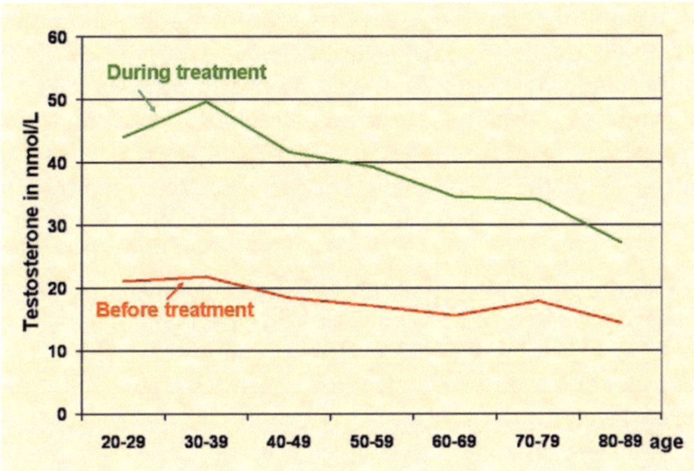

Fig. 4. Testosterone levels in different age groups before (the lower, red line) and during hCG treatment (the upper, green line).

Testosterone concentrations in different age groups have risen for 908 patients under hormone therapy (testosterone endosynthesis induction treatment through the administration of hCG) by an average of between 88 percent and 128 percent. At the same time, it has been found that under hCG stimulation the prospects of endosynthesis decrease linearly with age in the age group 30-89 years. This is consistent with physiology (Figure 5). The prospects of testosterone endosynthesis decrease with age. The age group 30-39 years had an average 128% increase in testosterone levels; the age group 40-49 years - an average 126% increase in testosterone levels; the age group 50-59 years - an average 129% increase in testosterone levels; the age group 60-69 years - an average 121% increase in testosterone levels; the age group 70-79 years - an average 99% increase in testosterone levels; the age group 80-99 years - an average 88% increase in testosterone levels. The full range of values of parameters determining the prospects of testosterone endosynthesis in different age groups has been shown in Table 5.

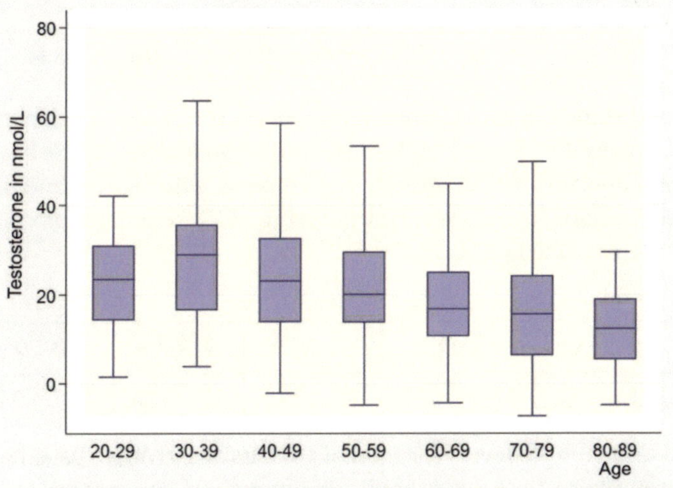

Fig. 5. The prospects of testosterone endosynthesis in different age groups.

On the basis of the findings of the analysis of testosterone concentrations that occur physiologically, without treatment, during testosterone endosynthesis stimulation, it was decided to measure standard physiological testosterone levels correlated with age. During testosterone endosynthesis stimulation, testosterone concentrations obtained ade it possible for the patients to exhibit significantly better mood ratings, to develop improved physical fitness, and to increase libido and potency. The testosterone concentrations obtained also had the following positive impacts on blood pressure and biochemical parameters: normalization of the lipid profile and the reduction in HbA1c levels. Therefore, the testosterone concentrations obtained were adopted as normative in different age groups. Standard deviations of testosterone level increase while inducing testosterone endosynthesis by administering hCG varies by age group. This situation has been taken into account in measuring standard testosterone levels in different age groups. It has been assumed that normal testosterone levels in a particular age group is a number between the highest average value of testosterone while inducing testosterone endosynthesis by administering hCG and one standard deviation in the age group. These standards are illustrated graphically in Figure 6, and entered in Table 6.

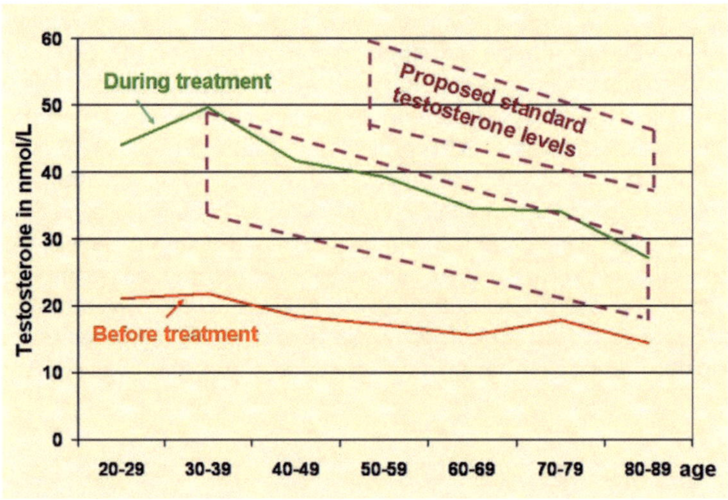

Fig. 6. The proposed standard testosterone levels for men of various age groups, based on the physiological capabilities caused by testosterone endosynthesis. The bottom line - the serum testosterone concentration in different age groups, prior to treatment; top line - testosterone concentrations in each age group during hCG treatment; box - proposed age-related standard testosterone levels.

Age	30-39 y	40-49 y	50-59 y	60-69 y	70-79 y	80-89 y
T (nmol/lL)	33.5 ÷ 49.6	27.3 ÷ 41.7	26.6÷39.2	21 ÷ 34.4	19.2 ÷ 34.0	16.7 ÷ 27.1

Table 6. Standard testosterone levels for men of various age groups, based on the analysis of potential testosterone endosynthesis capabilities among 908 patients treated by inducing testosterone endosynthesis by administration of hCG.

A very important question arises: if testosterone levels are so high, as the authors propose, are they not harmful? However, since these concentrations have been obtained by endosynthesis, it is obvious that they are in accordance with the body's physiological ability to synthesize testosterone. In addition, it has been known for more than 20 years that long-term high-dose testosterone therapy does not give significant metabolic side effects (Matsumoto, 1990). The correct threshold for proper testosterone functioning and for proper testosterone effects also increases with age (Schiavi, et al., 1993). Therefore the proposed age-related standards for testosterone must be much higher than those observed previously. A retrospective analysis of material possessed has suggested that the hormonal balance in today's young men is significantly worse than the hormonal balance for their fathers when they were in their youth. It has been shown in fact that the total testosterone level in today's young men is roughly two-thirds of their fathers' testosterone level. If we draw a line in parallel with the decline in serum testosterone levels with age for the age group of 35 to 70 years, and then draw it backwards, from the age of 90 to the earlier years, it will appear that the fathers, aged 30-35, exhibited significantly higher testosterone levels than their descendants at comparable ages (Fig. 7).

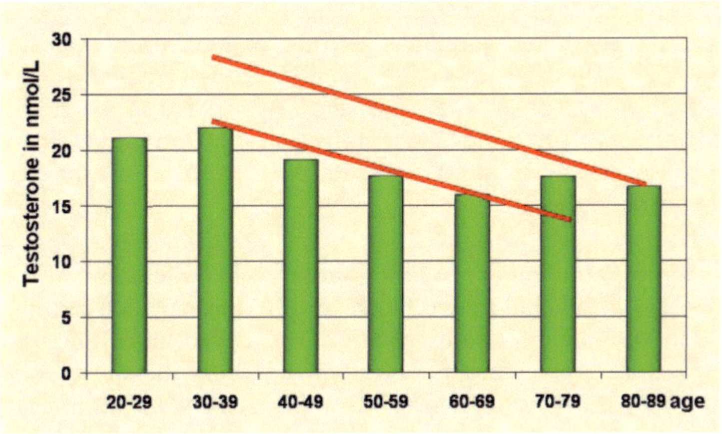

Fig. 7. Concentrations of testosterone in men aged 20-90 years and the line aptly showing their fathers' testosterone levels in the past.

Figure 7 shows that the concentration of testosterone in today's young men aged 30-35 is, on average, 23 nmol/L Concentrations of testosterone of their ancestors aged 85-89 averaged 17.2 nmol/L Therefore, standard values in the testosterone concentration range - the dispersion of values previously ranging to 31 nmol/L- have now narrowed to such an extent that the difference in testosterone levels between younger and older men is only 5 nmol/L i.e. 16% of normal range 10-42 nmol/L It practically means that young men now have testosterone levels about 35% lower than those of their ancestors. Therefore, it can be concluded that, on the one hand, the whole world population is aging. On the other hand, the biological condition of today's youth suggests that in such a metabolic-hormonal state the youth of today will not increase human life expectancy. It is highly likely that they will die at a much younger age than their ancestors did in the past. The reasons for these changes are more complex. Genetic factors, lifestyle habits, medications, toxins, free radicals, body weight, psychological and social aspects, chronic stress, mental health, and social position play a significant role.

3. Late - onset hypogonadism and other diseases

Testosterone levels in maturing man peak around age of 30 and then start to decline slowly. This decline in serum testosterone of aging men can lead to the development of many diseases (e.g. hypertension, ischemic heart disease etc.). The metabolic syndrome (defined as a combination of lipid abnormalities and cardiovascular risk factors), abdominal obesity, insulin resistance, arterial hypertension or raised blood pressure, are also associated with testosterone deficiency (Kalyani & Dobs, 2007). All men are at risk for erectile dysfunction and prostate diseases including Benign Prostatic Hyperplasia (BPH) and Prostate Cancer (PC), which occur in later years of life of men. Additionally, Alzheimer's disease and Parkinson's disease are both common in the elderly men, especially in those over 85. Low testosterone levels − a risk factor for development of visceral obesity − are associated with an acute decrease in circulating HDL cholesterol and increase of triglycerides. There may be a link between low testosterone levels in males and type 2 diabetes with elevated insulin levels. Some of these problems are due to the concentrations of total and free testosterone but there are also those that are associated with the derivatives of persistent testosterone deficiency. Late onset hypogonadism may result in the metabolic syndrome frequently leading to diabetes and/or to accelerated heart disease. When testosterone hormones in our body are balanced, the symptoms disappear. An increase in serum testosterone, results in normalization of lipid profile, improves glucose tolerance, decreases HbA1c, and produces the increase in bone mass observed in densitometry. Pharmacological correction of hormones results in marked improvements in the sexual health (increasing both libido and potency), removes depression symptoms, and reduces or completely removes all symptoms of BPH and of Parkinson's disease.

3.1 Late - onset hypogonadism is not just testosterone deficiency

So far the aging process and clinical and biochemical changes which cause aging have been linked to reduction in testosterone concentration. This approach is, however, too simplistic. Testosterone is the direct precursor to estradiol, which is the most potent endogenous estrogen, and to many other hormone derivatives which have a significant impact on the normal structure and on the function of the human body. Therefore therapy to increase testosterone is inextricably linked with estradiol supplementation. Here special attention should be paid to the fact that not all preparations of testosterone can be converted to estradiol and to other derivatives, which makes such supplementation seem not to improve, but, sometimes, to make the situation worse. Estrogen affects the skeletal bone and cardiovascular systems in many radical ways. The decline in estrogen is associated with osteoporosis, premature atherosclerosis, marked risk of myocardial infarction, and with loss of bone mass (Gooren & Bunck, 2004).

While testosterone can act directly on cells, it can also be converted to dihydroxytestosterone (DHT) by 5α-reductase. The same chemical reaction occurs which converts estradiol to 4-hydroxyestradiol. In addition to hormonal effects, this compound has the peculiarity of saturation binding for dopamine receptors widely distributed in the brain. If one compares the chemical structure of dopamine with that of 4-hydroxyestradiol, it is possible to find the key to the dopamine receptor − a benzene ring with two hydroxyl groups attached to the ring − which can be seen in Figure 8.

Dopamine receptors saturation in human brain has some very important implications of many physiological and pathological states. Dopamine deficiency causes Parkinson's disease. Dopamine plays a crucial role in our mental health. Also, male sexual fitness is closely related to hormonal balance nd especially to dopamine and 4-hydroxyestradiol. Outlined below are some of the entities associated with testosterone deficit or with the deficit of testosterone derivatives.

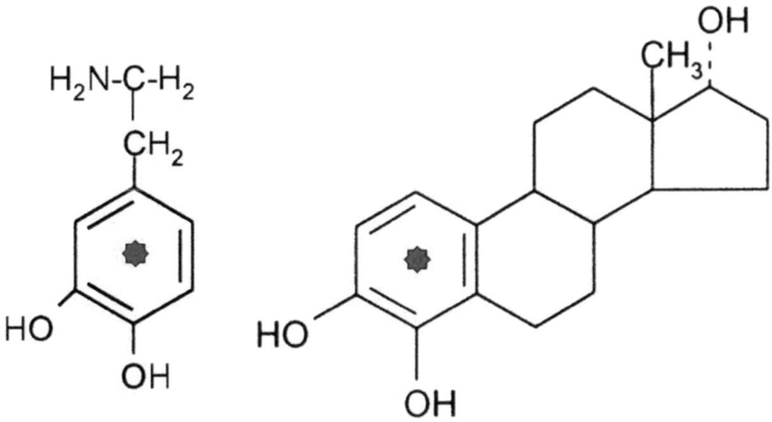

Dopamine 4-hydroxyestradiol

Fig. 8. The dopamine structure and the 4-hydroxyestradiol structure.

3.2 Late - onset hypogonadism and type 2 diabetes

Clinical trial results have shown that men with type 2 diabetes have a significantly greater testosterone deficiency (Zitzmann & Nieschlag, 2006). In a large population study of subjects aged over 20, men with total testosterone levels in the lowest quartile and men with free testosterone in the lowest quartile had a 4-fold higher prevalence of diabetes compared with men with testosterone levels in the first quartile /$p = 0.04$/ (Muller et al., 2005). Metabolic syndrome, defined as a combination of lipid disorders and cardiovascular risk factors: abdominal obesity, insulin resistance, and arterial hypertension, also increases the risk for late onset hypogonadism ((Kalyani & Dobs, 2007). In my own research, out of 1200 men with late onset hypogonadism treated with hCG, more than 10 percent had diabetes. Raising the serum testosterone levels in these patients as a result of hCG therapy significantly improved glucose tolerance. Increasing testosterone levels, the average level of output being 18.3 nmol/L-38.6 nmol/L, resulted in a reduction of HbA1c by an average of 1.75% ($p<0.001$). This effect is shown graphically in Figure 9.

Normalization of HbA1c followed in the not-previously-treated diabetic group, as well as in the group of patients taking their medication without changing the dose. In some patients previously treated for diabetes, at the time of hCG administration, it was necessary to lower the dose or even to discontinue antidiabetic therapy. Among patients without known diabetes (HbA1c<6.0%), as a result of hCG therapy, HbA1c reductions were observed by an average of 0.5%. In patients with diabetes, insulin level was also determined. Average output level was 16.55 mU/L, and with intensified hCG therapy the average calculated insulin level was 7.8 mU/L.

I believe that the term "insulin resistance" is overused. Insulin resistance does not cause diabetes. The inability to metabolize glucose (burn sugar), fully and continually is the cause of type 2 diabetes. An increase in the concentration of the glucose in the extracellular space induces the increase in insulin levels. But insulin does not move sugar into cells when the cell-glucose level is equally high. Acceleration of tissue metabolism after injection of testosterone causes excessively fast burning of glucose, which decreases cell-glucose levels. Then, according to the concentration gradient, glucose enters the cell and this reduces extracellular cell concentrations of glucose. With the reduction of glucose concentration in the extracellular space, blood insulin levels fall below a certain level. Therefore "insulin resistance" does not apply in this case.

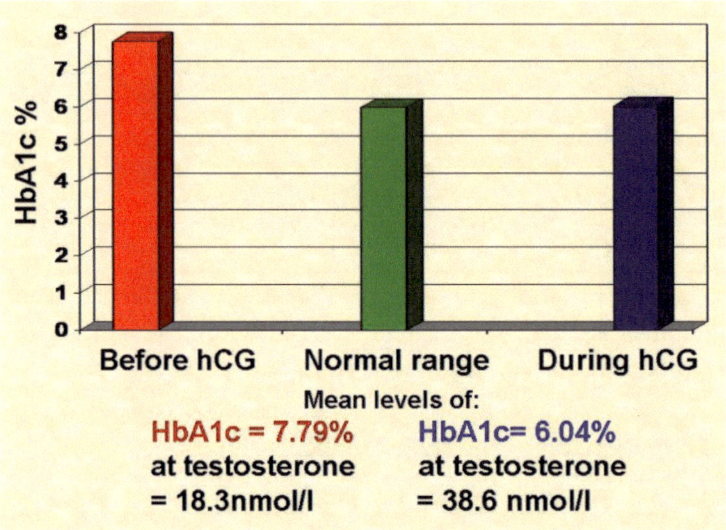

Fig. 9. HbA1c normalization as a result of hCG therapy.

3.3 Late - onset hypogonadism and hyperlipidemia

As men age, there is a dramatic decrease in testosterone production, with a corresponding decrease in the production of estradiol. Excess lipids in the blood lead to atherosclerosis. Cholesterol, which can be very annoying, is in fact absolutely necessary. Too high or too low a concentration thereof has a detrimental effect. LDL cholesterol serves as precursor for the synthesis of steroid hormones. Moreover, every cell in the body requires LDL cholesterol to maintain cell wall integrity. With age, cell turnover is reduced. What is more, there are lower cholesterol production rates to create new cells. An excessive reduction of cholesterol levels in the body results in the deficit of raw materials for cellular renewal and in the deficit in the synthesis of steroid hormones. Various formulations are present in the treatment for hypercholesterolemia. However, hypercholesterolemia can also be normalized only by accelerating the metabolic processes. Anabolic testosterone boost effectively corrects the moderate lipid metabolic disorders. The hCG hormone therapy, which results in a significant increase in testosterone concentration and in E2 concentration (in testosterone level – from 18.3 nmol/L to 38.6 nmol/L; in E2 level – from 138.6 pmol/L to 280.9 pmol/L), improves lipid profile. There is a 15 to 20% decrease in total cholesterol and its fractions. This effect is shown graphically in Figure 10.

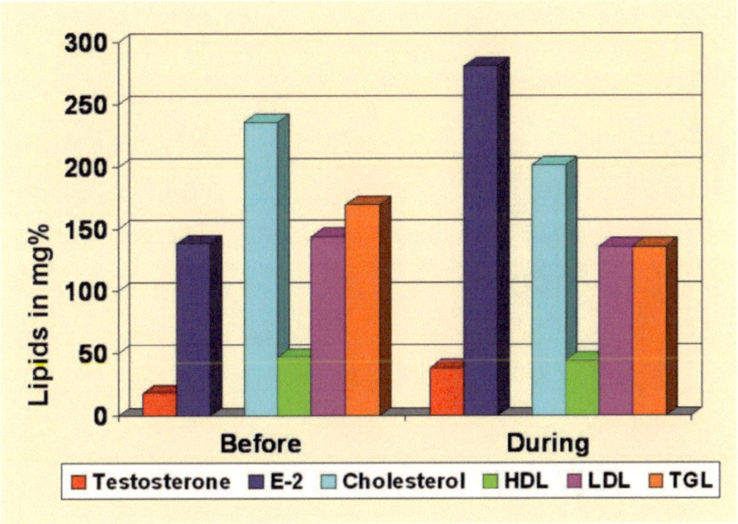

Fig. 10. Improved lipids during HCG-treatment hormonal treatment

3.4 Late - onset hypogonadism and osteoporosis

It is beyond discussion that women have osteoporosis as a direct result of ovarian hormone imbalance. In bone densitometry studies, 90% of those examined are females and only 10% are males; hence the great retardation of male endocrinology and of densitometric diagnosis of osteoporosis in men in relation to the same areas of medicine with regard to women. According to the recommendations of World Health Organisation, a woman should take hormone therapy early enough to avoid dangerous irreversible anatomical changes. What about a man? At puberty male estrogen can affect skeletal growth and bone mineralization. The study of men in the andropause also indicates a relation of estrogen level to bone mineral density (Riggs, et al. 2002). Studies have shown that two-thirds of the effects of testosterone replacement therapy (particularly with regard to increase in bone mineral) are due to excessive estrogen levels in aromatization of testosterone (Khosla, et al., 1998, Leder, et al., 2003). There is a clear relationship between the amount of androgens (bioavailable testosterone) and estrogens (bioavailable estradiol E2). In a large-scale study (data from 2623 men over 65, enjoying good health) levels of free and bioavailable testosterone and bioavailable estradiol levels correlated. Low levels of bioavailable estradiol were associated with age and with osteoporosis (Orwoll, et al. 2006). In our own panel of 1200 patients, it was found that raising man's testosterone levels to the values recommended for a given age was simultaneously accompanied by the increase of estradiol level. This caused the incorporation of calcium into bones, without any additional classical treatment of osteoporosis. The hormonal therapy used was to induce endogenous testosterone synthesis by human chorionic gonadotrophin (hCG). Please find below a depiction of the effects. A two year hCG therapy in a patient aged 60 years increased the bone density by 6.7% (Figure 11 and Figure 12); and a long-term therapy could help restore bone density to that of a fine young man. Figure 13 shows densitometric data of the chapter's author (age 62y). Bone density of a fine young man – Young Ref (%) = 92.7; bone density with reference to age – Age Match (%) = 118.1 Z-Score = 1.26)

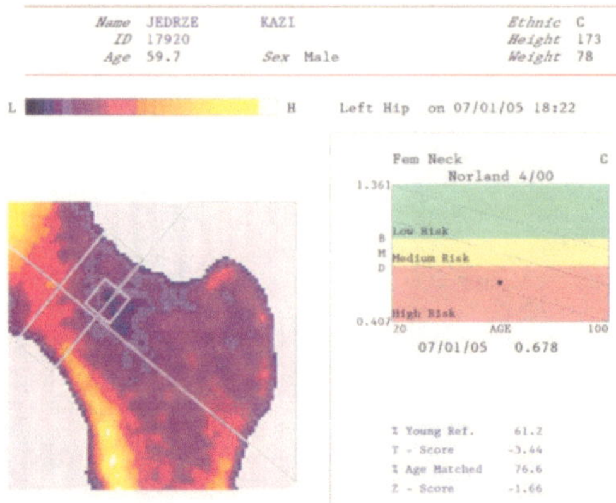

Fig. 11.

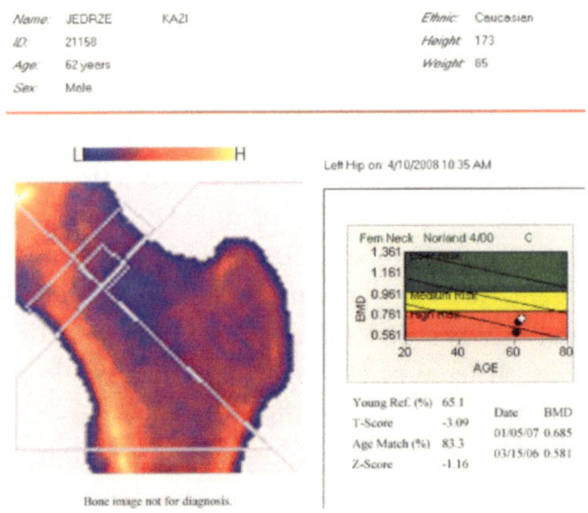

Fig. 12.

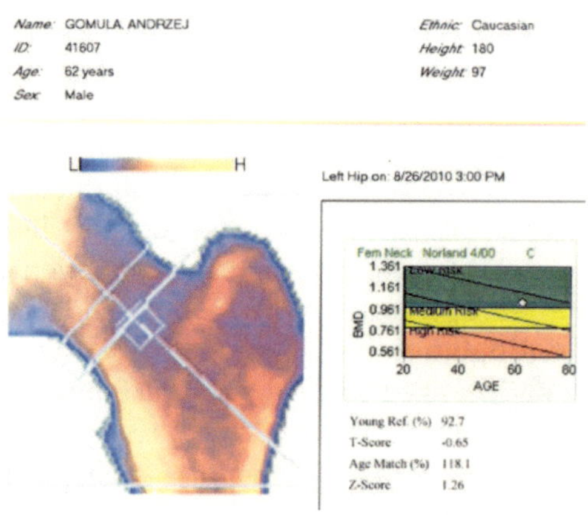

Fig. 13.

3.5 Late - onset hypogonadism, chronic prostatitis, BPH and prostate cancer

It should come as no surprise to anyone that chronic prostatitis, benign prostatic hyperplasia (BPH), and prostate cancer (PC) are consequences of hormonal deficits. Prostate-specific antigen (PSA), a marker that has been used for many years in early prostate cancer detection, turned out to be less than 100% accurate to diagnose prostate malignancy. PSA was originally supposed to be a unique marker for prostate cancer. It was supposed to be just what its name implies - a specific marker. Over the past few decades an enormous amount of material has been written about the role of PSA in diagnosis of prostate cancer. Doctors started to use other PSA values - such as PSA velocity, PSA density, and percent-free PSA - to get a more accurate idea of what was happening within the prostate. When the PSA reaches or exceeds the level of 0.5 ng/mL, it is strongly recommended to take all-out diagnostic measures, in order to ascertain the absence of PC (Gould, et al., 2006). Practically in such cases, the biopsy of the prostate should be done. After a prostate biopsy, the PSA continues to rise, so the biopsy is repeated. This method often cannot give definite confirmation of prostate cancer, which has been the first dilemma. The other dilemma: what if the blood tests detect much lower levels of PSA? What if the reduction amounts to 2-3 fold? Long-term clinical experience shows that a sudden significant increase in PSA level is possible with any surgery, after virus infection regardless of its location, or with regard to a severe exacerbation of chronic inflammatory diseases. A sudden increase in one's PSA level should not escape the attention, but it is not equivalent to the occurrence or the development of prostate cancer. Changes in the PSA levels may be the consequence of the high levels of prostaglandins, which induce non-specific inflammations of the prostate usually seen in urine samples under a microscope.

Harbitz stated over 30 years ago that male gonadal dysfunction (endocrine testicular failure) leads to adenomas and to the prostate cancer (Harbitz & Haugen, 1974). It is an undeniable fact that testosterone levels peak in a man at approximately age 30, but this does not yet cause BPH or prostate cancer. And the older the man, and the greater the chances of testosterone deficiency, the higher the prevalence of benign prostatic hyperplasia and of PC. It can no longer be doubted, questioned, whether BPH and PC are closely related to the hormonal changes in men, and practically to testosterone deficiency.

There are publications, which say that there was never any association between testosterone treatment, when subjects were all healthy men, and the increase of prostate volume and serum PSA level. They also say that in the treatment of men with hypogonadism, the therapy led to moderate prostate enlargement and to a 15% increase in PSA (Algarte-Genin, et al., 2004, Behre, et al., 1994, Gould & Kirby, 2006). Among my own 1200 patients under treatment for hypogonadism, more than two-fold increase in endogenous testosterone concentrations after 37 months of hCG therapy resulted in a 40% decrease in their PSA levels. The aforementioned decrease is closely related not only to concentration of testosterone, but to the level of estradiol, which stimulates LHRH mRNA synthesis and increases pituitary LH synthesis. Testosterone deficiency does not cause prostate pathology. However, the losses of testosterone and long-term E2 deficiency result in the situation in which the hypothalamus and pituitary gland can become prostate's greatest enemies. Therefore, modern hormonal medications used to treat BPH have self-stimulation points in the lateral hypothalamus (Oesterling, 1991, Reissmann, et al., 2000, Debruyne, et al., 2008).

3.5.1 Late - onset hypogonadism, BPH and chronic prostatitis

The symptoms of BPH are practically only recognized when there are irreversible anatomical changes in the prostate, causing LUTS. Patients with BPH often see the doctor when they already have symptoms of LUTS. Meanwhile, the symptoms of chronic prostatitis will be in place long before that. Antibiotic or other medications are rather ineffective in those patients and the hormone therapy can help to relieve clinical symptoms. The effects of hormonal disbalance, including testosterone deficiency, can be seen on transabdominal and transrectal ultrasound scans.

If hypoechoic areas in the transition zone of the prostate (marked with dots in Figures 14÷17) are noted in ultrasound, it is a common sign of deficient testosterone levels. Such changes are occasionally described as inflammation and are not paid due attention to.

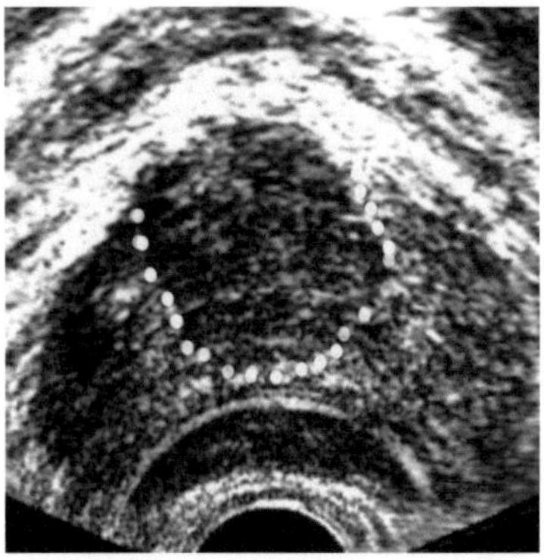

Fig.14.

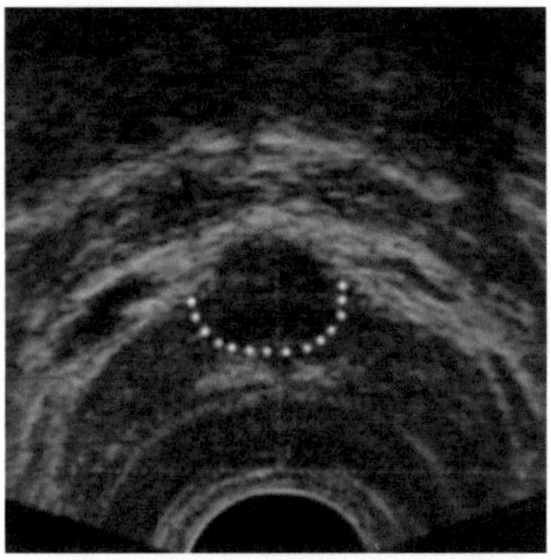

Fig. 15.

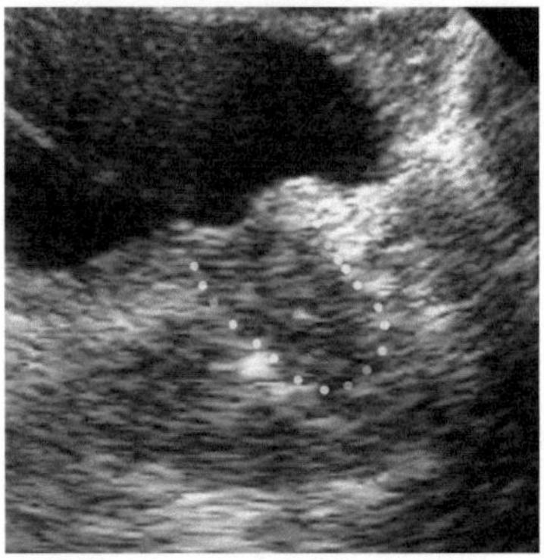

Fig. 16.

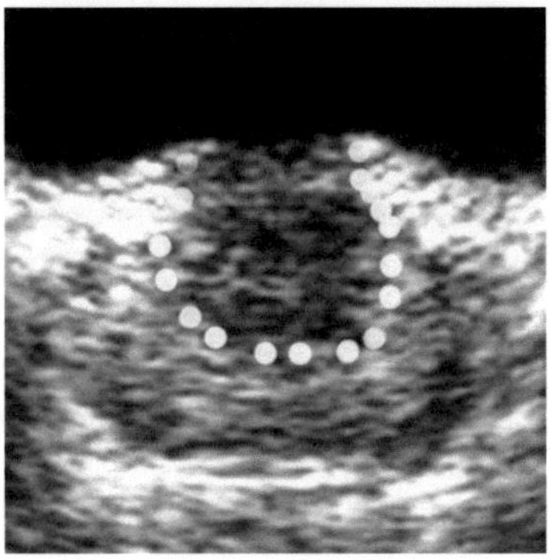

Fig. 17.

Figure 14.÷17. Ultrasound scan images of the prostate of testosterone deficiency patients. Figure 14 & 15. Transrectal ultrasonography. Figure 16 & 17. Abdominal examination. Hypoechoic area marked by dots.

In my 30 years of being an urologist, I have treated hundreds of men diagnosed with prostatitis by other physicians. Antibiotics treatment could last several weeks or even months. Worst of all, it was not effective. Treatment with hCG led to the freedom from symptoms within 1-3 weeks. These symptoms were associated with the spread of prostate adenoma which, as it can lift the bladder, causes prostate inflammation symptoms. During hCG therapy, there is a reduction in adenoma, as demonstrated by MRI (Figures 18÷20).

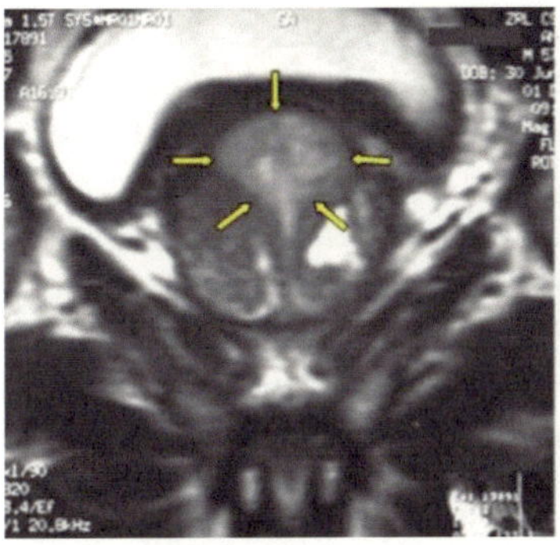
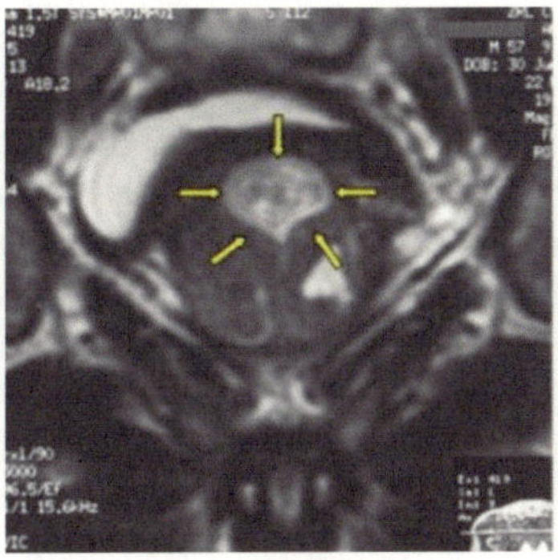
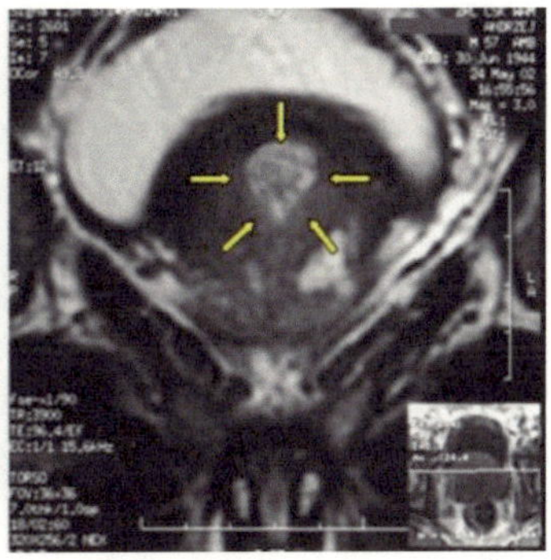

Fig. 18. Fig. 19. Fig. 20.

Fig. 18. – 20. Prostate MRI before hCG therapy (Fig. 18), after 3 months of hCG therapy (Fig. 19), and after 6 months of hCG therapy (Fig. 20). Arrows indicate regions of prostate adenoma – hyperplasia of the transition zone – which as a result of hCG treatment was markedly reduced.

Some experts now recommend alpha-blockers and hormones as first-line treatment for patients with moderate to severe BPH symptoms. It must be emphatically stated that alpha-blockers therapy appears to have no effect on the disease; it does not hinder its development; it only mitigates symptoms of BPH and facilitates urination. But after using alpha-blockers for a number of years adenoma can enlarge to the extent that surgical treatment becomes necessary. At the same time, there will be irreversible pathological changes of the bladder wall, which disrupt the normal function thereof. Thus, alpha-blockers do not solve the problem of treatment for BPH.

In hormonal therapy of BPH the agents used are: 1.- 5α-reductase inhibitors, and 2. - drugs, which inhibit LH synthesis or LHRH synthesis.

Ad. 1. 5-alpha reductase inhibitors block the conversion of testosterone to dihydroxytestosterone. Their effectiveness in the management of BPH is debatable. Laurie Barclay, MD (Pfizer), issued a statement used in Pfizer commercial that Finasteride was no better than placebo in treating BPH symptoms. In fact, 5 alpha reductase inhibitors may cause hot flashes, decreased libido and impotence (Oesterling, 1991).

In my opinion, this drug works, but its metabolic and functional consequences mean that the balance of potential profit versus loss can be harmful for men. Therefore I have not been using 5 alpha reductase inhibitors in the treatment of BPH.

Ad. 2. In the treatment of BPH, other drugs have been used as well to decrease LH synthesis for more than 20 years. This effect has been achieved by LHRH analogues or LHRH agonists (Oesterling, 1991, Reissmann, et al., 2000, Debruyne, et al., 2008). This therapy, however, has significant disadvantages. It blocks testosterone endosynthesis, which leads to metabolic and functional complications. A fundamental question arises: What kind of man will deprive himself of potency and disrupt his normal body chemistry and metabolism in order to improve the health of his prostate? And so, shall we provide such a treatment, if it can block LH synthesis, and, while at the same time, more than a twofold increase in testosterone undoubtedly can positively affect the biology of man?

3.5.2 LOH and prostate cancer

Half a century ago arose the bizarre notion that testosterone was really dangerous and that it could cause prostate cancer. Years later, it became clear that there was no credible scientific basis for the claim that high levels of testosterone accelerated development of prostate cancer. In fact, the opposite is true (Bonczyk, et al., 2008). The theory that testosterone may stimulate the growth of prostate cancer originates from 1941 when Huggins and Hodges reported that carcinoma was androgen-dependent. They demonstrated the importance of lowering testosterone levels in prostate cancer progression. Huggins and Hodges won the 1966 Nobel Peace Prize for their groundbreaking work revealing that castration causes regression of prostate cancer; while testosterone may cause its progression (Huggins & Hodges, 1941). It is now known that a multiplicity of data contradict Huggins and Hodges's contention that testosterone accelerates prostate cancer growth. Apparently it was negligent misinterpretation of one patient observation (Morgentaler, 2006). And they won the Nobel Prize. This caused a distorted look at the testosterone-prostate cancer link over the last half century. Even 15 years ago in Poland, testosterone was considered a carcinogen by Polish Ministry of Health and Social Welfare (Official Law Daily, 1996). There is no evidence that among men with prostate cancer, serum testosterone concentration is higher than in the rest of the population. On the other hand, low testosterone values coexisting with prostate cancer are associated with worse prognosis, a lower degree of differentiation, and a higher degree of severity of cancer (Morgentaler, 2006, Yano, et al., 2007). Moreover, there is no convincing evidence showing the effect of testosterone on the development of pre-cancerous prostate condition. Rhoden et al. determined that the risk of the development of prostate cancer in hypogonadal patients receiving testosterone, with and without accompanying HG-PIN, does not increase with hormone therapy. After twelve months, the risk was 1,2% in men without HG-PIN, and 5% in men with HGPIN detected. The aforementioned values do not exceed those in the general population (Rhoden & Morgentaler, 2003). At the same time, one can find statements that there are two classic contraindications for the administration of testosterone, namely suspected or histologically proven prostate cancer and symptomatic benign prostatic hyperplasia (Montorsi, 2007). While I understand precautions that most men with prostate cancer should avoid testosterone therapy, even though I use it for my patients, a total ban on the use of testosterone to treat BPH appears to be an anachronism.

25 years ago, Fowler and Whitmore proposed the concept of "saturation" in order to explain the relationship between prostate cancer and serum testosterone levels. It explains why the increase in serum testosterone levels in patients treated with that hormone does not cause the disease (Fowler & Whitmore, 1981). The correctness of this concept is confirmed by observations of patients, despite treatment with T, there was no increase in PSA or prostate volume. In men suffering from hypogonadism the treatment did not lead to excessive growth in prostate size, and it led to an only 15% increase in PSA (Algarte-Genin, et al., 2004, Gould & Kirby, 2006). Currently, it is believed that exogenous testosterone treatment in patients with PC, which does not follow androgen ablation, should not worsen prognosis of cancer (Bonczyk, et al., 2008). It has long been feared that the Late Onset Hypogonadism (LOH) treatment by administering testosterone may increase the risk of high-grade prostate cancer. Numerous studies show that there is no PSA increase during testosterone therapy. Among my own 1200 patients under treatment for hypogonadism, more than two-fold increase in endogenous testosterone concentrations after 37 months of hCG therapy resulted in a 40% decrease in their PSA levels. In each age group – and the older the man, the more severe it is – there are patients who present insufficient endosynthesis, but they constitute only a few percent of total number of patients. During the extended follow-up of these patients, it has been found that 14% of

them have had some form of prostate cancer within 3 to 36 months. The results clearly show that there is a greater decrease in endogenous testosterone synthesis, but at the same time there is an increased risk of prostate cancer. The patients in question had very high LH/PSA ratio. Therefore prostate cancer is not caused by testosterone, but, to the contrary, it is a consequence of the development of testosterone deficiency. Moreover, there is a correlation between testosterone levels and the degree of PC malignancy (Hoffman, et al., 2000). It has been known for years that patients diagnosed with prostate cancer and with high Gleason scores, have lower than normal levels of testosterone. Lower testosterone levels result in greater PC malignancy (Schatzl, et al., 2001). Patients with high Gleason score prostate cancer have lower testosterone and estradiol serum levels.
There is also no evidence that men with prostate cancer have a much higher testosterone concentration than the normal population. On the other hand, low testosterone values found in men with prostate cancer are associated with poorer prognosis, with a lower degree of differentiation of PC, and with a higher degree of PC severity (Hoffman, et al., 2000, Morgentaler, 2006, Yano, et al., 2007). In men treated with testosterone, prostate cancer was detected in biopsies of 1% of patients, while in men with the prevalence of hypogonadism – in 14.3%. There are some reports that testosterone therapy may reduce the risk of prostate cancer (Fowler & Whitmore, 1981, Prout & Brewer, 1967). Only some reports, because who would dare to publish anything incompatible with the study by Nobel laureates?

3.6 Late - onset hypogonadism, sexual drive, potency and libido

For many years, we have been reassured that only androgens have a key role in both stimulating and maintaining sexual function in men. It was believed that testosterone and the existence of a normal level of libido were inseparably connected (Shabsigh, 2003, Morales, et al., 2004). Nevertheless, sexual dysfunction in men is directly associated not only with testosterone but also with estradiol (E-2) and with other neurohormonal factors. Erectile dysfunction was linked to the development of benign prostatic hyperplasia (BPH), without even taking into account the fact that both benign prostatic hyperplasia (BPH) and erectile dysfunction (ED) were often caused by the hormone deficit. The effects of women's hormone replacement therapy on their psychological and sexual functioning are still the subject of the research in the borderline field between medicine and psychology. Female hormone therapy in treating menopause is common around the world. Meanwhile, several years ago it was stated that the effects of this therapy on men were not known. Hormone replacement therapy for men has been lagging for at least 20 years compared with hormone replacement therapy in women (Tenover, 1999). There is a decline in testosterone production in elderly men that can lead to a decrease in sexual desire (Kaufman & T'Sjoen, 2002). Androgen therapy can stop and even reverse this degenerating process (Hajjar, et al., 1997, Morales, et al., 2004). Information on the importance of testosterone in male sexuality is often divergent. It is known that surgical and pharmacological castration leads to impotence. On the other hand, it is recognized that testosterone deficiency is considered to be of little importance in the development of erectile dysfunction or in life force. (Anderson, 2003, Montorsi et al., 2003).
There was no sexual orientation change in men who underwent surgical castration. Sexual desire was preserved by the majority of the patients, but interest in sex decreased, which was associated with decreased frequency/intensity of orgasms (Zverina, et al., 1990). Testosterone replacement therapy suitable for men with primary testicular failure as a result

of surgery conduces to a return to good sexual health and to good psycho-social outcomes (Fossa, et al., 1999). A drop in men's testosterone levels results in reduced libido and sexual potency. The implementation of hormonal therapy in hipogonadal men at the time when testosterone levels increase significantly, approaching the upper limit for normal, causes regular nocturnal erections. It also increases the number of spontaneous erections and it increases sexual activity (Burries, et al., 1992, Tariq, 2002). Other authors also propose that libido is closely tied to testosterone levels and that hormone replacement therapy increases the frequency of sexual thoughts and significantly improves one's libido (Davidson, et al., 1982, Kwan, et al., 1983). Testosterone induces nitric oxide synthesis in vascular endothelium through its influence on arginase activity. This leads to the opening of vascular pathways; facilitates blood flow into the corpora cavernosa; and enhances penile erection. The same mechanism is used in treatment of erectile dysfunction (ED) with PDE-5 inhibitors. It is currently the primary means of treating ED.

However, such treatment might not be effective when there is a decrease in male libido (the decrease being one of the symptoms of andropause) as a result of a decrease in the level of testosterone which is a hormone produced in a man's testicles. The occurrence of erectile dysfunction causes an increase in depression. Meanwhile, the treatment of depression through the introduction of SSRIs (selective serotonin reuptake inhibitors) affects the deterioration of erectile function in a secondary way (Hsu & Shen, 1995, Keller, et al., 1997). Thus, Andropause Erectile Dysfunction Treatment and male depression treatment are often ineffective. It is worth remembering, however, that andropause can start from any age but generally around age 30, a relatively young age, when a man still has some 40 years of life. Erectile dysfunction, especially in young men, has not yet been linked with their hormonal status.

I have found that during hormone therapy my patients are affected by changes in their sexual health. A thorough analysis of the problem became the subject of the doctoral dissertation of one of my assistants (Czyżowska, 2009).

My research on 88 men aged 20-68 years, (mean age 45), clearly shows an increase in testosterone endosynthesis at the time of hCG Hormone Therapy, on average from 17.93 nmil/L to 40.86 nmol/L. At the same time, a significant increase in E-2 was found in those examined, on average from 168.72 pmol/L to the value of 332.44 pmol/L. The change in hormone levels of those examined resulted in a significant improvement in their sexual performance, in libido and in erectile potency, evaluated using the International Index of Erectile Function (IIEF-5) questionnaire. The average value of IIEF-5 before therapy was 13.4 points (SD = 5.0), and during therapy – 19.88 points (SD = 4.3). The data are shown in numbers in Table 7, and graphically in Figures 21÷22.

	Before therapy (average, SD)	During therapy (average, SD)	Significance
Testosterone	17.937 nmol/L, 7.11	40.89 nmol/L, 12.55	$p<0.0001$
Estradiol	168.72 pmol/L, 77.9	332.44 pmol/L, 141.72	$p<0.0001$
IIEF-5	13.4, 5.0	19.876, 4.3	$p<0.001$

Table 7. Average hormone concentrations and the IIEF-5 score before and during treatment

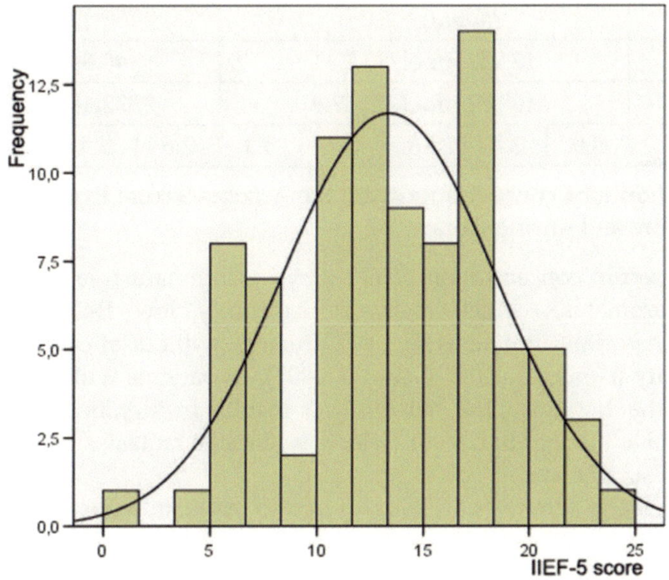

Fig. 21. Average IIEF-5 score before treatment

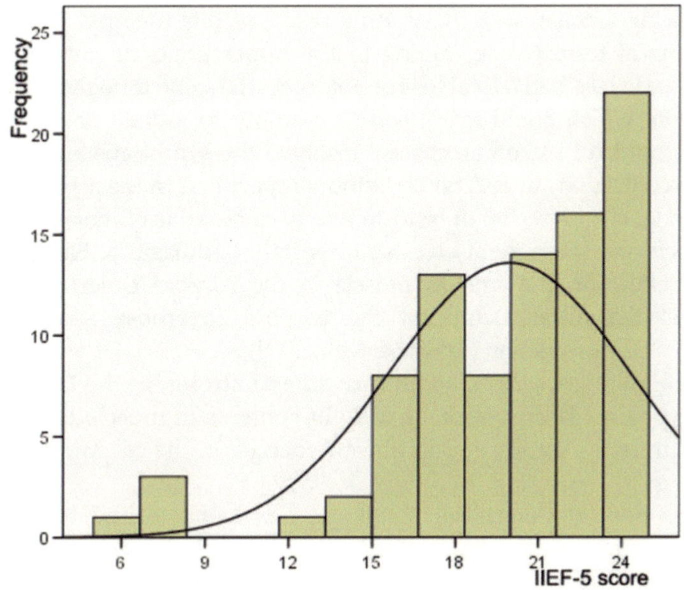

Fig. 22. Average IIEF-5 score during treatment

According to the Arizona Sexual Experiences Scale (ASEX), there was also a significant improvement in sexual health, from an average of 17.39 points (SD=4.24) before treatment to 12.45 points (SD=3.57). The average ASEX values distribution has been shown in Table 8.

	Before therapy (average, SD)					During therapy (average, SD)				
Testosterone	17.937 nmol/L, 7.11					40.89 nmol/L, 12.55				
Estradiol	168.72 pmol/L, 77.9					332.44 pmol/L, 141.72				
Scale – ASEX	3.9	3.4	3.6	3.1	3.3	2.6	2.3	2.6	2.5	2.5

Table 8. Average hormone concentrations and the Arizona Sexual Experiences Scale measurement before and during therapy.

As noted above, serum concentration of E-2 plays a dominant role in male sexual health. Low levels of aromatase, which result in extremely low E-2 concentrations, may, nevertheless, be important in male sexual performance without affecting sexual orientation and gender identity (Gomuła, 2006, Gomuła, 2007). In patients with congenital absence of aromatase only the low-dose E-2 substitution results in significant changes in sexual behavior. Estradiol administration leads to increased erotic fantasies, masturbation or sexual activity Carani, et al., 1999).

My own research clearly shows that E-2 is required to maintain sexual functions in adult men (Gomuła, 2007). The manifestations thereof have been observed after prolonged hormonal therapy. Androgen deficiency patients had their testosterone levels increased for therapeutic purposes. During the therapy, a parallel increase occurred in serum E-2 concentrations, as the effect of the all natural aromatase. Some patients had such high E-2 levels that they exceeded the normal physiological range. In order to reduce E-2 concentration, my patients received preparations blocking aromatase activity. As a result of this therapy, men characterized by high concentrations of testosterone (falling in the upper limits of normal), whose E-2 was detected at very low levels, had a total loss of libido. At the same time those men suffered from erectile dysfunction, which could even lead to inability to initiate or maintain an erection. Stopping the drug which blocked aromatase resolved the symptoms and resulted in a rapid return of high concentrations of E-2. Some authors report that in the activation of male sexual behavior the brain level conversion of testosterone to estradiol is of major importance and that testosterone's effects are not in themselves so important (Balthazar & Ball, 1998). Testosterone has a significant effect on the smooth muscle in the corpora cavernosa. Androgens may significantly affect the ultrastructure of the corpora cavernosa and these changes are responsible for erectile dysfunction (Traish & Kim, 2005).

In young men, the ratio between smooth muscle and stroma in the corpus cavernosum is 1:1. Long-term hypogonadism causes the ratio of contents in muscle tissue to be 1:5, which results in smooth muscle atrophy and in fibrotic changes of the corpora cavernosa (Yassin & Treish, 2004).

Fig. 23 represents normal cavernosal histological appearance and its loss as a result of testosterone deficiency, according to Yassin (Yassin & Treish, 2004).

Androgen replacement can lead especially in hypogonadism patients to recovery process within the trabecular tissue. This result means that testosterone therapy supports the "recovery process" not only in striated muscles in human body /reversible process/ (Yassin & Treish, 2004).

The basic question arises as to what should the first step be in a successful erectile dysfunction prevention and in a successful erectile dysfunction treatment? If the decrease in testosterone leads to penile tissue fibrosis, smooth muscle atrophy in corpora cavernosa, and damage to mechanisms blocking the blood flow from the corpora cavernosa, how do PDE-5 inhibitors pour the proverbial oil on the troubled waters? And at the same time testosterone restores penile smooth muscle.

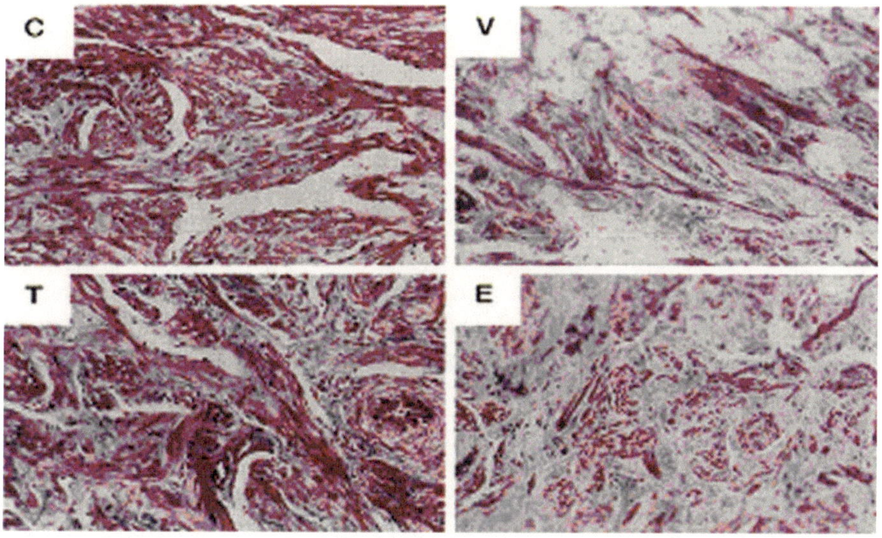

Fig. 23. Aging changes in the cavernosal tissue (Fig. 23-V) can also be induced by androgen deprivation (Fig. 23-E). The ratio of smooth muscle compartment to connective tissue which is normally 1:1 (Fig. 23 C & T) would suffer a shifting till 1:5 (Fig. 23 V & E) with a higher mRNA concentration as an expression of increasing number of alpha adrenoceptors according to Yassin (Yassin & Treish, 2004).

Testosterone deficiency is closely linked to the reduction in libido. And when one's libido is lowered, the effectiveness of PDE-5 inhibitors is also limited. In such situations, the preventive and curative procedure is to maintain adequate testosterone level in the body. What is more, in patients receiving PDE-5 inhibitors, the increase in the concentrations of testosterone can improve the penile vascular blood flow, which is yet another argument for using the aforementioned procedure.

It is also known that diabetes can increase the problem of erectile dysfunction. It was previously believed that diabetes lead to lower testosterone levels. In contrast, quite the opposite is happening. A drop in testosterone levels due to a decrease in glucose uptake facilitated by anabolism reduction causes diabetes. Increased levels of testosterone significantly improve glucose tolerance and reduce one's insulin levels and the HbA1c level. Testosterone deficit can thus affect sexuality, both at a particular moment and through changes in metabolic processes leading to vascular lesions. There may also be a significant delay in the increase/drop in testosterone, even for many years, which may lead to erectile dysfunction (Gomuła, 2006). Some argue that the very fact of the occurrence of erectile dysfunction, rather than the testosterone concentration level, is the main indication for hormone replacement (Shabsigh, 2003). But the mechanism of erection is based not only on testosterone levels. It is not based merely on the E-2 either. Because neither testosterone nor E-2 alone determine the adequacy of an erection. If the mechanisms of erection depended on changes in serum testosterone levels, one would have to wait many hours for an erection. Testosterone concentrations and E2 concentration increase as a result of natural endosyntesis. This lasts about 6 hours because that much time elapses from the original signals for spectral contrast in visual cortex during the first stage of sleep, rapid eye movement (REM). And the highest concentration of testosterone for a man is at approx. 4-5 am, after about six hours of sleep. The mechanisms of erection depend on such factors as the concentration of hormones, but they do not depend on them in a direct way. To obtain or maintain an adequate erection, one needs adequate levels of testosterone and of E-2. Therefore, aromatase, which converts testosterone to E-2, is also essential. Arginase, which induces the synthesis of nitric oxide in vascular endothelial cells, also plays an important role. 4-hydroxyestradiol derivative of estradiol is a substance that at the level of brain activity plays perhaps the most important role therein. 4-hydroxyestradiol has this property that it may saturate dopamine receptors in the brain. At high saturation level, dopamine stimulates these receptors, causing penile erection. Release of dopamine, which is one of many neurotransmitters, occurs rapidly. These two mechanisms are shown in Figure 24.

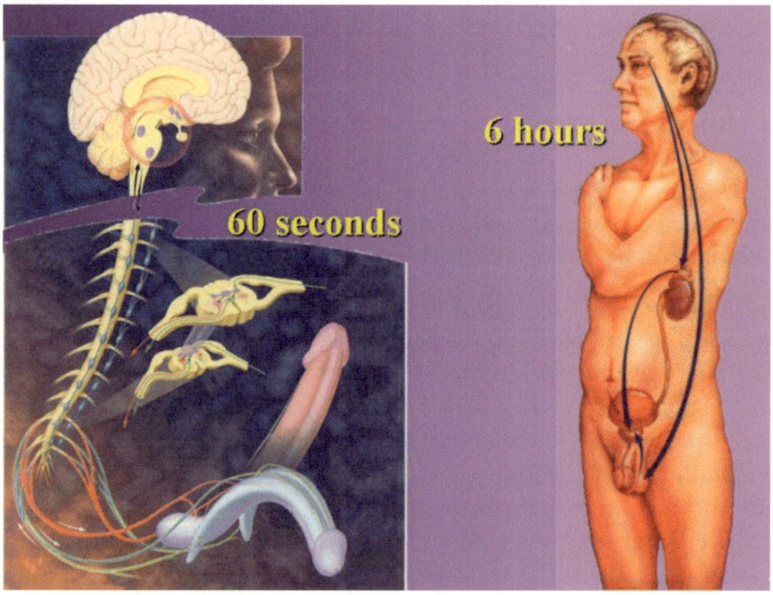

Fig. 24. Erection occurs as a result of the involvement of neurotransmiters, secreted at the time counted in seconds, and does not depend on hormonal changes, which can last for hours.

It clearly shows that we need to revise our views on the impact of hormones on our sexuality, potency, and libido, because not just hormones but also brain neurotransmitters have an impact on male sexuality.

3.7 Late - onset hypogonadism and depression

I have observed in my patients a change in their mental condition while they were under hormone therapy. A state of depression transformed itself into a state of joy. This gave enough reason to conduct a thorough analysis of the problem, which turned out to be the topic of the PhD dissertation of one of my assistants (Czyżowska, 2009).

Depression is a serious medical condition where a person may feel "down" or "hopeless" for weeks or more. According to the National Institute of Mental Health, the signs and symptoms of depression include: persistent sad, anxious, or "empty" mood; feelings of hopelessness, pessimism; feelings of guilt, worthlessness, helplessness; loss of interest or pleasure in hobbies and activities that were once enjoyed, including sex; decreased energy, fatigue, being "slowed down"; difficulty concentrating, remembering, making decisions; insomnia, early-morning awakening, or oversleeping; appetite and/or weight loss, or overeating and weight gain; thoughts of death or suicide, suicide attempts; restlessness, irritability; persistent physical symptoms that do not respond to treatment, such as headaches, digestive disorders, and chronic pain. Treatment of sexual disorders caused by depression with antidepressants based on Selective Serotonin Reuptake Inhibitor (SSRI) has a secondary detrimental effect on erection (Hsu & Shen, 1995, Keller, et al., 1997). It results in a vicious circle - antidepressants increase erection disorders, while sexual life disorders intensify depression. The circle is closed. How can it be broken?

Evidence proving therapeutical effect of estradiol in depression disorders has been found amongst women, however the research has not proven explicit relation between the estradiol level and depression among men (Studd & Panay, 2004). Neurosteroids produced in the central nervous system from cholesterol or other steroidal precursors are responsible for direct functioning within the brain, while alterations in their production typical for menopause in women and men cause certain aging symptoms. They directly influence, for example, body temperature regulation (hence the heat waves and cold sweats symptoms), memory function and emotions. Situational factors experienced by the given person, such as stress, secondarily disturb their secretions of hormones (Carruthers, 2004).

Research results demonstrated that hormone therapy for men, with hCG inducing testosterone endosynthesis causing over a double increase of testosterone and E-2 concentrations, result in substantial improvement of psychological condition and not only relieve depressive states, but also causes a progression from depression to the state of joy of life.

Based on the author's own research on 88 men aged between 20 and 68 years, (mean age 45 years), during the hormone therapy with hCG testosterone endosynthesis increase was achieved from E-2 average value 168.72 pmol/L up to 332.44 pmol/L. The change of hormonal state of the subjects resulted in substantial improvement of their psychological state assessed on the basis of extended Beck Depression Inventory /BDI/ (Beck, 1967).

The classic BDI evaluates exclusively depressive state. Condition above zero is not assessed, only depression is included. Accepting BDI as a good test however not designed to evaluate joy of life state, I have developed the questionnaire adding reflection towards opposite direction, i.e. towards joy of life. Implementing such a tool for analysis of patients' psychological state enabled the change of hormonal condition to be demonstrated as not only what causes relief from depression, but also progress to the state of joy of life.

Restoring man's normal concentration of testosterone and E-2 results in significant improvement of his mental health; depressive states subside. Furthermore, patients who prior to treatments were below state "0", in depression, during the therapy note states significantly above state "0"; they move to the joy of life state, as presented in Fig. 25.

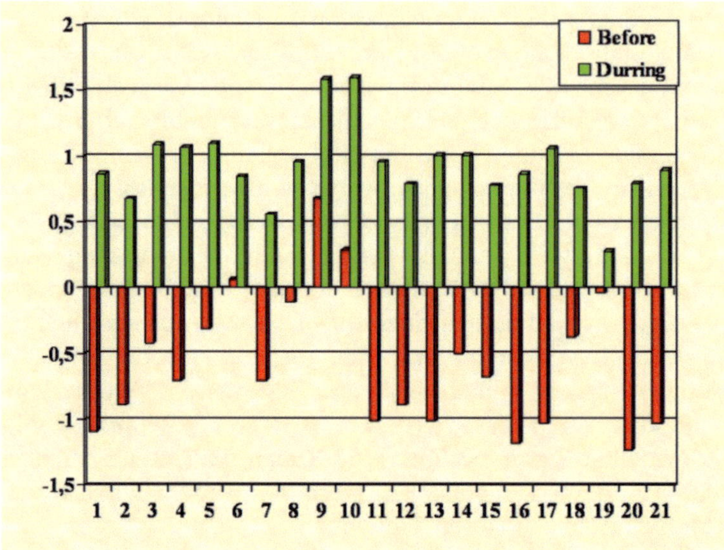

Fig. 25. Psychological state according to BDI: before the therapy - red, after the therapy - green. Patients who suffered from depression are in the joy of life area during the treatment.

The facts above presented explicitly demonstrate a close correlation between hormonal and psychological states of man.

3.8 Late - onset hypogonadism and Parkinson's disease

Although Parkinson's disease (PD) is diagnosed in only 0.1% of the total population, in the population older than 70 years of age its prevalence reaches 1%. The mean age of developing the disease is 58 years, and PD affects men more frequently than women /1.6:1/ (Edwards, et al., 2002, Nelson, 2002). The main cause of PD is the degeneration of dopaminergic neurons of substantia nigra in the nigro-striatal system of the brain. The development of the disease is believed to be triggered by both genetic and environmental factors. So far there have been very few reports in the literature, linking PD with the hormonal condition of a patient. Yet numerous symptoms resulting from the deficiency of such sex hormones as testosterone in men and progesterone-estrogen group in women, may co-exist with motor and other PD symptoms. These include impotence, lowered joy of life, lack of energy and mental depression (Edwards, et al., 2002, Nelson, 2002). Experimental studies have shown that estrogens can protect hippocampus neurons against beta-amyloid protein, which is implicated in the development of PD. The estrogens influence a creation of new synapses and improve the survival of neurons in hippocampus region (Serwin, 1994, Okun, et al., 2001).

Recent studies suggest the existence of morphogenic influence of estrogens on neurons and on plasticity of synapses. Estrogens appear to provoke synapsogenesis in hypothalamic cells. Apart from that, nonspecific systems activating brain neuroplasticity processes seem to be modulated as well (Skibińska & Kossuth, 2003).

The neuroprotective action of estradiol is connected with oxidation processes. Oxidative stress is known to be important in the process of dopaminergic neuronal degeneration in Parkinson's disease, whereas estrogens have neuroprotective effects in neurodegenerative disorders (Sawada, et al., 1998). HRT in men has been used only recently and never so widely as in women, thus we have less experience for HRT in men.

Regardless of the fact that the relation between dopamine and androgens at the level of the central nervous system is still not absolutely clear, on the basis of my own clinical observations it can be stated categorically that in men there exists a strong correlation between the hormonal system and PD symptoms. This statement is supported by the initial examinations and observation of PD patients who consider to undergo HRT.

The preliminary study comprised of 16 men suffering from PD and LOH, aged 64 -78 years. The hCG therapy used was to induce testosterone endosynthesis. The follow-up lasted from 1 to 4 years.

Following the therapy, the serum testosterone concentration increased from the mean baseline level of 12.3 nmol/l to 34.8 nmol/L. So far, the main parameter that has been considered for HRT in men has been the testosterone concentration. When the hCG was administered, though, the testosterone concentration increase was accompanied by simultaneous increase of estradiol level. In the analysed group of patients, the increase of the mean estradiol level was from the baseline of 46 pmol/L to 189 pmol/L.

The addition of the hormonal therapy was supplemental to the standard long-term pharmacological anti-PD treatment. As a result of this addition, a dramatic improvement of PD symptoms was observed.

Before the hormonal therapy began, the patients complained of motor latency and insufficiency, hand tremors, muscular tremor and rigidity in legs. During the treatment these symptoms clearly improved or completely disappeared.

Just stating the fact, though, without being able to document it, may justly be questionable. Numerical assessment and analysis of parameters from various questionnaires are ambiguous. That is why every possible effort has been made to present undeniable proof and evidence of beneficial changes in the clinical condition of PD patients. The first evidence for the relationship between LOH and clinical symptoms of PD is the film which was shown during ISSAM Seminar 'Androgen Deficiency in the Adult Male' at the 4th World Congress of The Aging Male in Prague.

Dr Malcolm Carruthers, a Congress participant, wrote in his book, published a few months after the Congress:"The results showed that after treatment, Parkinsonian symptoms greatly improved. Physical symptoms of slow, limited movement (bradykinesia), hand tremor, muscular tremor and rigidity of the legs clearly improved or disappeared, as did standing and walking alone, and ease of movement. Daily activities of living such as eating, dressing, personal hygiene and handwriting were all made easier. Clear improvements in many symptom areas were also documented by the film evidence" (Carruthers, 2004). An excerpt of the film can be seen on www.medan.pl.

The mental condition of the patients also improved substantially. The patients who had been slow, even dull, depressive, unwilling to contact with others, once the therapy commenced, changed dramatically.

After the hCG therapy was introduced, PD and other accompanying symptoms improved noticeably. Dyskinesis and involuntary body functions, being the adverse effects of treatment with L-dopa, discontinued or occurred sporadically.

If any patients had not been able to stand up, that problem disappeared. Now the patients could walk by themselves. They also reported that the way they moved had improved. Without any help of others, they could walk on an uneven ground or even stroll in woods.

The patients were able to eat their meals without any help, they could normally use a spoon, a knife and a fork because the hand tremor stopped. They could do their shirt and coat buttons up, and needed no help from others to get dressed or to wash themselves.

Another important objective element of improvement was the disappearance of sialosis. Their handwriting also improved, became clearer, with no traces of tremor or micrographism.

In 5 out of 16 patients described here, the improvement of their quality of life (QOL) also included the sexual function. Both their libido and potency improved. They resumed sexual activity, in which they had been inactive for a long time.

The hormonal therapy enabled them to live as before they fell ill, without having to be helped by others. Their quality of life benefited from that situation too. Their caregiving families felt extremely relieved. PD patients' families voluntarily admitted that the hormonal therapy was effective not only for PD sufferers but it improved quality of life of their families as well.

Initially, the PD-treatment regime had been kept. Neither the drugs nor their doses had been changed. After a few months of hCG administration, though, it was possible to lower the dosage or even withdraw certain anti-parkinsonism drugs, without aggravation of PD symptoms.

In the study presented, there was no control group. Yet, when the hormone-stimulation therapy was stopped, the patients' condition and symptoms clearly deteriorated, returning to what they had been like before the hormonal treatment was administered. Once the hormonal therapy was restarted, parkinsonian symptoms disappeared again. That fact was observed by patients and by their families as well.

Parkinson's disease and hormonal deficiency are inextricably linked. Both men and women suffer from Parkinson's disease because of deficit of estradiol, and more specifically because of the deficit of 4-hydroxyestradiol (dihydroxyestradiol), which is a derivative of estradiol. The molecular structure drawings, which illustrate how dopamine and 4-hydroxyestradiol are attached to the same key site to dopamine receptor in the brain, as given above, are in the subsection *2.1. Late Onset Hypogonadism is not just testosterone deficiency*. And it is only 4-hydroxyestradiol - a chemical compound, which due to its chemical structure, may saturate dopamine E-2 receptors in the brain. Therefore, in the treatment of Parkinson's disease special attention should be paid not only to testosterone levels, but particularly to the concentration of E-2. The desirable concentration of E-2 is approximately 250-300 pmol/l. This implies, however, maintaining also excessively high levels of testosterone, which cause hyperactivity in patients. In such cases, apart from hCG injections, I resort to microdoses of transdermal E-2 treatment in order to obtain the desired physiological serum levels of testosterone.

3.9 LOH and mortality & morbidity from coronary artery disease

Cardiovascular diseases, which include CAD, are now the biggest killer in the developed countries. The mortality rate from CAD varies by a factor of five in different populations in the world. Yet, in spite of such a high range in mortality rate, the ratio of male-to female deaths is relatively constant at more than three-to-one (Tunstall-Pedoe, 1999). This cannot be explained solely by differences in the risk factors for cardiovascular disease, between the sexes (Rayner, et al., 1998). The remarkably lower prevalence of CAD is particularily prominent in pre-menopausal women, but increases slightly after the menopause (Kalin, & Zurnoff 1990).

These facts led to the notion that diminishing levels of testosterone in aging men, which lead to late onset hypogonadism (LOH), are responsible for such differences and higher mortality of men. Indeed, the nested case-control study on 11'600 men aged 40 to 79 years (EPIC-Norfolk UK) showed inverse relationship of endogenous testosterone concentration and mortality due to cardiovascular disease and all causes including CAD and cancer. This study clearly suggested that high endogenous testosterone concentrations appear to lower mortality rates of men due to all causes, cardiovascular disease and cancer (Khaw, K.T., et al., 2007).

In the "Hypogonadism in Males (HIM)" study (Mulligan, et al. 2006) on 2162 male patients over 45 years of age and visiting their primary care physicians for general reasons, it was found that 38.7% of them were hypogonadal and 3.7% of them were receiving testosterone. Among men not receiving testosterone, odds ratios for having hypogonadism were significantly higher in men with arterial hypertension (1.84), hyperlipidemia (1.47), diabetes (2.09), obesity (2.38). Conversely, late onset hypogonadism (LOH) and the Testosterone Deficiency (TD) connection with cardiovascular disease is evident from TD associations with diabetes (Dhindsa, et al. 2010) and metabolic syndrome (Kalyani & Dobs, 2000) and such findings as an inverse relationship between testosterone level and aortic atherosclerosis, which was seen among middle-aged and older men in the Rotterdam Study (Hak, et al., 2002).

Low free testosterone has also been associated with abdominal aortic aneurysm in community-dwelling men aged 70-88 years (Yeap et al., 2010). Furthermore, for men aged 50 to 91 years of age who were followed for 20 years in the Rancho Bernardo Study (Barrett-Connor et al., 1999), serum testosterone levels were inversely related to weight, body mass index, arterial blood pressure, serum insulin and plasma glucose. Nevertheless, as these factors may be relevant to mortality there was clear evidence that men with serum testosterone concentration below 25th percentile had a 40% higher risk of death, independent of obesity, lifestyle choices (eg. exercise, smoking) and age (Laughlin, et al., 2008, Tivestena et al., 2009). Another 5-year retrospect study on male veterans (N=858), compared mortality of men with normal (± 450 ng/dL) T levels to those with low (<250 ng/dL) total testosterone and low (< 0.75ng/dL) free testosterone levels (Shores, et al., 2006). The results showed that mortality for subjects with low T was almost twice as high (34.9%) as for those with normal T levels was 20.1%. There is an obvious link between mortality and morbidity due to coronary CAD and other cardiovascular diseases and LOH due to low free testosterone levels in serum of aging men (Wu & von Eckardstein, 2003, Wu, et al., 2010). This is due to existing strong correlation of testosterone defficiency with glucose tolerance, visceral obesity, serum lipid disorders and elevated arterial pressure (Kalyani & Dobs, 2007). These factors usually lead to vascular disorders. The clinical studies (English, et al., (1997) showed that low natural androgen concentration can cause deletorious changes in atherogenic lipid profile, high fibrinogen and a hypercoagulable state, an increase in insulin resistance and hyperinsulinemia, higher systolic and diastolic blood pressures. The biologically plausible mechanism of testosterone protective action against cardiovascular disorers can be explained by the fact that testosterone has direct vasoactive properties (English, et al., (1997). In animal models of isolated coronary, femoral and pulmonary arteries testosterone showed a dose-dependent vasodilatory effect (Channer & Jones, 2003). It is caused by a direct effect on the vascular smooth muscle, by either an effect on potassium or calcium channels (Deenadayalu, V.P., et al. 2001, English, K.M., 2002). In man, testosterone has been shown to cause dose-dependent vasodilation both in vitro and in vivo. During cardiac surgery on man, the coronary artery diameter and subsequent

coronary flow immediately increased when testosterone was injected via intracoronary indwelling catheter (Webb, C.M. et al., 1999).
During the non-invasive therapy of LOH when the increased T concentration levels can be sustained for longer periods. T can not only protect man against atherogenic factors but also may cause long-term coronary dilatation. This is due to testosterone interaction with arginase activity, which results in increased synthesis of nitric oxide in endothelial cells in the entire vascular system. Nitric oxide is a well known vasodilator, which acts systemically. The synthesis of NO is also used in the treatment of erectile dysfunction (ED) by applying fosfodiesterase 5 inhibitors (PDE-5-I). Interestingly, nowadays these PDE-5 inhibitors become popular as a treatment of choice for some cardiovascular diseases.
Large scale clinical studies on long term effects of treatment of LOH with hCG on CAD were not yet reported, but case reports from my colleagues in cardiology who clinically follow some of my patients with exercise tests, are positive, including diminshing or disappearance of so called angina pectoris pain.

3.10 Late - onset hypogonadism and immune resistance

I have no scientific evidence to support any representation of a change in the immunity in my patients undergoing hormone therapy. Conducting such research is practically very difficult, perhaps impossible. Antibiotics, aspirin, and anti-inflammatory drugs should not be taken for at least a year by patients who have their immune status tested. This is impossible!!! But I can say with conviction that men whose testosterone levels increased 2-fold during hCG therapy as well as those already experiencing androversion (for androversion see 3.3 LOH and androversion) claimed that they did not get colds and that they had no infections, which they had had quite often before.

4. The treatment of late - onset hypogonadism

Now, the most widely practiced therapy for men with LOH are injections of testosterone esters or transcutaneous applications of 1% and 2% testosterone gel preparations. This is because many years ago it was erroneously believed that, with age, all men lose their ability for endo-synthesis of testosterone.
Another method known over the past 50 years, presently gaining "renaissance" of recognition, has been the stimulation of testosterone endo-synthesis by administering hCG (Gould, 1951, Gomula, 2001, Gomuła, 2002-a, Gomuła, 2002-b, Gomuła & Twarkowski, 2002, Gomuła, 2006, Gomuła, 2007).
The serum testosterone concentrations observed in patients treated with hCG increased by at least 150% and up to 200% (Gould, 1951, Janczewski, et al., 1966, Gomuła, 2001, Gomuła, 2002-a, Liu et al., 2002, Gomuła, 2007, Gomuła & Rabijewski, 2010).
Yet, if applying hCG makes it possible to almost double testosterone concentration, why to inject testosterone esters to men when they still have the ability for endo-synthesis of their own, natural testosterone?
The hCG therapy improves testicular function, while treatment with synthetic testosterone inhibits it. Years ago, there was a trend to produce oral contraceptives for men but this idea was soon abandoned. That oral contraceptive for men was supposed to be testosterone ester pill. The information that taking synthetic testosterone not only inhibits spermatogenesis, but also inhibits male's own testosterone endo-synthesis, is now almost labeled as "classified". In fact, after three months of taking synthetic testosterone, a man becomes

totally infertile (WHO, 1990, Wallace, et al., 1993, Anderson & Wu, 1996, Zhang et al., 1999, Baird, 2002, Anderson & Waites, 2003, Si-Tian, et al., 2004). Furthermore, long-time testosterone therapy may result in irreversible testicular atrophy. From this moment on, a man becomes dependent on taking testosterone. The discontinuation of testosterone intake leads to metabolic disorders, which may cause many other diseases to develop.

4.1 Late - onset hypogonadism and hCG therapy

The effect of the treatment of 908 patients taking hCG was described in 2010 (Gomula & Rabijewski, 2010). Below, I present a further study of 1200 men (age range 20-89 years; mean, 54). Mean follow-up period of the patients was over 37 months.

During the therapy with hCG (2 x 5000 i.u. per week) there was an average increase in serum concentrations of total testosterone from 18.4 nmol/L to 38.59 nmol/L. It was noted that during the hCG therapy, there was no increase of SHBG. To the contrary, the SHBG concentrations even showed a slight decrease. This meant that as the result of hCG treatment, free and bioavailable testosterone concentrations increased. The rise was proportional to that in total testosterone, as was reported (Fiers & Kaufman, 1999).

There was an average increase in free testosterone concentrations from 0.0829 ng/mL (1.98%) to 0.201 ng/mL (2.29%) The bio-available testosterone concentration also increased: – on average from 1.94 ng/mL (46.4%) to 4.71 ng /mL (53.6%). At the same time, there was a steady increase in the average concentration of estradiol, from 138.6 pmol/L to 280.9 pmol/L. In paralel, the average PSA level decreased by 40% (from 3.09 ng/mL to 1.83 ng/mL) after 37 months of therapy. These results are shown in Table 9, below.

	T	T-f	T-ba	E-2	SHBG	PSA-t
Before	18.4	0.0829 (1.98%)	1.94 (46.4 %)	138.6	35.1	3.09
During	38.59	0.201 (2.29%)	4.71 (53.6 %)	280.9	34.86	1.83

T= total testosterone (in nmol/L), T-f = free testosterone (in ng/mL), T-ba = bioavailable testosterone (in ng/mL), E-2=estradiol (in pmol/L), SHBG=sex hormone binding globulin (in nmol/L), PSA-t = total Prostate-Specific Antigen (in ng/mL).

Table 9. Testosterone (total, free, bioavailable), estradiol, SHBG & PSA before and during/after 3 years of hCG therapy

During LOH treatment with testosterone there was also no significant PSA increase, which was regarded as evidence further supporting the safety of this therapy (Wang, et al., 2009). But achieving a 40% reduction in PSA during the hCG therapy, with a simultaneous increase of more than 2-fold in serum testosterone levels as reported above show for the first time that the hCG therapy is not only highly effective for all age groups, but quite safe as well.

There is clear evidence now that hCG therapy is safe and effective as a treatment of choice for men with late onset hypogonadism. During many years of continuous use of preparations, where hCG was the active ingredient, for LOH therapy, none of untoward side-effects were observed nor reported. It has also been confirmed by the files at the Division for Monitoring of Adverse Actions of the High Authority for Registration of Drugs and other Medical Products in Poland. The reports in these files have shown that in the last 14 years there has not been any case reporting a man showing the potential side effects of preparations used in the treatment, in which the hCG is the active ingredient (Reports from the years 1996-2009). This applies to 1200 patients treated by my and to the thousands of other patients treated by other physicians across Europe.

4.2 LOH and the possibility to restore testosterone endosynthesis

Stimulation of hormonal balance with hCG in LOH men, in most cases does increase endosynthesis of natural testosterone. This is true also for all age groups. In young men the increase can be even as high as 300%. With age, the induction of endosynthesis with hCG therapy gets relatively weaker, but still effective enough to eradicate manifestations of the Testosterone Deficiency Syndrome (TDS). The analysis of the findings of the author's studies show that the opinions about the Testosterone Deficiency Syndrome etiology, so far reported in medical publications were erroneous. The author's studies on the material of 908 males treated with the hCG preparations for inducing testosterone endosynthesis, has proved that such induction is possible in any age group, but physiologically it diminishes with man's age. (Gomuła & Rabijewski, 2010). Yet, effective endosynthesis is maintained until late senility, which is in the contrast to the belief that Leydig's cells completely cease to function with age. In men aged 30–39 years, the mean increase of serum testosterone concentration resulting from hCG therapy was 128%, in those aged 40 - 49 years - 126%, in age group of 50 - 59 years - 129%, aged 60 - 69 years - 121%, aged 70 - 79 years - 99%, and in those aged 80 - 99 years it was 88%.

A statistical analysis has revealed that the effectiveness of hCG therapy depends mainly on the LH/F ratio, and to a lesser extent on the patient's age (where: LH = luteinizing hormone in the IU/L, and F = free PSA (expressed as free PSA/total PSA in %).

The data showing the relationship of the decrease in the ability of testosterone endosynthesis with the LH/F ratio, rather than age, are provided in Table 10, below.

	LH:F= 0.1	LH:F= 0.15	LH:F= 0.20	LH:F= 0.25	LH:F= 0.3	LH:F= 0.35
30-40y	175%	160%	145%	130%	115%	100%
40-50y	164%	149%	134%	119%	104%	89%
50-60y	153%	138%	123%	108%	93%	78%
60-70y	142%	127%	112%	97%	82%	67%
70-80y	131%	110%	109%	89%	72%	52%
80-89y	119%	98%	84%	81%	60%	41%

Table 10. Ability of testosterone endosynthesis versus the LH/F ratio and age

Knowing the LH/F ratio helps to predict the outcome of the hCG treatment. When the LH/F ratio is lower than **0.15,** a patient is still able to rebuild the synthesis of endogenic testosterone. Once LH/F ratio increases above **0.30**, a patient is much less likely to be able to achieve that. Another very important correlation. The serum LH and free PSA levels are essential for the health of prostate. In the recent studies of drugs for treatment of benign prostatic hyperplasia (BPH), there is an emphasis on lowering LH. For many years the LHRH analogues have been used to treat prostate cancer.

When the LH/F index in a patient with late onset hypogonadism exceeds 0.5, there is an indication for particularly thorough detection of prostate cancer.

The results of my follow-up of these 1200 patients show clearly that the decrease in the ability of testosterone endosynthesis is synonymous with increased risk of prostate cancer.

4.3 Late - onset hypogonadism and androversion

The effect of HRT with exo-testosterone is that after the treatment is discontinued, the patient's testosterone concentration level is lower than that which was when the treatment was initiated. In contrast to this, when hCG therapy is discontinued, the abilities for testosterone endo-synthesis are the same as they were before the treatment. Around 30% of patients developed a phenomenon, which can be called androversion - no need nor willingness to continue the hCG therapy, once an increase of 50–150% of testosterone levels was reached by natural endosynthesis.

The long term hCG treatment (6-24 months) can cause permanent increase (i.e. saturation) in testosterone endosynthesis, so the further induction by hCG administration will be not indicated. Is it possible to predict whether a man has the chance of achieving such a state of androversion? The answer is still uncertain. When a man, in his initial blood tests, has a very high concentration of LH and low testosterone levels, the prognosis for him to reach a state of androversion is negative. In such cases, the thorough prostate cancer detection tests are highly indicated, as such a patient belongs to the high-risk group. What is more, there is no increased PC risk associated with the continuing of hCG therapy for such a patient. Importantly, however, there may be an increased risk of prostate cancer, if and when the hCG therapy is discontinued. In case when there is a decrease in SHBG, this indicates that hCG therapy can be safely discontinued. The concentrations of LH, testosterone, SHGB, E-2, and PSA must be measured after one month and then again after two months. If for a period of two months, the concentrations of testosterone are high, in excess of those in the previous therapy, it is the proof of the onset of androversion. Furthermore, it is the sign of the end of indications for further hCG treatment. The aforementioned parameters should be monitored every 6 months. If, after 6 months, one notices a drop in serum testosterone, it is advisable to renew regular hCG treatment. If, however, a low concentration of testosterone, high LH levels, and elevated PSA reccur in the subsequent blood tests, this should be a signal to do further diagnostic tests, in order to be able to exclude or to undertake measures to treat prostate cancer.

4.4 Recomendation for Late - onset hypogonadism therapy – discussion

The problem with therapy of LOH in men, is the long-standing notion that andropause is like mirror image of menopause. Commonly, by the term « menopause » we understand the period when amenorrhea sets in for many years to follow, and women may even undergo HRT. A rather correct term for this period of women's life is « post-menopause ». The medically defined « menopause » lasts for only few months during which, the menstrual cycle gradually comes to a stop. This is due to the rapid decay and eventually total cessation of synthesis capacity of hormones in ovaries.

In men, such a phenomenon does not take place. A man loses his hormonal capacity, fertility and sexuality gradually over a period of many, many years. There are no such things in men, like such rapid, almost dramatic drops in concentrations of gonadal hormones.

The official recommendations of the National Health Service of Poland for treatments of men with LOH, recommend the use of both: either Testosterone or hCG therapies with no emphasis on either one. This well-balanced approach merits recognition.

Testosterone preparations – hormone replacement therapy (HRT) – are recommended in a series of guidelines for the LOH treatment established by the world renowned doctors and scientists. In their work, there is also reference to the HCG treatment: « Human chorionic gonadotropin (hCG) stimulates testosterone production of Leydig cells, albeit at a lower rate in older men, than in younger men. Since insufficient information exists about the therapeutic and adverse effects of hCG treatment in older men and its higher cost, this treatment cannot be recommended in LOH, except when fertility is an issue » (Wang, et al., 2009).

Over the last almost 50 years there have been many studies published on the effectiveness of hCG to induce endosynthesis of testosterone. They showed increases of testosterone concentrations from 150% to over 200% resulting from hCG therapy (Gould, 1951, Gomuła, 2001, Gomuła, 2002-a, Liu, et al., 2002, Gomuła, 2007, Gomuła & Rabijewski, 2010).

Own prospective study of 1200 patients aged from 20 to 89 y and monitored for >10 years undeniably showed hCG effectiveness in inducing endosynthesis of T. In effect, the hCG-therapy resulted in the increase of serum testosterone from a mean of 18.4 nmol/L initially, to mean 38.59 nmol/L during therapy (Gomuła & Rabijewski, 2010). There is clear evidence that hCG therapy is safe and effective as a treatment of choice for men with late onset hypogonadism. It has also been confirmed by the reports on file at the Division for Monitoring of Adverse Actions of the High Authority for Registration of Drugs and other Medical Products in Poland. The reports have shown that in the last 16 years there has not been any case reporting a man showing the potential side effects of preparations used in the treatment, in which the hCG is the active ingredient (Reports from the years 1996-2011).

This applies to 1200 patients treated by me and to the thousands of other patients treated by other doctors across Europe.

On the economic side, the treatment cost of LOH when using hCG is lower than the cost of the newly available T preparations. In the UE countries, it amounts to about 50 Euro/month.

It is beyond any doubt that some authors of such consensus statement are aware of the negative impact of testosterone replacement therapy on fertility of men. They are the authors who published on the contraceptive action of **T** in men (Wallace, et al., 1993, Anderson & Wu, 1996, Weinbauer, et al, 2001).

Furthermore, many peer reviewed papers, including the report from World Health Organization, confirmed that after up to three months of HRT with testosterone, from 40% to 90% male patients developed azoo-spermy or significant oligo-spermy - clearly a contraceptive situation - leading to a permanent pharmacological sterilization of men! (WHO, 1990, Wallace, et al., 1993, Anderson & Wu, 1996, Zhang et al., 1999, Baird, 2002, Anderson & Waites, 2003, Si-Tian, et al., 2004).

These facts have been known for over 20 years, but are still suppressed from information available to the general public. Just to the contrary, the mandatory information for physicians and patients attached to each box of the products, does not even mention the infertility/sterilization as a possible side-effect action of HRT with testosterone! Even in the newest-generation testosterone product ANDROTOP, the attached leaflet lists only the following warning: « The Androtop medication is not intended for treatment of male infertility or impotence.. » .

When comparing the two facts:

1. treatment of men with exo-applied synthetic testosterone may cause not only infertility but also anatomical and functional destruction of testicles and eventually leads to their complete atrophy including disappearance;

2. treatment with hCG improves functioning of testicles, with corresponding increase of secretion of « good », natural testosterone, the conclusion is simple: the treatment of LOH with naturally secreted testosterone is better, safer and more economical then it is a case synthetic exo-applied testosterone!

The superiority of the hCG treatment over the testosterone treatment has already been described (Gould, 1951).

This information, however, did not receive universal recognition. Yet hCG therapy has been proven to be effective and safe. Moreover, as a result of testosterone treatment, permanent sterilization of men follows. Other risks, which mainly occur with long-term use include irreversible testicular atrophy. And then only successful marketing of pharmaceutical companies remains. Patients seem condemned to a lifetime use of testosterone. Otherwise their cellular metabolism drops so low that they are vulnerable to many diseases and to early death.

I want to apologize to the guideline authors - some of whom are my friends – but I cannot accept the fact that not having conducted any studies on hCG treatment they ruled that the method was uncertain. They claimed that perhaps it was even dangerous. Is the lack of experience concerning the effects of hCG in the LOH treatment a sufficient reason to reject this alternative safe, effective and affordable therapy?

5. Conclusions

This has turned out to be the most troublesome section…

Not because I had objective problems, no, but because of my ethical issues.

Among the authors of LOH therapy guidelines, which were established at international levels, there are my long-time friends. I do not want to upset them because I strongly believe that what they did was acting in good faith, but I cannot exclude the fact that they had been insidiously stimulated by the pharmaceutical industry. Yet, the ultimate aim of a physician's actions is acting for the good of a patient, so in such context, the friendship takes a second place. Consequently, the conclusions that are listed below are very delicate ethically but unambiguously to the point.

1. There is no doubt now that testosterone deficit, which grows with age, negatively affects the man's biology in its broad meaning.
2. The own material presented in the paper allows the author to conclude that the minimal reference values for testosterone concentration levels, at which testosterone therapy should be initiated, which are accepted universally so far, are definitely too low.
3. Introducing a therapy to increase testosterone levels only when for many years testosterone deficit has inflicted irreversible anatomical changes, seems to be clearly delayed, and is harmful for the man's health.
4. Applying testosterone replacement therapy to a man with LOH makes sense only when it is impossible to provoke the man's own testosterone endosynthesis. If a man is still able to rebuild his own testosterone endosynthesis, the treatment with hCG is recommended, otherwise the testosterone replacement therapy will soon make him infertile. Moreover applying testosterone replacement therapy for a long time, will result in testicular atrophy.
5. Consequently, the guidelines and recommendations on LOH treatment should be verified and modified as soon as possible.

6. Acknowledgements

I wish to express my sincere gratitude to my close friend - Dr Bruno Lunenfeld - for inspiring me to work in the field of the Aging Male for many years, as especially to conduct studies in the effectiveness of hCG therapy in inducing testosterone endosynthesis. I received a similar support from Prof. Alvaro Morales, for which I am very grateful too. During performing my studies, I felt a constant support from Dr. Malcolm Carruthers, Prof. Assam Yashin, Prof. Peter Sheplev, Prof. Nykola Boiko, Prof. Stefan Zgliczynski - thank you all, my friends. Walking the steep path of a professional career in science, where I have attempted to prove the safety and effectiveness of hCG therapy, I have encountered numerous enemies. I want to thank them too - their activities have made me fight for the scientific truth even more tenaciously.

7. References

Algarte-Genin, M., Cussenot, O., Costa, P. (2004) Prevention of prostate cancer by androgens: experimental paradox or clinical reality. *Eur Urol*, 46, 285-295.

Anderson, J. (2003) The role of antiandrogen monotherapy in the treatment of prostate cancer. *BJU*, 91, 455–462.

Anderson, R.A., Wu, F.C. (1996) Comparison between testosterone enanthate-induced azoospermia and oligozoospermia in a male contraceptive study. II. Pharmacokinetics and pharmacodynamics of once weekly administration of testosterone enanthate. *J Clin Endocrinol Metab*, 81, 896-901.

Anderson, R.A., Waites, G.M.H. (2003) Development of methods of male contraception: impact of the World Health Organization Task Force. *Fertil. Steril.*, 80, 1–15.

Baird, D.T. (2002) Male contraception. *Endocr Rev*, 23, 735–762.

Balthazar, J., Ball, G.F. (1998) New insights into the regulation and function of brain estrogen synthase (aromataze). *Trends Neurosci*, 21, 243–249.

Bancroft, J. (1989) Androgens, sexuality and the aging male. in: F. Labrie, L. Proulx (edit.), *Endocrinology* (p. 913-916). Amsterdam: Elsevier.

Barrett-Connor, E., Von Mühlen, D.G., Kritz-Silverstein, D. Bioavailable testosterone and depressed mood in older men: the Rancho Bernardo Study. *J Clin Endocrinol Metab*, 84,,(2), 573-7.

Beck, A. (1967) *Depression. Clinical, experimental, and theoretical aspects*. London, Staple Press.

Behre, H.M., Bohmeyer, J., Nieschlag, E. (1994) Prostate volume in testosterone-treated and untreated hypogonadal men in comparison to age-matched normal controls. *Clin Endocrinol*, 40, 341-349.

Bonczyk, M., Zdrojowy, R., Makota, D., Kołodziej, A. (2008) Testosterone and prostate cancer. *Urol Pol*, 61, 19–23.

Burries, A., Banks, S., Carter, C. et al. (1992) A long-term, prospective study of the physiologic and behavioral effects of hormone replacement in untreated hypogonadal men. *J Androl*, 13, 297–304.

Carani, C., Rochira, V., Faustini-Fustini, M. et al. (1999) Role of oestrogen in male sexual behaviour: insights from the natural model of aromatase deficiency. Clin Endocrinol (Oxf), 51, 517–524.

Carruthers, M. (2004) *Androgen deficiency in the adult male*. Taylor & Francis, London, Oxforshire and New York.

Channer, K.S., Jones, T.H. (2003) Cardiovascular effects of testosterone: implications of the „male menopause" *Heart*, 89, 121-122.

Czyżowska, A. (2009) The importance of hormone replacement therapy in sexual health and in depression for men. PhD thesis. *Department of Psychology, University of Warsaw.*

Davidson, J., Kwan, M., Greenleaf, W. (1982) Hormonal replacement and sexuality. *Clin Endocrinol Metab*, 11, 599–614.

Debruyne, F., Gres, A.,A., Arustamov, D.,L. (2008) Placebo-Controlled Dose-Ranging Phase 2 Study of Subcutaneously Administered LHRH Antagonist Cetrorelix in Patients with Symptomatic Benign Prostatic Hyperplasia. *Eur Urol*, 54, 170–180.

Deenadayalu, V.P., White, R.E., Stallone, J.N. et al. (2001) Testosterone relaxes coronary arteries by opening large-conductance calcium-activated potassium channel. *Am J Physiol*, 281, 1720-7.

Deslypere, J.,P., Vermulen, A. (1984) Leydig cell function in normal men: effects of aging, life-style, residence, diet, and activity. J Clin Endocrinol Metab, 59, 955-62.

Dhindsa, S., Miller, M.G., McWhirter, M,L,, et al. 2010 Testosterone concentrations in diabetic and nondiabetic obese men. *Diabetes Care,* 33, 1186-1192.

Edwards, E.,Ch., Kitt, E., Oliver, J. et al. (2002) Depression and Parkinson's Disease: a new look at an old problem. *Depression and Anxiety*, 16, 39-43.

English, K.M, Steeds, R.P., Jones, T.H. et al. (1997) Testosterone and ischemic heart disease-is there a link? *QJM*, 90, 787-91.

English, K.M., Jones R.D., Jones, T.H. et al. (2002) Testosterone acts as a coronary vasodilator by a calcium-channel antagonist action. *J Endocrinol Invest*, 25, 455-8.

Feldman, H.A., Longcope, C., Derby, C. et al. (2002) Age trends in the level of serum testosterone and other hormones in middle-aged men: longitudinal results from Massachusetts Male Aging Study. *J Clin Endocrinol Metab*, 87, 589–598.

Ferrini, M., Wang, C., Hakim, A.S. et al. (2001) Age-related increased expression of inducible NDS and cytotoxic markers in T2T hypothalamic regions. *Neuroendocrinology*, 74, 1-8.

Ferrini, R.L., Barrett-Connor, E. (1998) Sex hormones and age: a cross-sectional study of testosterone and estradiol and their bioavailable fractions in community dwelling men. *American Journal of Epidemiology*, 147, 750-754.

Fiers, T., Kaufman J.M. (1999) A critical evaluation of simple methods for the estimation of free testosterone in serum. *J Clin Endocrinol Metab*, 84, 3666-3672.

Fossa, S., Opjordsmoen, S., Haug, E. (1999) Androgen replacement and quality of life in patients treated for bilateral testicular cancer. *Eur J Cancer* , 35, 1220–1225.

Fowler, J.E., Whitmore, Jr W.F. (1981) The response of metastatic adenocarcinoma of the prostate to exogenous testosterone. *J Urol*, 126, 372-375.

Gomula, A. (2001) The influence of chorionic gonadotropin on the endogenic testosterone synthesis. 1st Asian ISSAM Meting on the Aging Male. Kuala Lumpur. 1–4.03. 2001. *Aging Male*, 3: 85.

Gomula, A. (2002-a) Clinical effects of hCG treatment – new method of hormonal repleacement therapy. 3th World Congress on the Aging Male, Berlin 2002. *Aging Male*, 2002, 4, 260.

Gomuła, A. (2002-b) The deficit of androgens and aging men. *Urol Pol*, 55, 13–22.

Gomuła, A., Twarkowski P. (2002) Effect of hormone replacement therapy for benign prostatic hyperplasia. XXXII Congress of Polish Urological Association, *Urol Pol*, 55, 41.

Gomula, A. (2006) The influence of sex hormones and neurotransmitters on sexual function and behaviour. *Polish Sexology*, 4, 21–33.

Gomuła, A. (2006) The influence of sex hormones and neurotransmitters on sexual function and behaviour. *Polish Sexology*, 4, 21–33.

Gomuła, A. (2007) *When a man ages*. Medan, Warszawa, ISBN 83-911373-2-5

Gomuła, A., Rabijewski, M. (2010) Testosterone deficiency syndrome - diagnosis and treatment - based on age-related testosterone referent levels. *Polish Sexology*, 8, 1-16.

Gooren, L.J.G. (2000) Quality-of-life issues in the aging male. *Aging Male*, 3, 185-189.

Gooren, L.J.G., Bunck, M. C. M. (2004) Androgen replacement therapy. *Drugs*, 64, 1861-1891.

Gould, W. (1951) The male climacteric. *Medical Time*, 79, 154–161.

Gould, D.C., Kirby, R.S. (2006) Testosterone replacement therapy for late onset hypogonadism: what is the risk of inducing prostate cancer? *Prostate Cancer and Prostatic Diseases*, 9, 14-18.

Gould, D.C., Feneley M.R., Kirby R.B. (2006) Prostate-specyfic antigen testing in hypogonadism: implications for the safety of testosterone replacement therapy. *BJU International*, 98, 1-9.

Hajjar, R., Kaiser, F., Morley, J. (1997) Outcomes of long-term testosterone replacement therapy in older hypogonadal males: a retrospective study. *J Clin Endocrinol Metab*, 82, 3793–3796.

Hak, A.E., Witteman, J.C., de Jong, F.H. et al. (2002) Low levels of endogenous androgens increase the risk of atherosclerosis in elderly men: the Rotterdam study. *J Clin Endocrinol Metab*, 87, 3632-3639.

Harbitz, T.B., Haugen, O.A. (1974) Endocrine disturbances in men with benign hyperplasia and carcinoma of the prostate. A morphological study in an autopsy series. *Acta Path Microbiol Scand*, 244, (suppl.), 1-13.).

Harman, S.M., Metter, E.J., Tobin, J.D. et al. (2001) Longitudinal effects of aging on serum total and free testosterone levels in healthy men: Baltimore Longitudinal Study of Aging. J Clin Endocrinol Metab, 86, 724–731.

Hijazi, R.A., Cunningham, G.R. (2005) Andropause: is androgen replacement therapy indicated for the aging male? *Annual Review of Medicine*, 56, 117-137.

Hoffman, M.A., DeWolf, W.C., Morgentaler A. (2000) Is low serum free testosterone a marker for high grade prostate cancer? *J Urol*, 163, 824-827.

Hogervorst, E. (2004) Testosterone and Alzheimer's disease. *Aging Male*, 7, 31. Abstracts of the 4th World Congress of the Aging Male.

Hsu, J.H., Shen, W.W. (1995) Male sexual side effects associated with antidepressants: a descriptive clinical study of 32 patients. *International Journal of Psychiatry in Medicine*, 25, 191-201.

Huggins, C., Hodges, C.V. (1941) Studies on prostatic cancer, I: the effect of castration, of estrogen and of androgen injection on serum phosphatases in metastatic carcinoma of the prostate. *Cancer Res*, 1, 293-297.

Janczewski, Z., Bablom, L., Czaplicki, M. (1966) Treatment of andropause. *Polish J Endocrinol* 17, 443-447.

Kalin, M.F., Zurnoff, B. (1990) Sex hormone and coronary disease: a review of the clinical studies. *Steroids*, 55, 330-52.

Kalyani, R.R., Dobs, A.S. (2007) Androgen deficiency, diabetes and metabolic syndrome. *Curr Opin Endocrino. Obes*, 2007; 14: 226–234.

Kaufman, J., T'Sjoen, G. (2002) The effects of testosterone deficiency on male sexual function. *Aging Male*, 5, 242–247.

Kaufmann, J.M., Vermeulen, A. (2005) The decline of androgens levels in elderly men and its clinical and therapeutic implications. *Endocr Review*, 26, 833–876.

Keller, A., Hamer, R., Rosen, R.C. (1997) Serotonin reuptake inhibitor-induced sexual dysfunction and its treatment: a large-scale retrospective study of 596 psychiatric outpatients. *Journal of Sex and Marital Therapy*, 3, 165-175.

Khaw, K.T., Dowsett, M., Folkerd, *Circulation* 2007.

Khosla, S., Melton, L.J., Atkinson, E.J. et al. (1998) Relationship of serum sex steroid levels and bone turnover markers with bone mineral density in men and women: a key role for bioavailable estrogen. *J Clin Endocrinol Metab*, 83, 2266–2274.

Kwan, M., Greenleaf, W., Mann, J. (1983) The nature of androgenom men sexuality: A combinated laboratory/self reporter study oh hypogonadal men. *J Clin Endocrinol Metab*, 57, 557–561.

Laughlin, G.A., Barrett-Connor, E., Bergstrom, J. Low serum testosterone and mortality in older men. *J Clin Endocrinol Metab*, 93, 68-75.

Lazarou, S., Reyes-Vallejo, L., Morgentaler, A. (2006) Wide variability in laboratory reference values for serum testosterone. *Journal of Sexual Medicine*, 3, 1085-1089.

Leder, B.Z., LeBlanc, K.M., Schoenfeld, D.A. et al. (2003) Differential effects of androgens and estrogens on bone turnover in normal men. *J Clin Endocrinol Metab*, 88, 204–210.

Liu, P.Y. Wishart, S.M., Handelsman, D.J. (2002) A double-blind, placeb-controlled, radndomized clinical trial of recobinant human chorionic gonadotropin on muscle strenght and physical function and activity in older men with partial ege-related androgen deficiency. *J Clin Endocrinol Metab*, 87 (7), 3125-35.

Lunenfeld, B., Gooren, L. (2002) *Textbook of men's health*. New York: The Parthenon Publishing Group. ISBN 18-421401-1-6

Lunenfeld, B., Saad, F., Hoesl, C.E., (2005) ISA, ISSAM and EAU recommendations for the investigation, treatment and monitoring of late-onset hypogonadism in males: scientific background and rationale. *Aging Male*, 8, 59–74.

Matsumoto, A.M. (1990) Effects of chronic testosterone administration in normal men: safety and efficacy of high dosage testosterone and parallel dose-dependent suppression of luteinizing hormone, follicle-stimulating hormone, and sperm production. *J Clin Endocrinol Metab*, 70, 282-287.

Montorsi, F., Salonia, A., Deho, F., Cestari, A., Guazzoni, G., Di Silverio, F. (2003) Pharmacological management of erectile disfunction. *B J Urol Int*, 91, 446–454.

Montorsi, F. (2007) Testosterone and the Prostate: The Evidence So Far. *Eur Urol*, suppl., 6, 874–878.

Morales, A., Buvat, J., Gooren, L. et al. (2004) Endocrine aspects of sexual dysfunction in men. *J Sex Med*, 1, 69–83.

Morales, A., Schulman, C.C., Tostain, J. et al (2006) Testosterone deficiency syndrome (TDS) needs to be named appropriately – the importance of accurate terminology. *Eur Urol*, 50, 407–449.

Morgentaler, A. (2006) Testosterone and prostate cancer: an historical perspective on a modern myth. *Eur Urol*, 50, 935-939.

Morley, J.E., Perry, III H.M. (2003) Andropause – an old concept in new clothing. *Clin Geriatr Med*, 19, 507–528.

Mosby's Medical, *Nursing and Allied Health Dictionary*. 5th Ed., Mosby (1998), USA.

Muller, M., Grobbee, D.E., den Tonkelaar, I. et al. (2005) Endogenous sex hormones and metabolic syndrome in aging men. *J Clin Endocrinol Metab*, 90, 2618–2623.

Mulligan, T. Et al. (2006) Prevalence of hypogonadism in males aged at least 45 years: the HIM Study. *Int J Clin Pract*, 60, 762-769.

Nelson, K. (2002) Research for environmentol triggers of Parkinson's disease. *The Lancet Neurol*, 1, 333-41.

Nieschlag, E., Swerdloff, R., Behre, H.M. et al. (2005) Investigation, treatment and monitoring of hypogonadism in males: ISA, ISSAM and EAU recommendations. *Int J Androlog*, 28, 125–127.

Oesterling, J.E. (1991) LHRH Agonist. A nonsurgical treatment for Benign Prostatic Hyperplasia. *J Andrology*, 12, 381-388.

Official Law Daily (1996) number 121, September 11, par. 571 by Polish Ministry of Health and Social Welfare.

Okun, M.S., Walter, B.L., McDonald, W.M. (2002) Beneficial effects of testosterone replacement for the nonmotor symptoms of Parkinson disease. *Arch Neurol*, 11, 1750-3.

Orwoll, E., Lambert, L.C., Marshall, L.M. et al. (2006) Testosterone and estradiol among older men. *J Clin Endocrinol Metab*, 91, 1336-1344.

Prout, G. R., Brewer, W. R. (1967) Response of men with advanced prostatic carcinoma to exogenous administration of testosterone. *Cancer*, 20, 1871-1878.

Rayner, M, Mockford, C. Boaz, A. (1998) *Coronary heart disease statistics*. London, British Heart Foundation.

Reissmann, T., Schally, A.V., Bouchard, H et al. (2000) The LHRH Antagonist Cetrorelix: a review. *Human Reproduction Update*, 6, 322-331.

Reports from the years 1996-2011 the Division for Monitoring of Adverse Actions of the High Authority for Registration of Drugs and other Medical Products in Poland - held by the author.

Rhoden, E.L., Morgentaler, A. (2003) Testosterone replacement therapy in hypogonadal men at high risk for prostate cancer: results of 1 year of treatment in men with prostatic intraepithelial neoplasia. *J Urol*, 170, 2348-2351.

Riggs, B.L. et al. (2002) Sex steroids and the construction and conservation of the adult skeleton. *Endocrinological Review.*, 23, 279-302.

Sawada, H., Ibi, M., Kihara, T. et al. (1998) Estradiol protects mesencephalic dopaminergic neurons from oxidative stress-induced neuronal death. *J Neurosci Res*, 54 (5), 707-19.

Schatzl, G., Madersbacher, S., Thurridl, T. et al. (2001) High-grade prostate cancer is associated with low serum testosterone levels. *Prostate*, 47, 52-58.

Schiavi, R.C. et al. (1993) Hormones and nocturnal penile tumescence in healthy aging men. Archives of Sexual Behavior, 22, 207-215.

Serwin, B.B. (1994) Estrogenic effects on memory in women. *Ann NY Acad, Sci*, 743, 213-31.

Shabsigh, R. (2003) Hypogonadism and erectile dysfunction: the role for testosterone therapy. *Int J Impot Res*, 1 (supl. 4), 9–13.

Shores, M.M,, Matsumoto, A.M., Sloan, K.L.. et al., 2006 Low testosterone and mortality in male veterans. *Arch Intern Med*, 166, 1660–1665.

Si-Tian, L., You-Lun, G., Cui-Hong, L., Chang-Hai, H. (2004) Hormonal contraception in Chinese men: variations in suppression of spermatogenesis with injectable testosterone undecanoate and levonorgestrel implants. *Asian J Androl*, 6, 41–46.

Skibińska, A., Kossuth, M. (2003) Estrogens and plasticity of synapses. *Neurol Neurochir Pol*, Suppl. 4, 379-92.

Snyder, P., Peachey, H., Berlin, J. et al. (2000) Effects of testosterone replacement in hypogonadal men. *J Clin Endocrinol Metab*, 85, 2670-2677.

Snyder, P.J. (2001) Effects of age on testicular function and consequences of testosterone treatment. *J Clin Endocrinol Metab*, 86, 2369-2372.

Studd, J., Panay, N. (2004) Hormones and depression in women. *Climacteric*, 7, 338-346.

Tariq, S. (2002) Changes in libido/sex life. in: *Textbook of men's health*. Lunenfeld B., Gooren L. (edit.). The Parthenon Publishing Group, London, 381–388. ISBN 18-421401-1-6.

Tenover, J.L. (1997) Testosterone and the aging male. *Journal of Andrology*, 18, 103-106.

Tenover, J.L. (1999) Testosterone replacement therapy in older adult men. *International Journal of Andrology*, 22, 300-306.

Tivesten, A., Vandenput, L., Labrie, F., et al. Low serum testosterone and estradiol predict mortality in elderly men. *J Clin Endocrinol Metab*, 2009, 94,,2482-2488.

Traish, A.M., Kim, N. (2005) The physiological role of androgens in penile erection: regulating of corpus cavernosum structure and function. *Journal of Sexual Medicine*, 2, 759-770.

Trinick, T.R, Feneley M.R., Carruthers M. (2011) International web survey shows high prevalence of symptomatic testosterone deficiency in men. The Aging Male, 14, 10–15.

Tunstall-Pedoe, H., Kuulasmaa, K., Mahonen, M., et al. (1999) Contribution of trends in survival and coronary event rate to change in coronary heart disease mortality. 10-year results WHO MONICA *Lancet*, 353, 1547-57.

Vermeulen, A. (2001) Androgen replacement therapy in the aging male - a critical evaluation. *J Clin Endocrinol Metab*, 86, 2380-2389.

Vermeulen, A., Kaufman, J.M., Giagulli, V.A. (1996) Influence of some biological indexes on sex hormone binding globulin and androgen levels in aging or obese males. *J Clin Endocrinol Metab*, 81, 1821-1826.

Wallace, E.M., Gow, S.M., Wu, F.C. (1993) Comparison between testosterone enanthate-induced azoospermia and oligozoospermia in a male contraceptive study. I. Plasma luteinizing hormone, follicle stimulating hormone, testosterone, estradiol, and inhibin concentrations. *J Clin Endocrinol Metab*, 77, 290–293.

Wang, C., Alexander, G., Berman, N. et al. (1996) Testosterone replacement therapy improves mood in hypogonadal men — a clinical research center study. *J Clin Endocrinol Metab*, 81, 3578–3583.

Wang, C., Nieschlag, E., Swerdloff, R. et al. (2009) Investigation, Treatment and Monitoring of Hypogonadism in Males: ISA, ISSAM, EAU, EAA and ASA Recemendation. *Eur Urol*, 55, 121-130.

Webb, C.M., MacNeil, J.G., Hayward C.S. et al. (1999) Effects of testosterone on coronary vasomotor regulation in men with coronary heart disease. *Circulation*, 100, 1690-6.

Weinbauer, G.F., Schlatt, S., Walter, V., Nieschlag, N. (2001) Testosterone-induced inhibition of spermatogenesis is more closely related to suppression of FSH than to testicular androgen levels in the cynomolgus monkey model (Macaca fascicularis). *J Endocrinol*, 168, 25–38.

World Health Organization Task Force on Methods for the Regulation of Male Fertility. Contraceptive efficacy of testosterone-induced azoospermia in normal men. *Lancet* (1990), 336, 955–959.

Wu, F.C., von Eckardstein, A. (2003) Androgens and coronary artery disease. *Endocr Rev*, 24, 183–217.

Wu, F.C., Tajar, A., Beynon, J.M., et al. (2010) EMAS Group. Identification of late-onset hypogonadism in middle-aged and elderly men. *N Engl J Med*, 363, 123-135.

Yano, M, Imamoto, T, Suzuki, H et al. (2007) The clinical potential of pretreatment serum testosterone level to improve the efficiency of prostate cancer screening. *Eur Urol*, 51, 375-380.

Yassin A., Treish A. (2004) LUTS/BPH, alpha-adrenoreceptors and erectile function. *Arab Journal of Urology*, 2, 8-12.

Yeap, B B , Hyde, Z., Norman, P.E., Chubb, S.A.P., Golledge, J. (2010) Associations of total testosterone, sex hormone-binding globulin, calculated free testosterone, and luteinizing hormone with prevalence of abdominal aortic aneurysm in older men. *J Clin Endocrinol Metab*, 95, 1123-1130.

Zgliczyński, S. & Zgliczyński, W. (2002) *Standards of Endocrinology*. Studio PIN, Warszawa, ISBN: 83-915669-1-9.

Zhang, G.Y., Gu, Y.Q., Wang, X.H., Cui, Y.G., Bremner ,W.J. (1999) A clinical trial of injectable testosterone undecanoate as a potential male contraceptive in normal Chinese men. *J Clin Endocrinol Metab*, 84, 3642–3647.

Zitzmann, M., Nieschlag, E. (2006) Testosterone substitution: current modalities and perspectives. *J Reproduktionsmed Endokrinol*, 3 (2), 109–116.

Zverina, J., Hampl, R., Sulocava, J., Starka ,L. (1990) Hormonal status and sexual behaviour of 16 men after surgical castration. *Arch Ital Urol Nefrol Androl*, 62, 55–58.

7

Hypogonadism After Childhood Cancer Treatment

Lorna Zadravec Zaletel[1], Ljupčo Todorovski[2] and Berta Jereb[1]
[1]Institute of Oncology,
[2]University of Ljubljana, Faculty of Administration
Slovenia

1. Introduction

Long-term survival of children with cancer has greatly improved in the last decades due to effective treatment, especially multiagent chemotherapy (ChT). The chief concern is now being directed toward the late effects of treatment. Endocrine glands, gonads in particular, are very susceptible to damaging effects of anticancer therapy. The damaging effect of both ChT and radiotherapy (RT) on gonads is well known (Cohen 2003, Diamond et al. 2001, Spoudeas 2002). In a study of 2283 long-term survivors of childhood cancer Byrne and colleagues found that RT below the diaphragm depressed fertility in both sexes for about 25%, ChT with alkylating agents (AA) with or without RT below the diaphragm depressed fertility by 60% in men, in women, however, AA therapy administered alone had no apparent effect on fertility (Byrne et al. 1987). Hypogonadism is most often due to direct damage by ChT, RT and/or surgery, rarely is due to damage to the hypothalamus and/or pituitary gland (Cicognani et al. 2003, Müller 2003).

The gonads have two main functions, the production of sex hormones (estrogens and testosterone) and germ cells (ova and sperm). Both of them depend on a normal function of the hypothalamic-pituitary-gonadal axis. Long term survivors of childhood cancer are at risk of hypogonadism related to gonadotropin secretion, but more frequently hypogonadism is caused by direct damage of testes or ovaries. In human testis two functions are combined: sex steroid production and sperm production. Germ cells form sperm, Sertoli cells support and nurture the developing germ cells and Leydig cells produce testosterone. These three cell types are organized into two functional compartments: germ cells and Sertoli cells form the seminiferous tubules where spermatogenesis takes place, and the network of Leydig cells are responsible for the production of testosterone, which is necessary for normal spermatogenesis. These two compartments are under separate controls and affected in different ways by cancer treatments (Meistrich 2009, Shalet 2009, Sklar 1999).

In the ovary, follicle is the site where the production of sex hormones and germ cells takes place. As a result, when ovarian failure occurs, both sex hormone production and fertility are disrupted. Germ cells in the ovary unlike spermatogonial cells lack the ability of repopulation. Preliminary stages of oogenesis are completed shortly after birth, the dominant part of the cell population in ovary being oocytes in the stationary stage of prophase. Older age is an important risk factor for ovarian failure following childhood cancer and its treatment, given the progressive decline in oocyte reserve with increasing age (Johnston & Wallace 2009, Sklar 1999). If ovarian function is lost prior to the onset of puberty, it results in delayed puberty and primary amenorrhea. If ovarian function is lost during or after pubertal maturation, arrested puberty, secondary amenorrhea, and premature maenopause are observed. In the adolescent and young adults with ovarian failure increased plasma concentrations of gonadotropins and reduced levels of estradiol are typically found.

1.1 Toxic effects of ionizing radiation on testes

1.1.1 Germ cell epithelium

The sperm-producing cells are more vulnerable to cancer treatment than Leydig cells, and are frequently impaired by radiotherapy and different types of chemotherapy. Even small doses of ionizing radiation can damage germinal epithelium of testes. Among the germ cells, type A spermatogonial cells are the most sensitive (especially more differentiated stages A2-4, which are at the stage of mitosis) and type B spermatogonial cells (Ash 1980, Greiner 1985, Lu & Meistrich 1979, Meistrich et al. 1982, Rowley et al. 1974). These sensitive cells can be destroyed with a single dose of radiation as low as 15 cGy. Germ cells in later stages of spermatogenesis, eg. spermatocytes, and spermatides, are less sensitive to ionizing radiation (destroyed by a single dose of 200 cGy or more) (Ash 1980, Lushbaugh & Casarett 1976). After irradiation, the surviving germ cells (early type A spermatogonial cells) develop into more radiosensitive germ cells. Therefore, fractionated RT (administered in several small doses) may be more harmful because it empties the storage of germ cells (Ash 1980, Greiner 1982). Only type A spermatogonial cells can repopulate. If a sufficient number of these cells survive, there is recovery of spermatogenesis, even after several years (Hahn et al. 1982). The rate of damage of spermatogenesis and time in which there's a full recovery depends on the size of RT dose to the testes. Duration of azoospermia is likely to depend on the number of destroyed germ cells. After a single dose of less than 100 cGy to the testes, recovery of spermatogenesis occurs in 9-18 months, after a dose of 200 to 300 cGy in 30 months and after a dose of 400 to 600 cGy in more than 5-years (even after more than 10-years) (Lushbaugh & Casarett 1976, Sandeman 1966, Sanders et al. 1991, Rowley et al. 1974). Single doses greater than 600 cGy cause irreparable damage of spermatogenesis. After fractionated RT a total dose of more than 150 to 200 cGy cause irreversible azoospermia (Greiner 1982, Sandeman 1966). Oligospermia or azoospermia may occur during treatment with RT or mostly during the 2- 3-months from the start of RT (Sandeman 1966). During radiation treatment testes are rarely directly exposed to ionizing radiation, but they are exposed to indirect radiation (e.g. abdominal RT). Several studies reported radiation doses the testes receive at the spillage of ionizing radiation during RT of areas under the diaphragm. This dose to the testes following RT of abdominal areas may be as high as 7 to 13% of the total dose (i.e. the order of 100 to 300 cGy) (da Cunha et al. 1984, Kinsella et al. 1989, Lushbaugh & Casarett 1976, Whitehead et al. 1982). The dose of this size can cause irreversible azoospermia (Greiner 1982, Sandeman 1966). This dose to the testes can be reduced by an additional lead shielding of testis to the level bellow 50cGy, which is not harmful for spermatogenesis (Kovač et al. 1990, Whitehead et al. 1982). Germ cell dysfunction with azoospermia is present in essentially all males treated with TBI (Sanders et al. 1991). Recovery of germ cell function has occurred rarely and primarily following single-dose irradiation (Sanders et al. 1991, Sklar et al. 1984). Germ cell dysfunction with resultant infertility is often associated with reduced testicular volume, increased FSH concentrations, and reduced plasma concentrations of inhibin B.

1.1.2 Leydig cells

Leydig cells are less sensitive for damaging effect of RT than germ cells, requiring higher dose of ionizing radiation (more than 1500 cGy) for failure, therefore only direct testicular irradiation can cause significant damage of LC. LC are the most sensitive for damaging effect of RT in prepubertal period (Castillo et al. 1990, Shalet et al. 1985). The probability of radiation induced Leydig cell failure is directly related to the dose delivered and inversely related to age at treatment (Leiper et al. 1986, Sarafoglou et al. 1997, Shalet et al. 1989). In the majority of males who receive 2000 cGy fractionated radiation to the testes there is no impairment of testosterone production, but after 2400 cGy of fractionated irradiation as therapy for young males with testicular relapse of ALL there is a very high risk for Leydig cell damage (Sklar 1999). The majority of boys who are prepubertal at the time of treatment, will develop Leydig cell failure after 2400 cGy testicular irradiation and require androgen replacement (Leiper et al. 1986, Shalet et al. 1985). Low doses of ionizing radiation but above 75 cGy can lead to dysfunction of the LC (compensated insufficiency of LC with normal levels of testosterone) (Rowley et al. 1974).

Unlike germinal epithelium LC impairment may develop several years after RT and is usually irreparable (Shalet et al. 1985). Treatment-induced Leydig cell failure and testosterone insufficiency following cancer tretament are relatively uncommon compared with germ cell dysfunction and infertility. Leydig cell failure results in delayed/arrested puberty and lack of secondary sexual characteristics if it occurs before onset of puberty. If it occurs following the completion of normal pubertal development, it can result in reduced libido, erectile dysfunction, decreased bone mineral density, decreased muscle mass, and other metabolic disturbances (Sklar 1999). Increased plasma concentrations of LH combined with low levels of testosterone are characteristic for Leydig cell dysfunction, but these changes may not become apparent until the individual has reached mid-adolescence (Shalet et al. 1985).

1.2 Toxic effects of cytostatic agents on testes

1.2.1 Germ cell epithelium

The chemotherapeutic agents most commonly associated with impaired male fertility are alkylating agents (AA). These citostatic agents are used in the treatment of many types of childhood cancer. Agents in this group are: cyclophosphamide (CY), busulfan, melphalan, nitrogen mustard (NM), DTIC, nitrosoureas (CCNU, BCNU), procarbazine, chlorambucil, ifosfamide. Alkylating agents damage especially late (differentiating) spermatogonial cells and early spermatocytes, and less mature spermatozoa (Meistrich et al. 1982). In the treatment of childhood cancer many cytostatic agents are used at the same time, making it difficult to identify gonadotoxic effect of individual cytostatic. The toxic effect of CY has been studied most. After the cumulative dose of CY of less than 7.5 g/m2 males may retain normal sperm production, after a dose between 7.5 and 22.5 g/m2 oligo-and azoospermia are observed, but the dose greater than 25 g / m 2 causes azoospermia (Kenney et al. 2001). It seems that the threshold dose of CY for azoospermia is around 10 g / m2 (Aubier et al. 1989, Casteren et al. 2009, Relander et al. 2000). Patients treated in prepubertal period have a lower risk for germ cell damage than those treated in postpubertal period (Aubier et al. 1989, Brämswig et al. 1990, Pennisi et al. 1975). Procarbazine, another alkylating agent, commonly used in the treatment of

Hodgkin's disease, can also induce impaired sperm production in a dose-dependent fashion. MOPP (mechlorethamine, vincristine, procarbazine, and prednisone) or MOPP-like combinations, such as MVPP (mechlorethamine, vinblastine, procarbazine and prednisone) induce azoospermia in 90-100 % of pts with a 10-20% chance of recovery even 10 years after treatment (Chapman et al. 1979, Diamond & Bercu 2001, Viviani et al. 1985, Whitehead et al. 1982). Recovery of spermatogenesis following MOPP therapy appears to be dose-related, 3 courses of MOPP representing a limiting gonadal exposure for recovery, suggesting only a partial killing of germinal stem cells (da Cunha et al. 1984). Patients with Hodgkin's disease who received three cycles of MOPP alternating with three cycles of ABVD (doxorubicin, bleomycin, vinblastine and dacarbazine) suffer less testicular damage than patients who received 6 cycles of MOPP (Berg et al. 2004, Mackie et al. 1996). Chemotherapy with COPP (CY, VCR, PBZ, prednisone) or OPPA (VCR, prednisone, procarbazine and adriamycin) can cause azoospermia in 50% of patients. ABVD (Adriamycin, bleomycin, vinblastine,DTIC) protocol is less gonadotoxic, usually causing transient germ cell impairment with total recovery (Berg et al. 2004, Santoro et al. 1987, Viviani et al. 1985). CY and cytarabine were reported the most damaging antileukemic drugs for spermatogenesis (Lendon et al. 1978). There has been a report that cytarabine in cumulative doses greater than 1 g/m^2 is correlated with a decreased tubular fertility index in boys (Lendon et al. 1978). There are reports that vincristine also might have important role in causing azoospermia, when administered in childhood or adolescence (Waxmann et al. 1982).

Chemotherapy regimens containing cisplatin or carboplatin can induce germ cell damage with a different rate of recovery of spermatogenesis (Lampe et al. 1997). Recovery of spermatogenesis may be lower in those who received ChT with vinca alkaloids (vincristine and vinblastine) as well. Antimetabolites usually do not cause irreversible damage to testes, but can cause temporary oligospermia. (Sussman & Leonard 1980).

1.2.2 Leydig cells

Leydig cells are less vulnerable to damage from cancer therapy than germ cells, and chemotherapy-induced dysfunction of Leydig cells requiring testosterone replacement therapy is rare (Blatt et al. 1981, Sklar 1999). Leydig cell dysfunction may be observed following treatment with alkylating agent regimens. Ten to 57% of male patients can develop elevated serum concentrations of LH following treatment, but chemotherapy-induced Leydig cell dysfunction is generally subclinical (Bramswig et al. 1990, Kenney et al. 2001, Mackie et al. 1996, Relander et al. 2000, Romerius et al. 2009, Sklar 1999).

1.3 Toxic effects of ionizing radiation on ovaries

Ionizing radiation causes ovarian function impairment as a function of cumulative dose and age. Ovaries are frequently inside RT field or in its immediate vicinity during pelvic or abdominal RT. Preservation of ovarian function depends on the ability of single oocyte to repair damage. That is why RT with multiple small fractions is less toxic for ovaries than RT with one larger fraction, due to greater potential of damage repair during two smaller fractions (Greiner 1985). Females receiving abdominal, pelvic, or spinal irradiation are at increased risk of ovarian failure, especially if both ovaries are within the treatment field (Hamre et al. 1987, Horning et al. 1981, Sklar et al. 2006, Thibaud et al. 1992, Wallace 2005). However, when ovarian transposition is performed prior to RT, ovarian function is retained in the majority of young girls and adolescent females (Ortin et al. 1990, Sklar 1999, Thibaud et al. 1992). In women over 40 years of age radiation dose of 400 to 700 cGy is sufficient for the sterilization, in younger women the dose from 1250 to 1500 cGy is necessary for sterilization (Ash 1980), and for those treated at the age of 10 years or less even dose of 2000 cGy is necessary for permanent ovarian damage (Lushbaugh & Casarett 1976, Sanders et al. 1991, Wallace et al. 2005). Nevertheless doses of less than 1000 cGy are capable of inducing ovarian damage in patients who have additional risk factors, such as concomitant exposure to alkylating agents and older age at diagnosis. In a report from the CCSS, doses of radiotherapy to the ovary of at least 2000 cGy were associated with the highest risk of ovarian failure; more than 70% of patients exposed to such doses developed ovarian failure, with higher rates in older individuals (13–20 years) when compared with those who were younger (0–12 years) at the time of treatment (Chemaitilly et al. 2006). Moreover, if radiation is given in association with alkylating agents, ovarian dysfunction may occur despite the use of lower doses. In the report from CCSS acute ovarian failure occurred in 6.3% of eligible survivors, exposure of the ovaries to high-dose radiation (especially over 1000 cGy), alkylating agents and older ages being significant risk factors for ovarian failure (Chemaitilly et al. 2006). Premature nonsurgical menopause occurred in 8% of participants versus 0.8% of siblings. Risk factors for premature menopause included attained age, exposure to increasing doses of radiation to the ovaries, increasing alkylating agent score, and the diagnosis of Hodgkin's lymphoma. The cumulative incidence of premature menopause in individuals treated with both alkylating agents and abdominal- pelvic radiation was in the range of 30% (Sklar et al. 2006). Offspring of women who received uterine radiation doses of more than 500 cGy were more likely to be small for gestational age, but there was no evidence for an increased risk of congenital malformations (Green et al. 2002). These studies demonstrated that women treated with pelvic irradiation and/or high alkylating agent doses were at risk for acute ovarian failure, premature menopause, and small-for-gestational-age offspring.

1.4 Toxic effects of cytostatic agents on ovaries

Ovaries are less sensitive to harmful effect of cytostatics than germ cells of testes. Biopsy of the ovary in girls after treatment with chemotherapy showed decreased number of primordial and antral follicles (even more pronounced after treatment with multiagent ChT and RT), decreased follicular maturation, cortical and stromal fibrosis, with / without proliferation and thickening of blood vessels (Chapman et al. 1979, Nicosia et al. 1985). Most sensitive for damaging effect of ChT are growing and preovulatory follicles, therefore ovaries of prepubertal girls are less sensitive to injury after ChT exposure (Stillman et al. 1982). Another reason for higher resistance of ovaries of prepubertal girls to ChT is their greater follicular reserve when compared with the ovaries of adults (Chemaitilly et al. 2006, Grigg et al. 2000). Among chemotherapeutic agents, alkylating agents, which prevent cell division by interacting with DNA, are known to be associated with the occurrence of ovarian failure (Brydøy et al. 2007, Chematilly et al. 2006, Green et al. 2009, Ortin et al. 1990, Zacharin et al. 2010), ovarian failure being dependent on the cumulative dose of cytostatic and age of patients during treatment. In CCSS-study, it was reported that alkylating agents cyclophosphamide and procarbazine were significant risk factors for ovarian failure (Chematilly et al. 2006). Although exposure to procarbazine was an independent risk factor for ovarian failure, regardless of age at treatment, cyclophosphamide significantly increased that risk only in subjects treated at an older age. As the number of oocytes declines with

advancing age, the ovaries of older individuals become more vulnerable to gonadal toxins compared with that seen in younger subjects (Sarafoglou et al. 1997, Sklar 1999). In the study of Ortin and colleagues 10% of girls were amenorrhoic after receiving 6 or more cycles of MOPP and none of those who received other regimes of ChT (e.g. MOPP / ABVD, ABVD). After combined treatment with ChT (6 or more cycles of MOPP) and pelvic RT at a dose of 2000 to 4400 cGy (with or without ovaropeksy) incidence of ovarian failure was about 50%. None of the girls who received 3 or less cycles of MOPP had ovarian failure (Ortin et al. 1990). Females who received, both before and after pubertal development, high-dose myeloablative therapy with alkylating agents such as busulfan, melphalan, and thiotepa in preparation for bone marrow transplantation are at high risk of developing ovarian failure (Michel et al. 1997). Recovery of function has been recorded only rarely (Michel et al. 1997, Thibaud et al. 1998). However, the majority of girls receiving standard chemotherapy maintain or recover ovarian function during the immediate posttreatment period (Horning et al. 1981, Sklar 1999). Histologic examination of ovarian tissue in prepubertal and postpubertal girls treated for solid tumors or leukemia nevertheless revealed a decreased number of ovarian follicles and inhibition of follicular growth compared with age-matched controls (Himelstein- Braw et al. 1978, Larsen et al. 2003). Therefore, among women who retain or recover ovarian function following treatment with ChT, a subset will experience premature menopause when they reach their 20s and 30s (Byrne et al. 1992, Sklar et al. 2006). In a report from the CCSS, female survivors with a history of exposure to high doses of alkylating agents, to lomustine or to cyclophosphamide were less likely to become pregnant when compared with sibling controls (Green et al. 2009). No adverse pregnancy outcomes were identified, however in a large study conducted within the framework of the CCSS (Green et al. 2002).
The aim of our study was: to establish the incidence of hypogonadism and the risk factors for its developement in childhood-cancer survivors in Slovenia and define the highest respective the lowest risk groups.

2. Patients and methods

2.1 Patients

In Slovenia, 1474 children were treated for cancer under the age of 16 years from 1.1.1965 to 31.12.1995 at the University Clinical Hospital Ljubljana and/or Institute of Oncology Ljubljana. At the time of our study 712 patients were alive, 460 of them were more than 16 years of age and were at least 3 years off treatment. Of those patients 390 were regularly followed at the outpatient clinic at the Institute of Oncology in Ljubljana (Jereb 2000, Zaletel 2004). We included in our study 297 consecutive patients in whom endocrinological evaluation was performed until 1.1.2003. Ninety-three patients refused examinations. There were 115 females and 182 males. They were 0-16 (median 9 yrs) years of age at the diagnosis of malignancy and had endocrinological evaluation 3-32 (median 11,5) years after the end of treatment at age of 14-42 (median 20) years. All pts were pubertal or postpubertal when studied. Distribution of diagnosis among patients included in our study is shown in table 1.
The majority (90%) of patients had combined treatment including 2-3 modalities, surgery (S), ChT, RT, a quarter of them had all 3 modalities, while 41% had combined ChT and RT. To evaluate the risk factors for hypogonadism after treatment for childhood cancer, we used a multivariate analysis method of the classification trees.

DIAGNOSIS	Males	Females	All
	n	n	n (%)
Leukemia	30	37	67 (22.5)
Hodgkin's disease	40	24	64 (21.5)
Brain tumor	30	18	48 (16)
NHL	35	3	38 (13)
Soft tissue sarcoma	16	8	24 (8)
Wilms' tumor	11	7	18 (6)
Bone sarcoma	6	6	12 (4)
Germ cell tumor	4	6	10 (3.5)
Neuroblastoma	4	1	5 (1.5)
Retinoblastoma	2	3	5 (1.5)
Carcinoma of nasopharynx	2	1	3 (1)
Other ♣	2	1	3 (1)
All	182	115	297 (100)

♣ retroperitoneal paraganglioma, hepatoblastoma, invasive adenoma of suprarenal gland, one each

Table 1. Diagnosis in 297 patients

2.2 Methods

2.2.1 Assessment of gonadal function

The patient´s data regarding diagnosis and treatment were collected from medical files, information concerning quality of life including attained educational level, marital status, employment and social life, past and present menstrual histories, the course of puberty and fertility histories was ascertained by interview. General physical examination was performed in terms of recording height, weight, clinical abnormalities and Tanner stages of pubic hair and genital development were recorded. Each patient´s blood samples were analysed for basal concentrations of testosterone (RIA, IMUNOTECH), estradiol (DELFIA-LKB) and prolactin (DELFIA-LKB). Concentrations of LH (DELFIA-LKB) and FSH (DELFIA-LKB) were determined before and 10, 20, 30, 60 minutes after i.v. administration of gonadotropin releasing hormone (50 mcg/m^2) (LH-RH). Primary hypogonadism (PH) was defined as basal serum FSH and/or LH level above the normal upper limit and exaggerated response after stimulation with LH-RH. In men, elevated basal serum FSH levels indicated germinal epithelium damage (GE-DA), while elevated LH levels (with/without reduced testosterone levels) indicated Leydig cells (LC) damage (LC-DA). Normal basal values of LH and/or FSH and exaggerated response after LH-RH stimulation were considered as subclinical impairment (SIG). Exaggerated response of FSH after LH-RH was considered as dysfunction of germinal epithelium (GE-dys), while exaggerated response of LH after LH-RH was considered as dysfunction of LC (LC-dys). PH and SIG together were named gonadal impairment (GI). Low serum basal FSH and LH levels with poor response after i.v. bolus of LH-RH was considered as secondary hypogonadism.

2.2.2 Classification tree analysis

Classification tree analysis is a multivariate analysis method that allows for studying of simultaneous influence of a series of independent variables on a single dependent variable (Jereb 1973). The output of the analysis is a classification tree, read from the root node, through the internal nodes all the way to the leaves. In each internal node, a test on the value of a single independent variable for the given case is being performed. Based on the outcome of the test, we follow one of the branches originating from the node. Following the branches in that manner, we arrive in one of the leaf nodes of the tree that provides a classification, i.e., the predicted value of the dependent variable, of the case at hand. In addition to predicting the value of the dependent variable for a given case, the structure of the classification tree also reveals the influence and relative importance of the values of independent variables on the dependent one.

Classification tree is being constructed by successive divisions of the original group of cases into pairs of subgroups, where each division is based on the value of a single independent variable. For each division (often referred to as a split), the variable is being selected that produces "pure" subgroups; the purity being measured as a fraction of cases with the same value of the dependent variable. In ideal case, a completely "pure" group of cases that share the same value of the dependent variable is obtained. Each of the subgroups generated in the process becomes a parent group in the next step of the analysis and is further divided in the same way. The division of cases stops when the group of cases is completely pure or when it contains less than a user-defined minimal number of cases. In our study, the C4.5 (Quinlan 1993) program for constructing classification trees was used. C4.5 allows the setting of several parameters that influence branching and quality of the final classification tree: most notably there is one parameter that determines the smallest number of cases to be included in a single group, and another parameter that determines the degree of the tree post-pruning performed. For details please refer to the description in (Quinlan 1993). The optimal values of these parameters were determined using a standard cross-validation method (Jazbec et al. 2007, Macedoni-Lukšič et al. 2003, Velensek et al. 2008). The usual performance measure for classification trees is the accuracy of the tree when predicting the outcome (the value of the dependent variable) on samples not seen during the process of tree building.

Note finally, that since we use an alternative performance criterion, the classification tree obtained the cross-validation procedure outlined above is not expected to provide accurate classification of cases into hypogonadism and non-hypogonadism classes. Instead of using the tree as an accurate predictor, we were interested in analyzing the tree structure and identifying the risk group where incidence of hypogonadism is significantly higher than the one observed in the population of 297 patients included in the study. Multivariate analysis with classification tree was not done when specific abnormalities were found in less than ten percent of examinated childhood cancer survivors.

Multivariate statistical analysis with classification tree analysis was performed with two groups of independent variables and their values. The first group included six independent variables:

- gender (female, male)
- age at diagnosis (in years),
- type of malignancy (1-12, see Table 1),
- surgery (yes, no)
- radiotherapy (yes, no)
- chemotherapy (yes, no).

In the second group of independent variables, variables from the first group were further broken down (type of surgery, parts of the body, which was irradiated, type of ChT), because we wanted to determine the effect of various treatments on the gonadal function. The observation time, i.e. the time from the end of treatment to the gonadal evaluation, was added as a new variable. Variables of the second groups were:

- gender (female, male)
- age at diagnosis (in years),
- type of malignancy (1-12, see Table 1),
- surgery (no, outside the abdomen, abdominal surgery, orchidectomy, ovariectomy),
- radiotherapy (no, brain RT, RT above the diaphragm except the brain, RT of the upper abdomen, pelvic RT, testicular RT)
- chemotherapy (no, ChT without AA, ChT with AA),
- observation time.

We analyzed the influence of both groups of independent variables to each of the two dependent of PH and GI (i.e., PH and/or SIG) in three different groups of patients: all patients, females and males (impairment of LC, LC-DA and LC-dys as well as impairment of germinal epithelium, GE-DA and GE-dys).

3. Results

Primary hypogonadism was found in 76 (26%) adolescents, in 62 (34%) males and 14 (12%) females. Gonadal impairment was found in 114 (38%) adolescents, in 89 (49%) males and 25 (22%) females (Table 2).

Diagnosis	Males		Females		All	
	All (n)	Pts with PH n (%)	All (n)	Pts with PH n (%)	All (n)	Pts with PH n (%)
Leukaemia	30	5 (16.5)	37	1 (2.7)	67	6 (9)
Hodgkin's disease	40	26 (65)	24	6 (25)	64	32 (50)
Brain tumor	30	3(10)	18	2 (11)	48	5 (10)
NHL	35	12 (34)	3	0	38	12 (32)
Soft tissue sarcoma	16	7 (44)	8	1 (12.5)	24	8 (33)
Wilms' tumor	11	2 (18)	7	0	18	2 (11)
Bone sarcoma	6	2 (33)	6	1 (16.5)	12	3 (25)
Germ cell tumor	4	2 (50)	6	3 (50)	10	5 (50)
Neuroblastoma	4	2 (50)	1	0	5	2 (40)
Retinoblastoma	2	1 (50)	3	0	5	1 (20)
Carcinoma of nasopharynx	2	0	1	0	3	0
Others ♣	2	0	1	0	3	0
All	182	62 (34)	115	14 (22)	297	76 (26)

♣ retroperitoneal paraganglioma, hepatoblastoma, invasive adenoma of suprarenal gland, one each
PH - primary hypogonadism

Table 2. Primary hypogonadism versus diagnosis and gender in 297 patients.

All but one male subjects with PH had damage of germinal epithelium (15 of them at the same time damage of LC, 30 of them at the same time dysfunction of LC), with one failure, we found LC and DKE. In 12 of the 61 patients with germinal epithelium damage semen analyses was performed; in 11 patients azoospermia was found, one had normal spermiogram. Dysfunction of LC was detected in 54 patients (in 21 patients the only finding), dysfunction of germinal epithelium was found in 9 patients. All 14 female patients with PH had elevated basal FSH and FSH after stimulation, 5 of them had elevated basal LH and LH after stimulation, four had increased LH after stimulation, 6 had decreased levels of estradiol. Among 4 patients with PH who were treated in prepubertal period, two had delayed puberty. Ovarian dysfunction was detected in 11 patients, all had elevated levels of LH after stimulation, 6 had elevated FSH after stimulation as well. All had normal serum estradiol. The highest incidence (50%) of PH was found in those patients treated for Hodgkin's disease (HD) or germ cell tumor (GCT), the lowest incidence (10%) was found in those treated for brain tumors, leukemia and Wilms' tumor (Table 2). The incidence of PH depended on type of treatment as well. The highest proportion of PH (26 - 40%) was found in patients treated with combined treatment, t.i. ChT and RT with / without surgery (Table 3).

Type of treatment	All	Pts with PH n (%)
RT + ChT	121	31 (26)
S + RT+ ChT	76	31 (40.5)
OP + RT	38	4 (10.5)
OP + ChT	31	5 (16)
ChT	14	2 (14)
S	9	0
RT	8	2 (22)
All	297	76 (26)

PH - primary hypogonadism, RT - radiotherapy, ChT- chemotherapy, S – surgery

Table 3. Primary hypogonadism versus type of treatment in 297 patients.

Secondary hypogonadism was found in 6 patients. Three of them had panhypopituitarism after treatment of hypothalamic tumor (2 patients) or orbital tumor (one patient) with surgery and RT (from 4400 to 5000 cGy), 2 patients were treated for brain tumors with surgery and RT (5500 or. 6500 cGy), 1 patient was treated for leukemia with ChT and brain RT (3000 cGy).
Sixty-seven patients had whole brain irradiation with a dose of 1200 - 4000 (median 2400) cGy in prepubertal period. Six patients had precocious puberty; 5 girls after treatment of leukemia and 1 boy after treatment of NHL. Those 6 patients were treated with ChT and brain RT at the age of 5 to 8 years. In all 6 the dose of ionizing radiation to the brain was equal to or greater than 2400 cGy (2400 - 3400, med. 2400 cGy).

3.1 Results of classification tree analysis
3.1.1 First group of independent variables
3.1.1.1 Dependent variable – primary hypogonadism, all patients

PH was found in 76 (26%) of 297 patients. The most important risk factor for PH, which divided the basic group into two subgroups, was diagnosis of HD (Figure 1). The second most important factor which divided a group of adolescents, treated for HD, was gender, and the next still important independant variable was therapy with ChT. Other independent variables from the first group didn't emerged as important risk factors for PH. Therefore, with this analysis we defined a group of 33 (11% of all) patients with the highest (72%) risk of PH; these are men treated for HD with ChT. Two hundred thirty-three patienst, who did not have HD, had low (19%) risk of PH. Low risk (25%) of PH was found also in the group of female patients, treated for HD.

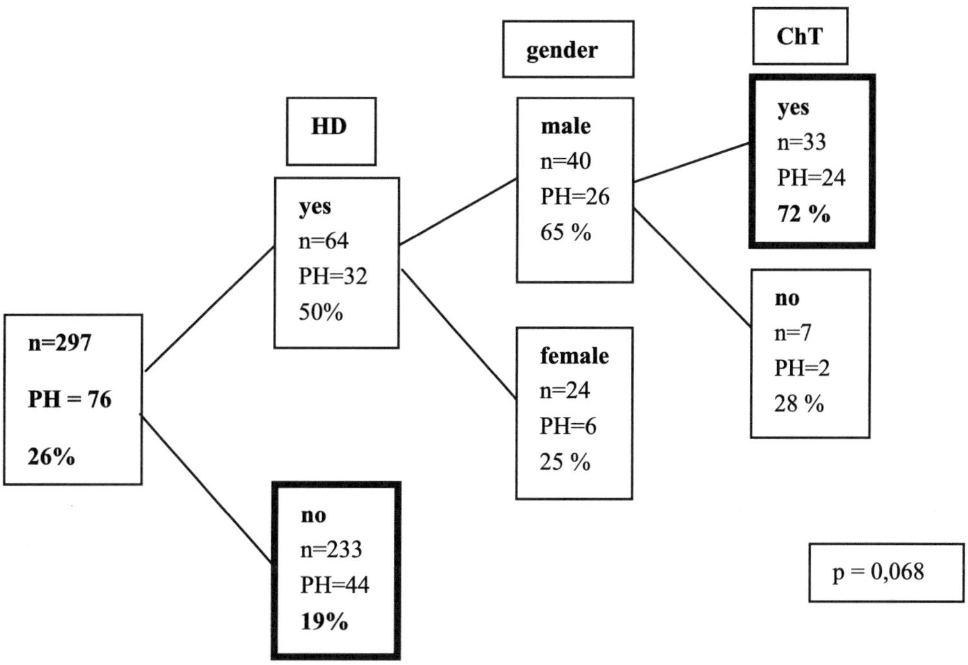

PH - primary hypogonadism, ChT - chemotherapy, HD - Hodgkin's disease

Fig. 1. Classification tree analysis with first group of independent variables and PH as dependent variable in 297 patients

Statistical significance of this analysis was borderline (p = 0,068). We performed the analysis with the same independent variables only for males and it confirmed the results of previous analysis with statistically significance p = 0.045 (Figure 2). Namely, once again in the group of patients with the highest risk of PH (72%) were those treated for HD with ChT. Patients treated for other types of cancer, had a risk of PH of only 25%. Of the seven male patients treated for HD without ChT, only two had PH. Both were treated with pelvic RT.

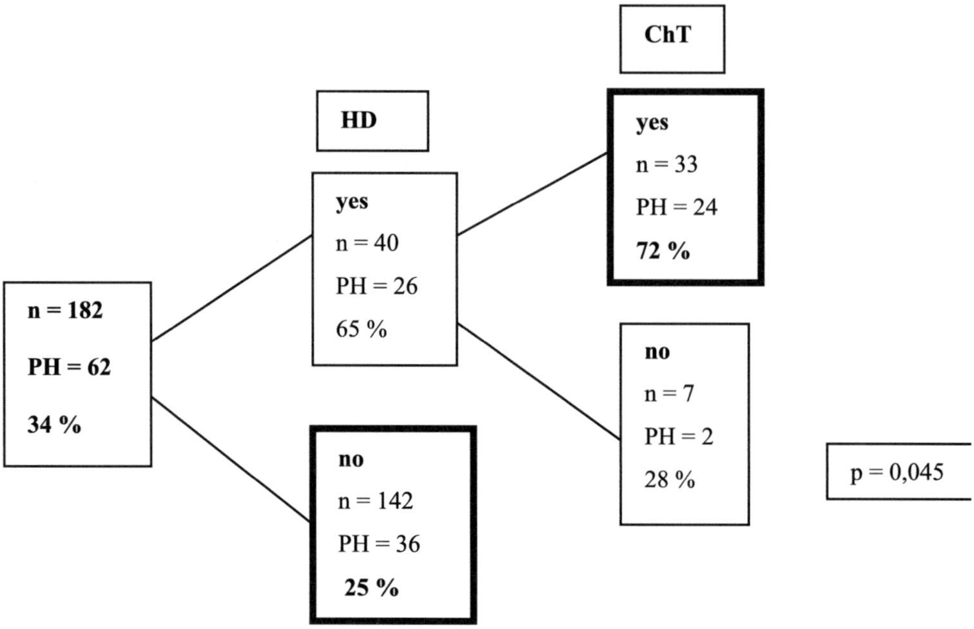

PH - primary hypogonadism, ChT - chemotherapy, HD - Hodgkin's disease

Fig. 2. Classification tree analysis with first group of independent variables and PH as dependent variable in 182 male patients

3.1.1.2 Dependent variable - gonadal impairment (GI, gonadal damage and subclinical impairment) in all patients

GI was found in 114 (38%) adolescents. Independent variable type of diagnosis, germ cell tumor, turned out as the most important risk factor for GI. Namely, 9 out of 10 patients treated for GCT had GI. In the remaining 287 patients the most significant risk factor for GI stood gender (Fig. 3). Males had 48% and females had 18% risk of GI. The group of male patiens further divided by important risk factors for GI: ChT, RT and diagnosis of cancer other than leukemia. With this analysis, we therefore defined the group of patients at highest, 68%, risk of GI: 92 male patients who were treated with ChT and RT for cancer other than leukemia. The lowest, 18%, risk of GI, had two groups of patients; group of females (excluding GCT) and group of 34 male patients who did not receive ChT.
In this multivariate analysis the highest (90%) risk of GI had a group od 10 patients (4 males, 6 females) treated for GCT; 5 patients had PH, 3 females after bilateral ovariectomy abdominal RT (one) and 2 males, one after unilateral orchidectomy and ChT with AA for testicular GCT, and the second after ChT with AA for mediastinal GCT. Four patients (2 females and 2 males) had SIG - all having been treated by unilateral removal of the ovary or testis and ChT with AA. The only patient of this group with normal function of the gonads was a female treated for GCT by unilateral ovariectomy and ChT (including bleomycin, etoposide, cisplatin and ifosfamide) at the age 13. Cumulative doses of AA were comparable to those received by the girls with GI following unilateral ovariectomy (ages 9 and 14 years). So, in this group of patients at high risk of GI gonadal surgery and ChT with AA seems to be important risk factors for gonadal impairment.

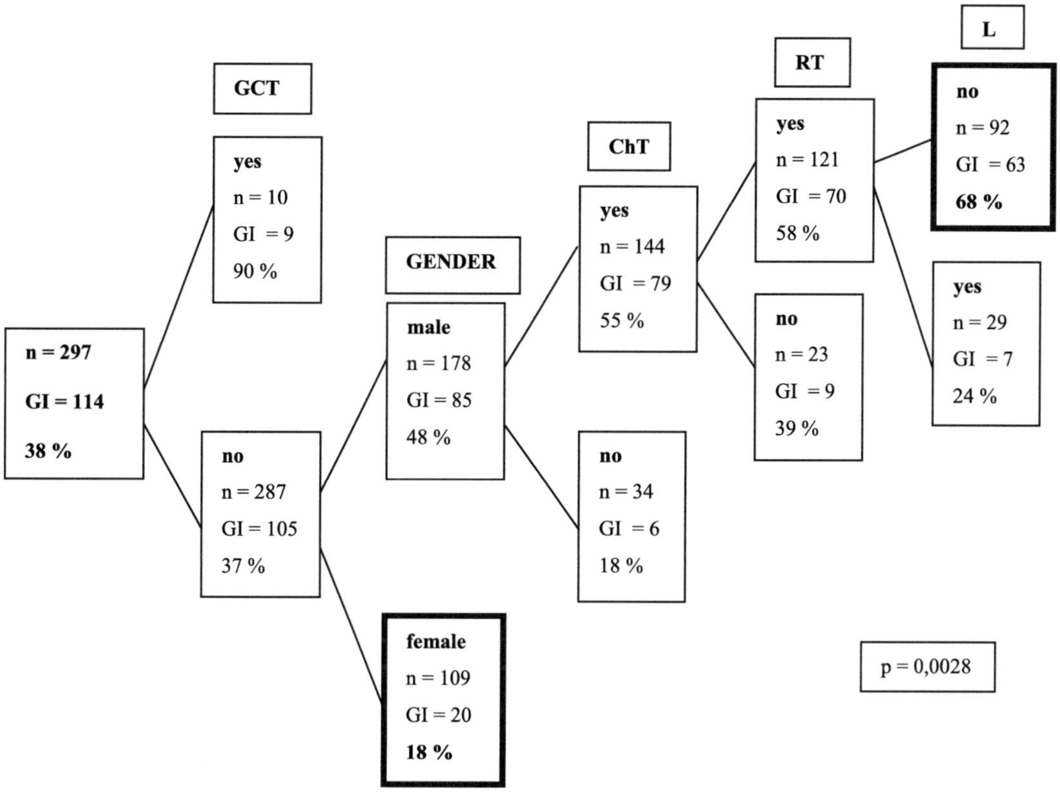

GI - gonadal impairment, GCT - germ cell tumor, L - leukemia, ChT - chemotherapy, RT - radiotherapy

Fig. 3. Classification tree analysis with first group of independent variables and GI as dependent variable in 297 patients

We looked more in detail at the group of 29 male patient, after the last division in the classification tree analysis, the risk factor being diagnosis: leukemia. Less than half of them received ChT with AA, two of them had testicular RT, none had pelvic RT. In 5 patients PH was diagnosed; 2 after testicular RT, 3 after ChT with AA - 2 received the highest cumulative dose of CY and cytarabine in their group (7 g/m2 and 9.5 g/m2). Two patients had subclinical gonadal impairment (SIG) after ChT with AA and/or cytarabine. On the contrary, in the other group of 92 patients, treated for other malignancies, with the highest proportion of GI, as many as 90% received ChT with AA and a quarter of them had pelvic RT. Thirty-one of 46 patients with PH received ChT with AA, 14 ChT with AA and pelvic RT (1500 to 4000 cGy), one was treated with ChT without AA and RT to the whole abdomen (1400 cGy). Fourteen out of 17 patients with SIG received ChT with AA (one pelvic RT as well), 3 patients received ChT without AA, but had RT of the whole abdomen. Therefore the most significant risk factors for GI in our patients were beside the diagnosis of GCT male gender and therapy with ChT and RT. In the group with the highest risk of GI among risk factors has stood out ChT with AA and pelvic RT (and gonadal surgery and ChT with AA in the group of patients with GCT). In the group with low risk of GI mainly ChT with AA and testicular RT emerged as risk factors.

3.1.1.3 Dependent variable - gonadal impairment (GI) in male patients

The analysis confirmed the results of the previous analysis. The largest, 68%, risk of GI, had a group of men, who were treated for cancer other than leukemia with ChT and RT (Fig. 4).

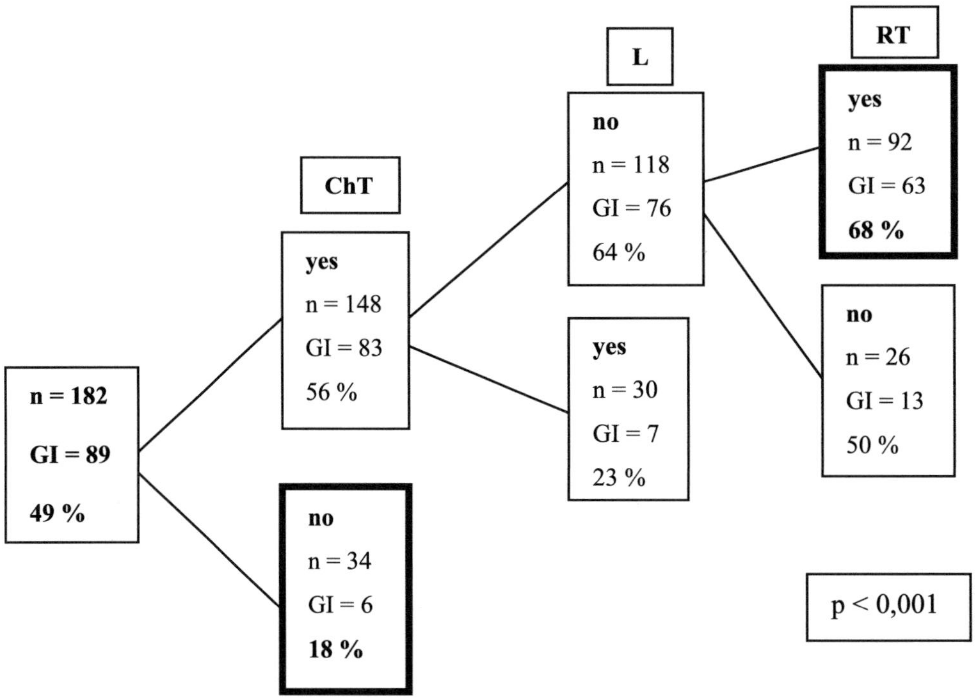

GI - gonadal impairment, L - leukemia, ChT - chemotherapy, RT - radiotherapy

Fig. 4. Classification tree analysis with first group of independent variables and GI as dependent variable in 182 male patients

We looked more in detail at the group of 34 males who did not receive ChT. Six patients had GI. Three of them had PH, all after pelvic RT (3000 - 4000 cGy). Three patients had SIG after being treated for brain tumors, 2 with surgery only, one with brain RT. Of the remaining 28 patients of this group (with normal gonadal function six had pelvic RT (2800 to 4800 cGy). Therefore, in the group of patients with low risk of GI (without therapy with ChT) mainly pelvic RT emerged as risk factor.

3.1.1.4 Dependent variable - gonadal impairment (GI) in female patients

Classification tree analysis with first group of independent variables and GI as dependent variable was performed for the cohort of 115 female patients as well. It had only one division, the only risk factor being diagnosis GCT. Six patients treated for GCT were at high risk (83%) for GI. The other group of 109 patients was not further divided (Fig. 5). This tree was not significantly different from random predictions, probably because of a very small number of positive outcomes and some other independent variables relevant for ovarian failure, which are not yet known.

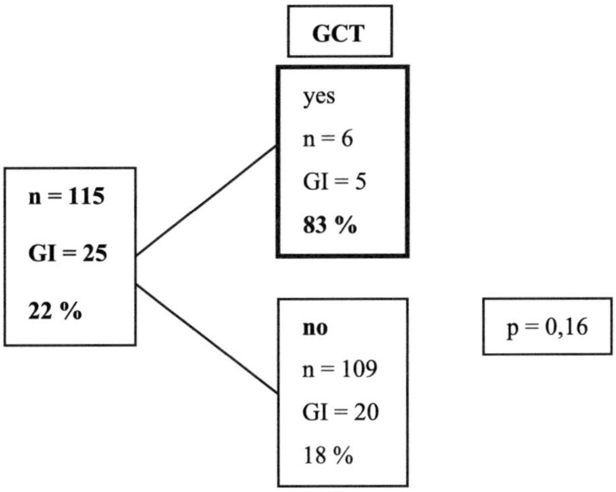

GI - gonadal impairment, GCT-germ cell tumor

Fig. 5. Classification tree analysis with first group of independent variables and GI as dependent variable in 115 female patients

3.1.2 Second group of independent variables

3.1.2.1 Dependent variable - primary hypogonadism in all patients

Again, all patients were included in the analysis.. The most important risk factor for PH turned out to be pelvic RT (Fig. 6). Risk for PH in patients, treated with pelvic RT, was 55% and 19% only in the other group. The second most important factor which divided the group of 51 patients, who had pelvic RT, was type of diagnosis, and the third one treatment with ChT.
We defined a group of 29 patients with the highest, 79%, risk of PH, namely those who had pelvic RT, didn't have diagnosis of brain tumor and were treated with ChT including AA or did not receive ChT at all. In the group of 246 patients who didn't have pelvic RT, ChT with AA emerged as the most important risk factor for PH, followed by male gender and diagnosis of HD. Similar to the analysis with the first group of independent variables (Fig.1) we identified a group of 24 patients with the highest risk of PH (66%) among those patients who didn't have pelvic RT; t.i. males treated for HD with ChT including AA. We defined a group of patients with the lowest, 1%, risk of PH. Those were 87 patients who had neither pelvic RT nor ChT with AA (PH was found in one patient only after being treated with testicular RT). Low risk of PH (7%) had as well a group of 56 females who received ChT with AA, but didn't have pelvic RT. Males treated with ChT with AA but without pelvic RT, had much higher risk of PH (42%), suggesting that ChT with AA presented greater risk factor of PH in males than in females.
The highest risk for PH (79%) had the group of patients treated for cancer other than brain tumor, with pelvic RT and ChT with AA (23 patients) or without ChT (6 patients). Only 6 patients in this group didn't develop PH; 2 females treated with unilateral RT to iliaco-inguinal region (2400 cGy) and ChT with AA for HD (one female with 2 relapses 6 cycles of LOPP (chlorambucil, vincristine, procarbazine and prednisone), 6 cycles of MOPP-ABV and 6 cycles of ABVD). Among 4 males without PH one received RT to both iliacal regions (3000 cGy) and 2 cycles of MOPP ChT, one received RT to the left femur and iliac bone (4800 cGy) for hondrosarcoma of the iliac bone, and 2 were treated for NHL of the caecum with

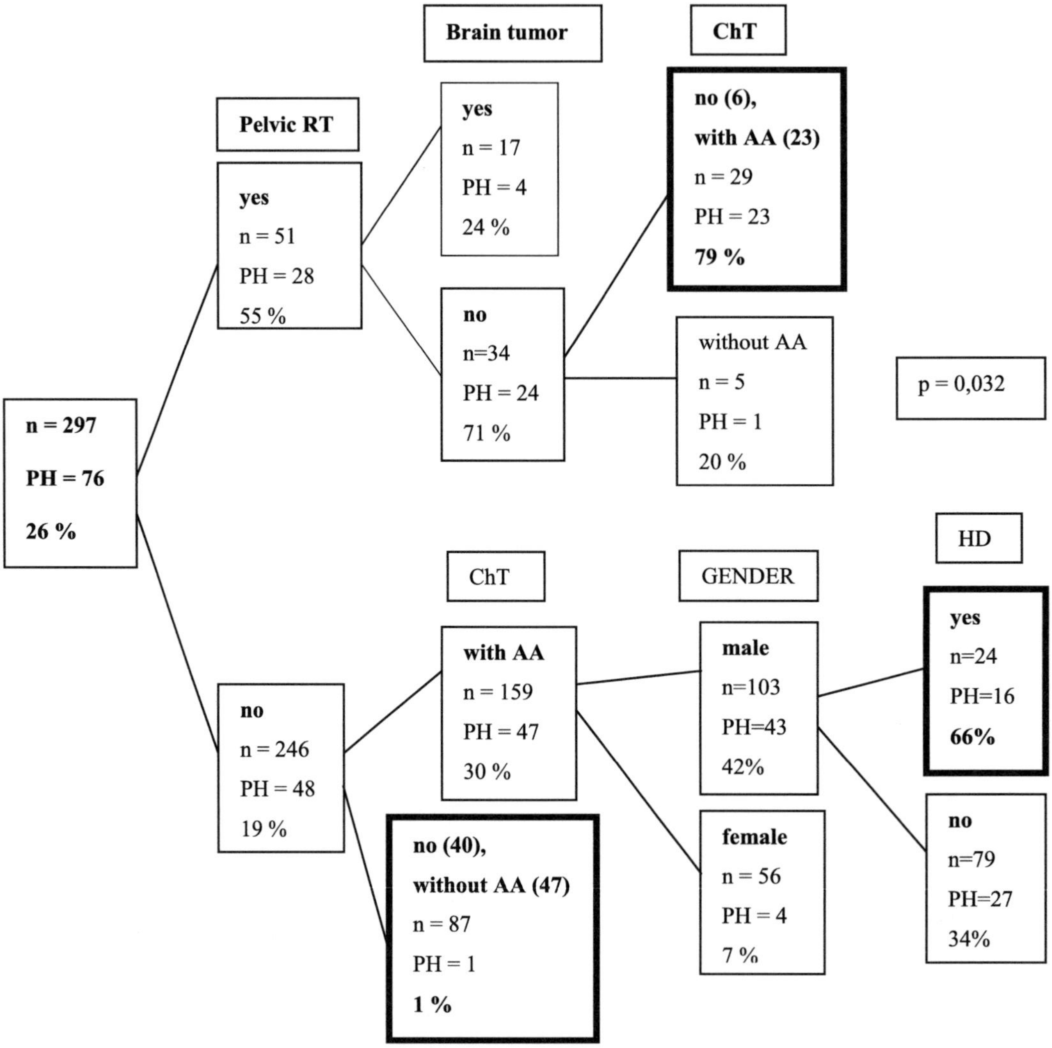

PH - primary hypogonadism, AA - alkylating agents, ChT - chemotherapy, RT - radiotherapy, HD - Hodgkin's disease

Fig. 6. Classification tree analysis with second group of independent variables and PH as dependent variable in 297 patients

surgery, ChT with AA and RT (one had 900 cGy to the whole central nervous system, the other had abdominal RT with 3000 cGy). Of the 6 patients in the group not receiving ChT with AA, as many as five had PH; 3 of them had whole abdominal RT, 2 RT of bilateral iliacoinguinal regions. Among patients who had pelvic RT, a group of 17 patients with low proportion of PH emerged. They were treated for brain tumor by craniospinal RT (600-4400 cGy), 7 of them also received ChT with AA. All 4 patients with PH were treated for medulloblastoma, 3 of them received, in addition to craniospinal RT, ChT with Procarbazine or CCNU. The risk of PH in patients treated with craniospinal RT and ChT with AA was therefore 43%, while in those treated with craniospinal RT without ChT with AA, was only

10%. With this statistical analysis we found that the significant risk factors for PH were pelvic RT, ChT with AA, male gender and diagnosis of HD. In the group with a lower risk of PH craniospinal RT and ChT with AA emerged as important risk factors for PH.

3.1.2.2 Dependent variable - gonadal impairment (GI) (t.i. gonadal damage and subclinical impairment)

Gonadal impairment was found in 114 (38%) adolescents. The most significant risk factor for GI was RT (Fig. 7). The group of 100 patients who had brain RT only had the lowest (15%) risk of GI, in the group of the remaining 197 patients, who were irradiated to any other part of the body or had no RT, the risk of GI was 50%. Similar to the analysis of the first set of variables male patients treated with ChT and RT stood out as a group with the highest (75%) risk of GI.

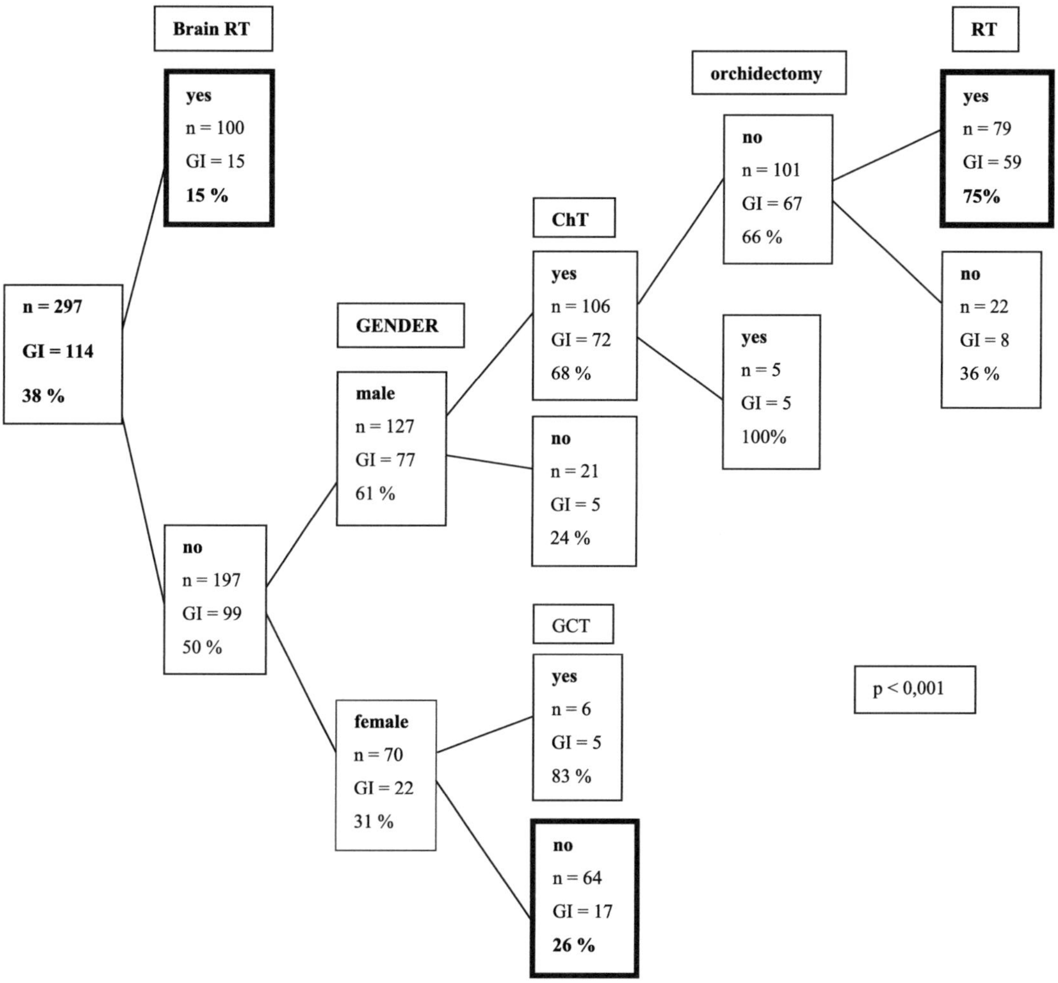

GI - gonadal impairment, AA - alkylating agents, GCT - germ cell tumor, ChT - chemotherapy, RT - radiotherapy

Fig. 7. Classification tree analysis with second group of independent variables and GI as dependent variable in 297 patients

We looked more in detail at the group of 100 (63 males, 37 females) patients with the lowest risk of GI who had only brain RT; 69% of them were treated for ALL, 27% for brain tumors, 9% for NHL, 4% for soft tissue sarcoma. Only 45% of this group of patients received ChT with AA. All 7 males who had PH, received ChT with AA, as did also 6 of 8 patients (3 females, 5 males) with SIG. In the second division of decision tree the subgroup of male patients had 61% risk of GI and the subgroup of females only 31%, although a similar proportion of patients in both subgroups received ChT with AA (72%: 75%) or did not receive ChT (28%: 25%) and the same (27%) proportion of patients had pelvic RT.
Therefore, in this statistical analysis the most important risk factors for GI turned out to be: male gender, treatment with ChT with AA and RT and orchidectomy.

3.1.2.3 Dependent variable - impairment of germinal epithelium GEI, t.i. germinal epithelium damage (GE-DA) and germinal epithelium dysfunction (GE-dys) in male patients

In this analysis as the most important risk factor for GEI emerged ChT with AA (Fig. 8). Only 10% of males who didn't receive ChT with AA had GEI (all 6 patients in this group who had GEI, had pelvic or testicular RT). The second most important factor that divided the group of 121 males who received ChT with AA, was pelvic RT. The risk of GEI in the group of 18 patients who had pelvic RT was as high as 89%. The next most important risk factor, which divided the group of patients who received ChT with AA and didn't have pelvic RT, was diagnosis HD. It is the same result as above when analyzing all patiens (with dependent variable PH), a group of 24 patients treated for HD with ChT with AA but without pelvic RT (71% risk of GEI). In the other group of patients treated for other malignancies than HD were at greater risk of GEI those who had RT above the diaphragm and were at the age of 10 years or less at the time of treatment (83% risk of GEI). In this analysis the most important risk factors for GEI turned out to be: ChT with AA and pelvic RT.
In the group of 18 patients who received ChT with AA and had pelvic RT, only 2 patients had normal gonadal function; one patient received 2 cycles of MOPP and RT of iliac regions with a dose of 3000 cGy for HD, the other had craniospinal RT with 900 cGy and ChT following BFM protocol (including 7 g/ m 2 of CY and 3, 2 g/m2 of cytarabine) for NHL. High, 71% the risk of GEI, had a group of 24 patients with HD treated with ChT with AA without pelvic RT. Seven patients of this group didn't have GEI. They received ChT following protocol LOPP (6 cycles), MOPP (1 to 4 cycles) or OPPA (2 cycles).
At the last division of this tree patients age at treatment emerged as risk factor for GEI. The group of 25 patients who were treated for HD with ChT with AA and RT above the diaphragm, was divided into those who were 10 or less years of age at diagnosis (83% risk of GEI), and into the group of older patients (31% risk of GEI). The younger patients received a slightly higher cumulative dose of CY (2.8 - 40, med. 10 g/m2) than the group of older patients (1.4 - 16, med. 5 g/m2), doses of cytarabine were approximately equal in both groups. Among patients without GEI in the group of younger patients there was one who received CY 15 g/m2. Taking in account that the two age groups have different cumulative doses of AA, we can not consider patient's age at treatment as an important risk factor for GEI.
Therefore, in this analysis the most important risk factors for damage or dysfunction of germinal epithelium were ChT with AA, pelvic RT, diagnosis HD and orchidectomy.

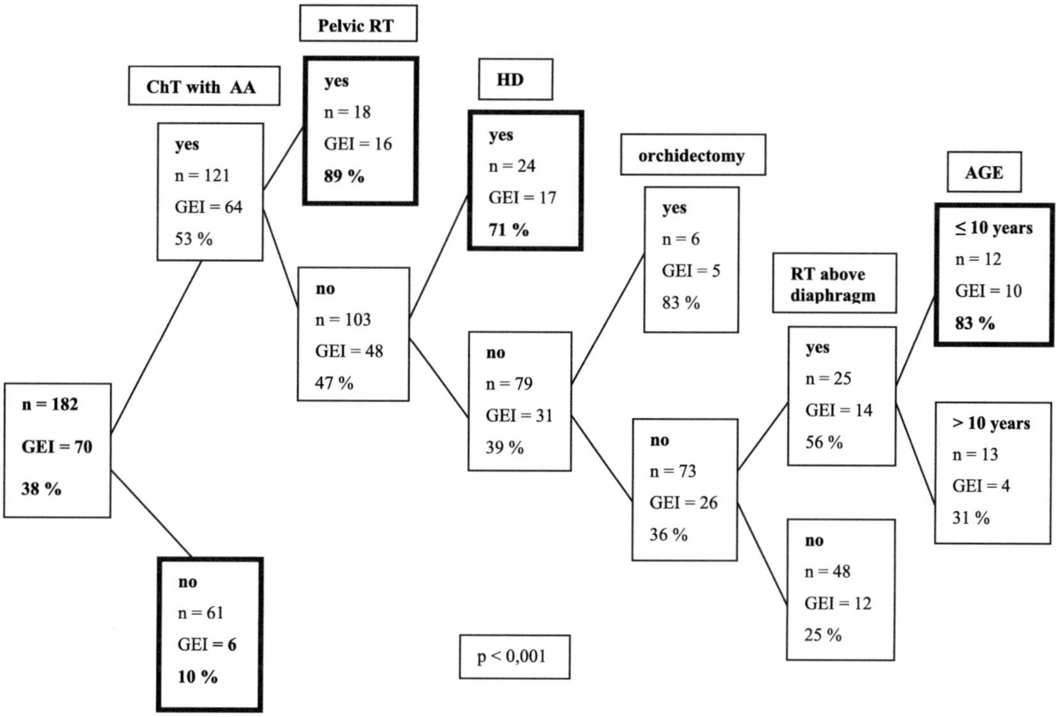

GEI - impairment of germinal epithelium, AA – alkylating agents, ChT – chemotherapy, RT – radiotherapy, HD – Hodgkin's disease

Fig. 8. Classification tree analysis with second group of independent variables and GEI (impairment of germinal epithelium) as dependent variable in 182 male patients

3.1.2.4 Dependent variable - impairment of Leydig cells (LCI), t.i. damage of LC (LC-DA) and dysfunction of LC (LC-dys) in male patients

In this analysis as the most important risk factor for LCI stood out treatment with ChT (Fig. 9). All but three patients with LCI received ChT. In the group of 148 patients who received ChT, 67 patients had LCI; all but the 6 of them received ChT with AA (13 of them also had pelvic RT, one testicular RT). Five of the 6 patients not receiving ChT with AA had abdominal RT.

The highest, 83%, risk of LCI was in the group of patients, who received ChT and had orchidectomy. Similar to the above analysis (GI in all patients), we defined a group of 79 patients with high risk for LCI (61%); namely patients treated with ChT and RT of other regions than brain. Eleven patients in this group had both, damage of GE and damage of LC (2 after testicular RT, 3 after ChT with AA and pelvic RT, 6 after the ChT), 37 patients had dysfunction of LC; 24 of them with the damage of GE as well (15 after ChT with AA, 8 after ChT with AA and pelvic RT, one after pelvic RT), 13 patients had an isolated finding (10 after ChT with AA, 3 following abdominal RT).

In the group of 22 patients treated with ChT, but without RT (with 23% risk of LCI), all 5 patients with LCI had only dysfunction of LC and all received ChT with AA. In the group of 34 patients with the lowest, 9%, risk of LCI, patients didn't receive ChT; only 3 patients had LCI (one patient following abdominal RT, 2 patients after brain RT).

Therefore, in this analysis orchidectomy and therapy with ChT and RT emerged as the most important risk factors for LCI.

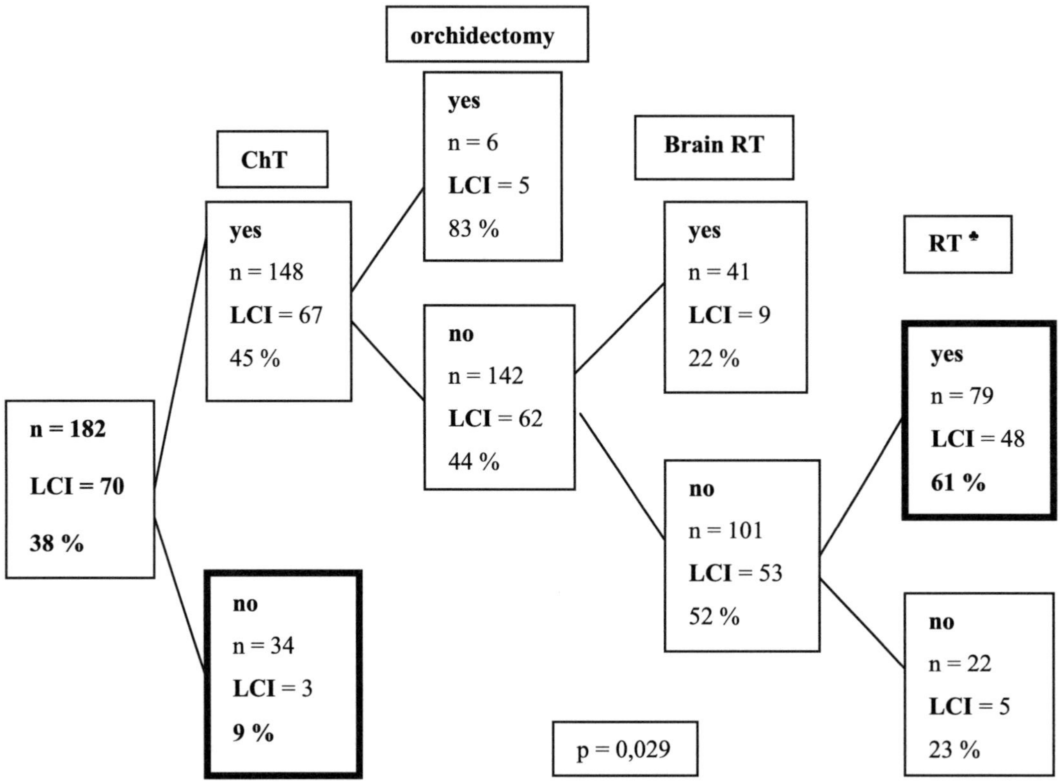

LCI - impairment of Leydig cells, ChT – chemotherapy, RT♣ – radiotherapy to other region than brain

Fig. 9. Classification tree analysis with second group of independent variables and impairment of Leydig cells (LCI) as dependent variable in 182 male patients

3.1.2.5 Dependent variable –gonadal impairment (GI) in female patients, t.i. damage of ovarian function and dysfunction of ovarian function in female patients

The decision tree with the second group of independent variables (Fig. 10) was more branched than the one using the first group of independent variables (Fig. 5), although this tree was not significantly different from statistical random predictions. Similar to the previous tree the highest risk for GI was observed in the group of females treated for GCT (GI in 5 out of the 6 patients). The remaining group of 109 patients with 18% risk of GI, treated for other malignancies, was further divided by the most important risk factor - pelvic RT. In the group of 16 patients treated with pelvic RT risk of GI was 50%. As many as 7 out of the 8 patients with GI had damage of ovarian function, t.i.PH (one following RT of the whole abdomen (2000 cGy) and ChT with AA for leukemia, 2 after craniospinal RT (3400 and 3600 cGy) and ChT with AA (only one) for medulloblastoma, 2 after RT of unilateral iliac region (3000 and 2400 cGy) and ChT with AA for HD, 2 following pelvic RT (3000 and 4000 cGy) and ChT with AA for sarcoma. One of the patients in this group had only ovarian dysfunction after craniospinal RT (2400 cGy) and ChT without AA for leukemia. The risk of

GI in the subgroup of 93 female patients without pelvic RT was as low as 13%. Only 4 out of 12 patients with GI in this group had damage of ovarian function (all after ChT with AA), 8 patients had only ovarian dysfunction (4 following ChT with AA).
In the group of 6 females treated for GCT at the age of 9 to 15 (med. 13) years, 5 had GI; 2 female patients had bilateral ovariectomy, one had ovarian damage after unilateral ovariectomy and abdominal RT, two females had dysfunction of ovarian function after unilateral removal of the ovary and ChT with AA.
In females, therefore, the most important risk factors for ovarian failure turned out to be pelvic RT, ChT with AA and ovariectomy.

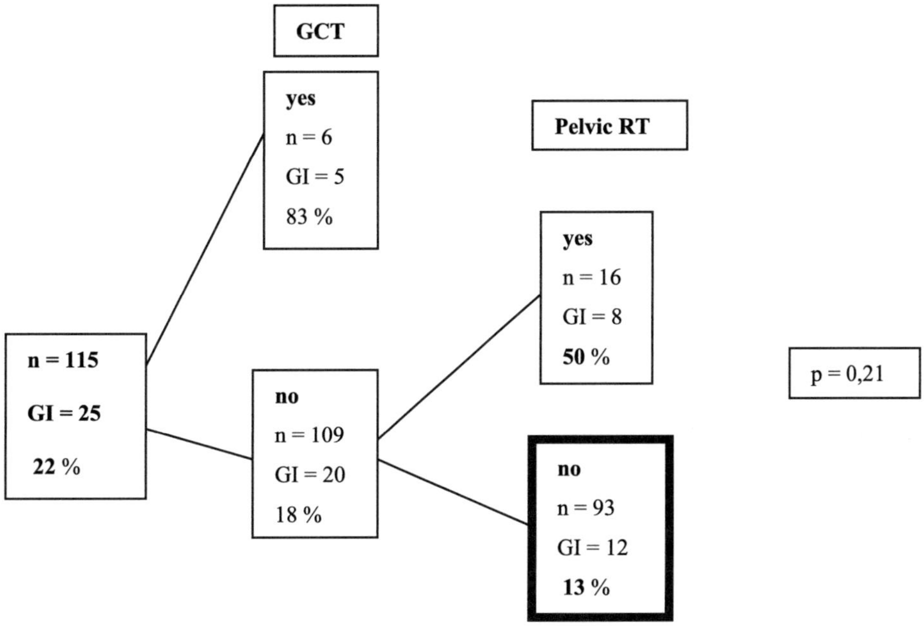

GI - gonadal impairment, GCT - germ cell tumor, RT - radiotherapy

Fig. 10. Classification tree analysis with second group of independent variables and gonadal impairment as dependent variable in 115 female patients

General observations

Forty-six patients (21 males, 25 females) in our study had no PH, despite treatment with either ChT including AA or pelvic or testicular RT. Thirty-four (19 males, 15 females) of them were treated with ChT, which contained the antimetabolites methotrexate and 6-mercaptopurine, VCR, corticosteroids with or without L-asparaginase and adriamycin. Eleven patients (2 males and 9 females) received ChT containing actinomycin D (AMD) and vincristine (VCR) with or without adriamycin. One girl received ChT with vinblastine. Six patients (3 males and 3 females) out of 46 in this group of patients had subclinical impairment of the gonads (males had dysfunction of LC only) and as many as 4 patients (2 males and 2 females) had ChT with AMD and VCR. The impact of antimetabolite cytarabine on gonadal function could not be assessed because this cytostatic was administered to patients as part of ChT protocols, which contained AA (especially CY). So, we can conclude on the basis of our cohort of patients that ChT with antimetabolites (other

than cytarabine), antibiotics and vinca alkaloids wasn't toxic to germinal epithelium of testes, but primarily AMD and VCR may cause mild failure of ovaries and LC.
Chemotherapy regimens usually include several cytostatics, to study the toxic effect of each one on the gonads was therefore not possible. In our study, one male patient received the largest cumulative dose of cyclofosfamide 24 g/m2 at the age of 5 for retinoblastoma by ChT protocol containing vincristine and Adriamycin as well. In this patient we discovered damage of GE and LC-dysfunction. On the other hand male patient treated at the age of 9 years with ChT containing cumulative dose of CY 20 g/m2 for bone sarcoma had normal gonadal function. Normal functioning of the testes after treatment with combined ChT was found in another male patients after receiving a cumulative dose of CY of 15 g/m2, and other 3 males after receiving 11 -12 g/m2.
One male patient received the highest cumulative dose of cisplatinum (1 g/m2) at the age of 16 years for nasopharyngeal cancer with local RT and ChT, containing platinol, vinblastine, methotrexate and bleomycin. He maintained normal gonadal function.

4. Discussion

We found primary hypogonadism (PH) in 76 (26%) long-term survivors, 62 (34%) males and 14 (12%) females. High incidence (50%) of PH was found in those treated for Hodgkin's disease (HD) or germ cell tumor (GCT). A group of males, treated for HD with ChT was at high risk (72%) for PH as was a group treated with RT to the pelvis and ChT with AA, 79% (Fig. 1). At high risk of damage to and dysfunction of the germ epithelium of the testes were those treated with pelvic RT and ChT with AA. At high risk for damage to and dysfunction of ovaries were those treated for GCT (89%) and those treated with pelvic RT (50%).

4.1 Gender

Primary hypogonadism was detected in one third of males and in 12% females, indicating a greater susceptibility of male gonads for the deleterious effects of cancer treatment in childhood. In the multivariate analysis, 3 trees showed gender as the second most important risk factor for PH or GI (Fig.1,3,7); in the analysis of risk factors for PH in patients treated for HD the risk for PH in males was 65%, in females 25% (Fig. 1), in the analysis of risk factors for GI after exclusion of patients treated for GCT, the risk for GI in males was 48%, in females 18% (Fig. 3) and in the analysis of risk factors for GI (the second group of independent variables) in patients who had brain RT the risk of GI was 61% in males and 31% in females (Fig. 7). This is consistent with observations of other authors (Byrne et al. 1987, Kinsella et al. 1989, Rivkees & Crawford 1988).

4.2 Age at diagnosis

In multivariate analysis, age at treatment did not turned out as a significant risk factor for hypogonadism. Only in the analysis of risk factors for germ epithelium impairment at the last division patients age at diagnosis emerged as a risk factor for GEI. Namely, the group of 25 patients who were treated for HD with ChT with AA and RT above the diaphragm, was divided into those who were 10 or less years of age at diagnosis (83% risk of GEI), and into the group of older patients (31% risk of GEI). But the cumulative doses of AA were different in the two age groups and we can not consider patient's age at treatment as an important risk factor for GEI.

In our study, therefore, we didn't observe the impact of age at diagnosis or pubertal status of patient during treatment on severity of gonadal damage. The results of various studies regarding age of male patients at diagnosis as independent variable are contradictory. Some authors reported lesser degree of testicular damage in those patients treated in prepubertal period in comparison with those treated in postpubertal period (Rivkees & Crawford 1988, Waxman et al. 1982), while others didn't confirm that observation (Aubier et al. 1989, Casteren et al. 2009, Hoorweg -Nijman et al. 1992, Lendon et al. 1978, Mustieles et al. 1995). However, in very few studies took into account the size of cumulative doses of AA, that patients in different age groups received (Lendon et al. 1978, Rivkees & Crawford 1988).
On the other hand there are numerous studies reporting reduced susceptibility of ovaries to deleterious effects of cancer therapy in prepubertal period, when the number of oocytes is larger and they are in the "peaceful" phase (Chapman et al. 1979, Chemaitilly at al. 2006, Lushbaugh & Casarett 1976, Sanders et al. 1991, Wallace et al. 2005, Waxman et al. 1982).

4.3 Type of malignancy

The largest, 50%, incidence of PH was observed in patients treated for HD and germ cell tumors and the lowest, 9-11 %, in those treated for leukemia, brain tumors and Wilms' tumor (Table 2). In multivariate analysis diagnosis of GCT and HD repeatedly turned out to be important risk factors for PH and GI (Fig. 1,2,3,5,8,10). This is related to the nature of the disease (germ cell tumors of the gonads) and the type of treatment. Majority of patients with HD were treated with combination therapy (ChT and RT with / without surgery), in which the largest, 26 to 40%, proportion of patients with PH was observed (Table 3). In addition, ChT for HD usually contains more than one gonadotoxic AA simultaneously in the same protocol. As many as 65% of male subjects with diagnosis of HD had PH (Fig. 1,2).
Another reason for high incidence of PH in males treated for HD is preexistent impairment of spermatogenesis before treatment. Indeed, some authors have observed reduced number and / or reduced sperm motility in the ejaculate in as many as one third of adult males with HD prior to treatment (Vigersky et al. 1982, Whitehead et al. 1982). On the contrary, in adult women ovarian biopsy did not reveal any abnormalities prior to treatment of HD (Chapman et al. 1979).

4.4 Surgery

As for surgery in the multivariate analysis only orchidectomy stood as important risk factor for GI as well as germinal epithelium impairment (GEI) and LC impairment (LCI) (Fig. 7-9). In 6 of our male patients unilateral orchidectomy was performed during treatment (3 had testicular GCT, 2 paratesticular rhabdomyosarcoma, one leukemia). In all 6 gonadal impairment was observed, namely 4 had damage of germ cell epithelium and LC , one had dysfunction of germ cell epithelium and LC and one had dysfunction of LC only. It is true that all those 6 patients received ChT with AA as well but probably surgery itself also contributed to the testicular damage. Nijman et al. (1987) observed elevated levels of FSH, LH, and decreased levels of testosterone in adult patients undergoing unilateral orchidectomy. These findings were attributed to the LC insufficiency in the remaining testis.
Unilateral ovariectomy as independent variable itself didn't stand as an important risk factor in the analysis, but the diagnosis GCT was the most important risk factor for ovarian damage and dysfunction (Fig. 5, 10). In all 6 females with GCT ovariectomy was performed, in 3 bilateral, in 3 unilateral. All 3 girls with unilateral ovariectomy received also ChT with

AA without pelvic RT; in 2 ovarian dysfunction was observed, the third one had normal gonadal function. Unilateral ovariectomy is therefore compatible with normal gonadal function, which was also observed by other authors (Perrin et al. 1999).
In 12 patients within diagnostic procedures for HD staging laparotomy with transposition of ovaries to the posterior wall of the uterus was performed. Only 2 of these patients had pelvic RT (unilateral iliac region), all but one received ChT with AA. Ovarian damage was observed in 3 of those 12 females, namely in one following unilateral iliac RT with 2400 cGy and 6 cycles of LOPP at the age of 6 years (primary amenorrhea), the other 2 after RT of the upper abdomen with 3000 and 3600 cGy and 6 cycles of MOPP at the age of 11 and 14 years (both delivered healthy children). The remaining 9 patients had no signs of ovarian failure, six of them gave birth to healthy babies. Therefore, it seems that transposition of ovaries itself does not reduce the fertility. Indeed Thomas et al. (1976) didn't observe neither worsening of ovarian function nor interrupted gamets transfer after ovarian transposition in their patients with HD. Nevertheless, possible complications of this surgery, among others, are tubal obstruction and ovarian failure due to vascular damage (Thibaud et al. 1992).

4.5 Radiotherapy (RT)

RT has emerged as an important risk factor in the analysis of GI in males (Fig. 3,4) and pelvic RT was a major risk factor for PH in all subjects (Fig. 6). Risk for PH after pelvic RT was as high as 55%. With another division we identified a group of 17 patients treated with craniospinal RT for brain tumors, with low, 24%, incidence of PH. Addition of ChT with AA (mostly CCNU and PBZ) to RT, increased incidence of PH to 43% (being only 10% in those without ChT including AA). So, ChT with CCNU or PBZ in our subjects markedly increased risk of PH, especially in men, as 2 of the 3 males after craniospinal RT and ChT with AA had PH and none of the 6 males after only craniospinal RT had PH. One of 4 females had PH after RT alone. Higher gonadotoxicity of craniospinal RT in girls than in boys is in concordance with reports of other authors (Hamre et al. 1987, Sklar et al. 1990).
In the analysis of risk factors for ovarian impairment (Fig. 10) as the most important risk factor emerged GCT and in the second division pelvic RT. Similarly, other authors observed that pelvic RT is the most important risk factor for ovarian failure (Hamre et al. 1987, Stillman et al. 1981) observed that the only risk factor for ovarian failure in 182 long-term survivors of childhood cancer was ovarian position relative to the RT field and not ChT. Of course, ovarian failure may be caused by ChT with AA (Chapman et al. 1979, Nicosia et al. 1985, Ortin et al. 1990, Siris et al. 1976), what was observed in our study as well, namely all females with PH without receiving pelvic RT had ChT with AA.
Four females in our series had unilateral pelvic RT. Two had evidence of PH, but all received ChT with AA and PBZ as well. After RT of paraaortic lymph nodes the estimated ovarian dose is about 6 % of the prescribed dose (in the range of 100 cGy) and this dose of radiation can cause transient disturbances of menstrual cycle. Haie-Mader and colleagues (1993) analyzed ovarian function in 134 females treated for HD or gynecological cancer and showed that the age over 25 years, MOPP ChT and total dose to the ovaries higher than 500 cGy are important risk factors for ovarian castration.
In the analysis of risk factors for impairment of germ cell epithelium (GEI) the highest, 89%, risk of GEI, was observed in the group of males who received ChT with AA and had pelvic RT (Fig. 8). Only two of the 18 patients in this group did not have GEI, namely one patient after RT of bilateral iliac regions (3000 cGy) and two cycles of MOPP and the other following craniospinal RT (900 cGy) and ChT with AA (incl. 7 g/m2 CY).

This observation is consistent with reports of other authors (Byrne et al.1987, Casteren et al. 2009). In the group of 61 male patients who didn't receive ChT with AA, all 6 patients with GEI had pelvic or testicular RT (Fig.8).

By the last division in the analysis of risk factors for PH (Fig. 1), a group of 7 male patients, treated for HD without ChT, was identified. PH was observed in 2 patients only, in both following pelvic RT with 4000 cGy. Only one of our male patients had additional shielding of testes during pelvic RT (3600 cGy to bilateral iliacoinguinal regions) by a lead capsule, he received 6 cycles of LOPP. In spite laboratory testing showing damage of germinal epithelium and LC dysfunction he fathered 2 children, suggesting only a partial impairment of spermatogenesis. This is consistent with the study of Kovač et al. (1990) in which authors reported about significant reduction of testicular dose by an additional lead shielding of testis (Kovač et al. 1990).

4.6 Chemotherapy (ChT)

ChT emerged as an important risk factor in all multivariate analysis using the first set of variables. In the analysis of risk factors for PH as well as GI in male patients ChT turned out to be very important risk factor, immediately after the type of malignancy (GCT or HD) (Fig. 2,4). In the analysis of risk factors for PH using a second set of independent variables (Fig. 8), a group of 246 patients who didn't have pelvic RT divided further by therapy with ChT. So, we identified a group of 87 patients neither receiving ChT with AA nor pelvic RT, with the lowest, 1%, risk of PH. The only one patient with PH in this group had testicular RT. Using multivariate analysis we, therefore, identified a group of childhood cancer survivors in whom gonadal testing could be omitted.

We observed greater impact of ChT with AA on gonadal function in boys than girls, as 42% males and only 7% females treated with ChT with AA without pelvic RT, had PH (Fig. 6). Similar conclusions were drawn in the study of Byrne et al. (1987) analyzing 2283 long-term survivors of childhood cancer and showed that RT under the diaphragm decreased fertility in both sexes for 25%, ChT with AA (with or without abdominal RT) decreased fertility only in boys for 60%, but not in girls.

This reflects in the analysis of risk factors for impairment of germ cell epithelium (Fig. 8) where the most important risk factor for GEI was ChT with AA, followed by pelvic RT. Males who received ChT with AA for HD without having pelvic RT, had incidence of GEI as high as 71%. Only 7 of 24 patients in this group of patients had normal testicular function, 4 patients after 6 cycles of LOPP cycles, 2 patients after 1 to 4 cycles of MOPP, one after 2 cycles of OPPA. On the other hand none of the male subjects after 6 or more cycles of MOPP ChT had normal function of germ cell epithelium. Our findings are in concordance with data from other studies establishing that MOPP or MOPP-like combinations, such as MVPP (mechlorethamine, vinblastine, procarbazine and prednisone) and COPP induce azoospermia in 90-100 % of pts with a 10-20% chance of recovery even 10 years after treatment (Chapman et al. 1979, Diamond& Bercu 2001, Viviani et al. 1985, Waxmann et al. 1982, Whitehead et al. 1982, Zaletel 2010). Recovery of spermatogenesis following MOPP therapy appears to be dose-related with 3 courses of MOPP representing a limiting gonadal exposure for the recovery, suggesting only partial killing of germinal stem cells (da Cunha et al. 1984). Indeed, in our study we found normal gonadal function in two males after having received 1 and 2 cycles of MOPP ChT. We found ChT according to the protocol LOPP less damaging for testicular function than MOPP, causing GEI in 5 of 10 males having received 6 cycles, a finding not published elsewhere to our knowledge. It seems that chlorambucil inside LOPP protocol is more gonadotoxic than nitrogen mustard in MOPP protocol. Our subjects received many different chemotherapy regimens, so the comparison with the results of other studies is difficult.

Among patients who didn't receive pelvic RT, the highest incidence of PH was observed in the group of males treated for HD with ChT including AA (66%) (Fig. 6). Those males who were treated with ChT including AA for other malignancies, had much lower incidence of PH (34%). This finding is consistent with other studies reporting that ChT used in treatment of HD is more gonadotoxic from other ChT regimens (Müller 2003).

In women, in the analysis of risk factors for ovarian impairment pelvic RT emerged as the most important risk factor, immediately after diagnosis GCT (Fig. 10). But 6 of the 8 patients who had pelvic RT received ChT with AA as well. On the other hand, all females with ovarian impairment, who didn't receive pelvic RT, were treated with ChT with AA. So, we can conclude that ChT with AA contributed to development of ovarian impairment. ChT according to MOPP protocol is more toxic to the ovaries than other types of ChT. There are data of adverse effects of ChT that is in use for HD, on ovarian function in adult females, but very little on ovarian function in girls. In the study of Ortin and colleagues 2 of 18 girls were amenorrhoic after having received 6 or more cycles of MOPP (Ortin et al. 1990). In our study none of the 6 females was amenorrhoic after 6 or more cycles of MOPP, but 2 had evidence of ovarian damage while retaining fertility Probably in girls younger than 16 years ChT is less gonadotoxic because relative quiescence of stromal cells and oocytes in prepubertal period protects ovaries from cell cycle specific cytotoxic agents (Siris et al. 1976, Stillman et al. 1981).

Forty-six patients didn't receive neither testicular or pelvic RT nor ChT with AA. They were treated with ChT containing antimetabolites (except cytarabine), antibiotics and vinca alkaloids. None of them had PH. Other authors as well, didn't observe important role of this type of ChT in pathogenesis of gonadal failure (Blatt et al. 1981, Müller 2003), although they reported on transient oligospermia in adult patients following treatment with methotrexate (Sussman & Leonard 1980) and on possible role of VCR in pathogenesis of germ cell epithelium damage in childhood and adolescence (Rautonen et al. 1992). In the group of patients treated with ChT containing AMD and VCR, 2 female patients had ovarian dysfunction and 2 males had LC dysfunction, suggesting that therapy with these 2 chemotherapy agents can cause mild degree of ovarian or LC damage. To our knowledge there is no article reporting on the potential gonadotoxicity of AMD.

4.7 Observation time

In none of the multivariate analysis observation time emerged as a significant risk factor for gonadal impairment. This is in accordance with expectations, as normally gonadal failure develops during or shortly after administration of toxic therapy and correction of gonadal damage eventually takes place within the first decade thereafter or so (Mustieles et al. 1995, Rowley et al. 1974, Viviani et al. 1985, Waxman et al. 1982). In 73 patients, we performed gonadal testing twice. Indeed, in 3 males the second testing showed normal functioning of the germ cell epithelium, after first testing showing damage of germ cell epithelium (4 to 16 years earlier). In female subjects as well the correction of the ovarian function was found. One of them had secondary amenorrhea after treatment and after 5 years menstrual cycle restored. The second one had primary amenorrhea till 16 years of age and then restored normal menstrual cycle. In contrast to the germ cell failure, damage of LC can develop within a few years after treatment, and usually there is no correction of LC damage (Shalet et al. 1985). Indeed, in 4 male patients in our cohort we found LC impairment at the second testing 3 to 10 years after their first testing, when they had normal function or only dysfunction of LC.

4.8 Leydig cell damage

LC damage was detected in 16 adolescents. All who were on treatment in prepubertal period (10 patients) had normal pubertal development. Lowered testosterone level was observed only in one patient, who received ChT with AA and RT above the diaphragm at the age of 10 years for HD. At relapse, 5 years later, he had additional ChT with AA and RT to the upper abdomen (3400 cGy). So, the majority of these 16 patients had clinically insignificant impairment of LC function. Two of these patients had testicular RT (1200 cGy in 4 fractions). Other authors did neither observe clinically significant impairment of LC after the testicular dose of this size (Brauner et al. 1983, Castillo et al. 1999). Of the remaining 14 patients with LC damage, only 4 had pelvic RT with / without ChT with AA, 10 patients had ChT with AA without pelvic RT. So, failure of LC in these adolescents was not simply a consequence of RT, but was mainly caused by ChT with AA. Most studies after ChT with AA observed compensatory insufficiency of LC (normal testosterone level and elevated basal level of LH and / or elevated level of LH after stimulation) (Brämswig et al . 1990, Kenney et al. 2001, Meistrich 2009, Romerius at al. 2009, Sherins et al. 1978, Whitehead et al. 1982). However, in two studies LC dysfunction following ChT with AA was not identified (Pennisi et al. 1975, Shalet et al. 1981). The likely cause of this discrepancy lies in the fact that in one of these studies LC function was evaluated only by basal LH levels without GnRH-test, but LC dysfunction can reflect in increased LH response to GnRH (Pennisi et al. 1975). All our 16 patients with LC damage had damage of germinal epithelium as well.

LC dysfunction was observed in 54 patients. All but 6 received ChT with AA (9 of them had pelvic RT as well). Again, this result confirms that ChT with AA contributes in the pathogenesis of compensatory LC damage.

Incidence of LC damage is increasing in the years after treatment, therefore, patients with elevated basal or stimulated LH require annual monitoring of LH and testosterone and the timely introduction of hormone replacement therapy when reduced secretion of testosterone is discovered.

4.9 Secondary hypogonadism

Secondary hypogonadism was detected in two female patients with panhipopituitarism after combination therapy of GCT of hypothalamus, in three patients after treatment of brain tumors located outside the hypothalamus or pituitary gland with surgery and postoperative RT (5000 - 6500 cGy) and in one female after whole brain RT with 3000 cGy for leukemia. All patients with secondary hypogonadism had hiposomatotropism as well, which corresponds to reports of others (Constine et al. 1993, Gleeson & Shalet 2004).

4.10 Classification tree analysis

We analyzed our data by multivariate analysis method, classification tree model, which allows for studying of simultaneous influence of a series of independent variables on a single dependent variable. The main advantage of this method is its ability to detect the mutual effect of independent variables. The decision tree determines groups of subjects with a set of specific values of independent variables, in which the risk of gonadal damage is the highest or the lowest. So, in analysis where we took damage and dysfunction of germinal epithelium of testes as dependent variable we identified a group of patients at highest risk of this outcome, namely males who were treated with ChT with AA and pelvic RT. In analysis of risk factors for primary hypogonadism (PH), we identified a group of patients with very low risk, 1%, for this outcome, namely, males who had neither ChT with AA nor pelvic or testicular RT as their treatment.

Classification trees in our study were mostly significantly different from random prediction, with the exception of those trees constructed on data from female patients, due to the low number of patients with "positive" outcomes (e.g. PH). Predictive accuracy of the trees was high and it would be even higher if the analysis included other independent variables that might further explain the difference between groups of subjects with different outcome regarding dependent variable. In our analysis, we wanted to include more independent variables, or several different values for independent variables (e.g. cumulative doses of various cytostatics), but, despite the relatively large number of subjects, we could not do it. Each multivariate analysis restricts the number of independent variables and their values. On the other hand, other risk factors for gonadal damage can exist which we haven't identified yet.

Maybe, a limitation of this method is that in some analysis, a larger group of patients is not further divided, e.g. a group of 233 patients who were treated for cancer other than HD (Fig. 1) and a group of 109 female patients who was not treated for GCT (Fig. 5). The reason for this was the small number of subjects with observed outcome (e.g. PH) in these groups of patient. So we could loose some information on potential risk factors for impaired gonadal function in these patients. Decision trees, which we got using the second group of independent variables, were more diversified and gave also more information (Fig. 6-10).

In the published articles studying gonadal function after childhood cancer treatment different multivariate analysis for analyzing risk factors were used, mainly logistic regression (Chematilly et al. 2006, Haie-Mader et al. 1993, Rautonen et al. 1992, Romerius et al. 2009, Stillman et al. 1981), linear regression (Siimes & Rautonen 1990), Cox regression analysis (Byrne et al. 1987). But no one used the decision tree classification model, therefore, not been able to identify links between risk factors for impaired gonadal function. But there are a number of articles published in medicine, in which a classification tree method was used (Jazbec et al. 2004, Jereb & Eklund 1973, Macedoni-Lukšič et al. 2003, Velensek et al. 2008).

4.11 Assessment of gonadal function

For assessment of gonadal function in long-term survivors of childhood leukemia we used, beside clinical evaluation, hormonal testing, which is an indirect measure of testicular and ovarian function. Several studies showed that in men basal FSH level and FSH response to GnRH correlate well with sperm production (Aubier et al. 1989, Hoorweg-Nijman et al. 1992, Kinsella et al.1989, Kirkland et al. 1976, Mustieles et al. 1995, Siimes & Rautonen 1990). An increased FSH response to GnRH can be the first manifestation of testicular damage, although normal FSH levels do not rule out the possibility of azoospermia (Aubier et al. 1989, Kenney et al. 2001). All our male patients with PH were advised to perform analysis of spermiogram, but only 12 of them decided to do so. In 11 of them azoospermia was found, confirming that GnRH-testing offers a good estimate of spermatogenesis. On the other hand 6 male patients with documented PH became fathers, suggesting that elevated levels of FSH do not rule out fertile ability. But on the other hand normal FSH levels do not exclude the possibility of impaired spermatogenesis (Aubier et al. 1989, Kenney et al. 2001). We couldn't confirm that observation because none of our male patients with normal laboratory findings performed spermanalysis. But none of them had problems with fertile capability. We didn't use testicular volume for evaluation of gonadal function in male subjects. Indeed, some studies reported that testicular volume is not a reliable indicator of spermatogenesis (Kenney et al. 2001, Relander et al. 2000). There are reports on Inhibin B as a good serum marker which correlate well with sperm concentration (Beek at al. 2007, Casteren et al. 2009).

GnRH-test served us for the evaluation of LC function as well. Good test for the evaluation of LC function is HCG test, which measures testosterone levels after repeated administration of chorionic gonadotropin (Brauner et al. 1983). However, this test is difficult to implement as it lasts for several days. Anyway, Brauner (1983) found good correlation between GnRH-test and HCG-test in males if performed in postpubertal period. Actually, our subjects were tested in postpubertal period.

Five of 24 males with germ cell epithelium damage fathered children indicating that they are not azoospermic but possibly oligospermic and fertile. Hoorweg-Nijman and colleagues found elevated levels of FSH compatible with normospermia (Hoorweg-Nijman et al. 1992). FSH levels may provide an estimate of possible impaired spermatogenesis, however only semen analysis is confirmatory assessment of male gonadal function.

We used GnRH-test for evaluation of ovarian function as well. Primary hypogonadism was detected in 14 females, but only 6 of them are amenorrhoic, 3 after bilateral ovariectomy for GCT. Interestingly, one of our patients in spite of being amenorrhoic and having levels of gonadotropins in menopausal range, gave birth to a healthy boy. Of the remaining 8 female patients with PH, one had transient, secondary amenorrhea lasting for 5 years, one is in early menopause (at 38 years of age) after 2 deliveries, 6 of them have irregular periods, 2 after 1 to 2 deliveries. Indeed, in most studies the term ovarian failure was used in patients with amenorrhea, elevated levels of gonadotropins and lower levels of estradiol (Stillman et al. 1981, Chapman et al. 1979). Thus, ovarian failure, defined in such a way, was diagnosed in 6 of our female patients only. So we, maybe, slightly overestimated the rate of PH in female patients (as well as in male patients) taking under the cover of ovarian damage more subtile, clinically insignificant gonadal damage as well. But it is likely that these patients are at risk of early menopause which already happened in one of our female patients. After cancer therapy, indeed, the number of primordial follicles decreases further, increasing the "age" of ovaries and shortening fertile period (Larsen et al. 2003). Hyperexcitability of gonadal axis (elevated LH / FSH after stimulation with GnRH), t.i. ovarian dysfunction, was detected in 11 of our female patients. All have regular menstrual cycles and five of them gave birth to healthy children. However, ovarian hyperexcitability may indicate mild impairment of ovarian tissue and higher risk of early menopause in most subjects but does not appear to be clinically significant. Other comparable studies of ovarian function after cancer treatment in childhood authors have not reported on hyperexcitability.

5. Conclusions

With the presented population based study we confirmed several already known results of other studies, such as :

- a greater susceptibility of male gonads for the deleterious effects of cancer treatment in childhood,

- RT is an important risk factor for GI in males and pelvic RT as a major risk factor for PH in all, male as well as in female survivors,
- unilateral orchidectomy is an important risk factor for germinal epithelium impairment as well as LC impairment , which is attributed to the LC insufficiency in the remaining testis,
- unilateral ovariectomy is compatible with normal gonadal function,
- gonadal failure develops during or shortly after administration of toxic therapy and correction of gonadal damage eventually takes place in male as well as in female survivors. In contrast to the germ cell failure, damage of LC can develop within a few years after treatment, and usually there is no correction of LC damage therefore. Therefore, patients with elevated basal or stimulated LH levels require annual monitoring of LH and testosterone and the timely introduction of hormone replacement therapy when reduced secretion of testosterone is discovered.

But there was no multivariate analysis using the decision tree classification model, which is able to identify links between risk factors for impaired gonadal function. With this model we could also identify a group of patients with the lowest risk of gonadal impairment those who had neither pelvic or testicular RT nor ChT including AA. In those hormonal testing could be omitted.

6. Acknowledgements

The research was supported by Ministry of science and Ministry of health in Slovenia.

7. References

[1] Ash, P. (1980). The influence of radiation on fertility *in man. Br J Radiol,* Vol. 53 No. 628: 271-8.

[2] Aubier, F., Flamant, F., Brauner, R., Caillaud, JM., Chaussain, JM. & Lemerle, J. (1989). Male gonadal function after chemotherapy for solid tumors in childhood. *J Clin Oncol,* Vol, 7, No. 3: 304-9.

[3] van Beek, RD., Smit, M., van den Heuvel-Eibrink, MM., de Jong, FH., Hakvoort-Cammel, FG., van den Bos, C., van den Berg, H., Weber, RF., Pieters, R. & de Muinck Keizer-Schrama, SM. (2007). Inhibin B is superior to FSH as a serum marker for spermatogenesis in men treated for Hodgkin's lymphoma with chemotherapy during childhood. *Hum Reprod,* Vol. 22, No 12:3215-22..

[4] Berg, H., Furstner, F., Bos, C. & Behrendt, H. (2004). Decreasing in number of MOPP courses reduces gonadal damage in survivors of childhood Hodgkin disease. *Pediatr Blood Cancer,* Vol.42, No. 3: 210-5.

[5] Blatt, J., Poplack, DG. & Sherins, RJ. (1981).Testicular function in boys after chemotherapy for acute lymphoblastic leukemia. *N Engl J Med,* Vol. 304 No. 19: 1121-4.

[6] Brämswig, JH., Heiermann, E. & Nieschlag, E. (1990). The effects of different cumulative doses of chemotherapy on testicular function. *Cancer,* Vol. 65, No. 6: 1298-1302.

[7] Brauner, R., Czernichow, P., Cramer, P., Schaison, G. & Rappaport, R.(1983). Leydig-cell function in children after direct testicular irradiation for acute lymphoblastic leukemia. *N Engl J Med* , Vol. 309:25-8.

[8] Brydøy, M., Fossa, SD., Dahl, O. & Bjøro, T. (2007). Gonadal dysfunction and fertility problems in cancer survivors. *Acta Oncologica*, Vol. 46, No. 4: 480-489.

[9] Byrne, J., Fears, TR., Gail, MH., Pee, D., Connelly, RR., Austin, DF., Holmes, GF., Holmes, FF., Latourette, HB. & Meigs, JW. (1992). Early menopause in long-term survivors of cancer during adolescence. *Am J Obstet Gynecol*, Vol. 166, No. 3: 788-93.

[10] Byrne, J., Mulvihill, JJ., Myers, MH., Connelly, RR., Naughton, MD., Krauss, MR., Steinhorn, SC., Hassinger, DD., Austin, DF. & Bragg, K. (1987). *Effects* of treatment on fertility in long-term survivors of childhood or adolescent cancer. *N Engl J Med*, Vol. 317, No. 21:1315-21.

[11] Casteren, NJ., van der Linden, GHM., Hakvoort-Cammel, GAJ., Hahlen, K., Dohle, GR.& van den Heuvel-Eibrink, MM. (2009). Effects of childhood cancer treatment on fertility markers in adult male long-term survivors. *Pediatr Blood Cancer*, Vol. 52: (108-112).

[12] Castillo, LA., Craft, AW., Kernahan, J., Evans, RG. & Aynsley-Green, A. (1990). Gonadal function after 12-Gy testicular irradiation in childhood acute lymphoblastic leukaemia. *Med Pediatr Oncol*, Vol. 18 No. 3: 185-9.

[13] Castillo, LA., Craft, AW., Kernahan, J., Evans, RG. & Aynsley-Green, A. (1990). Gonadal function after 12-Gy testicular irradiation in childhood acute lymphoblastic leukaemia. *Med Pediatr Oncol*, Vol. 18:185-9.

[14] Chapman, RM., Rees, LH., Sutcliffe, SB. Edwards, CR. & Malpa,s JS. (1979). Cyclical combination chemotherapy and gonadal function. *Lancet,* Vol.1, No. 8111.. 285-9.

[15] Chemaitilly, W., Mertens, AC., Mitby, P., Whitton, J., Stovall, M.,Yasui, Y., Robison, LL. & Sklar, CA. (2006). Acute ovarian failure in the childhood cancer survivor study. *Journal of Clinical Endocrinology and Metabolism*, Vol 91, No. 5: 1723–1728.

[16] Cicognani, A., Pasini, A., Pession, A., Pirazzoli, P., Burnelli, R., Barbieri, E., Mazzanti, L. & Cacciari, E. (2003). Gonadal function and pubertal developement after treatment of childhood malignancy. *J Pediatr Endocrinol Metab,* Vol. 16, Suppl. 2: 21-6.

[17] Cohen, LE. (2003) Endocrine late effects of cancer treatment. *Curr Opin Pediatr*, Vol. 15, No 1: 3-9.

[18] Constine, LS., Woolf, PD., Cann, D., Mick, G., McCormick, K., Raubertas, RF. & Rubin P. (1993). Hypothalamic-pituitary dysfunction after radiation for brain tumors. *N Engl J Med*, Vol. 328:87-94.

[19] da Cunha MF, Meistrich ML, Fuller LM Cundiff JH, Hagemeister FB, Velasquez WS, McLaughlin P, Riggs SA, Cabanillas FF & Salvador PG (1984). Recovery of spermatogenesis after treatment for Hodgkin's disease: limiting dose of MOPP chemotherapy. *J Clin Oncol*, Vol. 2, No 6: 571-7.

[20] Diamond FB & Bercu BB (2001). Endocrine sequelae of cancer therapy in childhood. *J Endocrinol Invest*, Vol. 24, No 9: 648-58.

[21] Gleeson, HK. & Shalet, SM. (2004). The impact of cancer therapy on the endocrine system in survivors of childhood brain tumours. *Endocr Relat Cancer*, Vol. 11(No. 4): 589-602.

[22] Green, DM., Kawashima, T., Stovall, M., Leisenring, W., Sklar, CA., Mertens, AC., Donaldson, SA., Byrne, J. & Robison, LL. (2009). Fertility of female survivors of childhood cancer: a report from the Childhood Cancer Survivor Study. *Journal of Clinical Oncology*, Vol 27, No 16: 2677–2685.

[23] Green, DM., Whitton, JA., Stovall, M., Mertens, AC., Donaldson, SS., Ruymann, FB., Pendergrass, TW. & Robison, LL. (2002). Pregnancy outcome of female survivors of childhood cancer: a report from the Childhood Cancer Survivor Study. *Am J Obstet Gynecol,* Vol. 187, No 4.: 1070–1080.

[24] Greiner, R. (1982). Die erholung der spermatogenese nach fraktionierter, niedrig dosierter bestrahlung der männlichen gonaden. *Strahlentherapie,* Vol. 158, No.6: 342-55.

[25] Greiner, R. (1985). Wirkung der strahlen- und chemotherapie auf die gonadenfunktion. *Münch Med Wochenschr,* Vol 127, No. 37: 870-4.

[26] Grigg, AP., McLachlan, R., Zajac, J. & Szer, J. (2000). Reproductive status in long-term bone marrow transplant survivors receiving busulfan-cyclophosphamide (120 mg/kg). *Bone Marrow Transplantation,* Vol 26, No 10: 1089–1095.

[27] Hahn, EW., Feingold, SM., Simpson, L. & Batata, M. (1982). Recovery from aspermia induced by low-dose radiation in seminoma patients. *Cancer,* Vol. 50, No. 2: 337-40.

[28] Haie-Meder, C., Mlika-Cabanne, N., Briot, E., Michel, G., Briot, E., Gerbaulet, A., Lhomme, C., Cosset, JM., Sarrazin, D., Flamant, F. & Hayat, M. (1993). Radiotherapy after ovarian transposition: ovarian function and fertility preservation. *Int J Radiat Oncol Biol Phys,*Vol. 25: 419-24.

[29] Hamre, MR., Robison, LL., Nesbit, ME., Sather, HN., Meadows, AT., Ortega, JA., D'Angio, GJ. & Hammond GD. (1987), Effects of radiation on ovarian function in long-term survivors of childhood acute lymphoblastic leukemia: A report from the Children Cancer Study Group. *J Clin Oncol,* Vol 5, No. 11:1759-65.

[30] Himelstein-Braw, R., Peters, H. & Faber, M. (1978). Morphological studies of the ovaries of leukaemic children. *British Journal of Cancer.* Vol. 38, No. 1: 82–87.

[31] Hoorweg-Nijman, JJG., Delemarre-van, de Wall HA., de Wall, FC. & Behrendt, H. (1992) Cyclophosphamide- induced disturbance of gonadotropin secretion manifesting testicular damage. *Acta Endocrinologica,* Vol 126, No.2: 143-148.

[32] Horning, SJ., Hoppe, RT., Kaplan, HS. & Rosenberg, SA. (1981) Female reproductive potential after treatment for Hodgkin's disease. *N Engl J Med,* Vol.304, No. 23:1377-82.

[33] Jazbec, J. Todorovski, L. & Jereb B. (2007). Classification tree analysis of second neoplasms in survivors of childhood cancer. *BMC Cancer,* Vol. 7, No. 7: 27.

[34] Jereb, B. (2000). Model for long-term follow-up of survivors of childhood cancer. *Med Pediatr Oncol.,* Vol. 34, No 4:256-8.

[35] Jereb, B.& Eklund, G. (1973). Factor influencing the cure rate in nephroblastoma. *Acta Radiologica Therapy Physics Biology,* Vol. 12, No. 2: 84-106.

[36] Johnston, RJ. & Wallace, WH. (2009). Normal ovarian function and assessment of ovarian reserve in the survivor of childhood cancer. *Pediatr Blood Cancer,* Vol.53, No. 2: 296-302.

[37] Kenney, LB., Laufer, MR., Grant, FD., Grier, H., Diller, L. (2001). High risk of infertility and long term gonadal damage in males treated with high dose cyclophosphamide for sarcoma during childhood. *Cancer,* .Vol. 91, No. 3: 613-21.

[38] Kinsella, T., Trivette, G., Rowland, J., Sorace, R., Miller, R., Fraass, B., Steinberg, SM., Glatstein, E. & Sherins RJ. (1989). Long.term follow-up of testicular function following radiation therapy for early-stage Hodgkin's disease. *J Clin Oncol,* Vol. 7, No. 6: 718-24.

[39] Kirkland RT, Bongiovanni AM, Cornfeld D et al. (1976). Gonadotropin responses to luteinizing releasing factor in boys treated with cyclophosphamide for nephrotic syndrome. The Journal of Pediatrics, Vol. 89, No. 6:941-944.

[40] Kovač, V., Umek, B. & Marolt, F. (1990). The influence of radiotherapy on spermatogenesis in patients with testicular seminoma in relation to protection from scattered radiation. *Radiol Iugosl*, Vol 24: 191-4.

[41] Lampe, H., Horwich, A., Norman, A., Nicholls, J. & Dearnaley DP. (1997). Fertility after chemotherapy for testicular germ cell cancers. *J Clin Oncol*, Vol 15, No 1: 239-45.

[42] Larsen, E., Muller, J., Schmiegelow, K., Rechnitzer, C. & Andersen, AN. (2003). Reduced ovarian function in long-term survivors of radiation and chemotherapy treated childhood cancer. *J Clin Endocrinol Metab*, Vol 388, No. 11: 5307–5314.

[43] Leiper, AD., Grant, DB. & Chessels, JM. (1986). Gonadal function after testicular radiation for acute lymphoblastic leukemia. *Arch Dis Child*, Vol 61, No.1: 53–56.

[44] Lendon, M., Hann, IM., Palmer, MK., Shalet, SM. & Jones PH. (1978). Testicular histology after combination chemotherapy in childhood for acute lymphoblastic leukaemia. *Lancet*, Vol. 2 No. 8087: 439-441.

[45] Lu CC & Meistrich ML. (1979). Cytotoxic effects of chemotherapeutic drugs on mouse testis cells. *Cancer Res*, Vol. 39, No. 9: 3575-82.

[46] Lushbaugh, CC. & Casarett, GW. (1976). The effects of gonadal irradiation in clinical radiation therapy: a review. *Cancer*, Vol.37, Suppl 2: 1111-20.

[47] Macedoni-Lukšič, M., Jereb, B. & Todorovski, L. (2003). Long-term sequelae inchildren treated for brain tumors: impairments, disability and handicap. *Pediatr Hematol and Oncol*, Vol. 20, No. 2: 89-101.

[48] Mackie, EJ., Radford, M. & Shalet, SM. (1996) Gonadal function following chemotherapy for childhood Hodgkin's disease. *Med Pediatr Oncol*, Vol. 27, No 2: 74-8.

[49] Meistrich, ML. (2009). Male gonadal toxicity. *Pediatr Blood Cancer*; Vol. 53, No. 2: 261-266.

[50] Meistrich, ML., Finch, M., da Cunha, MF., Hacker, U., Au, WW. (1982). Damaging effects of fourteen chemotherapeutic drugs on mouse testis cells. *Cancer Res*, Vol. 42, No. 1: 122-31.

[51] Michel, G., Socié, G., Gebhard, F. Bernaudin, F., Thuret, I., Vannier, JP., Demeocq, F., Leverger, G., Pico, JL., Rubie, H., Mechinaud, F., Reiffers, J., Gratecos, N., Troussard, X., Jouet, JP., Simonin, G., Gluckman, E. & Maraninchi D.(1997) Late effects of allogeneic bone marrow transplantation for children with acute myeloblastic leukemia in first complete remission: the impact of conditioning regimen without total-body irradiation-a report from the Société Française de Greffe de Moelle. *J Clin Oncol*, Vol.15, No. 6: 2238-46.

[52] Müller, J.(2003). Impact of cancer therapy on the reproductive axis. *Horm Res*, Vol. 59: Suppl 1: 12-20.

[53] Mustieles, C., Munoz, A., Alonso, M., Ros, P., Yturriaga. R,, Maldonado, S. & Otheo E, Barrio R. (1995) Male gonadal function after chemotherapy in survivors of childhood malignancy. *Medical and Pediatric Oncology*, Vol. 24. No. 6: 347-351.

[54] Nicosia, SV., Matus-Ridley, M. & Meadows, AT. (1985). Gonadal effects of cancer therapy in girls. *Cancer*, Vol. 55, No. 10: 2364-72.

[55] Nijman, JM., Schraffordt, H., Kremer, J. & Sleijfer, DTh. (1987). Gonadal function after surgery and chemotherapy in men with stage ll and lll nonseminomatous testicular tumors. *J Clin Oncol*, Vol. 5:651-656.

[56] Ortin, TTS., Shostak, CA. & Donaldson, SS. (1990). Gonadal status and reproductive function following tratment for Hodgkin's disease in childhood:the Stanford experience. *Int J Radiat Oncol Biol Phys*, Vol 19:No. 4:873-80.

[57] Pennisi, AJ., Grushkin, CM. & Lieberman, E. (1975) Gonadal function in children with nephrosis treated with cyclophosphamide. *Am J Dis Child 1975*, Vol. 129; No.3: 315-8.

[58] Perrin, LC., Low, J., Nicklin, JL. , Ward, BG. & Crandon, AJ. (1999). Fertility and ovarian function after conservative surgery for germ cell tumours of the ovary. *Aust N Z J Obstet Gynaecol*, Vol 39 (No. 2):243-245.

[59] Quinlan, JR. (1993). C4.5: Programs for Machine Learning. San Mateo,CA: Morgan Kaufmann.

[60] Rautonen, J., Koskimies, A.& Siimes, MA. (1992). Vincristine is associated with risk of azoospermia in adult male survivors of childhood malignancies. *Eur. J. Cancer*, Vol. 28A:1837-41.

[61] Relander, T., Cavallin-Ståhl, E., Garwicz, S., Olsson, AM. & Willén M. (2000). Gonadal and sexual function in men treated for childhood cancer. *Med Pediatr Oncol*, Vol. 35, No 1:52-63.

[62] Rivkees, SA. & Crawford, JD. (1988).The relationship of gonadal activity and chemotherapy-induced gonadal damage. *JAMA*, Vol. 259:2123-2125.

[63] Romerius, P., Stahl, O., Moell, C., Relander, T., Cavallin-Stahl, E.,Wiebe, T., Giwercman, YL. & Giwercman A. (2009). Hypogonadism risk in men treated for childhood cancer. *Journal of Clinical Endocrinology and Metabolism*, Vol. 94. No.11: 4180–4186.

[64] Rowley, MJ., Leach, DR., Warner, GA. & Heller, CG. (1974). Effect of graded doses of ionizing radiation on the human testis. *Radiat Res*, Vol. 59, No. 3: 665-678.

[65] Sandeman, TF. (1966). The effects of X irradiation on male human fertility. *Br J Radiol*, Vol. 39, No.468: 901-7.

[66] Sanders, JE & Seattle Marrow Transplant Team (1991). The impact of marrow transplant preparative regimens on subsequent growth and development. *Semin Hematol*, Vol. 28, No. 3: 244-9.

[67] Santoro, A., Bonadonna, G., Valagussa, P. Zucali, R., Viviani, S., Villani, F., Pagnoni, AM., Bonfante, V., Musumeci, R. & Crippa F. (1987). Long-term results of combined chemotherapy- radiotherapy approach in Hodgkin's disease: Superiority of ABVD plus radiotherapy versus MOPP plus radiotherapy. *J Clin Oncol*, Vol. 5, No. 1: 27-37.

[68] Sarafoglou, K., Boulad, F., Gillio, A. & Sklar, C. (1997) Gonadal function after bone marrow transplantation for acute leukemia during childhood. *J Pediatr*, Vol. 130, No. 2: 210-6.

[69] Shalet, SM. (2009) Normal testicular function and spermatogenesis. *Pediatr Blood cancer*, Vol. 53, No. 2: 285-288.

[70] Shalet, SM., Hann, IM., Lendon, M., Morris Jones, PH., & Beardwell, CG. (1981).Testicular function after combination chemotherapy in childhood for acute lymphoblastic leukemia. *Arch Dis Child*, Vol. 56:275-8.

[71] Shalet, SM., Horner, A., Ahmed, SR. & Morris-Jones, PH. (1985). Leydig cell damage after testicular irradiation for lymphoblastic leukaemia. *Med Pediatr Oncol,* Vol 13, No 2: 65-68.

[72] Shalet, SM., Tsatsoulis, A., Whitehead, E. & Read, G. (1989). Vulnerability of the human Leydig cell to radiation damage is dependent upon age. *Journal of Endocrinolog,* Vol. 120, No. 1: 161–165.

[73] Sherins, RJ., Olweny, CLM.& Ziegler, JL. (1978). Gynecomastia and gonadal dysfunction in adolescent boys treated with combination chemotherapy for Hodgkin's disease. *N Engl J Med,* Vol. 299, No. 1: 12-6.

[74] Siimes, MA. & Rautonen, J. (1990) Small testicles with impaired production of sperm in adult male survivors of childhood malignancies. *Cancer;* Vol. 65, No 6: 1303-1306.

[75] Siris, ES., Leventhal, BG. & Vaitukaitis, JL. (1976). Effects of childhood leukemia and chemotherapy on puberty and reproductive function in girls. *N Engl J Med, Vol.* 294:1143-6.

[76] Sklar, C. (1999). Reproductive physiology and treatment-related loss of sex hormone production *Med Pediatr Oncol,* Vol. 33, No.1: 2-8.

[77] Sklar, CA., Kim, TH.& Ramsay, NK (1984). Testicular function following bone marrow transplantation performed during or after puberty. *Cancer,* Vol.53, No. 7: 1498-501.

[78] Sklar, CA., Mertens, AC., Mitby, P., Whitton, J., Stovall, M., Kasper, C., Mulder, J., Green, D., Nicholson, HS., Yasui, Y.& Robison, LL. (2006). Premature menopause in survivors of childhood cancer: a report from the Childhood Cancer Survivor Study. *Journal of the National Cancer Institute,* Vol 98, No. 13: 890–896.

[79] Sklar, CA., Robinson, LL., Nesbit, ME., Sather, HN., Meadows, AT., Ortega, JA., Kim, TH. & Hammond, GD.(1990). Effects of radation on testicular function in long-term survivors of childhood acute lymphoblastic leukemia: A report from the Children Cancer Study Group. *J Clin Oncol,* Vol.8: 1981-7.

[80] Spoudeas, HA. (2002) Growth and endocrine function after chemotherapy and radiotherapy in childhood. *Eur J Cancer,* Vol. 38, No. 13: 1748-59.

[81] Stillman, R.J, Schinfeld, JS., Schiff, I., Gelber, RD., Greenberger, J., Larson, M., Jaffe, N. & Li, FP. (1981). Ovarian failure in long-term survivors of childhood malignancy. *Am J Obstet Gynecol,* Vol. 139:62-66.

[82] Stillman, RJ., Schiff, I. &t Schinfeld, J. (1982) Reproductive and gonadal function in the female after therapy for childhood malignancy. *Obstet Gynecol Surv,* Vol. 37. No. 6: 385-93.

[83] Sussman, A. & Leonard, JM. (1980). Psoriasis, methotrexate and oligospermia. *Arch Dermatol,* Vol. 116, No 2: 215-217.

[84] Thibaud, E., Ramirez, M., Brauner, R., Flamant, F., Zucker, JM., Fékété, C.& Rappaport, R. (1992) Preservation of ovarian function by ovarian transposition performed before pelvic irradiation during childhood. *J Pediatr.*Vol 121, No. 6: 880-4.

[85] Thibaud, E., Rodriguez-Macias, K., Trivin, C., Esperou, H., Michon, J. & Brauner, R. (1998). Ovarian function after bone marrow transplantation during childhood. *Bone Marrow Transplantation,* Vol. 21, No. 3: 287–290.

[86] Thomas, PR., Winstanly, D., Peckham, MJ., Austin, DE., Murray, MA. & Jacobs, HS. (1976). Reproductive and endocrine function in patients with Hodgkin's disease: Effects of oophoropexy and irradiation. *Br J Cancer,* Vol. 33: 226-231.

[87] Velensek, V., Mazic, U., Krzisnik, C., Demšar, D., Jazbec, J. & Jereb, B. (2008). Cardiac damage after treatment of childhood cancer: A long-term follow-up. *BMC Cancer,* Vol 8:141-148.

[88] Vigersky, RA., Chapman, RM., Berenberg, J. & Glass, AR. (1982). Testicular dysfunction in untreated Hodgkin' disease. *Am J Med,* Vol. 73: 482-6.

[89] Viviani, S., Santoro, A., Ragni, G., Bonfante, V., Bestetti, O.& Bonadonna, G (1985). Gonadal toxicity after combination chemotherapy for Hodgkin's disease. Comparative results of MOPP vs ABVD. *Eur J Cancer Clin Oncol,* Vol. 21, No. 5: 601-5.

[90] Wallace, WH., Thomson, AB., Saran, F. & Kelsey, TW. (2005). Predicting age of ovarian failure after radiation to a field that includes the ovaries. *Int J Radiat Oncol Biol Phys.* Vol. 62, No. 3: 738-44.

[91] Waxman, JHX., Terry, YA., Wrigley, PFM, Malpas, JS., Rees, LH., Besser, GM & Lister TA. (1982) Gonadal function in Hodgkin's disease: long-term follow-up of chemotherapy. *Br Med J,* Vol 285, No. 6355:1612-13.

[92] Whitehead, E., Shalet, SM., Blackledge, G., Todd, I., Crowther, D.& Beardwell, CG. (1982). The effects of Hodgkin's disease and combination chemotherapy on gonadal function in the adult male. *Cancer,* Vol 49, No. 3: 418-422.

[93] Zacharin, M. (2010). Disorders of ovarian function in childhood and adolescence: evolving needs of the growing child. An endocrine perspective. *BJOG,* Vol. 117, No. 2: 156-162.

[94] Zaletel, LZ., Bratanic, N. & Jereb, B.(2004). Gonadal function in patients treated for leukemia in childhood.*Leuk Lymphoma,* Vol. 45, No. 9:1797-802.

[95] Zaletel, LZ., Bratanic, N. & Jereb, B.(2010). Gonadal function in patients treted for Hodgkin's disease in childhood. *Radiol. Oncol.,* Vol. 44, No 3:187-193.

Osteoporosis in Men - A Crucial Role of Sex Hormones

Michał Rabijewski and Lucyna Papierska
Department of Endocrinology,
Medical Centre for Postgraduate Education, Warsaw,
Poland

1. Introduction

Osteoporosis is a disorder characterized by reduced bone mass, impaired bone quality and a propensity to fracture. Traditionally, osteoporosis has been viewed as a syndrome characterized by back pain and vertebral fractures. Osteoporotic fractures have long been regarded as a female ailment, but with the increasing longevity of men, it appears that the incidence and prevalence of osteoporotic fractures in men is not very different from the rate in women although it occurs approximately 10 years later in the lives of men. Morbidity and mortality associated with fractures and their (surgical) treatment is considerably greater than in women. A multitude of factors determine bone strength: genetic, nutritional (calcium), vitamin D, physical activity, and hormonal factors. Hormonal factors are significant throughout life, from puberty onwards. In adolescence they are indispensable for the formation of peak bone mass. Throughout life, sex steroids maintain bone formation. Surprisingly, in men estrogens appear to be more significant for the development of peak bone mass and the maintenance of bone mineral density than androgens. In men estrogens are derived from androgens and levels of both of them are strongly interrelated (adequate androgen levels imply adequate estrogen levels).

2. Qualities of bone in men

Fracture is the result of failure of the material composition and the structural design of bone to tolerate the loads imposed upon it. These properties, or bone 'qualities', are compromised with the emergence of age-related abnormalities in bone modelling and remodelling, the cellular machinery responsible for the attainment of peak bone strength during growth and its maintenance during adulthood. The abnormalities contributing to material and structural decay are: a negative bone balance produced by each basic multicellular unit (BMU), a sustained increase in remodelling intensity in midlife in women but not in men unless frankly hypogonadal, reduced periosteal apposition after completion of longitudinal growth and secondary hyperparathyroidism (Khosla et al. 2006). However, the most important cause of bone loss is the increase in the intensity of bone remodelling on the trabecular, intracortical and endocortical bone surfaces (Amin & Felson 2001; Benito et al. 2004). The trabecular bone loss proceeds mainly by thinning in men - see Figure 1. Remodelling on intracortical surfaces results in intracortical porosity, particularly in cortex adjacent to the marrow cavity, trabecularisation of the endosteal cortex and a decrease in cortical width. The effect is likely greater in women than in men. Periosteal apposition slows after completion of growth. Some studies suggest that men have greater periosteal apposition than women (Vanderschueren et al. 2004).

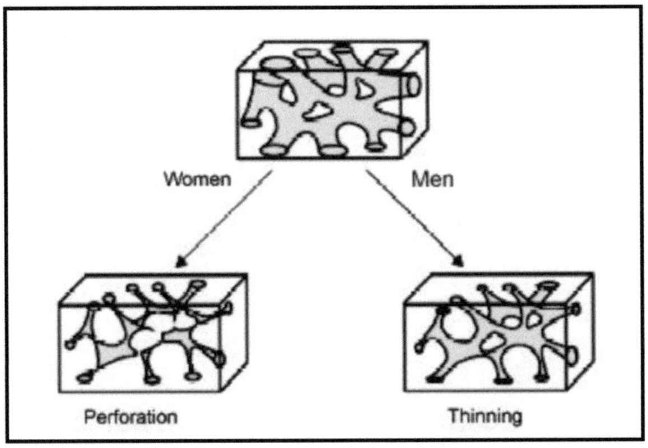

Fig. 1. Gender differences in pattern of trabecular bone loss resulting in trabecular thinning in men and increased cortical porosity and trabecular perforation in women.

Compared with women, men have greater bone strength not because of increased bone mineral density, but because of greater bone size, resulting from bone acquired at the periosteal surface. Periosteal bone formation is a result of two endocrine effects: androgen-mediated stimulatory effects on periosteal bone formation and estrogen induced inhibitory effects on periosteal expansion. So, greater periosteal bone expansion in men has been traditional assumed to result from exposure to higher levels of androgens and/or lower levels of estrogens (Vanderschueren et al. 2006).

3. Hormonal determinants of bone mass

3.1 Androgens and bone

Androgens are pivotal for the acquisition of bone mass in adolescence and the maintenance of bone mass in adulthood (Finkelstein et al. 1996). In men, chronically low androgen levels are associated with low bone mass, and testosterone replacement can enhance BMD. However, it is not yet precisely clear what role androgens play in the maintenance of bone mass in men. Peak bone mass is acquired between the ages of 12–16 years, and even beyond. It represents the sum of several processes including a marked increase in bone formation. Boys tend to reach peak 2 years later than girls and their BMD is higher than that in women at all skeletal sites. In part this relates to a greater cross-sectional bone area in males. The timing of gonadal steroid surges are critical for bone acquisition since there is a relatively short window of time in which bone formation is favored and matrix synthesis is markedly enhanced (Rochira et al. 2006). In adulthood normal testosterone levels are required for the maintenance of BMD. Hypogonadal men suffer from osteoporosis, and bone fractures in men in their forties or fifties may well be the first manifestation of undiagnosed hypogonadism (Vanderschueren et al. 2004). Variations of free testosterone within the normal range are an independent predictor of cortical bone density, and also of previous osteoporosis-related fractures. Elderly men and older men with a deficiency in total testosterone and estradiol are more likely to be osteoporotic and at greater risk of hip fracture. Men with a deficiency of total testosterone were more likely to have rapid bone loss from the hip or to suffer from hip fractures following minimal trauma. Also men with osteoporosis were more likely to have a deficiency of testosterone and estradiol (Khosla et al. 2006).

3.2 Estrogens and bone

Estrogens play also an essential role in maintaining bone mass in men.. Men with estrogens deficiency or impaired estrogens action have delayed epiphyseal closure and osteopenia (Monshima et al. 1991). It was shown that in men with aromatase deficiency the administration of estrogen had a significant beneficial effect on skeletal growth and bone maturation (Rochira 2000). In elderly men, estrogen seems to play a more dominant role than testosterone in regulating bone resorption. In elderly men, lower than normal levels of estrogen appeared to be associated with vertebral fractures (Rochira et al. 2006). Age-related decreases of estradiol, especially levels below 40 pmol/l, may be the major cause of bone loss (Barrett-Connor et al. 2000).

Estrogens in men are predominately the product of peripheral aromatization of androgens. Androgens (androstenedione, dehydroepiandrosterone produced by the adrenal gland, and testosterone produced by the testis) serve as precursors for chemical conversion to estrone and estradiol via the enzyme aromatase. The testis itself produce approximately 20% of the total estradiol. Adipose tissue is the most important source of estrogens in men. Plasma testosterone levels show an age-related decline while plasma estrogen levels in men remain relatively constant with aging resulting in an increased estrogen/androgen ratio. Estrogen deficiency in elderly men is tightly coupled to androgen deficiency since all estrogens are derived from androgens through aromatization. Restoring plasma testosterone to normal also normalizes plasma estradiol levels.

3.3 Current model of influence of sex hormones on bone in men

Recently data have challenged the traditional concept of stimulatory *vs.* inhibitory effects of androgens and estrogens. The role of androgens as the main determinant of male bone acquisition has been challenged by observations in men with aromatase deficiency (Carani et al. 1997; Rochira et al. 2000). These men, who have normal androgen concentrations, but undetectable levels of endogenous estrogen, have surprisingly low bone mass and areal density and respond very well to estrogen therapy. Reduced bone mass in these subjects is not due to reduced volumetric bone density, but reflects a deficit in bone size and the increase in bone mass during estrogen therapy was found to be driven primarily by an increase in bone size, without treatment effect on volumetric density. The enlargement of cortical bone reflected *periosteal apposition*. As evidenced in the aromatase-deficient adolescent androgens alone may not be sufficient to drive periosteal expansion. Moreover, the periosteal expansion observed in response to estrogen therapy demonstrates that estrogens stimulate rather than inhibit periosteal apposition. While, exposure to estrogens is essential for the process of periosteal bone expansion in men.

Thus, the interaction of estrogen with the periosteum has been studied. Animal data suggest that estrogens may decrease the set point of the mechanostat and thereby increase the sensitivity of bone for mechanical stimuli (Lee 2003). This may indirectly impact on the response of the bone to androgens, because androgens increase lean body mass and the mechanical loading of the male skeleton and this mechanical loading constitutes one of the main triggers for androgen induced periosteal apposition. Androgens indirectly induce mechanical loading through their anabolic action on muscle, and there is growing evidence that estrogens interact with this process. Exposure to estrogen may be critical to allow the increased loading to be translated into periosteal bone formation and radial expansion (Vanderschueren 2003).

Estrogen action on bone may reflect an interaction with GH and/or IGF-I, two main determinants of cortical bone growth (Bateman et al. 1998). Estrogens are known to have a biphasic effect on pubertal skeletal growth. During early puberty, low estrogen concentrations increase the secretion of GH and IGF-I synthesis. As a consequence, estrogens stimulate skeletal growth. Hence, sex steroid-related changes in GH and IGF-I secretion may impact on bone size and cross-sectional area. By the end of puberty, elevated concentrations of estrogen limit skeletal longitudinal growth through a direct effect on growth plate closure. By the end of puberty, estrogens may inhibit radial growth in men (Juul 2001). Estrogen-related changes in serum IGF-I may be more important than direct estrogen-mediated stimulation of the periosteal surfaces. Estradiol stimulates radial bone growth as a result of an up-regulation of hepatic IGF-I synthesis and secretion, but only ER activation results in changes in serum IGF-I, indicating that AR-mediated androgen action, is independent of GH and/or IGF-I.

Effects of estrogen on periosteal bone are dose dependent. Low levels of estrogen might increase the mechanical sensitivity of the periosteum and/or affect circulating IGF-I levels, while higher concentrations of estrogen might inhibit periosteal bone apposition and its interaction with mechanical loading, possibly through an ERβ effect (Moverare et al. 2003). The inhibitory effect of estrogen is not observed in men, because men are exposed to low endogenous estrogen concentrations. Also disruption of ERβ does not affect the male cortical phenotype. Men exhibit more periosteal expansion because they are more exposed to the stimulatory effects of androgens and less exposed to the inhibitory effects of estrogens. Androgens may primarily affect lean body mass and the loading of the male skeleton; exposure to low-dose estrogen may allow this loading to induce bone expansion.

In addition to the changes in trabecular and cortical morphology, abnormalities in bone remodelling produce changes in bone 'qualities' at higher levels of resolution. Advancing age is associated with a reduction in osteonal size, accompanied by an increase in haversian canal diameter due to the reduced bone formation by each BMU. Smaller osteons result in less resistance to crack propagation through interstitial bone (Khosla et al. 2006). Also, smaller osteons give rise to a greater proportion interstitial (rather than osteonal) bone which has a higher tissue mineralization density, fewer osteocytes and is liable to accumulate microdamage and offer less resistance to crack propagation. These phenomena are likely to occur in both sexes but in women, osteonal density (the number per unit volume) may increase because of the high intracortical remodelling; the osteons are smaller but there are more of them (Amin et al. 2001).

Sex differences in bone size are contributing to the lower incidence of fractures in men. Men also have larger muscle mass and higher body weight so that compressive stress (load/area) is similar in young adult men and women. Men and women have similar cortical thickness which confers a greater cortical area in men (because their bones have a larger perimeter). Peak trabecular number and thickness is similar in men and women at the iliac crest and vertebral bone. Men have thicker trabeculae at the distal radius which may be more resistant to perforation. Reasons for sex differences in bone fragility are multifaceted: sex differences in trabecular morphology (thinning in men and perforation in women), less cortical porosity, endocortical remodelling and thinning in men, particularly and possibly greater periosteal apposition in men. Other factors that may contribute to sex differences in bone fragility include differences in osteonal morphology, tissue mineralisation and matrix composition (Amin et al. 2001; Seeman et al. 2002;Vanderschueren et al. 2004). Model of sex hormones action on bone is shown on Figure 2.

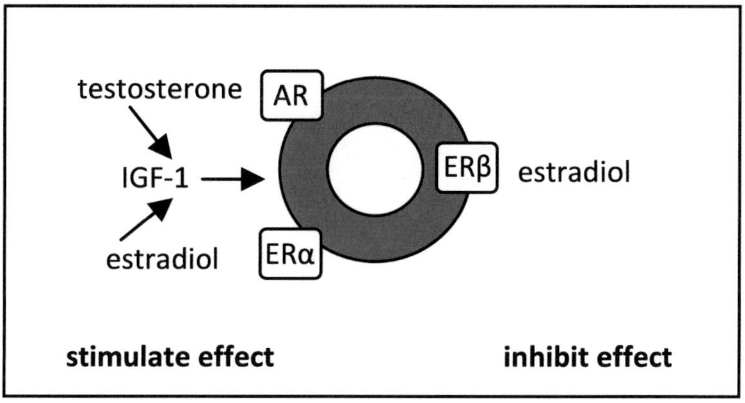

Fig. 2. Model of sex hormones action on bone: testosterone stimulates periosteal expansion, whereas estradiol has a double action on periosteal bone apposition. Estrogen action on the periosteum may be also result of indirectly changes in IGF-I.

4. Epidemiology of osteoporosis in men

It is agreed that the life-time risk of osteoporotic fracture in men is around one-third of that in women About 4 to 6 percent of men older than 50 have osteoporosis, and 33 to 47 percent have osteopenia. The prevalence of osteoporosis is 7 percent in white men, 5 percent in black men, and about 3 percent in Hispanic-American men. Because men have greater bone mass, they present with osteoporotic fracture about 10 years later than women. Thus, starting at about age 75, the incidence of hip fracture increases rapidly. The life-time risk of a hip fracture in Caucasian men is 13 to 25% (Cooper et al.1992; Johnell et al. 2005). Because of the predicted growth in the number of elderly persons, the number of men with osteoporotic fracture is expected to increase.

5. Fractures in men

Fractures represent the primary clinical consequence of osteoporosis. The difference in fracture incidence observed between men and women is due not only to a difference in their bone strength but also to the type and frequency of trauma experienced by men over life. Fractures of the hip, vertebrae and forearm are more likely to occur after minimal trauma in aging men. Of these fractures, those involving the hip and vertebrae are associated with some of the greatest morbidity and mortality for men (Anderson et al.1999). The fracture incidence in men follows a bimodal distribution tending to peak in adolescence and with advanced age. Although women have a greater incidence of fractures with aging, men are actually more likely than women to sustain a fracture at younger ages, what is related, in part, to the greater frequency of severe trauma associated with their fractures. The incidence rate for a work-related fracture for male employees is more than twice that for female employees, These fractures appear to be related to high-energy trauma events (Anderson & Cooper 1999). After the age of 50 yr, the trend reverses, with women tending to have a higher incidence of overall fractures than men. In both men and women, there is an exponential rise in fracture incidence after age 75 yr, particularly for hip fractures; however, the absolute incidence tends to be lower in men. Osteoporotic fractures in men appear to involve fractures of the hip, vertebrae, forearm, and humerus, although fragility fractures at other sites, including the pelvis, ribs, and clavicle, also occur in aging men. Of all the hip, forearm and clinical vertebral fractures, approximately 30, 20, and 40% occur in men, respectively. The lower absolute incidence in osteoporotic fractures in older men may be due to the an increased frequency of falls in women (Bilezikian 1999; Campion & Maricic 2003).

5.1 Hip fractures

Among all osteoporotic fractures, hip fractures account for the greatest morbidity and mortality for men. Overall, the incidence of hip fractures in men is uncommon until after the age of 75 yr, when the risk increases exponentially. The age-adjusted female to male ratio for hip fractures has been observed to be highest for whites, with a ratio up to 3–4:1 (Maggi et al.1991). With the improving longevity of men and the increasing size of the population, the number of men with hip fracture worldwide is estimated to reach 1.8 million in 2050 (Khosla et al. 2006). The mortality and morbidity associated with hip fractures are greater for men than women (Forsens et al. 1999). Men are twice as likely to die in hospital after a hip fracture as women. Estimates for the 1-yr mortality rate after hip fracture ranges from 31–35% in men compared with 17–22% in women (Bass et al. 2007). Greater number of comorbid conditions at the time of fracture contribute to mortality risk and up to 50% of men may need institutionalized care after hip fracture. Men are less likely to return to autonomous living circumstances than women at 1 yr after hip fracture. In men ages 60–69 yr, the decrease in life expectancy after a hip fracture is 11.5 yr, compared with men ages 70–79 yr and age 80 yr or older, where the decrease in life expectancy is 5 and 1.5 yr, respectively (Center et al.1999). Despite these facts, men are less likely to be investigated or treated for osteoporosis after hip fracture.

5.2 Vertebral fractures

Vertebral fractures are not always associated with pain that would bring them to clinical attention. The true incidence of these fractures is often underestimated. The age-standardized prevalence of vertebral deformity in Europe is estimated to be the same for both men and women, either 12 or 20%, depending on the criteria used to define vertebral deformity (O'Neill et al.1996). Below age 65 yr, men had a higher prevalence of vertebral deformity than women, whereas after this age the trend was reversed. The prevalence of vertebral deformity increased with age. The age-adjusted incidence for radiographically defined vertebral fractures in men is half the rate of women. In a 10-yr study prevalent vertebral deformity was a predictor of mortality in men during the forthcoming decade (age-adjusted hazard ratio, 2.4) (Hasserius rt al. 2003). Severe vertebral deformity is related to functional impairment and the association between vertebral deformity and negative health outcomes appears to be even stronger in men than in women.

6. Risk factors for osteoporosis in men

Development of osteoporosis in men is primarily related to aging and genetic factors but30 to 60 percent of cases of osteoporosis are associated with one or more secondary risk factors. The three major causes of secondary osteoporosis in men are alcohol abuse, glucocorticoid glucocorticoid therapy and hypogonadism. Of these, glucocorticoid-induced osteoporosis is the most common.

6.1 Glucocorticoid therapy

Long-term oral glucocorticoid therapy accounts for nearly one in six cases of male osteoporosis. The extent of bone loss is related to the duration of therapy and the dosage of the steroid. Because of the high risk of bone loss, treatment of osteoporosis is recommended for any patient taking 5 mg or more of steroids per day for longer than six months. The recommended treatment is a bisphosphonate supplemented with calcium and vitamin D (Recommendation of American Collefe of Rheumatology 2001).

6.2 Tobacco and alcohol use

Tobacco use and excessive alcohol consumption are more prevalent in men than in women, and both are independently associated with an increased incidence of osteoporotic fractures (Anderson et al.1997). Tobacco-related bone loss is linked to smoking duration and quantity. The mechanism may be a combination of decreased body weight, decreased calcium absorption, decreased estradiol levels, and a direct toxic effect on bone metabolism. Alcohol in modest amounts may have a protective effect on bone density, but sustained high consumption causes bone loss. It is likely that alcohol has a direct toxic effect on osteoblastic function. Excessive alcohol consumption is also often associated with poor nutrition and decreased physical activity, both of which are associated with bone loss (Seeman et al. 1983). Further studies are needed to determine the quantity of alcohol above which the protective effect ceases and bone loss occurs.

6.3 Hypogonadism

Hypogonadism induces a state of high bone turnover with accelerated bone loss and increased fracture risk which results from combined deficiency of testosterone and estradiol (Goderie-Plomp et al. 2004). Symptomatic hypogonadism is an indication for testosterone substitution in all causes (primary and secondary hypogonadism). .Also in men with history of delayed poberty peak bone mass in significant lower than in healthy men, what can be the reason of greater risk of fracture and high incidence of osteoporosis in this population (Finkelstein et al. 1996).

Aging is accompanied by progressive moderate decrease in the population mean serum concentration of total testosterone. A marked age-related increase of serum sex hormone-binding globulin (SHBG) levels is also found which results in a decrease in the non-SHBG-bound fractions of testosterone available for biological action, i.e. decreased free- and bioavailable testosterone, as well as a moderate decrease of free- and bioavailable estradiol (Araujo 2004)/ . Aging in men is also accompanied by increasing prevalence of signs and symptoms, including osteoporosis, that are reminiscent of those observed in young hypogonadal men, but which in the elderly are at most only in part related to the decline of testosterone production. With age, both low serum testosterone and symptoms and signs consistent with hypogonadism become increasingly prevalent but also less specific (Zitzmann et al. 2006). The minimal testosterone levels needs in the elderly are not clearly established and may to vary between individuals. In this elderly population, effects of testosterone treatment on BMD have been inconsistent, with the most convincing effects being observed in men with very low serum testosterone (Katznelson et al. 1996; Snyder et al. 2000; Wang et al. 2001). In elderly men, testosterone treatment may have additional beneficial effects on muscle mass and strength, which may help decrease fracture risk through a reduced propensity to fall (Snyder et al.1999).

6.4 Estradiol deficiency

Declining levels of estrogens levels with age contribute to bone loss and fracture risk in men. Estrogen plays an important role in regulating bone density, bone resorption and bone loss in elderly men as well as in the acquisition of peak bone mass. It seems, that free estradiol and SHBG, but not free testosterone, are independently associated with fracture risk, clinical vertebral fractures, non-vertebral osteoporotic fractures and hip fractures. Specifically, the yearly incidence of fractures was inversely associated with serum estradiol levels at estradiol levels less than 16 pg/ml; above this level, there was no relationship between fracture incidence and estradiol levels (Amin et al., 2000, Barrett-Connor et al. 2000)

These findings have clinical implications: measurement of serum sex steroid levels, particularly estradiol levels, in men with osteoporosis and use of selective estrogen receptor modulators (SERMs) in preventing bone loss in aging men may be usefull.

6.5 Vitamin D deficiency

Vitamin D deficiency is a widespread condition and still poses a major problem to bone health in wide population. Vitamin D and its hydroxylated derivatives can be produced either endogenously after exposure to sunlight or gained from dietary intake. Vitamin D deficiency results in secondary hyperparathyroidism (elevated parathyroid hormone serum levels) followed by demineralization of bone. Secondary hyperparathyroidism usually arises from hypocalcemia, as seen in chronic renal failure or vitamin D deficiency (Campion & Maricic 2003). Significant correlations between low spinal bone mineral density and low vitamin D levels can be observed. Vitamin D represents a key regulator of intestinal calcium absorption and its association with bone metabolism and osteoporosis - osteomalacia - is clear. Aging in males is connected with decreased renal hydroxylation of 25OH-vitamin D to calcitriol what is associated with low action of 1-alpha hydroxylase and may lead to low serum levels of active vitamin D derivatives . In patients with osteomalacia the material properties of properly mineralized bone are not reached and these patients are predisposed to fractures (Bilezikian 1999; Khosla et al. 2006).

6.6 Others risk factors and causes of secondary osteoporosis in men

Others risk factors which also could be associated with idiopathic osteoporosis in men (Harper & Weber 1998) and the more common others medical conditions which could lead to osteoporosis are listed in Table 1.

Secondary causes of osteoporosis should be excluded before the diagnosis of idiopathic osteoporosis can be made. Low bone mass and falls are both determinants of osteoporotic fracture in men. The following are a list of risk factors which could be associated with idiopathic osteoporosis in men.

High risk causes
History of nontraumatic fracture (hip, vertebrae or wrist)
Osteopenia seen on plane radiograph
Glucocorticoid use of 5mg of more for longer than six months
Hypogonadism
Hyperparathyroidism
Medium risk causes
Anticonvulsant grug use
Excess alcohol consumption and tobacco use
Rheumatoid and other inflammatory arthritis
Multiple myeloma ot lymphoma
Hyperthyroidism and hypothyroidism
Family history of osteoporosis
Prolonged immobilization, lack of physical activity
Conditions associated with increased risk of falling
Infrequent causes
Chronic renal and liver diseases
Cushing's disease
Low body mass index
Gastric or bowel resection, celiac disease

Table 1. Risk factors for osteoporosis in men.

7. Diagnosis

Osteoporosis can be defined as "a skeletal disease" characterized by low bone mass and micro-architectural deterioration of bone tissue, leading to enhanced bone fragility and a consequent increase in fracture risk. The World Health Organization has definitions for osteopenia and osteoporosis in women, but not in men. In women, osteopenia is defined as a T score of between -1 and -2.5, and osteoporosis as a T-score of -2.5 or more. The T-score is the number of standard deviations by which the bone mineral density of an individual person differs from that of the young, normal mean of the same population. A strength of this diagnostic threshold has been the fashioning of a common approach to describe the disease. The WHO have supported the use of a single reference population (white women aged 20-29 years), a single reference site (the femoral neck) and a single technology (DXA) (Kanis et al. 2008).

Osteoporosis in men would be defined as a BMD value at the femoral neck that lay 2.5 SD or more below the average value of young healthy women The many studies that have examined fracture risk in men have come to disparate conclusions concerning the relationship between fracture risk and BMD. The relation between BMD and fracture risk changes with age, so that age-adjustment is required. The comparative studies show that the risk of hip fracture is similar in men and women for any given absolute value for BMD measured mainly at the hip. In the meta-analysis described above the relationship between hip fracture incidence and BMD at the proximal femur was identical in men and women at any given age (Johnell 2005). These studies indicate that a similar cut-off value for femoral neck BMD that is used in women should be used in the diagnosis of osteoporosis in men. The implementation of probability based fracture risk assessment (e.g. FRAX) will decrease the clinical utility of the T-score but diagnostic criteria remain of value in diagnostic of osteoporosis in men (Orwoll 2000).

Osteoporosis in men commonly presents with vertebral body fracture or hip fracture, whereas in women it is often diagnosed by routine bone density screening, but osteoporosis can be identified in men before fractures occur. Men with history of nontraumatic fracture, particularly of the hip, vertebral body, or distal wrist; radiographic evidence of osteopenia (because 30 to 50 percent of bone mass must be lost before evidence of loss is seen on a plain radiograph); long-term glucocorticoid use; hypogonadism; hyperparathyroidism; and other risk factors for osteoporosis, including disease states, medications affecting bone metabolism, or gait disorder, should be considered for formal osteoporosis testing (Khosla et al.2006).

Physicians might consider routinely screening men aged 70 or older, because this is the age when fracture rates increase most rapidly. Men with asymptomatic vertebral body fractures, who are at substantially increased risk of future fractures, can be identified using serial measurements of height. A man with a loss of height or whose distal ribs touch the pelvic brim should be considered for thoracic and lumbar spine radiographs to look for vertebral fractures. Screening measures include diagnostic radiologic studies using dual-energy x-ray absorptiometry (DXA) of the hip and spine, heel ultrasonography, or quantitative computed tomography. In men, declining BMD and T scores (the comparison with peak BMD adjusted for sex and race) correlate with an increased risk of hip and other fractures similar to that occurring in women.

Once osteoporosis is diagnosed, the cause should be determined, if possible, to identify the various risk factors and medical conditions causing secondary osteoporosis. The search for risk factors should include review of the history and physical examination findings plus a laboratory evaluation. Routine laboratory tests include complete blood cell count, liver and kidney panels, and measurement of calcium, phosphorus, alkaline phosphatase, thyroid-stimulating hormone level, and total testosterone levels - table 2.

Initial screening	Additional tests
Complete blood cell cunt	Serum protein
Calcium	24+hour urine calciuria
Phosphorus	Estradiol level
Alkaline phosphatase	Parathyroid hormone level
Kidney and liver function tests	
25-hydroxyvitamin D	
TSH	
Total testosterone	

Table 2. Laboratory evaluation for osteoporosis in men

8. Treatment of osteoporosis in men

Few randomized controlled clinical trials on drug treatment for osteoporosis have been conducted in men. This is due to the fact that data from earlier trials on mixed female-male populations are not accepted as a source of guidelines for men and only a few of the requested randomized controlled studies on purely male cohorts have been performed. Older drugs were approved for osteoporosis in general without the need for separate trials in men (e.g. calcium, fluoride, calcitonin, alfacalcidol) and, therefore, these are still available for treating men. It was suggested that significant differences in bone biology might exist between the sexes. This is a severe therapeutic disadvantage for men with osteoporosis. Interestingly, so far, for all drugs that have also been studied in men, similar therapeutic results, in terms of BMD and fracture reducing potency, have been reported in men and women, disproving the argument of significant differences in bone biology of the female and male skeleton.

8.1 General measures for prevention of osteoporosis in men.

Calcium and vitamin D intake probably provide beneficial effects on bone mass and fractures. Reducing modifiable individual risk factors of diet and lifestyle, including alcohol and nicotine intake, remain important throughout life. For men suffering from one or more diseases or medical conditions with a high risk for the development of secondary osteoporosis (see early detectionand counteractionmeasures are important, e.g. reduction of glucocorticoid dosage if possible, androgen therapy in cases of hypogonadism, thiazides for idiopathic hypercalcuria and early surgical treatment of primary hyperparathyroidism. In the elderly who are at risk for falls (e.g. those with reduced muscle strength, poor balance, previous falls) attempts to increase strength and balance or the use of a hip protector may be beneficial. Table 3 summarises general recommendations for the prevention of osteoporotic fractures in men.

Long-term regular physical activity and exercise
Maintenance of adequate calcium and vitamin D intake (total intake 1000–1500 mg calcium and 600–800 IU vitamin D per day)
Routine calcium/vitamin D supplementation after age 70 years
Limit alcohol intake and smoking
Recognize and treat testosterone deficiency
Identify other risk factors and consider specific prophylactic measures

Table 3. General measures for the prevention of osteoporotic fractures in men

8.2 Aetiological therapy in secondary osteoporosis

Since about 50% of men are diagnosed with secondary osteoporosis, an aetiology-adapted treatment is more important in male than in female. The treatment in such cases is often complicated. eg: glucocorticoids cause bone lose in dose-dependent manner, in corticotherapy of rheumatic disease however, too great a reduction in corticoids may increase the risk of osteoporosis, since an insufficient immunosuppressive effect will allow further degradation of bone tissue by proinflammatory cytokines. Furthermore, insufficient disease control is associated with less mobility. For a number of mono-aetiolgical, and for the majority of polyaetiological, secondary osteoporoses no aetiological therapies are available, i.e. the therapeutic strategy is no different from that used in idiopathic osteoporosis.

8.3 Treatment of idiopathic osteoporosis

In men with secondary osteoporosis, with no options for aetiology-related treatment, and in all cases of primary or idiopathic osteoporosis, an individually adapted therapeutic strategy has to be planned. Since osteoporosis is a chronic disease that has to be treated over several years, it is important to inform the patient carefully about modifiable risk factors, future fracture risk, chances of improving pain, therapeutic mechanism of the selected medications and their possible side effects. With the exception of estrogen and raloxifen, the same specific drugs as those used with women can be adopted in men. However, not all are approved for this application in men. Calcitonin, alfacalcidol and fluoride do not exclude male osteoporosis and they are listed as second-line treatments. Bisphosphonates, strontium ranelate and teriparatide are firstline treatments, but only alendronate and risedronate have been approved for men. Teriparatide is not approved for men in the European Union countries.

8.4 Calcitonin and fluoride

There are only small studies on these two treatments in men with osteoporosis. There is one double blind, placebo-controlled study with the physiological osteoclast inhibitor calcitonin. In this study 28 men with osteoporosis received either 200 IU of salmon calcitonin nasal spray plus 500 mg calcium per day or a placebo nasal spray plus calcium. Lumbar spine BMD increase of 7.1% in the calcitonin group vs. 2.4% in the controls, in parallel with a higher decrease in bone resorption markers (Trovas et al.2002). In prospective controlled, 3-year trial of 60 men with primary osteoporosis a significantly lower vertebral fracture rate with low-dose-intermittent fluoride therapy compared to controls receiving only calcium plus vitamin D was found (Ringe et al. 1998).

8.5 Bisphosphonates

Bisphosphonate therapy has been shown to be effective in increasing BMD in men with primary osteoporosis, as well as in men with secondary osteoporosis, including hypogonadism and glucocorticoid-induced osteoporosis. The results of a randomized, controlled clinical trial showed that alendronate, given with calcium and vitamin D, was effective in preventing bone loss in men. The BMD increased by 7.3% at the lumbar spine and 2.5% at the femoral neck in the treatment group. Moreover, vertebral fracture risk was significantly reduced (0.8% in the treatment group compared with 7.1% in the placebo group). The efficacy of alendronate in treating osteoporosis in men has been confirmed (Orwoll et al.2000; Miller et al. 2004; Ringe et al. 2004) .

Risedronate is a potent bisphosphonate that has been demonstrated to reduce vertebral fractures in patients with glucocorticoid-induced osteoporosis within 1 year. Risedronate 35 mg once weekly has been approved recently as a second bisphosphonate for the treatment of men with a high fracture risk (Boonen et all.2006, Harrington et al.2004; McClung et al. 2001; Ringe et al. 2006).

Zoledronic acid is a potent intravenously administered bisphosphonate whose effects on fracture risk been assessed in a recent randomized placebo-controlled trial involving elderly men and women who had recently suffered a hip fracture. Yearly administration of 5 mg of zoledronic acid for a median of 1.9 years within 3 months of the fracture reduced the occurrence of overall new clinical fractures and mortality, but not hip fractures (Orwoll et al. 2010).

Bisphosphonates increased BMD and reduced fracture risk in men with glucocorticoid or leuprolide-induced bone loss. They are currently the treatment of choice for idiopathic osteoporosis in men.

Bisphosphonates are generally well tolerated. However, both intravenous and oral bisphosphonates have been linked in rare cases to osteonecrosis of the jaw, although current limited data suggest no clear increase in the risk of this complication in patients with osteoporosis. Rare case reports of atypical femoral diaphyseal fractures in patients on bisphosphonate therapy have also recently emerged in the literature and raise concerns about the long-term safety of this treatment in some individuals. However, more data are required on these atypical fractures

Although most trials of oral bisphosphonates in men have been either underpowered or not primarily designed to assess their effect on fracture incidence, some trials showed a significant 60%–88% reduction in the occurrence of new radiologic vertebral fractures. Although the increase in BMD with bisphosphonate therapy is similar in men and women and could therefore theoretically translate into a reduction of fracture risk similar to the one observed in women, more data are required to ascertain the benefits of oral bisphosphonates on non-vertebral and hip fractures in men (Orwoll et al. 2004).

8.6 Calcium and vitamin D

In two recent studies, injections of vitamin D2 (ergocalciferol) in men living in nursing homes resulted in reduced appendicular fractures. On the other hand, the antifracture efficacy of D3 (calciferol) 1,25 (OH)2D3 (calcitriol) in men without serious D3 deficiency remains controversial (Heikinheimo et al. 1992; Orwoll et al.1992).

Calcium intake should be 1,000 to 1,500 mg per day, and vitamin D intake should be 400 to 800 IU per day. Only 50 to 60 percent of older adults meet recommendations for calcium intake (Amin & Felson 2001). Older adults also have decreased vitamin D levels because skin synthesis, oral intake, and gastrointestinal absorption are diminished. Skin synthesis of vitamin D decreases because older patients tend to remain indoors and incur less exposure to sunlight.

8.7 Strontium ranelate

Strontium ranelate exerts dual - antiresorptive and anabolic action in bone. In recent study in men with primary osteoporosis it produced even significantly greater mean increases in BMD over 12 months compared with alendronate (Meunier et al.2004). However, the antifraxture effect of SR in men must be proved in further studies.

8.8 Androgen replacement therapy

Symptomatic hypogonadism is considered an indication for testosterone substitution at all ages (Wang 2009). In clinical trials in patients with Klinefelter syndorme and hypogonadism hypogonadotropic with low bone mineral density testosterone replacement therapy was associated with increase of BMD and decreasing of resorptions markers (Finkelstein et al. 1989). These effects may probably reduce the risk of fracture in part of patients. Also in

patiens witj primary and secondary hypogonadism due to testis diseases or hypothalamo-pituitary disriders, testosterone replacement therapy may reduce bone turnover and prevent further bone loss, and even increase BMD, at least in some patients (Behre et al.1997; Snyder et al. 2000). Effects on fracture risk have not been assessed.
In the case of low serum testosterone due to long-term treatment with systemic glucocorticoid administration, beneficial effects of testosterone treatment on BMD were observed (Crawford et al. 2003). In view of the lack of documentation of antifracture efficacy of testosterone, treatment of osteoporosis should include bisfosfonates or other antiosteoporotic agents, whether or not on testosterone substitution (Khosla et al.2006). In men with profound hypogonadism due to androgen deprivation therapy for prostate cancer, treatment with testosterone is contraindicated and the other therapeutic options should be considered such as SERMs, bisphosphonates and denosumab, can effectively reduce bone turnover, prevent bone loss and reduce fracture risk (Adlet et al. 2011; Khosla rt al. 2006).
As noted above, aging is accompanied by progressive moderate decrease in the population mean serum concentration of testosterone and increasing prevalence of men with serum (free, bioavailable) testosterone levels that lie below the range for young men (Araujo et al.2004). In this elderly population, effects of testosterone treatment on BMD have been inconsistent, with the most convincing effects being observed in men with very low serum testosterone (Katznelson et al.1996; Snyder et al. 2000; Wang et al 2001). In elderly men, testosterone treatment may have additional beneficial effects on muscle mass and strength, which may help decrease fracture risk through a reduced propensity to fall (Snyder et al. 1999). Nevertheless, the effect of testosterone treatment on fracture risk is unknown. By contrast, treatment with bisphosphonates and teriparatide has been shown to be effective in men with low baseline serum testosterone in subgroup analysis of clinical trials of treatment.
In this context, hypogonadism in older men requires a conservative approach and testosterone treatment should be considered only for men with frankly low serum testosterone, in the presence of unequivocal signs and symptoms of hypogonadism, In view of the lack of documentation of anti-fracture efficacy of testosterone, treatment of osteoporosis should include established osteoporosis treatments whether or not on testosterone substitution. Nevertheless, the effect of testosterone treatment on fracture risk is unknown and the long-term risk-benefit ratio of prolonged treatment in elderly men is not yet established. The potential adverse effects on haematocrit, prostate and cardiovascular risk requires alertness.

9. Teriparatade

A favourable effect of treatment with parathyroid hormone (PTH) on BMD in men with advanced osteoporosis has also been demonstrated in a small pilot study with daily injections of 400 IU PTH (1–34) [Teriparatide]. After 18 months, the average lumbar spine BMD had increased by 13.5% in the PTH-group and was unchanged in placebo group. In a larger trial of 437 men with osteoporosis (daily dose of 20 mg or 40 mg rhPTH or placebo, subcutaneously) over 11 months plus 18 months follow-up similar effects on BMD and a significantly lower rate of vertebral fractures for the pooled PTH groups were found. The similarity of those effects on BMD with the effects observed in clinical studies of women where the influence of the treatment on fracture incidence was assessed, clearly indicates the therapeutic usefulness of teriparatide in both sexes (Kaudman 2001; Kurland 2000)

10. Conclusion

In conclusion, osteoporosis is a prevalent health problem in men. An evidence-based approach should be adopted in the clinical investigation and drug treatment for this condition. Further research into the validity of diagnostic criteria, risk factors and emerging therapeutic agents for osteoporosis in men is however urgently required.

11. References

Adler SA. Management of osteoporosis in men on androgen deprivation therapy. Maturitas. 2011;68:143-147

Amin S, Zhang Y, Sawin CT et al. Association of hypogonadism and estradiol levels with bone mineral density in elderly men from the Framingham study. Ann Intern Med 2000;133:951-963

Amin S, Felson DT. Osteoporosis in men. Rheum Dis Clin North Am 2001;27:19-47.

Anderson FH, Cooper C. Hip and vertebral fractures. In: Orwoll ES, ed. Osteoporosis in men. San Diego, Calif.: Academic, 1999:29-49

Araujo AB, O'Donnell AB, Brambilla DJ et al. Prevalence and incidence of androgen deficiency in middle-aged and older man: estimates from the Massachusetts Male Aging Study. J Clin Endocrinol Metab 2004;89:5925-5926

Bass E, French DD, Bradham DD et al. Risk adjusted mortality rates of elderly veterans with hip fractures. Ann Epidemiol 2007;17:514–519

Barrett-Connor E. Mueller JE, von Muhlen DG et al. Low levels of estradiol are associated with vertebral fractures in older men, but not women: the Rancho Bernardo Study. Journal of Clinical Endocrinology and Metabolism 2000 85 219–223

Bateman TA, Zimmerman RJ, Ayers RA et al. Histomorphometric, physical, and mechanical effects of spaceflight and insulin-like growth factor-I on rat long bones. Bone 1998;23:527–535

Bilezikian JP. Osteoporosis in men. J Clin Endocrinol Metab 1999;84:3431-3434

Behre HM, Kliesch S, Leifke E et al. Long-term effect of testosterone therapy on bone mineral density in hypogonadal men. Journal of Clinical Endocrinology and Metabolism 1997;82:2386–2390

Benito M, Gomberg B, Wehrli RH et al. Deterioration of trabecular architecture in hypogonadal men. Journal of Clinical Endocrinology and Metabolism 2003;88:1497–1502

Boonen S, Delmas PD, Wenderoth D et all. Risedronate shown to be safe and effective in men with osteoporosis in a 2-year, double-blind, randomized, placebo-controlled, multicenter study. Osteoporos Int 2006;17(Suppl 2):S230–1

Campion JM, Maricic MJ. Osteoporosis in men. Am Fam Physician 2003;67(7):1521–6.

Carani C, Qin K, Simoni M et al. Effect of testosterone and estradiol in a man with aromatase deficiency. N Engl J Med 1007;337:91–95

Center JR, Nguyen TV, Schneider D et al. Mortality after all major types of osteoporotic fracture in men and women: an observational study. Lancet 1999;353(9156):878–882

Cooper C, Campion G, Melton LJ 3d. Hip fractures in the elderly: a worldwide projection. Osteoporos Int 1992;2:285-289

Cooper C, Melton LJ 3d. Epidemiology of osteoporosis. Trends Endocrinol Metab 1992;3:224-229

Crawford BAL, Liu PY, Kean MT et al. Randomized placebo-controlled trial of androgen effects on muscle and bone in men requiring long-term systemic glucocorticoid treatment. Journal of Clinical Endocrinology and Metabolism 2003 88 3167–3176

Finkelstein JS, Klibanski A, Neer RM et al. Increases in bone density during treatment of men with idiopathic hypogonadotropic hypogonadism. Journal of Clinical Endocrinology and Metabolism 1989 69 776–783

Finkelstein JS, Klibanski A & Neer RM. A longitudinal evaluation of bone mineral density in adult men with histories of delayed puberty. Journal of Clinical Endocrinology and Metabolism 1996;81:1152–1155

Forsen L, Sogaard AJ, Meyer HE et al. Survival after hip fracture: short- and long-term excess mortality according to age and gender. Osteoporos Int 1999;10:73-78

Goderie-Plomp HW, van der Klift M, de Ronde W et al. Endogenous sex hormones, sex hormone-binding globulin, and the risk of incident vertebral fractures n elderly men and women: the Rotterdam Study. Journal of Clinical Endocrinology and Metabolism 2004;89: 3261–3269

Harper KD, Weber TJ. Secondary osteoporosis: diagnostic considerations. Endocrinol Metab Clin North Am 1998;27:325-48

Hasserius R, Karlsson MK, Nilsson BE et al. European Vertebral Osteoporosis S. Prevalent vertebral deformities predict increased mortality and increased fracture rate in both men and women: a 10-year population-based study of 598 individuals from the Swedish cohort in the European Vertebral Osteoporosis Study. Osteoporos Int 2003;14:61–68

Heikinheimo RJ, Inkovaara JA, Harju EJ et al. Annual injection of Vitamin D and fractures of aged bones. Calcif Tissue Int 1992;51:105–10

Harrington T, Ste-Marie LG, Brandi ML et al. Risedronate rapidly reduces the risk for nonvertebral fractures in women with postmenopausal osteoporosis. Calcif Tissue Int 2004;74:129–35

Johnell O, Kanis JA, Oden A et al Predictive value of bone mineral density for hip and other fractures. Osteoporos Int 2005;20;1185-1194.

Juul A. The effects of oestrogens on linear bone growth. Hum Reprod Update 2001;7:303–313

Kanis JA, McCloskey EV, Johansson H et al. A reference standard for the description of osteoporosis. Bone, 2008;42:467-475

Katznelson L, Finkelstein J, Schoenfeld D et al. Increase in bone density and lean body mass during testosterone administration in men with acquired hypogonadism. J Clin Endocrinol Metab 1996;81:4358-4365

Kaufman JM, Scheele WH, Orwoll E et al. Recombinant human parathyroid hormone (1–34) therapy increases bone mineral density and may decrease the risk of fractures in men with low bone density. Osteoporos Int 2001;12(Suppl.2):S13.

Khosla S, Amin S, Orwoll E. Osteoporosis in men. Endocrine Reviews, 2006;29:441–464

Kurland ES, Cosman F, McMahon DJ et al. Parathyroid hormone as a therapy for idiopathic osteoporosis osteoporosis in men: effects on mineral density and bone markers. J Clin Endocrinol Metab 2000;85:3069–3076

Lee K, Jessop H, Suswillo R et al. Endocrinology: bone adaptation requires oestrogen receptor. Nature 2003;424:389-395

Maggi S, Kelsey JL, Litvak J, Heyse SP. Incidence of hip fractures in the elderly: a cross-national analysis. Osteoporos Int 1991;1:232–241
Meunier PJ, Roux C, Seeman E et al. The effects of strontium ranelate on the risk of vertebral fracture in women with postmenopausal osteoporosis. N Engl J Med 2004;350: 459–468
McClung MR, Geusens P,Miller PD et al. Effect of risedronate on the risk of hip fracture in elderly women. Hip Intervention Program Study Group. N Engl J Med 2001;344:333–40
Miller P, Schnitzer T, Emkey R et al. Weekly alendronate acid in male osteoporosis. Clin Drug Investig 2004;24:333–341
Morishima A, Grumbach MM, Simpson ER et al. Aromatase deficiency inmale and female siblings caused by a novel mutation and the physiological role of estrogens. J Clin Endocrinol Metab 1995;80:3689–98.
Moverare S, Venken K, Eriksson AL et al.Differential effects on bone of estrogen receptor _ and androgen receptor activation in orchidectomized adult male mice. Proc Natl Acad Sci USA 2003;100:13573–13578
O'Neill TW, Felsenberg D, Varlow J. et al. The prevalence of vertebral deformity in European men and women: the European vertebral osteoporosis study. J Bone Miner Res 1996;11:1010–1018
Orwoll ES, Oviatt SK, McClung MR et al. The rate of bone mineral loss in normal men and the effects of calcium and cholecalciferol supplementation. Ann Intern Med 1990;112:29–34
Orwoll E. Assessing bone density in men. J Bone Miner Res 2000;15:1867-70.
Orwoll E, Ettinger M, Weiss S et al. Alendronate for the treatment of osteoporosis in men. N Engl J Med 2000;343:604-610
Orwoll ES, Scheele WH, Paul S et al. The effect of teriparatide [human parathyroid hormone (1-34)] therapy on bone density in men with osteoporosis. J Bone Miner Res 2003;18:9-17
Orwoll EC. Treatment of osteoporosis in men. Calcif Tissue Int. 2004;75(2):114-119.
Orwoll ES, Miller PD, Adachi JD et al. Efficacy and safety of a once-yearly i.v. Infusion of zoledronic acid 5 mg versus a once-weekly 70-mg oral alendronate in the treatment of male osteoporosis: a randomized, multicenter, double-blind, active-controlled study. J Bone Miner Res. 2010;25:2239-2250
Recommendations for the prevention and treatment of glucocorticoid- induced osteoporosis. 2001 Update. American College of Rheumatology Ad Hoc Committee on Glucocorticoid-Induce Osteoporosis. Arthritis Rheum 2001;44:1496-1503
Ringe JD, Dorst A, Kipshoven C et al. Avoidance of vertebral fractures in men with idiopathic osteoporosis by a three year therapy with calcium and lowdose intermittent monofluorophosphate. Osteoporosis Int 1998;8:47–52
Ringe JD, Dorst A, Faber H et al. Alendonate treatment of established primary osteoporosis in men: 3-year results of a prospective, comparative, two-arm study. Rheumatology Int 2004;24:110–3.
Ringe JD, Faber H, Farahmand P et al. Efficacy of risedronate in men with primaryand secondary osteoporosis. Results of a 1- year study. Rheumatol Int 2006;26:427–31
Rochira V, Faustini-Fustini M, Balestrieri A et al. Estrogen replacement therapy in a man with congenital aromatase deficiency: effects of different doses of transdermal

estradiol on bone mineral density and hormonal parameters. J Clin Endocrinol Metab 2000;85:1841–1845

Rochira V, Balestrieri A, Madeo A et al Osteoporosis and male age-related hypogonadism: role of sex steroids on bone (patho)physiology. European Journal of Endocrinology 2006;154:175–185

Seeman E, Melton LJ 3d, O'Fallon WM, et al. Risk factors for spinal osteoporosis in men. Am J Med 1983;75:977-983

Seeman E Pathogenesis of bone fragility in women and men. Lancet 2002;359:1841–1850

Snyder PJ, Peachey TW, Hannoush P et al. Effects of testosterone treatment on body composition and muscle strength in men over 65 years old. J Clin Endocriniol Metab 1999;84:2647-2653

Snyder PJ, Peachey H, Berlin JA, et al. Effects of testosterone testosterone replacement in hypogonadal men. J Clin Endocrinol Metab 2000; 85(8):2670–2567

Trovas GP, Lyritis GP, Galanos A et all. A randomised trial of nasal spray salmon calcitonin in men with idiopathic osteoporosis: effects on bone mineral density and bone markers. J Bone Miner Res 2002;17:521–527

Wang C, Swerdloff RS, Iranmanes A et al. Effects of transdermal testosterone gel on bone turnover markers and bone mineral density in hypogonadal men. Clin Endocrinol 2001;54:739–750.

Wang C, Nieschlag E, Swerdloff R et al. ISA, ISSAM, EAU, EAA and ASA recommendations: investigation, treatment and monitoring of late-onset hypogonadism in males. The Aging Male 2009;1:5-12

Vanderschueren D, Vandenput l, Boonen S et al. Androgens and bone. Endocrine Rev 2004;25:389-425

Vanderschueren D, Venken K, Ophoff J. et al Sex steroids and the periosteum - reconsidering the roles of androgens and estrogens in periosteal expansion. J Clin Endocrinol Metab, 2005;91:378–382

Vanderschueren D, Vandenput L, Boonen S et al. Androgens and Bone Endocrine Reviews 2004;25:389–425

Zitzmann M, Faber S, Nieschlag E, Association of specific symptoms and metabolic risks with serum testosterone in older men. J Clin Endocrinol Metab 2006;91:4335-4343

Zitzmann M, Nieschlag E. Testosterone substitution: current modalities and perspectives. J Reproduktionsmed Endokrinol 2006;3:109-116.

9

Testosterone Deficiency Linked to Lower Urinary Tract Symptoms

Sae Chul Kim
Department of Urology College of Medicine Chung-Ang University Seoul, Korea

1. Introduction

Over the past decade, it has become clear many of the age-related health problems of men, that have hitherto been treated using different medical disciplines, are actually inter-related and require a more integrative approach in the aging male. Lower urinary tract symptoms (LUTS) may serve as an example. LUTS consists of storage, voiding, and post micturition symptoms affecting the lower urinary tract. Storage symptoms (daytime frequency, nocturia, urgency, incontinence) are experienced during the storage phase of the bladder. Voiding symptoms (weak stream, splitting or spraying, abdominal straining, hesitancy, intermittency, terminal dribble) are experienced during the voiding phase. Post-micturition symptoms (feeling of incomplete emptying, post micturition dribble) are experienced immediately after micturition. Individuals with LUTS often experience urinary incontinence (UI) or overactive bladder (OAB) symptoms. OAB is a subset of storage LUTS defined as urgency, with or without urgency UI, usually with frequency and nocturia. Men may report one or any combination of the symptoms and LUTS, including UI and OAB, have detrimental effects on health-related quality of life.

The prevalence of LUTS increases from 8% in the fourth decade of life to more than 70% in the seventh decade. In a large population-based cross-sectional survey the prevalence of storage LUTS (men, 51.3%; women, 59.2%) was greater than that for voiding (men, 25.7%; women, 19.5%) and post micturition (men, 16.9%; women, 14.2%) symptoms combined (Irwin et al., 2008).

Once symptoms arise, their progress is variable and unpredictable with about one third of patients improving, one third remaining stable and one third deteriorating. LUTS may point to serious pathology of the urogenital tract but are often nonspecific and large studies of patients have failed to show any correlation between LUTS and a specific diagnosis. An all-encompassing view of LUTS that focuses on the lower urinary tract as an integrated functional unit, but simultaneously reflects pathophysiology in the body as a whole, is more likely to improve a clinician's ability to manage the symptoms and therefore improve patient outcomes. Benign prostatic hyperplasia (BPH), which occurs more frequently with aging, is the most common cause of LUTS in middle-aged and elderly men, although many other diseases such as detrusor muscle weakness and/or instability, urinary tract infection, chronic prostatitis, urinary stone, prostate cancer, bladder cancer, neurological disease, e.g. multiple sclerosis, spinal cord injury, cauda equina syndrome, and cardiac and renal diseases may accompany LUTS.

The role of testosterone in voiding function remains obscure, although it plays a definite role in the etiopathogenesis of BPH. The indirect relation could obscure an interrelation between circulating levels of testosterone and symptoms of LUTS at a statistically significant level which nevertheless is biologically plausible. This chapter will discuss possible relationships between androgens and LUTS

2. Sex hormone involvement in the etiopathognesis of BPH

The two factors that are generally accepted to play a role in the etiopathogenesis of BPH are aging and androgen. While serum testosterone level steadily decreases after 40 years of age, the prevalence of histologic BPH in autopsy studies rises from approximately 20% in men aged 41-50 to 50% in men aged 51-60, and to over 90% in men older than 80 (Berry et al., 1984). An enlarged prostate (BPE) is detectable in approximately on half of the patients with histologic evidence of BPH. The gradual reduction of plasma testosterone in middle-aged and older men from mid-life onwards coincides paradoxically with the time when there is progressive growth of the prostate, a highly androgen-dependent organ. In the prostate, testosterone is converted into the more potent androgen, dihydrotestosterone (DHT) by 5α reductase. It is thought that DHT has a central role in BPH development and maintenance because the inhibition of 5α reductase activity is associated with decreased serum DHT concentration and decreased prostate size (Figure 1).

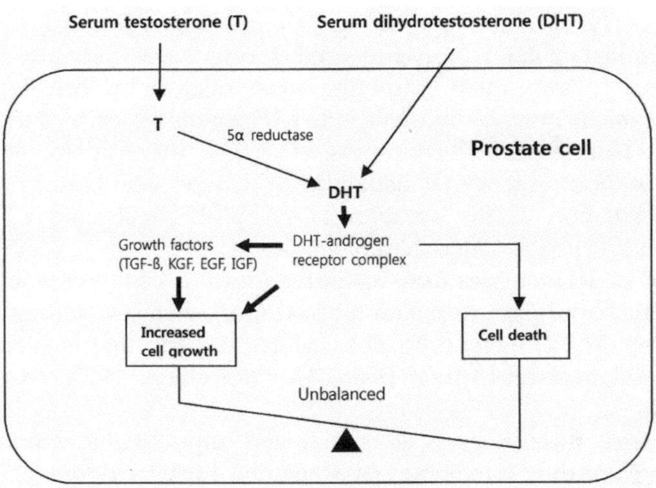

Fig. 1. Androgen regulation of cell growth in the prostate cell

Observations and clinical studies in men have clearly demonstrated that BPH is under endocrine control. Men castrated before puberty (eunuchs) develop neither BPH nor BPE, and individuals with an inherited deficiency of 5α reductase have only a vestigial prostate gland. Castration results in the regression of established BPH and improvement in urinary symptoms. Administration of a gonadotropin releasing hormone (GnRH) analog in men reversibly shrinks established BPH, resulting in objective improvement in urinary flow rate and subjective improvement in symptoms. Finally, clinical experience with finasteride, a 5α reductase type II inhibitor has documented the relevance of DHT on prostate size (Marberger, 1998). Despite these convicting data, the correlation between androgens and prostate volume in elderly men is less pronounced. Joseph et al. (2002) reported that a large prostate volume was marginally associated with increased total testosterone level in African-American men, but Meikle et al. (1997) found an inverse correlation between prostate volume and total testosterone level in 214 male twins based on white populations. Others have not found a significant association between total testosterone level and prostate volume. Partin et al. (1991) correlated 23 hormonal factors, including total testosterone/free testosterone to BPH volume assessed histologically. After correcting for age, the BPH volume correlated significantly with free testosterone, but not total testosterone. If not corrected for age, neither testosterone nor free testosterone correlated with BPH volume.

It has been demonstrated that 5 alpha-reductase activity (Bruchovsky et al., 1998), and androgen receptor levels (Barrack et al., 1983) increase with aging, which means that prostatic cells may gradually become more sensitive to DHT during aging, and that this stimulates cell replication in the prostate. Estradiol has been hypothesized to potentiate the effects of androgens in inducing BPH by inducing the androgen receptor, which thereby sensitizes the prostate to free testosterone. In dogs, estrogens have been shown to induce the androgen receptor, alter steroid metabolism resulting in higher levels of intraprostatic DHT, inhibit cell death when given in the presence of androgens, and stimulate stromal collagen production. Schatzl et al. (2000) found hypogonadism in approximately one fifth of elderly men with LUTS but it had no impact on LUTS status, PSA level, prostate volume, uroflowmetry, or endocrine parameters. In contrast to testosterone, they observed an age-related increase in estradiol (+0.86 pg/mL per decade), the only hormone to correlate with prostate volume, thus suggesting its significance for BPH and BPE. Gann et al. (1995) assessed the relation of steroid hormone levels with subsequent surgical treatment for BPH among participants in the Physicians Health Study and found a strong correlation for increasing risk and serum estrogen levels. The relevance of estrogens is underscored by the fact that, within the prostate, the highest concentrations have been detected in the stroma, the predominant tissue found in BPH. The rate-limiting step in estrogen biosynthesis is the conversion of androgens to estrogens, which is catalyzed by the enzyme aromatase. This enzyme is expressed in the human prostate and is regulated by follicle-stimulating hormone (FSH). The recent demonstration of a coexpression of gonadotropin hormones and their corresponding receptors in the human prostate suggests that FSH receptor activation acts in an endocrine fashion by way of age-dependent, elevated FSH (Schatzl et al., 2000). Alternatively, FSH might act in a para-autocrine fashion by way of locally produced FSH, potentially stimulating aromatase activity.

From the above mentioned facts, the age-related growth of the prostate cannot be explained by a mere increase or decrease in serum androgens. Schultheiss et al. (2004) reviewed previous studies and concluded that the link between androgens and age-related growth of the prostate might be explained by a shift of the hormonal ratio (e.g. the androgen/estrogen ratio), the changing intraprostatic hormonal level, or a modified action of hormones and their respective receptors, as well as of intraprostatic enzymes (e.g. 5α reductase). Additional large studies are needed to evaluate the above mechanisms.

3. Testosterone deficiency linked to LUTS

Historically, bladder outlet obstruction (BOO), LUTS, and BPH has been considered to be almost synonymous, however, an increasing number of studies now demonstrate that the correlations between these parameters are weak and symptoms may arise from many different etiologies. Although LUTS is commonly attributed to BOO caused by BPE, LUTS is not associated with BOO in a third to a half of men (Figure 2) and furthermore, the severity of LUTS secondary to BPH is not necessarily correlated with prostate volume (Chang et al., 2009). Some men with greatly enlarged glands may have little obstruction and few symptoms while others with prostate glands less enlarged have more outlet obstruction and severe symptoms. Asian men have a smaller prostate than Caucasians, but may have similar or higher symptom scores and a more impaired quality of life (Homma et al., 1997).

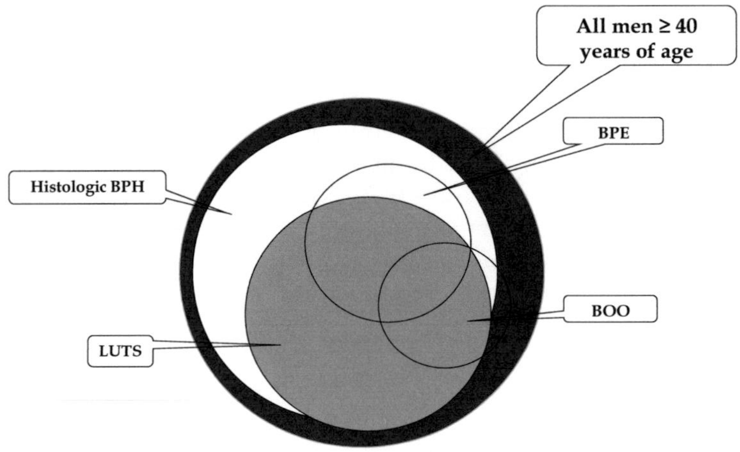

Fig. 2. Correlation between lower urinary tract symptoms (LUTS) and histologic benign prostatic hyperplasia (BPH), benign prostatic enlargement (BPE) and bladder outlet obstruction (BOO)

Many studies have tried to establish a relationship between sex steroids and BPH, but a few studies have analyzed the relationship between circulating testosterone and LUTS. At the epidemiological level, an association between central obesity in adulthood, the metabolic syndrome, erectile dysfunction (ED) and LUTS has been established (Rohrmann et al., 2007). A common denominator of the ailments is lower-than-normal testosterone levels occurring in a significant proportion of elderly men. However, there is no consensus on possible effects of testosterone on LUTS. Schatzl et al. (2003) found that hypogonadism was seen approximately one-fifth of elderly men with LUTS, but it had no impact on symptom status. Litman et al. (2007) found an inverse correlation between symptoms of LUTS and plasma total and bioavailable testosterone but this relationship disappeared after statistical adjustment for age. Roberts et al. (2004) reported a negative association between total testosterone and American Urological Association Symptom Index (AUA-SI) but not with bioavailable testosterone. Miwa et al. (2008) noted an inverse association of free testosterone, but not total testosterone, to International Prostate Symptom Score (IPSS). Recently, author (2009) found free and bioavailable testosterone had significant negative relationships with IPSS total scores and subscores for voiding symptoms even after adjusting for age, prostate total volume and transitional zone volume, high sensitivity C-reactive protein (CRP) and homeostasis model assessment of insulin resistance (HOMA-IR). In addition, free and bioavailable testosterone were significantly related to the presence of severe LUTS (IPSS

≥20) even after adjusting for confounding factors (Figure 3). However, the odds ratio of bioavailable testosterone was lower than that of free testosterone on multivariable analysis (Figure 4).

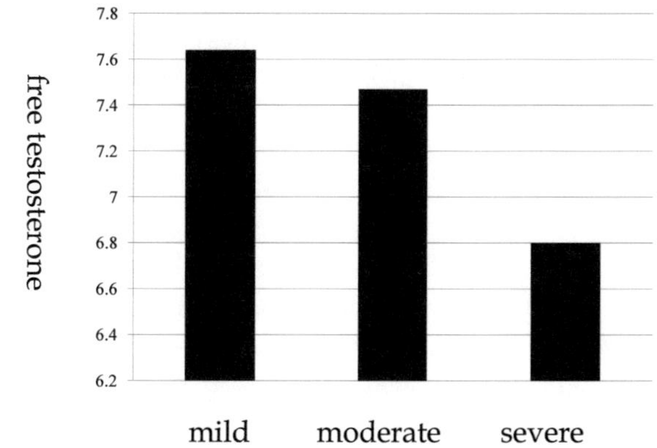

Fig. 3. Blood levels of free testosterone (pg/ml) depending on degree of LUTS severity (Adopted from Chang, et al., 2009)

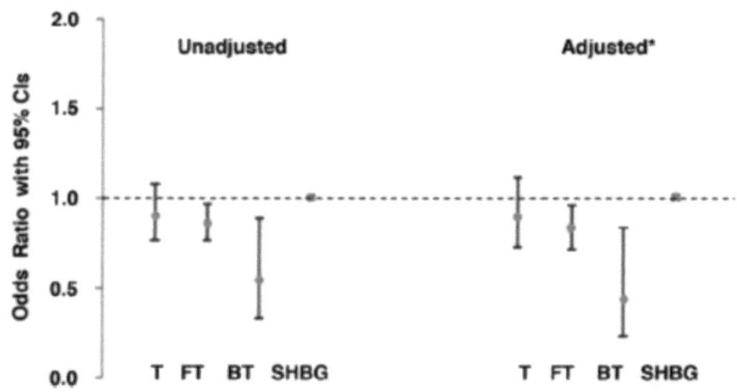

Fig. 4. Odds ratios (95% Cl) of total (T), free (FT) and bioavailable (BT) testosterone, and sex hormone binding globulin (SHBG) on log scales for prediction of severe LUTS (Adopted from Chang, et al., 2009)

A few studies have investigated serum DHT and LUTS. Of the studies examining this association, DHT has not been related with LUTS or BPH in prospective (Meigs et al., 2001; Gann et al., 1995) or cross sectional studies (Platz et al., 1999; Litman et al., 2007). Trifiro et al. (2010) found there was a weak (and unadjusted) association only, suggesting an increase in mean serum DHT concentration among men with LUTS compared with those without. However, serum DHT may not be an ideal measurement of intraprostatic androgen concentrations, as serum DHT does not necessarily correlate to prostate tissue concentrations of DHT. Because of this observation, the serum DHT metabolites 17 beta-diol-glucuronide and androrstanediol glucuronide (AAG) are often used to estimate DHT activity. A cross sectional and a prospective study showed higher levels of the DHT metabolites and testosterone to DHT metabolite ratios to be directly associated with LUTS or BPH (Kristal et al., 2008; Platz et al., 1999). Kristal et al (2008) showed stronger associations as a ratio suggesting that the testosterone : DHT metabolite or testosterone : DHT ratio may therefore be a more sensitive marker of LUTS/BPH than either hormone individually. Platz et al. (1999) estimated the risk of BPH and severe LUTS in relation to testosterone, DHT, estradiol and AAG in 300 men with severe LUTS. There was a positive relation with AAG and an inverse one with estradiol for the risk of BPH surgery/LUTS, the correlations persisting even after adjusting for steroid hormones and sex hormone binding globulin (SHBG).

A study showed at the 105th Annual Scientific Meeting of the AUA that as testosterone levels decreased, LUTS severity increased and maximum flow rate decreased, while prostate volume remained the same as hormone levels decreased (Sauver, et al., 2010). In another study to determine the relationship between androgens, LUTS and urodynamic variables of BOO in patients with LUTS/BPH, free testosterone was negatively correlated with detrusor pressure at the end of urinary flow (closure detrusor pressure) and pressure at the maximum urinary flow rate (Qmax) (Koritsiadis et al., 2008). Mean closure detrusor pressure and detrusor pressure at Qmax differed significantly between patients with low and normal free testosterone levels. Detrusor overactivity (DO) was noted in patients who had significantly lower free testosterone levels than those with no DO. Although several cross-sectional and prospective studies showed no consensus of association of testosterone with LUTS or BPH, it is notable that no studies have as yet reported an increased risk of LUTS with higher testosterone.

In the rabbit bladder outlet obstruction study, bladder dysfunction is mainly mediated by three cellular processes; 1) progressive denervation, 2) cellular mitochondria malfunction, 3) dysregulation of intracellular calcium storage and release from the sarcoplasmic reticulum (SR). Biomarkers for these three functions are calcium adenosine triphosphatase (ATPase) for calcium release, citrate synthase for mitochondrial function, and choline acetyl-transferse for cholinergic innervations (Juan et al., 2007). Bladder contraction can be divided into phasic and tonic period. The phasic response depends on the adenosine triphosphate (ATP) concentration in the bladder wall, whereas the tonic phase requires mitochondrial oxidative activity to generate energy. Castration of adult male rabbits resulted in a significant decrease in the activities of the mitochondria specific enzyme, citrate synthase of the bladder body and base, muscle and mucosa, urethra and corpora, while choline acetyl-transferse activity and calcium ATPase activity showed different responses depending on the sites (Juan et al., 2007).

Preliminary evidence indicates that men with LUTS benefit from testosterone treatment, and pilot studies have also shown that testosterone therapy has a positive effect on LUTS in late-onset hypogonadism. A study found that the higher plasma levels of testosterone generated with oral testosterone undecanoate than with testosterone gel (50mg/day) were more effective in reducing the score on the IPSS, probably indicating that there is a relationship between plasma levels of testosterone and their effects on LUTS (Yassin et al., 2008). Although this inverse association is contrary to the commonly held clinical opinion that higher serum androgen levels may worsen clinical LUTS and BPH, the risk would not applicable to normalization of the serum testosterone levels in late onset hypogonadism. Clinical trials are needed to confirm that testosterone replacement therapy in older men does not increase the risks of LUTS or clinical BPH. It would also be significant to explore whether normalization of plasma testosterone has an adjunctive therapeutic effect to the more established pharmacological treatment modalities of LUTS as in an adjunctive therapeutic effect of testosterone supplement to phosphodiesterase type 5 (PDE5) inhibitors for ED treatment accompanied by the testosterone deficiency (Buvat et al., 2011; Blute et al., 2009).

There is ample evidence from many epidemiological studies that LUTS and ED are strongly linked, independently of age. ED assessed by a questionnaire, International Index of Erectile Function (IIEF) score was strongly related to LUTS severity. When controlling for age, LUTS severity was by far the strongest predictor of erectile function, with an odd ratio for severe vs mild LUTS of 8.99 followed by diabetes, 3.01; cardiac disease, 2.17; hypertension, 1.83 and hyperlipidemia, 1.57 (McVary., 2006). The fact that LUTS severity is the strongest predictor of ED suggests that LUTS and ED may share their underlying causes and the underlying causes may explain the reasons why severity of LUTS does not correlates with prostate size. Although a direct causal relationship is not established yet, four pathophysiological mechanisms can explain the relationship. These include 1) insulin resistance and autonomic hyperactivity, 2) alteration in nitric oxide bioavailability, 3) Rho-kinase activation/endothelin pathway, 4) pelvic atherosclerosis, all of which are known to be androgen-dependent.

4. Insulin resistance and autonomic hyperactivity

It was proposed that LUTS is a part of the metabolic syndrome which includes hyperglycemia, obesity, dyslipidemia and hypertension. Recently, testosterone deficiency has captured attention to be a possible risk factor of metabolic syndrome. The basis of this concept came from increased insulin resistance found in both hypergonadotropic and hypogonadotropic hypogonadism. Patients of un-treated Klinefelter's syndrome, compared with control subjects, showed a significantly higher prevalence of metabolic risk factors (Bojesen et al., 2006). GnRH agonist-treated men with prostate cancer also showed significantly decreased insulin sensitivity (Smith et al., 2006). Long-term survivors of testicular cancer have an increased risk for cardiovascular events 10 or more years after chemotherapy (Huddart et al., 2003). Nuver et al. (2005) found lower testosterone associated with a higher body mass index (BMI) pretreatment and a larger BMI increase during follow-up in testicular cancer survivors following cisplatin-based chemotherapy than controls, suggesting testosterone may play a role in the development of the metabolic syndrome.

Plasma testosterone levels decline with aging in healthy men and features of the metabolic syndrome also show age-related deteriorations, suggesting that testosterone is an important regulator of insulin sensitivity in men. There are lots of evidences that late onset hypogonadism is associated with metabolic syndrome. Blouin et al. (2006) investigated whether this decline or the aging process per se accounts for the risk of metabolic syndrome. They observed that patients with a high testosterone level were more likely to have fewer than three components of metabolic syndrome than those with a low testosterone level. Author (2009) also found that HOMA-IR correlated negatively with serum total, free and bioavailable testosterone. Studies showed that blood levels of insulin and metabolic risk factors increased with lower testosterone levels in middle aged men (Laaksonen, et al., 2003). And patients with metabolic syndrome had significantly lower serum testosterone level than those without metabolic syndrome. Men who developed both metabolic syndrome and diabetes mellitus at 11-year follow-up were especially likely to have low testosterone levels already at baseline (Laaksonen, et al., 2004). Pitteloud et al (2005a) demonstrated men with hypogonadal testosterone levels were twice as insulin resistant as their eugonadal counterparts and 90% fulfill criteria for the metabolic syndrome.

Recent studies provide insight into the role of mitochondrial function in the pathogenesis of insulin resistance. Mitochondria have a critical role in Ca^{2+} buffering in bladder smooth muscle. Pitteloud et al. (2005a) demonstrated testosterone levels were positively correlated not only with insulin sensitivity but also with genetic (oxidative phosphorylation gene expression) and functional (maximal aerobic capacity) markers of mitochondrial function, suggesting a novel molecular mechanism whereby testosterone might modulate insulin sensitivity in men. Pitteloud et al. (2005b) found in another study that insulin resistance was associated with a decrease in Leydig cell testosterone secretion by evaluating the hypothalamic-pituitary-gonadal axis in men with a spectrum of insulin sensitivity.

The most common cause of ED is penile vascular insufficiency. This is usually part of a generalized endothelial dysfunction and is related to several conditions, including type 2 diabetes mellitus, hypertension, hyperlipidemia, and obesity, of which conditions underlie the pathophysiology of metabolic syndrome. There is evidence from multiple epidemiological studies that LUTS and ED are correlated, independent of age or comorbidities as diabetes or hypertension. The prevalence of LUTS was 72% in men with ED versus 38% in those without ED. And the presence of LUTS was a risk factor of ED. Therefore, men seeking care for one condition should always be screened for complaints of the other condition.

Metabolic risk factors induce testosterone deficiency. Obesity-related conditions such as obstructive sleep apnea, insulin resistance and type 2 diabetes mellitus are independently associated with decreased plasma testosterone. Possible mechanisms include decreased LH pulse amplitude, inhibitory effects of estrogen at the hypothalamus and pituitary and the effects of leptin and other peptides centrally and on Leydig cells. Diabetes induces testicular oxidative stress and damage,

Summing up, metabolic syndrome is a risk factor of LUTS and ED and may reduce the blood level of testosterone. Contrariwise, testosterone deficiency may be a causative factor of metabolic risk factors and may accompany LUTS and ED. LUTS is a risk factor of ED and vice versa. This interrelationship suggests that these ailments may be a symptom complex and may share the underlying causes (Figure 5).

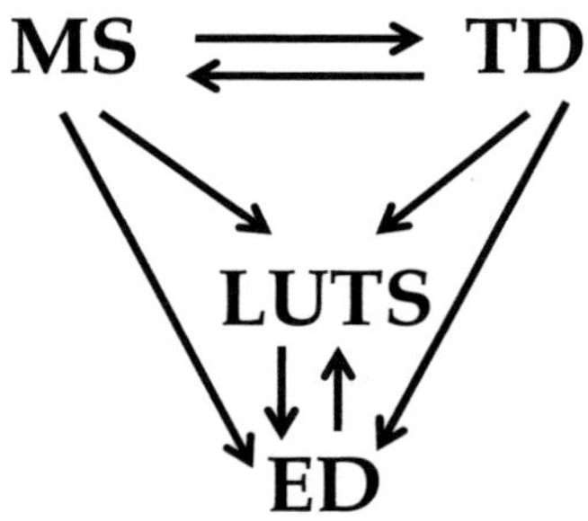

Fig. 5. Interrelationship between metabolic syndrme (MS) testosterone deficiency (TD) lower urinary tract symptom (LUTS) and erectile dysfunction (ED)

However, previous studies on the relationship between androgens and insulin sensitivity in men gave conflicting results depending on whether total or free testosterone levels were used. One explanation for this discrepancy is the SHBG is mediating the link between testosterone and insulin sensitivity. Proponents of the use of free testosterone argue that it is the best index of androgenicity in insulin-resistant men given the low SHBG levels that pertain in this setting (Plymate et al., 1988). Another explanation is that the assays used to measure free testosterone have serious methodological limitations (Matsumoto & Bremner, 2004).

In a recent study of the epidemiological relationship between metabolic syndrome and LUTS, it was hypothesized that metabolic syndrome is associated with overactivity of the autonomic nervous system, and that insulin resistance, a key element of metabolic syndrome, might be responsible. Hyperinsulinemia promotes endothelin-1 (ET-1) secretion through mitogen-activated protein (MAP)-kinase pathway leading to increase in smooth muscle contraction. In addition, it activates sympathetic nerve system contributing to further increase in the contraction. Overactivity of the autonomic nervous system is supposedly not responsible for the development of LUTS, but rather is believed to play a key role in increasing LUTS severity above an intrinsic basal intensity (McVary et al., 2005; Kasturi et al., 2006).

The studies of Meusburger & Keast (2001) and Keast et al. (2002) have provided elegant demonstrations on the potential role of androgens in maintaining the structure and function of many pelvic ganglion neurons. Giuliano et al. (1993) suggested that testosterone acting peripherally to the spinal cord enhances the erectile response of the cavernous nerve. Traish et al. (2007) showed that testosterone treatment of castrated animals restored the cavernosal nerve fibers and myelin sheath structure, similar to that observed in the sham group. Considering these reports and the hypothesis that noradrenaline and α1-AR that mediate adrenergic contraction of smooth muscles in the prostate, bladder neck, urethra and corpus cavernosum, contribute to the common link, testosterone deficiency could be a causative factor of LUTS via autonomic hyperactivity.

Another possible mechanism includes a direct relaxation effect of testosterone on smooth muscle cells, a change in the number of receptors for sympathetic affecter molecules or a change in sensitivity of smooth muscle cell α-adrenergic receptors (ARs). Comparative binding and functional studies of lower genitourinary tissues have demonstrated that α1-ARs are abundant in the bladder base and prostate but spare in the bladder body (Lepor & Shapiro, 1984). In certain human arteries, α1-AR expression increases and the relative proportion of α1-AR subtypes is modulated by aging (Rudner et al., 1999). These changes might be happening as well in the human prostatic, bladder and erectile tissue. The contractile response of the cavernosal strips of older men with ED was greater than for those isolated from younger men with ED, suggesting that aging has a role in adrenergic sensitivity in patients with ED (Christ et al., 1991). It has also been suggested that α1-ARs are up-regulated in patients with LUTS associated with BPH, resulting in increased smooth muscle tone in the prostatic capsule and bladder neck (Medina et al., 1999).

Theoretically, selective α1-AR antagonists are ideally suited for the treatment of the dynamic component of bladder outlet obstruction, because the resistance along the bladder outlet can be selectively reduced without impairing detrusor contraction. Virtually, α1-AR antagonists have been widely used in practice for treating symptomatic BPH/LUTS. Despite the clinical availability of α1-AR antagonists for treating LUTS, as yet it is not possible to provide a comprehensive picture of the impact of testosterone on α1- ARs. While androgen effect on central and peripheral nervous system are well known, the local effect of androgen on bladder and urethra has not been extensively studied. Even reports on the density of α1-ARs after castration are not consistent. Takyu (1993) found the density of α1-ARs in rabbit proximal urethra decreased after castration and testosterone supplementation restored the densities of α1-ARs to control levels. Morita et al. (1992) reported that α1-adrenergic and muscarinic cholinergic receptor densities decreased significantly after castration. Yono et al (2006) found the density of α1-ARs in the rat prostate decreased with aging. Because the percent of muscle density shows no significant change throughout life in the rat prostate (Moriyama et al., 1995), the age related decrease in the density of α1-ARs appears to result from direct down-regulation of α1-AR protein. Auger-Pourmarin et al. (1998) presented that testosterone administration produced a 23% decrease of α1-AR density, likely by an increase of prostatic glandular epithelium and a decrease in the relative proportion of smooth muscle, thus of α1-AR density. Lacey et al. (1996) found there was an apparent increase in α1-AR density in dog prostate after castration which returned to baseline with testosterone replacement. However, the increase in α1-ARs density resulted from relative increases in the ratio of smooth muscle to epithelium rather from direct up-regulation of α1-AR protein.

Lastly, recent studies provided an evidence that the inflammatory infiltrates, which are frequently found in and around nodules of BPH (Rohrmann et al, 2005), elevate serum CRP concentration, a non-specific marker of inflammation. Furthermore, the presence of metabolic syndrome might mediate intraprostatic inflammation because of its association with an elevated serum CRP concentration, which would link metabolic syndrome to symptomatic BPH (Rohrmann et al., 2005).

5. Alteration in nitric oxide bioavailability

It is widely accepted that NO, which is synthesized from its precursor L-arginine via NO synthase (NOS), is important in the relaxation of corpus cavernosum smooth muscle and vasculature. By activating gualnylate cyclase, with resultant elevation of cyclic guanylate monophosphate (cGMP), NO results in a lowering of intracellular calcium and smooth muscle relaxation. cGMP is an important secondary messenger of NO involved in modulating the contractility of various smooth muscles. It stimulates protein kinase G, which in turn initiates phosphorylation of membrane-bound proteins at the potassium channels. This leads to potassium ion outflow into the extracellular space resulting in hyperpolarization. Hyperpolarization leads to closure of the L-type calcium channels subsequently resulting in a decrease in the intracellular Ca^{++} ion concentration and consequent smooth muscle cell relaxation. PDE plays important roles in this process by modulating the levels of cGMP and their duration of action (Traish et al., 2007) (Figure 6).

NO is also present in the human prostate and bladder and putatively modulates smooth muscle tone. NOS activity has been reported to be highest in the prostatic urethra, intermediate in the bladder neck, and less pronounced in detrusor muscle. It has been reported that NOS expression, and thus NO production, of the prostate is reduced in the transition zone of the prostate in BPH compared with normal prostate (Bloch et al., 1997). The proposed reduction in expression of NOS isoforms results in increased smooth muscle cell contractile forces at the bladder neck and prostatic urethra leading to the subsequent development of LUTS or LUTS without BPH. On the other hand, reduced NOS/NO results in smooth muscle cell proliferation and may result in structural changes in the prostate and simultaneously increased contraction and affects outlet resistance and bladder compliance (Figure 7). Histochemical staining and immunohistochemistry confirmed dense nitrinergic innervations of glandular epithelium, fibromuscular stroma and blood vessels in the normal human prostate. The nitrinergic innervations is also less in hyperplastic human prostate than in normal prostate, and this may also contribute to affect voiding function (Podlasek et al., 2003).

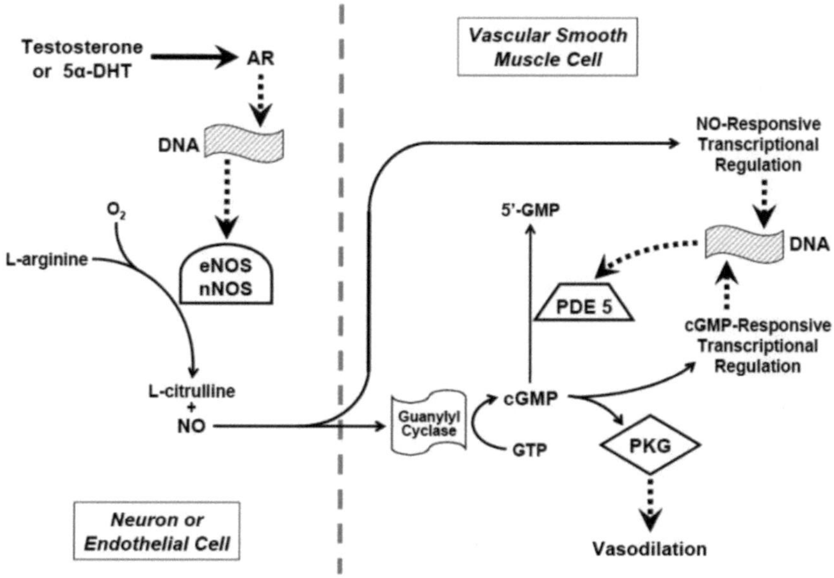

Fig. 6. Potential regulation of nitric oxide synthase (NOS) and hosphodiesterase type 5 (PDE5) by androgens (Adopted fromTraish, et al., 2007)

It is known that the lower urinary and genital tracts are embryologically and anatomically closely related, and that both are sensitive to sex steroids. A preponderance of evidence reports a role for androgens in regulating the expression and activity of NOS isoforms in the corpus cavernosum in animal models. In castrated animals, testosterone and DHT administration restored the erectile response and NOS expression in penis. It can be speculated that if testosterone participates in erectile mechanisms by modulating NOS and phosphodiesterase type 5 (PDE5), a similar interaction might be found in the lower urinary tract, given that the same enzymes and androgen receptors are also present.

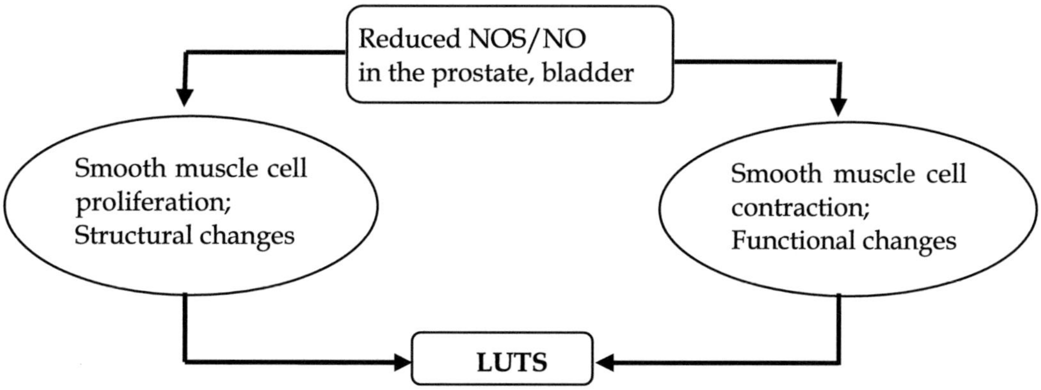

Fig. 7. NOS/NO theory for LUTS/ED (Adopted from McVary, et al., 2006)

Jones & Schoenberg (1985) suggested that aging itself might be an underlying cause of DO, besides BOO. In experimental studies, the inhibition of NO production causes bladder hyperactivity in rats in vivo (Persson et al., 1992), indicating a possible relation with changes in NOS activity in the lower urinary tract. Koritsiadis et al. (2008) found men with no DO had higher free testosterone levels, and all hypogonadal patients had DO, providing evidence that a decline in androgen levels might be a causative factor in DO, by triggering overactivity in an otherwise pathological bladder.

PDE5 hydrolyzes cGMP in vascular and cavernous smooth muscle into GMP. Activation of PDE5 terminates NO-induced, cGMP-mediated smooth muscle relaxation. In penile tissue, the balance between the intracellular levels of cGMP and GMP is primarily regulated by the activities of NOS and PDE5. Thus, it is likely that any disruption in the expression or activity of these enzymes will lead to pathophysiology. Castration has been shown to induce the expression and activity of PDE5 in rabbits and rats, and androgen supplementation has been shown to up-regulate the expression and activity of PDE5 (Zhang et al., 2005; Morelli et al., 2004). Further, administration of PDE inhibitor to castrated animals has little effect on the intracavernosal pressure in response to pelvic nerve stimulation (Zhang et al., 2005), suggesting that androgens are critical not only for regulating NOS activity, but also in modulating PDE5 activity. The presence of PDE in the urinary bladder was identified in studies of the rat (Qiu, et al., 2001) and the human (Werkstrom, et al., 2006).

A recent study, investigating PDE5 expression and activity in the human bladder, elegantly demonstrated that PDE5 regulates smooth muscles tone of the bladder. Vardenafil appeared to block PDE5 activity, and therefore, may be a possible therapeutic option for bladder dysfunction by ameliorating irritative LUTS. The study also found that castration decreased, and testosterone supplementation restored, PDE5 gene expression in rat bladder (Morelli, et al., 2009). Meanwhile, a large number of clinical studies have convincingly shown that PDE inhibitors have a beneficial effect on LUTS. Sairam et al (2002) found the overall trend in the IPSS was towards improvement after treatment with sildenafil. In a recent 12-week global dose-finding study conducted in 1058 men with BPH-LUTS, tadalafil was associated with statistically significant and clinically meaningful improvements in multiple measures of LUTS, including quality of life and ED improvement, compared to placebo (Roehrborn et al., 2008). Kim et al (2011) reported men with BPH-LUTS treated with tadalafil 5 mg once daily experienced a reduction in BPH-LUTS which was comparable to tamsulosin.

6. Rho-kinase activation/endothelin activity

Smooth muscle contraction has been attributed to an increase in the intracellular calcium concentration. However, some regulatory mechanisms can modify the sensitivity of contractile and regulatory proteins to calcium, leading to a smooth muscle contraction without changing intracellular calcium concentration (Somlyo A.P. & Somlyo A.V., 2000). One of these mechanisms is the Rho-kinase pathway, which is thought to be a major calcium-sensitizing mechanism in smooth muscle. The Rho-kinase is activated by a G-protein, RhoA, thought to be coupled to excitatory α1-adrenoceptors. The major contractile process in bladder is under acetylcholine control, through the activation of M3 muscarinic receptors. RhoA/Rho-kinase calcium sensitization pathway plays a major role in maintaining the contractile actions in bladder smooth muscle tone. Rees et al. (2003) found that a specific inhibitor of Rho-kinase, Y-27632, decreased the proliferation of human and rat prostatic smooth muscle cells, and inhibited noradrenergic contractions elicited by electrical field stimulation and exogenous phenylephrine in rat prostatic tissue.

In many pathological cases, hyperactivity of Rho/Rho-kinase signaling has been observed. Increased Rho-kinase activity, and consequently increased calcium sensitivity of the contractile machinery, can be found in the detrusor of rabbits with partial BOO (Bing et al., 2003) and in the corpus cavernosum smooth muscle of rabbits with partial BOO (Chang et al., 2005). Increased smooth muscle myosin basal phosphorylation necessary for smooth muscle contraction in the corpus cavernosum smooth muscle of partial BOO, mediated via an increase in Rho-kinase expression/activity, would be expected to make the corpus cavernosum smooth muscle more difficult to relax, which suggests that the RhoA/Rho-kinase pathway as being involved in the mechanism for LUTS-associated ED.

In various animal species estrogen receptors are shown to be expressed in central nervous structures involved in micturition (VanderHorst et al., 2001), as well as in the bladder and urethra (Williams & Papka, 1996; Makela et al., 2000). Chavalmane et al. (2010) found that estrogen supplementation significantly increased the relaxing response of carbacol-precontracted rat bladder strips to Y-27632, an inhibitor of Rho-kinase. On the contrary, testosterone administration in the same animal model did not increase responsiveness to Y-27632, but even reduced it. This was in apparent contrast with the observation in isolated human bladder cells, where testosterone mimicked estrogen effects. However, in human bladder cells co-incubation with letrozole, an inhibitor of aromatase, reverted all the testosterone-induced effects. In addition, DHT, a non-aromatizable androgen, did not substantially stimulate smooth muscle gene expression and cell motility. These findings suggest that active aromatization is operating in human bladder cells and that estrogen and not androgen receptors are involved in stimulating cell migration and expression of genes related to the smooth muscle phenotype. In contrast to human bladder, rat bladder does not express aromatase/CYP19A1 mRNA and testosterone presumably acts only through the androgen receptors. These data indicate that estrogen, more than androgen, receptors up-regulate Rho/Rho-kinase signaling and might have a role in calcium sensitization in human male bladder and androgens have the opposite effect. Clinical studies showing that androgen deficiency is associated with male bladder instability are in keeping with this view. Since an altered estrogen/androgen ratio characterizes several physiological and pathological conditions, often associated to bladder hyperactivity and LUTS, it is possible that a relative hyperesterogenism might induce bladder overactivity, through an activation of the Rho/Rho-kinase pathway.

The actions of several factors beside noradrenaline (e.g. endothelin-1, angiotensin II), possibly involved in the increased smooth muscle activity found in both LUTS/BPH and ED, are dependent on Rho-kinase activity that acts downstream from these receptors (Anderson, 2003). Although the exact mechanisms by which angiotensin II elicits its cellular effects are not known, the mechanism of action of angiotensin II in the cells is related to the Rho/Rho-kinase pathway. While estradiol did not change the number of human aortic endothelial cells secreting endothelin-1 but decreased the number of secreting cells stimulated with angiotensin-II, testosterone induced an increase in the number of cells secreting endothelin-1 and up-regulated endothelin-1 mRNA, indicating that testosterone, estradiol and angiotensin-II have parallel effects on the production of endothelin-1 (Pearson et al., 2008).

7. Pelvic atherosclerosis

Various studies show that bladder dysfunction can be caused by ischemia and suggest that atherosclerosis and hypercholesterolemia might be associated with LUTS. Ischemia in rabbit urinary bladder caused a marked reduction in the compliance and capacity of the bladder (Gill et al., 1988). Azadzoi et al. (1999) found that atherosclerosis-induced chronic bladder ischemia increased transforming growth factor-β1 expression in the bladder leading to fibrosis, smooth muscle atrophy and non-compliance. Hypercholesterolemia also interfered with bladder structure and compliance but to a significantly lesser extent compared with chronic bladder ischemia. It is known atherosclerosis and hypercholesterolemia are associated with low serum androgen levels. Bladder outlet obstruction results in bladder hypertrophy which induces ischemia. Levin et al. (1997) hypothesized that this leads to a release of intracellular calcium, leading to activation of specific enzymes and generation of free radicals. These then attack the membranes of nerves, sarcoplasmic reticulum and mitochondria.

In two cross-sectional studies of elderly men, intima-media thickness (IMT), an indicator of general atherosclerosis, was associated with lower testosterone levels (Hak et al., 2002; van den Beld et al., 2003). In a prospective population-based study, free but not total, testosterone levels were inversely related to IMT (Muller et al., 2004). In a logistic regression model adjusted for the confounding effect of cardiovascular risk factors, men with testosterone levels in the lowest quintile (<9.0 nmol L-1) had an independent OR =1.51 (P=0.015) of being in the highest IMT quintile (Svartberg et al., 2006). Besides the possible modulating effect of testosterone on cardiovascular disease risk factors, a few other possible explanations for the association between testosterone and atherosclerosis have been suggested. A direct beneficial effect of testosterone on plaque development, probably mediated by the vascular androgen receptor has been reported in an animal study (Hanke et al., 2001). Testosterone has also been shown to enhance endothelium-independent and endothelium-dependent vasodilation (Kang et al., 2002)

8. Conclusion

Many studies have tried to establish a relationship between sex steroids and BPH, but a few studies have analyzed the relationship between circulating testosterone and LUTS. Although there is no consensus on possible effects of testosterone on LUTS, endogenous testosterone may have a beneficial effect on the lower urinary tract function, and testosterone deficiency may provide a pathophysiologic basis for the link between LUTS. Preliminary evidence indicates that men with LUTS benefit from testosterone treatment. Four pathophysiological mechanisms can explain the relationship; insulin resistance and autonomic hyperactivity, alteration in NO/NOS/PDE activity, Rho-kinase activation/endothelin pathway, pelvic atherosclerosis, all of which are known to be androgen-dependent.

9. References

Andersson, KE. (2003). Erectile physiological and pathophysiological pathways involved in erectile dysfunction. *Journal of Urology*, 170:S6-S14.

Auger-Pourmarin, L.; Roubert, P. & Chabrier, PE. (1998). Alpha1-adrenoceptors in testosterone-induced prostatic hypertrophy. *European Journal of Pharmacology*, Vol.341, No.1, pp. 119-126.

Azadzoi, KM.; Tarcan T.; Siroky, MB. & Krane, RJ. (1999). Atherosclerosis-induced chronic ischemia causes bladder fibrosis and non-compliance in the rabbit. *Journal of Urology*, Vol.161, No.5, pp. 1626-1635.

Barrack, ER.; Bujnovszky, P. & Walsh, PC. (1983). Subcellular distribution of androgen receptors in human normal, benign hyperplastic, and malignant prostatic tissues: characterization of nuclear salt-resistant receptors. *Cancer Research*, Vol. 43, No. 3, pp. 1107-1116.

Berry, SJ.; Coffey, DS.; Walsh, PC. & Ewing, LL. (1984). The development of human benign prostatic hyperplasia with age. *Journal of Urology*, Vol. 132, No. 3, pp. 474-479.

Bing, W.; Chang, S.; Hypolite, JA.; DiSanto, ME.; Zderic, SA.; Rolf, L.; Wein, AJ. & Chacko, S. (2003). Obstruction-induced changes in urinary bladder smooth muscle contractility: a role for Rho kinase. *American Journal of Physiology- Renal Physiology*, Vol. 285, No. 5, pp. F990-997.

Bloch, W.; Klotz, T.; Loch, C.; Schmidt, G.; Engelmann, U. & Addicks, K. (1997). Distribution of nitric oxide synthase implies a regulation of circulation, smooth muscle tone, and secretory function in the human prostate by nitric oxide. *Prostate*, Vol. 15, No. 1, pp. 1-8.

Blouin, K.; Richard, C.; Brochu, G.; Hould, FS.; Lebel, S.; Marceau, S.; Biron, S,; Luu-The, V. & Tchernof, A. (2006). Androgen inactivation and steroid-converting enzyme expression in abdominal adipose tissue in men. *Journal of Endocrinology*, Vol. 191, No. 3, pp. 637-649.

Blute, M.; Hakimian, P.; Kashanian, J.; Shteynshluyger, A.; Lee, M. & Shabsigh, R. (2009). Erectile dysfunction and testosterone deficiency. *Frontiers of Hormone Research*, Vol. 37, pp.108-122.

Bojesen, A.; Kristensen, K.; Birkebaek, NH.; Fedder, J.; Mosekilde, L.; Bennett, P.; Laurberg, P.; Frystyk, J.; Flyvbjerg, A.; Christiansen, JS. & Gravholt, CH. (2006). The metabolic syndrome is frequent in Klinefelter's syndrome and is associated with abdominal obesity and hypogonadism. *Diabetes Care*, Vol. 29, No. 7, pp. 1591-1598.

Bruchovsky, N.; Rennie, PS.; Batzold, FH.; Goldenberg, SL.; Fletcher, T. & McLoughlin, MG. (1988). Kinetic parameters of 5 alpha-reductase activity in stroma and epithelium of normal, hyperplastic, and carcinomatous human prostates. *Journal of Clinical Endocrinology and Metabolism*, Vol. 67, No. 4, pp. 806-816.

Buvat, J.; Montorsi, F.; Maggi, M.; Porst, H.; Kaipia, A.; Colson, MH.; Cuzin, B.; Moncada, I.; Martin-Morales, A.; Yassin, A.; Meuleman, E.; Eardley, I.; Dean, JD. & Shabsigh, R. (2011). Hypogonadal men nonresponders to the PDE5 inhibitor tadalafil benefit from normalization of testosterone levels with a 1% hydroalcoholic testosterone gel in the treatment of erectile dysfunction (TADTEST study). *Journal of Sexual Medicine*, Vol. 8, No. 1, pp. 284-293.

Chang, IH.; Oh, SY. & Kim, SC. (2009). A possible relationship between testosterone and lower urinary tract symptoms in men. *Journal of Urology,* Vol. 182, No. 1, pp. 215-220.

Chang, S.; Hypolite, JA.; Zderic, SA.; Wein, AJ.; Chacko, S. & Disanto, ME. (2005). Increased corpus cavernosum smooth muscle tone associated with partial bladder outlet obstruction is mediated via Rho-kinase. *American Journal of Physiololgy- Regulatory, Integrative and Comparative Physiology,* Vol. 289, No. 4, pp. R1124-1130.

Chavalmane, AK.; Comeglio, P.; Morelli, A.; Filippi, S.; Fibbi, B.; Vignozzi, L.; Sarchielli, E.; Marchetta, M.; Failli, P.; Sandner, P.; Saad, F.; Gacci, M.; Vannelli, GB. & Maggi, M. (2010). Sex Steroid Receptors in Male Human Bladder: Expression and Biological Function. *Journal of Sexual Medicine,* Vol. 7, No. 8, pp. 2698-2713.

Christ, GJ.; Stone, B. & Melman, A. (1991). Age-dependent alterations in the efficacy of phenylephrine-induced contractions in vascular smooth muscle isolated from the corpus cavernosum of impotent men. *Canadian Journal of Physiology and Pharmacology,* Vol. 69, No. 7, pp. 909-913.

Gann, PH.; Hennekens, CH.; Longcope, C.; Verhoek-Oftedahl, W.; Grodstein, F. & Stampfer, MJ. (1995). A prospective study of plasma hormone levels, nonhormonal factors, and development of benign prostatic hyperplasia. *Prostate,* Vol. 26, No. 1, pp. 40-49.

Gill, HS.; Monson, FC.; Wein, AJ.; Ruggieri, MR. & Levin, RM. (1988). The effects of short-term in-vivo ischemia on the contractile function of the rabbit urinary bladder. *Journal of Urology,* Vol. 139, No. 6, pp. 1350-1354.

Giuliano, F.; Rampin, O.; Schirar, A.; Jardin, A. & Rousseau, JP. (1993). Autonomic control of penile erection: modulation by testosterone in the rat. *Journal of Neuroendocrinology,* Vol. 5, No. 6, pp. 677-683.

Hak, AE.; Witteman, JC.; de Jong, FH.; Geerlings, MI.; Hofman, A. & Pols, HA. (2002). Low levels of endogenous androgens increase the risk of atherosclerosis in elderly men: the Rotterdam study. *Journal of Clinical Endocrinology and Metabolism,* Vol. 87, No. 8, pp. 3632-3639.

Hanke, H.; Lenz, C.; Hess, B.; Spindler, KD. & Weidemann, W. (2001). Effect of testosterone on plaque development and androgen receptor expression in the arterial vessel wall. *Circulation,* Vol. 103, No. 10, pp. 1382-1385.

Homma, Y.; Kawabe, K.; Tsukamoto, T.; Yamanaka, H.; Okada, K.; Okajima, E.; Yoshida, O.; Kumazawa, J.; Gu, FL.; Lee C.; Hsu, TC.; dela Cruz, RC.; Tantiwang, A.; Lim, PH.; Sheikh, MA.; Bapat, SD.; Marshall, VR.; Tajima, K. & Aso, Y. (1997). Epidemiological survey of lower urinary tract symptoms in Asia and Australia using the international prostate symptom score. *International Journal of Urology,* Vol. 4, No. 1, pp. 40-46.

Huddart, RA.; Norman, A.; Shahidi, M.; Horwich, A.; Coward, D.; Nicholls, J. & Dearnaley, DP. (2003). Cardiovascular disease as a long-term complication of treatment for testicular cancer. *Journal of Clinical Oncology,* Vol. 21, No. 8, pp. 1513-1523.

Irwin,DE.; Abrams, P.; Milsom, I.; Kopp, Z.; Reilly, K.& EPIC Study Group. (2008). Understanding the elements of overactive bladder: questions raised by the EPIC study. *British Journal of Urology International.* Vol. 101, No. 11, pp. 1381-1387.

Jones, KW. & Schoenberg, HW. (1985) Comparison of the incidence of bladder hyperreflexia in patients with benign prostatic hypertrophy and age-matched female controls. *Journal of Urology,* Vol. 133, No. 3, pp. 425-426.

Joseph, MA.; Wei, JT.; Harlow, SD.; Cooney, KA.; Dunn, RL.; Jaffe, CA.; Montie, JE. & Schottenfeld, D. (2002). Relationship of serum sex-steroid hormones and prostate volume in African American men. *Prostate,* Vol. 53, No. 4, pp. 322-329.

Juan, YS.; Onal, B.; Broadaway, S.; Cosgrove, J.; Leggett, RE.; Whitbeck, C.; De, E.; Sokol, R.& Levin, RM. (2007) Effect of castration on male rabbit lower urinary tract tissue enzymes. *Molecular and Cellular Biochemistry,* Vol. 301, No. 1-2, pp. 227-233.

Kang, SM.; Jang, Y.; Kim, JY.; Chung, N.; Cho, SY.; Chae, JS. & Lee, JH. (2002). Effect of oral administration of testosterone on brachial arterial vasoreactivity in men with coronary artery disease. *American Journal of Cardiology,* Vol. 89, No. 7, pp. 862-864.

Kasturi, S.; Russell, S. & McVary KT. (2006). Metabolic syndrome and lower urinary tract symptoms secondary to benign prostatic hyperplasia. *Current Urology Report,* Vol. 7, No. 4, pp. 288-292.

Keast, JR.; Gleeson, RJ.; Shulkes, A. & Morris, MJ. (2002). Maturational and maintenance effects of testosterone on terminal axon density and neuropeptide expression in the rat vas deferens. *Neuroscience.* Vol. 112, No. 2, pp. 391-398.

Kim, SC.; Park, JK.; Kim, SW.; Lee, SW.; Ahn, TY.; Kim, JJ.; Paick, JS.; Park, NC.; Park, K.; Min, KS.; Kraus, SR.; Secrest, RJ.; Elion-Mboussa, A. & Viktrup, L. (2011). Tadalafil administered once daily for treatment of Asian men with lower urinary tract symptoms secondary to benign prostatic hyperplasia: Results from a placebo-controlled pilot study using tamsulosin as an active comparator. *Lower Urinary Tract Symptoms, in press*

Koritsiadis, G.; Stravodimos, K.; Mitropoulos, D.; Doumanis, G.; Fokitis, I.; Koritsiadis, S. & Constantinides, C. (2008). Androgens and bladder outlet obstruction: a correlation with pressure-flow variables in a preliminary study. *British Journal of Urology International,* Vol. 101, No. 12, pp. 1542-1546.

Kristal, AR.; Schenk, JM.; Song, Y.; Arnold, KB.; Neuhouser, ML.; Goodman, PJ.; Lin, DW.; Stanczyk, FZ. & Thompson, IM. (2008). Serum steroid and sex hormone-binding globulin concentrations and the risk of incident benign prostatic hyperplasia: results from the prostate cancer prevention trial. *American Journal of Epidemiology,* Vol. 167, No. 12, pp. 1416-1424.

Laaksonen, DE.; Niskanen, L.; Punnonen, K.; Nyyssönen, K.; Tuomainen, TP.; Salonen, R.; Rauramaa, R. & Salonen, JT. (2003). Sex hormones, inflammation and the metabolic syndrome: a population-based study. *European Journal of Endocrinology,* Vol. 149, No. 6, pp. 601-608.

Laaksonen, DE.; Niskanen, L.; Punnonen, K.; Nyyssönen, K.; Tuomainen, TP.; Valkonen, VP.; Salonen, R. & Salonen, JT. (2004). Testosterone and sex hormone-binding globulin predict the metabolic syndrome and diabetes in middle-aged men. *Diabetes Care,* Vol. 27, No. 5, pp. 1036-1041.

Lacey, JP.; Donatucci, CF.; Price, DT.; Page, SO.; Bennett, SA.; Tenniswood, MP. & Schwinn, DA. (1996). Effects of androgen deprivation on prostate alpha 1-adrenergic receptors. *Urology,* Vol. 48, No. 2, pp. 335-341.

Lepor, H. & Shapiro, E. (1984). Characterization of alpha1 adrenergic receptors in human benign prostatic hyperplasia. *Journal of Urology,* Vol. 132, No. 6, pp. 1226-1229.

Levin, RM.; Levin, SS.; Zhao, Y. & Buttyan, R. (1997). Cellular and molecular aspects of bladder hypertrophy. *European Urology,* Vol. 32, Suppl 1: pp. 15-21.

Litman, HJ.; Bhasin, S.; O'Leary, MP.; Link, CL. & McKinlay, JB. (2007). BACH Survey Investigators. An investigation of the relationship between sex-steroid levels and urological symptoms: results from the Boston Area Community Health survey. *British Journal of Urology International,* Vol. 100, No. 2, pp. 321-326.

Mäkelä, S.; Strauss, L.; Kuiper, G.; Valve, E.; Salmi, S.; Santti, R. & Gustafsson, JA. (2000). Differential expression of estrogen receptors alpha and beta in adult rat accessory sex glands and lower urinary tract. *Molecular and Cellular Endocrinology,* Vol. 170, No. 1-2, pp. 219-229.

Marberger, MJ. (1998). Long-term effects of finasteride in patients with benign prostatic hyperplasia: a double-blind, placebo-controlled, multicenter study. PROWESS Study Group. *Urology,* Vol. 51, No. 5, pp. 677-686.

Matsumoto, AM.& Bremner, WJ. (2004). Serum testosterone assays--accuracy matters. *Journal of Clinical Endocrinology and Metabolism,* Vol. 89, No. 2, pp. 520-524.

McVary, K. (2006). Lower urinary tract symptoms and sexual dysfunction: epidemiology and pathophysiology. *British Journal of Urology International, Vol.* 97, Suppl 2, pp. 23-28.

McVary, KT.; Rademaker, A.; Lloyd, GL. & Gann, P. (2005). Autonomic nervous system overactivity in men with lower urinary tract symptoms secondary to benign prostatic hyperplasia. *Journal of Urology,* Vol. 174, No. 4 Pt 1, pp. 1327-1433.

Medina, JJ.; Parra, RO. & Moore, RG. (1999). Benign prostatic hyperplasia (the aging prostate). *Medical Clinics of North America,* Vol. 83, No. 5, pp. 1213-1229.

Meigs, JB.; Mohr, B.; Barry, MJ.; Collins, MM. & McKinlay, JB. (2001). Risk factors for clinical benign prostatic hyperplasia in a community-based population of healthy aging men. *Journal of Clinical Epidemiology,* Vol. 54, No. 9, pp. 935-944.

Meikle, AW.; Stephenson, RA.; Lewis, CM. & Middleton, RG. (1997). Effects of age and sex hormones on transition and peripheral zone volumes of prostate and benign prostatic hyperplasia in twins. *Journal of Clinical Endocrinology and Metabolism,* Vol. 82, No. 2, pp. 571-575.

Sauver, J.; Jacobson, D.; McGree, M.; Girman, C.; Hill, C.; Lieber, M. & Nehra, A. (2010). Correlations between rates of decline in testosterone level and rates of change in lower urinary tract symptoms, prostatic enlargement, and maximum urinary flow rate. *Proceeding of the 105th Annual Scientific Meeting of the AUA,* #1633, San Francisco, May 2010.

Miwa, Y.; Kaneda, T. & Yokoyama, O. (2008). Association between lower urinary tract symptoms and serum levels of sex hormones in men. *Urology,* Vol. 72, No. 3, pp. 552-555.

Morelli, A.; Filippi, S.; Sandner, P.; Fibbi, B.; Chavalmane, AK.; Silvestrini, E.; Sarchielli, E.; Vignozzi, L.; Gacci, M.; Carini, M.; Vannelli, GB. & Maggi, M. (2009). Vardenafil modulates bladder contractility through cGMP-mediated inhibition of RhoA/Rho kinase signaling pathway in spontaneously hypertensive rats. *Journal of Sexual Medicine,* Vol. 6, No. 6, pp. 1594-1608.

Morelli, A.; Filippi, S.; Mancina, R.; Luconi, M.; Vignozzi, L.; Marini, M.; Orlando, C.; Vannelli, GB.; Aversa, A.; Natali, A.; Forti, G.; Giorgi, M.; Jannini, EA.; Ledda, F.& Maggi, M. (2004). Androgens regulate phosphodiesterase type 5 expression and functional activity in corpora cavernosa. *Endocrinology,* Vol. 145, No. 5, pp. 2253-2263.

Morita, T.; Tsuchiya, N.; Tsujii, T. & Kondo, S. (1992). Changes of autonomic receptors following castration and estrogen administration in the male rabbit urethral smooth muscle. *Tohoku Journal of Experimental Medicine,* Vol. 166, No. 403-405.

Moriyama, N.; Kurimoto, S.; Nagase, Y.; Inagaki, O.; Takanashi, M. & Kawabe, K. (1995). Age-related changes in alpha 1-adrenoceptors in rat prostate. *Urological Research,* Vol. 22, No.6, pp. 389-392.

Muesburger, SM. & Keast, JR. (2001).Testosterone and nerve growth factor have distinct but interacting effects on structure and neurotransmitter expression of adult pelvic ganglion cells in vitro. *Neuroscience*, Vol.108, No. 2, pp. 331-340.

Muller, M.; van den Beld, AW.; Bots, ML.; Grobbee, DE.; Lamberts, SW. & van der Schouw, YT. (2004). Endogenous sex hormones and progression of carotid atherosclerosis in elderly men. *Circulation,* Vol. 109, No. 17, pp. 2074-2079.

Nuver, J.; Smit, AJ.; Wolffenbuttel, BH.; Sluiter, WJ.; Hoekstra, HJ.; Sleijfer, DT. & Gietema, JA. (2005). The metabolic syndrome and disturbances in hormone levels in long-term survivors of disseminated testicular cancer. *Journal of Clinical Oncology.* Vol. 23, No. 16, pp. 3718-3725.

Partin, AW.; Oesterling, JE.; Epstein, JI.; Horton, R. & Walsh, PC.(1991). Influence of age and endocrine factors on the volume of benign prostatic hyperplasia. *Journal of Urology,* Vol. 145, No. 2, pp. 405-409.

Pearson, LJ.; Yandle, TG.; Nicholls, MG. & Evans, JJ. (2008) Regulation of endothelin-1 release from human endothelial cells by sex steroids and angiotensin-II. *Peptides,* Vol. 29, No. 6, pp.1057-1061.

Persson, K.; Igawa, Y.; Mattiasson, A. & Andersson, KE. (1992). Effects of inhibition of the L-arginine/nitric oxide pathway in the rat lower urinary tract in vivo and in vitro. *British Journal of Pharmacology,* Vol. 107, No. 1, pp. 178-184.

Pitteloud, N.; Mootha, VK.; Dwyer, AA.; Hardin, M.; Lee, H.; Eriksson, KF.; Tripathy, D.; Yialamas, M.; Groop, L.; Elahi, D. & Hayes, FJ. (2005). Relationship between testosterone levels, insulin sensitivity, and mitochondrial function in men. *Diabetes Care,* Vol. 28, No. 7, pp. 1636-1642.

Pitteloud, N.; Hardin, M.; Dwyer, AA.; Valassi, E.; Yialamas, M.; Elahi, D. & Hayes, FJ. (2005). Increasing insulin resistance is associated with a decrease in Leydig cell testosterone secretion in men. *Journal of Clinical Endocrinology and Metabolism,* Vol. 90, No. 5, pp. 2636-2641.

Platz, EA.; Kawachi, I.; Rimm, EB.; Longcope, C.; Stampfer, MJ.; Willett, WC. & Giovannucci, E. (1999). Plasma steroid hormones, surgery for benign prostatic hyperplasia, and severe lower urinary tract symptoms. *Prostate Cancer and Prostatic Disease,* Vol. 2, No. 5/6, pp. 285-289.

Plymate, SR.; Matej, LA.; Jones, RE. & Friedl, KE. (1988). Inhibition of sex hormone-binding globulin production in the human hepatoma (Hep G2) cell line by insulin and prolactin. *Journal of Clinical Endocrinology and Metabolism,* Vol. 67, No. 3, pp. 460-464.

Podlasek, C.; Zeiner, DJ. & McKenna, KE. (2003). Morphological changes and altered NOS isoform distribution in the BB/WOR diabetic rat prostate. *Journal of Urology,* Vol. 169, Suppl, pp. 285, A1108.

Qiu, Y.; Kraft, P.; Craig, EC.; Liu, X. & Haynes-Johnson, D. (2001). Identification and functional study of phosphodiesterases in rat urinary bladder. *Urological Research.* Vol. 29, No. 6, pp. 388-392.

Rees, RW.; Foxwell, NA.; Ralph, DJ.; Kell, PD.; Moncada, S. & Cellek, S. (2003). Y-27632, a Rho-kinase inhibitor, inhibits proliferation and adrenergic contraction of prostatic smooth muscles. *Journal of Urology,* Vol. 170, No. 6 pt 1, pp. 2517-2622.

Roberts, RO.; Jacobson, DJ.; Rhodes, T.; Klee, GG.; Leiber, MM. & Jacobsen, SJ. (2004). Serum sex hormones and measures of benign prostatic hyperplasia. *Prostate,* Vol. 61, No. 2, pp. 124-1231.

Roehrborn, CG.; McVary, KT.; Elion-Mboussa, A. & Viktrup, L. (2008). Tadalafil administered once daily for lower urinary tract symptoms secondary to benign prostatic hyperplasia: a dose finding study. *Journal of Urology,* Vol. 180, No. 4, pp. 1228-1234.

Rohrmann, S.; Nelson, WG.; Rifai, N.; Kanarek, N.; Basaria, S.; Tsilidis, KK.; Smit, E.; Giovannucci, E. & Platz, EA. (2007). Serum sex steroid hormones and lower urinary tract symptoms in Third National Health and Nutrition Examination Survey (NHANES III). *Urology,* Vol. 69, No. 4, pp. 708-713.

Rohrmann, S.; De Marzo, A.; M., Smit, E.; Giovannucci, E. & Platz, EA. (2005). Serum C-reactive protein concentration and lower urinary tract symptoms in older men in the Third National Health and Nutrition Examination Survey (NHANES III). *Prostate,* Vol. 62, No. 1, 27-33.

Rudner, XL.; Berkowitz, DE.; Booth, JV.; Funk, BL.; Cozart, KL.; D'Amico, EB.; El-Moalem, H.; Page, SO.; Richardson, CD.; Winters, B.; Marucci, L. & Schwinn, DA. (1999). Subtype specific regulation of human vascular alpha(1)-adrenergic receptors by vessel bed and age. *Circulation,* Vol. 100, No. 23, pp. 2336-2343.

Sairam, K.; Kulinskaya, E.; McNicholas, TA.; Boustead, GB. & Hanbury, DC. (2002). Sildenafil influences lower urinary tract symptoms. *British Journal of Urology International,* Vol. 90, No. 9, pp. 836-839.

Schatzl, G.; Madersbacher, S.; Temml, C.; Krenn-Schinkel, K.; Nader, A.; Sregi, G.; Lapin, A.; Hermann, M.; Berger, P. & Marberger, M. (2003). Serum androgen levels in men: impact of health status and age. *Urology,* Vol. 61, No. 3, pp. 629-633.

Schatzl, G.; Brössner, C.; Schmid, S.; Kugler, W.; Roehrich, M.; Treu, T.; Szalay, A.; Djavan, B.; Schmidbauer, CP.; Söregi, S. & Madersbacher, S. (2000). Endocrine status in elderly men with lower urinary tract symptoms: correlation of age, hormonal status, and lower urinary tract function. The Prostate Study Group of the Austrian Society of Urology. *Urology,* Vol. 55, No. 3, pp. 397-402.

Schultheiss, D.; Machtens, S. & Jonas, U. (2004). Testosterone therapy in the ageing male: what about the prostate. *Andrologia,* Vol. 36, No. 6, pp. 355-65.

Smith, MR.; Lee, H. & Nathan, DM. (2006). Insulin sensitivity during combined androgen blockade for prostate cancer. *Journal of Clinical Endocrinology and Metabolism,* Vol. 91, No. 4, pp. 1305-1308.

Somlyo, AP. & Somlyo, AV. (2000). Signal transduction by G-proteins, Rho-kinase and protein phosphatase to smooth muscle and non-muscle myosin II. *Journal of Physiology,* Vol. 522, No. Pt 2, pp. 177–185.

Svartberg, J.; von Mühlen, D.; Mathiesen, E.; Joakimsen, O.; Bønaa, KH. & Stensland-Bugge, E. (2006). Low testosterone levels are associated with carotid atherosclerosis in men. *Journal of Internal Medicine,* Vol. 259, No. 6, pp. 576-582.

Takyu S. (1993). Effects of testosterone on the autonomic receptor-mediated function in lower urinary tract from male rabbits. *Nippon Hinyokika Gakkai Zasshi.* Vol. 84, No. 2, pp. 330-338.

Trifiro, MD.; Parsons, JK.; Palazzi-Churas, K.; Bergstrom, J.; Lakin, C. & Barrett-Connor, E. (2010). Serum sex hormones and the 20-year risk of lower urinary tract symptoms in community-dwelling older men. *British Journal of Urology International.* Vol. 105, No. 11, pp. 1554-1559.

Traish, AM.; Goldstein, I. & Kim, NN. (2007). Testosterone and erectile function: from basic research to a new clinical paradigm for managing men with androgen insufficiency and erectile dysfunction. *European Urology,* Vol. 52, No. 1, pp. 54-70.

van den Beld, AW.; Bots, ML.; Janssen, JA.; Pols, HA.; Lamberts, SW. & Grobbee, DE. (2003). Endogenous hormones and carotid atherosclerosis in elderly men. *American Journal of Epidemiology,* Vol. 157, No. 1, pp. 25-31.

VanderHorst, VG.; Meijer, E. & Holstege, G. (2001). Estrogen receptor-alpha immunoreactivity in parasympathetic preganglionic neurons innervating the bladder in the adult ovariectomized cat. *Neuroscience Letters,* Vol. 298, No. 3, pp. 147-150.

Werkström, V.; Svensson, A.; Andersson, KE. & Hedlund, P. (2006). Phosphodiesterase 5 in the female pig and human urethra: morphological and functional aspects. *British Journal of Urology International,* Vol. 98, No. 2, pp. 414-423.

Williams, SJ. & Papka, RE. (1996). Estrogen receptor-immunoreactive neurons are present in the female rat lumbosacral spinal cord. *Journal of Neuroscience Research,* Vol. 46, No. 4, pp. 492-501.

Yassin, AA.; El-Sakka, AI.; Saad, F. & Gooren, LJ. (2008). Lower urinary-tract symptoms and testosterone in elderly men. *World Journal of Urology,* Vol. 26, No. 4, pp. 359-364.

Yono, M.; Foster, HE Jr.; Weiss, RM. & Latifpour, J. (2006). Age related changes in the functional, biochemical and molecular properties of alpha1-adrenoceptors in the rat genitourinary tract. *Journal of Urology,* Vol. 176, No. 3, pp. 1214-1219.

Zhang, XH.; Morelli, A.; Luconi, M.; Vignozzi, L.; Filippi, S.; Marini, M.; Vannelli, GB.; Mancina, R.; Forti, G.& Maggi, M. (2005). Testosterone regulates PDE5 expression and in vivo responsiveness to tadalafil in rat corpus cavernosum. *European Urology*. Vol. 47, No. 3, pp. 409-416.

10

Sex Hormones and Bacterial Infections

Marc Leone[1,2], Julien Textoris[1,2],
Christian Capo[1] and Jean-Louis Mege[1]
[1]*Unité de Recherche sur les Maladies Infectieuses Tropicales et Emergentes,
Centre National de la Recherche Scientifique Unité Mixte de Recherche 6236,
Faculté de Médecine, Marseille,*
[2]*Service d'Anesthésie et de Réanimation, Hôpital Nord,
Assistance Publique-Hôpitaux de Marseille,
Aix-Marseille Université, Marseille,
France*

1. Introduction

Epidemiological and experimental data suggest the association of gender and sex with susceptibility and severity of infectious diseases (Moss, 2005). Gender and sex likely affect viral and parasitic infectious diseases (Morales-Montor *et al.*, 2004; Fish, 2008; Snider *et al.*, 2009). Here we will review the effect of gender and sex on bacterial infectious diseases (sepsis, mycobacterial diseases and Q fever). We will differentiate gender and sex by considering that gender refers to differences determined by cultural and societal factors and sex refers to the biological differences between males and females (Fish, 2008). Indeed, variables such as poverty, occupational status and marital status affect differently men and women in different countries (Theobald *et al.*, 2006), leading to different risks of exposition to infectious pathogens and accesses to efficient treatment. This is illustrated by the decreased prevalence of tuberculosis in industrialized countries associated with socio-economic changes including reduced malnutrition and overcrowding, improved sanitary conditions in the workplaces before the use of chemotherapy (Davies *et al.*, 1999). Sex-based differences in the susceptibility to pathogens include what is due to chromosome effect and sex hormones. Thus, it is critical to delineate the respective roles of gender and sex on bacterial infections. The present review focuses on four features of the association between sex and bacterial infections with a special attention for bacterial sepsis, mycobacterial infections and *Coxiella burnetii* infection.

2. Epidemiological approach of susceptibility to bacterial infections

Epidemiological data show that the susceptibility to bacterial infectious diseases is unequally distributed in men and women. In sepsis, an infectious process associated with systemic inflammatory response syndrome, large-scale studies reported higher incidence in men than in women (Angus *et al.*, 2001; Martin *et al.*, 2003; Pietropaoli *et al.*, 2010). Men also develop more frequently sepsis episodes among patients with trauma (Osborn *et al.*, 2004; Wafaisade *et al.*, 2011) or acute kidney injury (Lopes *et al.*, 2010). In addition, men are over-represented among patients with respiratory infections (Esper *et al.*, 2006) or bloodstream infections (Laupland *et al.*, 2004) (Table 1).

Reference	**Number of patients**	**Patient selection**	**Sepsis incidence**	**Sepsis: Sex effect**	**Mortality: Sex effect**
Angus *et al.* 2001	6,621,559	All	3/1000	Men *vs.* Women 2.83 vs. 2.87 /1000	Men *vs.* Women 29.3 vs. 27.9%
Martin *et al.* 2003	750 million hospital admissions	All	1.3%	Men 1.28 [1.24 to 1.32]	Men *vs.* Women 22.0 vs. 21.8%
Osborn *et al.* 2004	30,303	Trauma	2%	Women 0.65 [0.49 to 0.86]	Women 0.76 [0.66 to 0.88]
Laupland *et al.* 2004	9,266	Positive blood culture	15.7/100,000 /year	Men *vs.* Women 17.7 vs. 13.5 / 100,000/year	No listed as independent risk factor
Esper *et al.* 2006	930 million hospitalizations	All	1.3% of all hospitalizations	Men 1.27 [1.24 to 1.30]	Men *vs.* Women 20.1 vs. 21.0%
Pietropaoli *et al.* 2010	Unknown	All	Unknown	Men *vs.* Women 54 vs. 46%	Men *vs.* Women 33 vs. 35% ($p = 0.01$)
Lopes *et al.* 2010	Unknown	Acute kidney injury	Unknown	Men *vs.* Women 72.5 vs. 27.5%	Men 1.1 [0.5-2.3]
Wafaisade *et al.* 2011	29,829	Trauma	10.2%	Men 1.81 [1.61 to 2.03]	Unknown

Table 1. Gender effect in epidemiological studies (Result are expressed as either absolute number, percentage, or relative risk and 95% confident interval as required (and available in the original study))

In the context of infectious diseases due to intracellular bacteria, such as tuberculosis (*Mycobacterium tuberculosis*) (Che & Antoine, 2011), Q fever (*C. burnetii*) (Tissot Dupont *et al.*, 1992; Anderson *et al.*, 2009) and Legionnaires' disease (*Legionella pneumophila)* (Campese *et al.*, 2011), men represent the majority of patients (Table 2).

Infection due to intracellular bacteria	**Sex ratio**	**Reference**
Tuberculosis	1.4	Che & Antoine, 2011
Q fever	2.4	Tissot-Dupont, 1992
Legionnaires' disease	2.9	Campese, 2011

Table 2. Epidemiological data show that males and females are differently affected by bacterial infections. The reasons that explain this difference in susceptibility to and/or severity of the disease may be multiple. They include different risks of pathogen exposure, social behavior associated with gender such as smoking or drinking and biological parameters such as sex hormones.

With respect to Q fever, the male-to-female ratio of patients admitted to hospital is 2.45 in adults (Tissot Dupont *et al.*, 1992). The rate of Q fever-related complications is higher in males than in females (Raoult *et al.*, 2000). Men represent 75% patients diagnosed as having *C. burnetii* endocarditis (Houpikian & Raoult, 2005), the most severe manifestation of chronic Q fever. Note that females have fewer symptoms during pregnancy (Tissot-Dupont *et al.*, 2007).

In contrast to susceptibility to bacterial infections, studying the role of sex in the mortality provided contrasting evidence. Some epidemiological studies did not report any gender differences in sepsis-related death (Crabtree *et al.*, 1999; Martin *et al.*, 2003; Laupland *et al.*, 2004; Esper *et al.*, 2006) whereas other found either increased mortality in men (Osborn *et al.*, 2004; Melamed & Sorvillo, 2009; Wafaisade *et al.*, 2011) or women (Combes *et al.*, 2009; Pietropaoli *et al.*, 2010; Nachtigall *et al.*, 2011). As men are also at increased risk of death due to trauma, cancer and cardiovascular diseases as compared with women, the analysis of epidemiological data should integrate these potential biases (Micheli *et al.*, 2009; Pinkhasov *et al.*, 2010; Coronado *et al.*, 2011).

The literature provides evidence that sex hormones may account for the differences of susceptibility to bacterial infections and their prognosis between men and women. The production of sex hormones evolves with aging, suggesting that susceptibility to infection will change along the life. In adults, the widest difference in sepsis incidence occurs between 25-30 years of age when sex hormones play a key role in the sexual dimorphism (Angus *et al.*, 2001). In elderly patients, sepsis tends to occur later in women than in men (Martin *et al.*, 2003). Most studies show that the infection distribution is similar in children independently of sex (Tissot Dupont *et al.*, 1992; Rose *et al.*, 2001; Odetola *et al.*, 2007). No difference is found in young boys and girls with Q fever (Maltezou & Raoult, 2002) or with tuberculosis (Che & Antoine, 2011).

Whether sex hormones govern the susceptibility to and the severity of bacterial infections, infection modulates the amounts of sex hormones. In patients with sepsis (Christeff *et al.*, 1988; Fourrier *et al.*, 1994; Majetschak *et al.*, 2000) or tuberculosis (Bottasso *et al.*, 2007; Rey *et al.*, 2007) circulating levels of estrogens are increased whereas those of testosterone dramatically fall. It has been also found that increased levels of estrogens are especially marked in males with sepsis (Fourrier *et al.*, 1994; Majetschak *et al.*, 2000). In addition, high circulating levels of estrogens seem efficient predictors of death in sepsis (Christeff *et al.*, 1988; Dossett *et al.*, 2008; May *et al.*, 2008). The mortality of elderly patients with severe infections is related to increased estradiol levels in both men and women, whereas increased testosterone levels are found in females who do not survive (Angstwurm *et al.*, 2005).

Pregnancy represents a remarkable model for investigating the effect of sex hormones on the development of infectious diseases. Indeed, the developing placenta produces human chorionic gonadotrophin that stimulates the ovaries to supply higher levels of estrogen and progesterone. It is well known that pregnancy is associated with listeriosis. Pregnant women with listeriosis account for 27% of all listeriosis cases and 60% of listeriosis cases among 10-40 years old persons (Lorber, 1997). Less spectacular is the case of Q fever. The primo-infection to *C. burnetii* during pregnancy increases the risk to develop a chronic evolution of the disease with potential fatal evolution (Carcopino *et al.*, 2009). The true incidence of sepsis or severe sepsis in parturient women is difficult to assess in part because the standard criteria used for sepsis identification are not effective to predict sepsis during pregnancy (Lappen *et al.*, 2010).

The analysis of epidemiological data indicates that male gender predisposes to develop sepsis and chronic bacterial infectious diseases whereas women are relatively protected. Although sex hormones seem to be critical in the sex dimorphism, we have to integrate other variables related to the host such as chromosomal factors and exposure to bacterial pathogens.

3. Sex hormones and experimental models of bacterial infection

The use of experimental models of infection was the easiest approach to study the role of sex hormones in bacterial infections; the availability of castrated animals with or without hormonal substitution has been largely contributive.

3.1 Experimental endotoxemia

Endotoxemia may be experimentally reproduced by the administration of lipopolysaccharide (LPS) to animals or human volunteers. LPS are present in the outer membrane of Gram-negative bacteria and act as endotoxins inducing strong inflammatory response in animals. Females produce a more vigorous pro-inflammatory response than males as demonstrated by higher circulating levels of Tumor Necrosis Factor (TNF) (Trentzsch *et al.*, 2003). The effect of sexual dimorphism in the outcome of endotoxemia depends on LPS dose. The intraperitoneal administration of low doses of LPS (5 mg/kg) to C57BL/6 mice leads to a lower survival of males compared to females (Laubach *et al.*, 1998) whereas the administration of higher doses (12.5 mg/kg) leads to similar mortality in males and females.

The study of the role of sex hormones in this dimorphism has benefited from the modulation of hormonal context. First, the circulating levels of TNF are higher in castrated C57BL/6 male mice than in intact males treated with LPS (Trentzsch *et al.*, 2003), suggesting that testosterone may reduce TNF production. Reinforcing this hypothesis, the LPS-induced response observed in castrated mice is reduced after testosterone treatment, regardless of sex (Spinedi *et al.*, 1992; Torres *et al.*, 2005). Second, the intraperitoneal injection of LPS in ovariectomized females is associated with reduced levels of TNF, interleukin (IL)-6, and IL-10 as compared with intact females. This is accompanied by the reduced macrophage expression of Toll-like receptor (TLR)-4, a pattern recognition receptor interacting with LPS (Rettew *et al.*, 2009). The role of estrogens in LPS response has been shown by complementation of castrated mice with sex hormones. Indeed, ovariectomized animals receiving exogenous 17β-estradiol showed higher TNF levels after endotoxin challenge than untreated gonadectomized or intact animals. In addition, peritoneal macrophages isolated from ovariectomized mice receiving 17β-estradiol replacement bind LPS more efficiently than untreated animals because of upregulated expression of CD14 and TLR-4 (Rettew *et al.*, 2009). Finally, the administration of 17β-estradiol to castrated C57BL/6J male mice increases the circulating levels of LPS-induced TNF production, as compared with control male or female mice (Trentzsch *et al.*, 2003). These findings should be analyzed according to the genetic background of the animals. Castrated males react differently according to the mouse strain (A/J, DBA/2J, AKR/J, BALB/cJ) (Trentzsch *et al.*, 2003; Torres *et al.*, 2005) after LPS challenge.

In contrast to estrogen treatment, the exogenous treatment of mice with progesterone-containing implants fails to increase circulating levels of LPS-binding protein, cell surface levels of CD14 on peritoneal macrophages or total TLR-4 content in macrophages (Rettew *et al.*, 2009). The role of testosterone appears variable according to the experimental conditions. Orchiectomy does not alter the mortality of wild-type male mice but, after orchiectomy, increased mortality is observed in knockout (KO) male mice that are phenotypically normal but lack the ability to produce increased nitric oxide during endotoxemia. This increased mortality in orchiectomized KO males is prevented by the administration of exogenous testosterone (Laubach *et al.*, 1998), demonstrating that exogenous testosterone is potentially protective for the host when nitric oxide production is deficient. This experiment also suggests that testosterone may play a different role in healthy individuals and patients in severe conditions.

In humans, 30 young volunteers including 15 males and 15 females received 2 ng/kg LPS. The females were studied in the follicular phase and nine of them used oral contraceptives. During endotoxemia, the decrease in blood pressure is more pronounced in females than in males. Norepinephrine sensitivity remains unchanged in females but decreases in males, suggesting that the clinical picture is more evident and the response to treatment is more effective in females than in males. The administration of LPS results in increased circulating levels of TNF, IL-6, interferon (IFN)-gamma and IL-10 in males and females, but TNF and IFN-gamma levels are significantly higher in females than in males (van Eijk *et al.*, 2007). This study suggests that the hypotension that likely occurs earlier in females than in males may be related to a more marked immune response to LPS administration.

Taken together, murine models of LPS-mediated inflammation and endotoxemia in humans highlight the role of estrogens, and testosterone to a lesser extent, in host responses to LPS and TLR-4 activation.

3.2 Mouse model of sepsis

The models of sepsis using cecal ligation and puncture (CLP) seem to be more accurate than those using LPS injection (Dyson & Singer, 2009). The most frequent scenario used to evaluate the effect of sex is a two-hit model consisting of hemorrhages followed by sepsis. Male and proestrus female C3H/HeN mice are subjected to hemorrhage or sham operation and to polymicrobial sepsis by CLP twenty-four hours after. Animals subjected to hemorrhage followed by CLP show depressed splenocyte and macrophage functions as compared with sham animals (Angele *et al.*, 1997). After CLP, females have lower mortality than males, irrespective of prior hemorrhage or sham operation. Unlike males, hemorrhages do not increase the mortality rate in females (Diodato *et al.*, 2001).

Female sex hormones likely play a major role in protection against CLP sepsis. Indeed, after CLP, the mortality of ovariectomized CBA/J mice is significantly higher than in intact mice. Ovariectomy results in a decreased production of IL-1 and IL-6 by splenic and peritoneal macrophages, but the production of IL-1 and IL-6 by macrophages from intact female mice is maintained after trauma-hemorrhage (Knöferl *et al.*, 2002). Thus, in septic conditions, female sex hormones protect female mice by producing increased levels of pro-inflammatory cytokines.

The modulation of estrogen receptors is a convenient way to study the role of estrogens in sepsis models. In a CLP model, multiple oral doses of a nonsteroidal selective estrogen receptor-beta agonist increase survival of mice, decrease systemic bacteremia, reduce peritoneal IL-6 and TNF levels. Interestingly, the estrogen receptor-beta agonist provides a comparable level of protection in both males and females (Cristofaro *et al.*, 2006). On another hand, the administration of an estrogen receptor alpha agonist entirely prevents the rise in plasma IL-6 and IL-10 levels induced by a sequence of trauma-hemorrhage whereas the administration of an estrogen receptor beta agonist is only in part effective. Similar conclusions can be drawn from experiments at the cell level. The effects of an estrogen receptor beta agonist on Kupffer cells, splenic macrophages, alveolar macrophages and peripheral blood mononuclear cells following trauma-hemorrhage are less pronounced than that of an estrogen receptor alpha agonist (Dienstknecht *et al.*, 2004). In all cases, the beneficial effects of 17β-estradiol are limited to tissue-fixed macrophages, suggesting the compartmentalization of host response (Suzuki *et al.*, 2007). In figure 1, we hypothesized possible mechanisms for explaining the dual role of estrogens in sepsis.

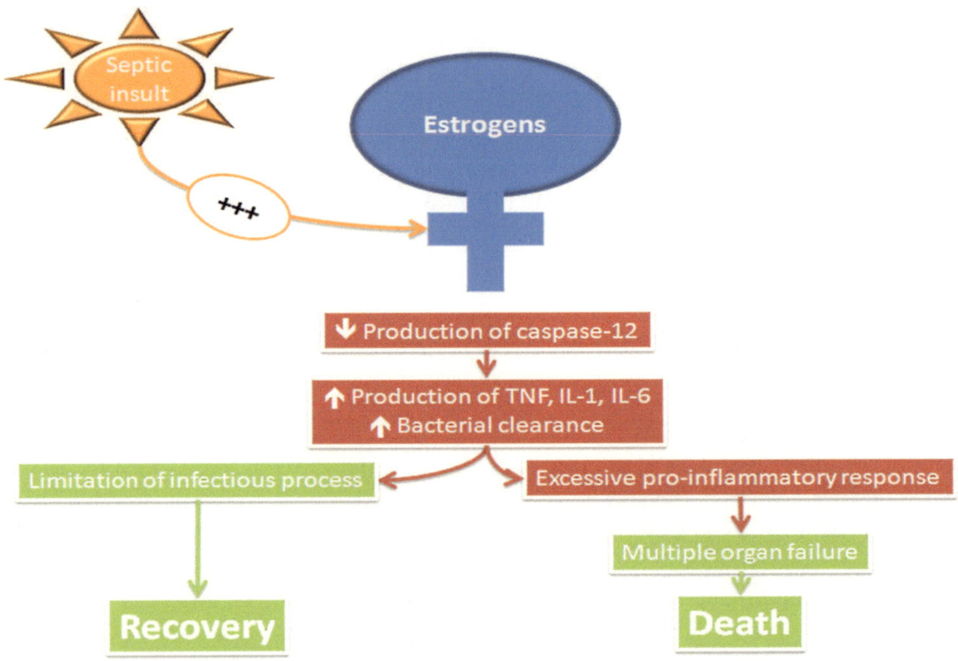

Estrogens reduce the production of caspase-12 and then increase that of pro-inflammatory mediators. This is associated either with a rapid limitation of the infectious process leading to fast recovery or with the occurrence of multiple organ failure related to an excessive pro-inflammatory response leading to death. Note that sepsis induces a positive feedback on estrogen production. (IL: interleukin, TNF: tumor necrosis factor).

Fig. 1. Interaction between estrogens and host response

Testosterone has detrimental effect on survival of male mice by attenuating immune response. Indeed, after CLP, the survival rate of male mice treated with flutamide, an androgen receptor blocker, is higher than that of vehicle-treated mice. Flutamide treatment also restores splenocyte proliferation and IL-2 release as well as the release of IL-1 by splenic macrophages (Angele *et al.*, 1997). The effect of testosterone on experimental sepsis may be controlled by IL-10. Indeed, after CLP early IL-10 treatment is associated with increased survival of males, but not of females (Kahlke *et al.*, 2000). In figure 2, we hypothesized possible mechanisms for explaining the role of testosterone in sepsis.

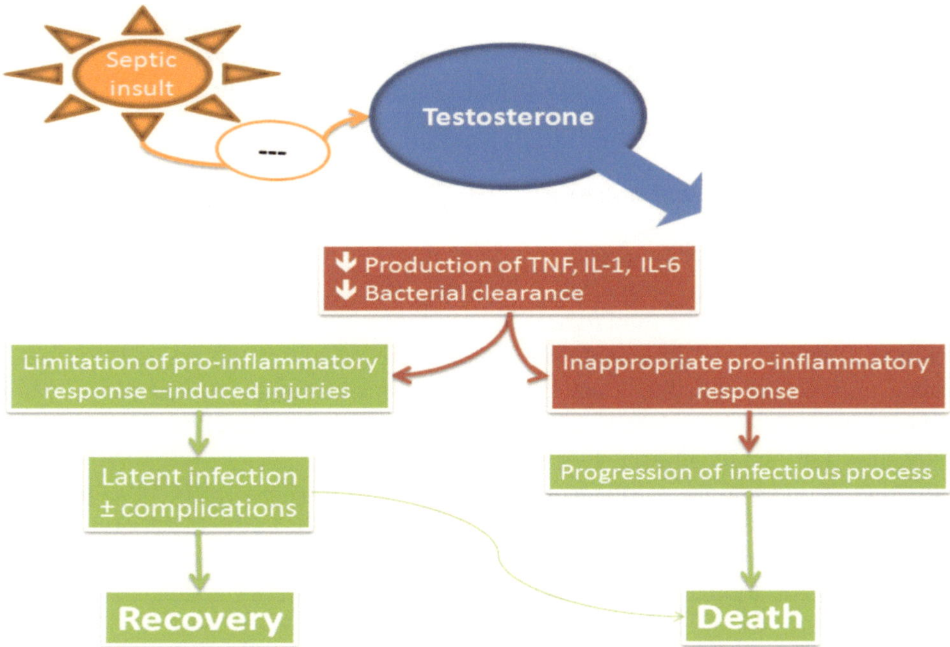

Testosterone decreases the intensity of the pro-inflammatory response, resulting in an inappropriate response to septic insult, progression of the infectious process and death. In some cases, the limitation of an excessive pro-inflammatory response may appear beneficial by limiting the occurrence of multiple organ failure. This can lead to a latent infection with infectious complications, resulting in either death or recovery. Note that sepsis induces a negative feedback on testosterone production. (IL: interleukin, TNF: tumor necrosis factor).

Fig. 2. Interaction between testosterone and host response

3.3 Infection by extracellular bacteria

Pseudomonas aeruginosa is one of the predominant Gram negative bacteria responsible for pulmonary infection in intensive care units (Leone *et al.*, 2007). The role of gender is not specifically reported in epidemiological studies although men are more prone to develop lung infection than women (Leone *et al.*, 2007). The importance of sex hormones has been assessed in a model of C57BL/6 mice challenged to pulmonary infection with *P. aeruginosa*. At variance with other models, the weight loss, bacterial load and inflammatory mediators in the lungs are higher in females than in males. The number of bacteria found in the lungs of IL-10-deficient males is higher than that observed in wild type males. These findings clearly show that female mice are more susceptible to *P. aeruginosa* lung infection than males and that IL-10 modulates host response to infection as described above in sepsis models (Guilbault *et al.*, 2002).

On the other hand, *P. aeruginosa* is the predominant bacterium found in the course of cystic fibrosis. Importantly, the outcomes are worse for cystic fibrosis women infected with *P. aeruginosa* as compared with men (Demko *et al.*, 1995). A mouse model has been dedicated to investigate the effect of gender on cystic fibrosis. The administration of exogenous estrogen to adult cystic fibrosis males with *P. aeruginosa* pneumonia leads to more severe manifestations of inflammation in both lung tissue and bronchial alveolar lavage fluid.

Inflammatory infiltrates are increased as determined by histological studies. The inflammatory response is accompanied by an increased lung tissue expression of both IL-23 and IL-17 (Wang *et al.*, 2010). Thus, sex hormones modulate *P. aeruginosa* infection with a marked inflammatory effect of estrogens.

3.4 Infections by intracellular bacteria

3.4.1 Mycobacterial infections

As tuberculosis occurs more frequently in males than in females, the effect of sex should be a common feature of mycobacterial infections. Male mice infected by *Mycobacterium marinum* are more susceptible than female mice in terms of mortality, incidence of gross skin lesions and bacterial load in lungs and spleen. The castration of males improves their resistance to infection and this effect is substantially reversed by continuous testosterone treatment. The testosterone treatment also increases the susceptibility of females to *M. marinum* infection, demonstrating that testosterone is partly responsible for the increased susceptibility of mice to *M. marinum* infection (Yamamoto *et al.*, 1991). In DBA/2 female mice infected with *Mycobacterium avium*, the number of bacilli in the lungs of infected mice increased after ovariectomy, suggesting a protective effect of female sex hormones. The treatment of ovariectomized mice with exogenous 17β-estradiol reduces the burden of bacilli to the level found in sham-operated mice. Estrogens enhance the bacteriostatic activity of IFN-gamma against *M. avium* via increased nitrite production by macrophages (Tsuyuguchi *et al.*, 2001). These findings show that estrogens enhance the host protection against mycobacterial infections but testosterone is detrimental.

3.4.2 *C. burnetii* infection

From the epidemiological data in which mature adult men are more at risk to develop Q fever than women (Tissot-Dupont *et al.*, 2007), we showed that sex hormones play a role in the occurrence and the severity of *C. burnetii* infection. In C57BL/6 mice infected with *C. burnetii*, bacterial load and granuloma numbers are lower in females than in males and are increased in ovariectomized females to levels similar to those found in males. The treatment of ovariectomized mice with 17β-estradiol reduces both bacterial loads and granuloma numbers (Leone *et al.*, 2004), demonstrating that estrogens control *C. burnetii* infection. To analyze the differences between males and females, intact and castrated mice have been infected with *C. burnetii* for 24 hours, and gene expression has been measured in liver cells using whole-genome microarrays. The expression of a total of 2,777 probes is specifically modulated by *C. burnetti* infection. Surprisingly, 86% of them are differentially expressed in males and females. Castration of males and females shows that sex hormones are responsible for more than 60% of the observed gene modulation, and this effect of sex hormones is most pronounced in males. Using functional annotation of modulated genes, four clusters have been identified as enriched in males. These clusters are related to cell-cell adhesion, signal transduction, defensins and cytokine/Jak-Stat pathways (Textoris *et al.*, 2010). A major cluster of modulated genes has been identified in females consisting of the circadian rhythm pathway with positive (Clock, Arntl) and negative (Per) limbs of a feedback loop. Clock and Arntl are down-modulated whereas Per is up-regulated. These changes may be associated with efficient bacterial elimination in females but not in males, in which the immune response would be inefficient.

4. Infectious diseases associated with pregnancy

The pregnancy is characterized by dramatic changes in sex hormones with decreased estrogen and increased progesterone levels. Estrogens and progesterone are known to affect the susceptibility to pathogens likely through the modulation of the immune responses. Indeed, pregnancy is a transient period of tolerance in which the prevention of fetus rejection increases the susceptibility to intracellular bacteria (Munoz-Suano *et al.*, 2011). Several examples of infectious diseases will illustrate this statement.

In humans, Q fever is frequently asymptomatic in pregnant women but it may result in increased risk to develop a chronic form of the disease (Carcopino *et al.*, 2009). Female BALB/c mice have been infected with *C. burnetii* through the intraperitoneal route before repeated pregnancies over a 2-year period. Persistent infection associated with abortion and perinatal death is observed in these mice. The occurrence of endocarditis on native valves, which characterize chronic Q fever following *C. burnetii* infection during pregnancy, has been observed in some infected pregnant mice (Stein *et al.*, 2000).

Pregnancy is a risk factor for typhoid infection (Olubuyide, 1992). After an infection challenge with *Salmonella enterica* serovar Typhimurium, the splenic bacterial load is markedly increased in pregnant mice compared with non-pregnant mice (Pejcic-Karapetrovic *et al.*, 2007). The increased bacterial load is related to sex hormones since a three-day treatment of virgin mice with 1 mg/day of estrogen increases their susceptibility to an intraperitoneal bacterial challenge as compared with control mice. In contrast, a three-day treatment of virgin mice with 1 mg/day of progesterone is associated with increased survival time (Kita *et al.*, 1989). It is likely that progesterone improves the resistance of mice by increasing the influx of peritoneal cells after infection whereas estrogen affects the acute inflammatory responses (Kita *et al.*, 1989).

Listeriosis is an infection that occurs in about 30% of cases in pregnant women (Lorber, 1997). The impact of sex hormones on the course of the disease has been especially well described. Exposure to diethylstilbestrol, a synthetic nonsteroidal estrogen, precipitates a dramatic increase in *Listeria* susceptibility. To assess the interplay between diethylstilbestrol, sex hormones and immune response, *L. monocytogenes* has been intravenously administered to C3H/HeSlc female and male mice treated with diethylstilbestrol. The delayed-type hypersensitivity response is suppressed in females treated with diethylstilbestrol but not in males. After castration, a diethylstilbestrol-induced suppression is also observed in males. Testosterone inhibits this diethylstilbestrol-induced suppression (Kato *et al.*, 1988). Another report shows that the administration of estradiol or diethylstilbestrol is associated with an increased mortality of female B6C3F1 mice infected with *L. monocytogenes*. This effect of estradiol or diethylstilbestrol is due to their estrogenic activity since compounds such as 5α-dihydrotestosterone or progesterone with little or no estrogenic activity do not affect the mortality of infected mice (Pung *et al.*, 1984). Female C3H/He mice treated with exogenous doses of estrogen have been inoculated with *L. monocytogenes* by the intraperitoneal route. On days 3, 5 and 7 after infection, the bacterial load in spleen and liver is higher in estrogen-treated mice than in control mice (Salem *et al.*, 1999). Note that the sensitivity of mice to infection is highly dependent on the genetic background since the C57BL/6 mice are 100 times more resistant to intravenously injected *L. monocytogenes* than BALB/c mice, due to the action of a single gene, Lr (Mandel & Cheers, 1980). Taken together, these experimental studies demonstrate the role of sex hormones in the context of materno-fetal tolerance and susceptibility to intracellular bacteria.

5. How sex hormones affect bacterial infection?

Although epidemiological analysis and experimental models of infection provide convincing evidence of the role of sex hormones in host susceptibility to bacterial pathogens, the mechanisms used by sex hormones to modulate the susceptibility of hosts to pathogens are poorly understood. It is likely that sex hormones target immune cells according to their critical role in host defense (Fish, 2008). It is known that estrogens, androgens and glucocorticoids influence a large proportion of cell transcriptome (Duma *et al.*, 2010) and interact with specific receptors on immune cells. Cell-mediated and humoral immune responses represent the adaptive part of the immunity and are usually associated with the clearance of intracellular pathogens. Females exhibit robust cell-mediated and humoral immune responses after infectious challenge or vaccination as compared with males (Bouman *et al.*, 2005). This is partly related to changes in T cell distribution. Women have higher $CD4^+$ T cells number than men, which accounts for the robustness of adaptive immune responses. In addition, the numbers of regulatory T cells (Treg) that shape immune responses vary during the ovarian cycle: the Treg number increases during the follicular phase of menstrual cycle when estrogens are high and decreases during the luteal phase when estrogens are low (Arruvito *et al.*, 2007). The increase in Treg number during the pregnancy is essential for materno-fetal tolerance but favors the occurrence of infectious diseases due to intracellular pathogens (Belkaid & Tarbell, 2009). Hence, estrogens appear as regulators of $CD4^+$ T cell subsets; they also affect the Th1/Th2 equilibrium known to be essential in the control of bacterial infections. Indeed, it is clearly demonstrated that estrogens and progesterone favor Th2 cell responses during the third trimester of pregnancy (Munoz-Suano *et al.*, 2011). Low doses of estrogens are associated with Th1 cell responses that support microbicidal responses via IFN-gamma production; the effect of estrogens seems to be related to increased expression of t-bet, a master regulator of Th1 differentiation. In contrast, high doses of estrogens promote Th2-cell responses known to interfere with antibacterial immunity (Fish, 2008). Estrogens affect antibody production via their action on B cells; they decrease the negative selection of immature B cells and increase the survival of autoreactive B cells and polyclonal activation of B cells (Grimaldi *et al.*, 2002; Verthelyi, 2001). This is consistent with increased levels of autoimmune diseases in women (McCombe *et al.*, 2009), but it is not demonstrated that estrogen-mediated increased humoral response to pathogens is due to a direct effect on B cells. In contrast to estrogens, the effects of androgens such as testosterone on adaptive immune response are suppressive, which accounts for decreased T- and B-cell proliferation, immunoglobulin and cytokine production (Fish, 2008). This may explain why men are more susceptible than women to infectious agents because of the inability to mount efficient adaptive immune response.

Sex hormones may also affect the innate immune response that is the first line of defense against pathogens and that is necessary to shape adaptive immune response. Monocytes and macrophages are cell effectors of innate anti-infectious immunity and support inflammatory responses. The number of circulating monocytes is higher in men and women after the menopause than in fertile women (Bouman *et al.*, 2004). The effects of estrogens on monocytes and macrophages are suppressive but have to be analyzed according to the context. They likely act on CD16 promoter, leading to downmodulated CD16 expression and decreased production of proinflammatory cytokines (Kramer *et al.*, 2004). Inflammatory cytokines such as TNF and IL-1 are modulated during the ovarian cycle: low doses of estrogens are associated with increased production of TNF and IL-1 as compared with high

doses of estrogens (Bouman *et al.*, 2005). The role of estrogens in inflammation has been assessed in sensitized mice with LPS. LPS elicits transcriptional activation of inflammatory genes in microglial cells. Their expression is inhibited in the brain from ovariectomized mice (Soucy *et al.*, 2005). On another hand, testosterone exerts a suppressive effect on monocytes and macrophages likely by decreasing the expression of TLR-4 (Rettew *et al.*, 2008). This is more ambiguous in vivo. Castration of male mice strikingly accelerates wound healing and dampens associated inflammatory response. Similarly, systemic treatment with flutamide depresses inflammatory response (Ashcroft & Mills, 2002). Other cells involved in the innate immune response are likely targeted by sex hormones. Indeed, the activity of neutrophils and natural killer cells is suppressed by estrogens (Fish, 2008). Estrogens regulate the differentiation of dendritic cells from bone marrow precursors to conventional dendritic cells producing IL-12. The treatment of mature splenic dendritic cells with estrogens leads to the expansion of IFN-gamma-producing dendritic cells (Bengtsson *et al.*, 2004).
The impact of sex hormones on adaptive immunity may explain the generally superior ability of females to deal with and to be protected from infections, but their effect on innate immunity clearly depends on hormone doses, explaining the differences between in vitro and in vivo data. This is related to the stress system that has potent action on inflammatory and immune responses (Chrousos, 2010).

6. Conclusion

Although it is difficult to separate biological factors from social and economic factors, the epidemiological studies have shown that the sexual dimorphism may explain the differences in the susceptibility to and/or the severity of bacterial infections between men and women. The use of experimental models of infection demonstrates the role of sex hormones in this sexual dimorphism. Sex hormones target the immune system known to be essential in the host response to infection and, in turn, can be modulated by infection. While estrogens induce efficient cell-mediated and humoral immune responses necessary to bacterial clearance, androgens are rather suppressive. The pregnancy is an excellent model of the interplay between hormonal and immune systems and it teaches us that hormonal control of immune responses varies with time. It would be essential in the future to examine the sex-based differences in immune responses in humans likely by using tissue bio-banks and high throughput methods.

7. References

Anderson, A. D.; Kruszon-Moran, D.; Loftis, A. D.; McQuillan, G.; Nicholson, W. L.; Priestley, R. A.; Candee, A. J.; Patterson, N. E. & Massung, R. F. (2009). Seroprevalence of Q fever in the United States, 2003-2004. *The American Journal of Tropical Medicine and Hygiene*, Vol.81, No.4, pp. 691-694, ISSN 1476-1645

Angele, M. K.; Wichmann, M. W.; Ayala, A.; Cioffi, W. G. & Chaudry, I. H. (1997). Testosterone receptor blockade after hemorrhage in males. Restoration of the depressed immune functions and improved survival following subsequent sepsis. *Archives of Surgery*, Vol.132, No.11, pp. 1207-1214, ISSN 0004-0010

Angstwurm, M. W. A.; Gaertner, R. & Schopohl, J. (2005). Outcome in elderly patients with severe infection is influenced by sex hormones but not gender. *Critical Care Medicine*, Vol.33, No.12, pp. 2786-2793, ISSN 0090-3493

Angus, D. C.; Linde-Zwirble, W. T.; Lidicker, J.; Clermont, G.; Carcillo, J. & Pinsky, M. R. (2001). Epidemiology of severe sepsis in the United States: analysis of incidence, outcome, and associated costs of care. *Critical Care Medicine*, Vol.29, No.7, pp.1303-1310, ISSN 0090-3493

Arruvito, L.; Sanz, M.; Banham, A. H. & Fainboim, L. (2007). Expansion of $CD4^{+}CD25^{+}$and $FOXP3^{+}$ regulatory T cells during the follicular phase of the menstrual cycle: implications for human reproduction. *Journal of Immunology*, Vol.178, No.4, pp.2572-2578, ISSN 0022-1767

Ashcroft, G. S. & Mills, S. J. (2002). Androgen receptor-mediated inhibition of cutaneous wound healing. *The Journal of Clinical Investigation*, Vol.110, No.5, pp. 615-624, ISSN 0021-9738

Belkaid, Y. & Tarbell, K. (2009). Regulatory T cells in the control of host-microorganism interactions. *Annual Review of Immunology*, Vol.27, 551-589, ISSN 0732-0582

Bengtsson, A. K. ; Ryan, E. J. ; Giordano, D. ; Magaletti, D. M. & Clark, E. A. (2004). 17beta-estradiol (E2) modulates cytokine and chemokine expression in human monocyte-derived dendritic cells. *Blood*, Vol.104, No.5, pp. 1404-1410, ISSN 0006-4971

Bottasso, O.; Bay, M. L.; Besedovsky, H. & del Rey, A. (2007). The immuno-endocrine component in the pathogenesis of tuberculosis. *Scandinavian Journal of Immunology*, Vol.66, No.2-3, pp. 166-175, ISSN 0300-9475

Bouman, A.; Heineman, M. J. & Faas, M. M. (2005). Sex hormones and the immune response in humans. *Human Reproduction Update*, Vol.11, No.4, pp. 411-423, ISSN 1355-4786

Bouman, A.; Schipper, M.; Heineman, M. J. & Faas, M. M. (2004). Gender difference in the non-specific and specific immune response in humans. *American Journal of Reproductive Immunology*, Vol.52, No.1, pp. 19-26, ISSN 1046-7408

Campese, C.; Bitar, D.; Jarraud, S.; Maine, C. ; Forey, F.; Etienne, J.; Desenclos, J. C.; Saura, C. & Che, D. (2011). Progress in the surveillance and control of *Legionella* infection in France, 1998-2008. *International Journal of Infectious Diseases: IJID: Official Publication of the International Society for Infectious Diseases*, Vol.15, No.1, pp. e30-37, ISSN 1878-3511

Carcopino, X.; Raoult, D.; Bretelle, F.; Boubli, L. & Stein, A. (2009). Q fever during pregnancy: a cause of poor fetal and maternal outcome. *Annals of the New York Academy of Sciences*, Vol.1166, 79-89, ISSN 1749-6632

Che, D. & Antoine, D. (2011). [Epidemiology of tuberculosis in France in 2008.]. *Medecine Et Maladies Infectieuses* [online],. Available from: http://www.ncbi.nlm.nih.gov/pubmed/21458935. [Accessed 2011-07-25], ISSN 1769-6690

Christeff, N.; Benassayag, C.; Carli-Vielle, C.; Carli, A. & Nunez, E. A. (1988). Elevated oestrogen and reduced testosterone levels in the serum of male septic shock patients. *Journal of Steroid Biochemistry*, Vol.29, No.4, pp. 435-440, ISSN 0022-4731

Chrousos, G. P. (2010). Stress and sex versus immunity and inflammation. *Science Signaling*, Vol.3, No.143, pp. 36, ISSN 1937-9145

Combes, A.; Luyt, C.-E.; Trouillet, J.-L.; Nieszkowska, A. & Chastre, J. (2009). Gender impact on the outcomes of critically ill patients with nosocomial infections. *Critical Care Medicine*, Vol.37, No.9, pp. 2506-2511, ISSN 1530-0293

Coronado, V. G.; Xu, L.; Basavaraju, S. V.; McGuire, L. C.; Wald, M. M.; Faul, M. D.; Guzman, B. R. & Hemphill, J. D. (2011). Surveillance for traumatic brain injury-related deaths-United States, 1997-2007. *MMWR. Surveillance Summaries: Morbidity and Mortality Weekly Report. Surveillance Summaries / CDC,* Vol.60, No.5, pp. 1-32, ISSN 1545-8636

Crabtree, T. D.; Pelletier, S. J.; Gleason, T. G.; Pruett, T. L. & Sawyer, R. G. (1999). Gender-dependent differences in outcome after the treatment of infection in hospitalized patients. *The Journal of the American Medical Association,* Vol.282, No.22, pp. 2143-2148, ISSN 0098-7484

Cristofaro, P. A.; Opal, S. M.; Palardy, J. E.; Parejo, N. A.; Jhung, J.; Keith, J. C., Jr & Harris, H. A. (2006). WAY-202196, a selective estrogen receptor-beta agonist, protects against death in experimental septic shock. *Critical Care Medicine,* Vol.34, No.8, pp. 2188-2193, ISSN 0090-3493

Davies R. P. O. ; Tocque, K. ; Bellis, M. A. ; Remmington, T. & Davies PDO (1999). Historical declines in tuberculosis in England and Wales: improving social conditions or natural selection? *Vesalius: Acta Internationales Historiae Medicinae,* Vol.5, No.1, pp. 25-29, ISSN

Demko, C. A.; Byard, P. J. & Davis, P. B. (1995). Gender differences in cystic fibrosis: *Pseudomonas aeruginosa* infection. *Journal of Clinical Epidemiology,* Vol.48, No.8, pp. 1041-1049, ISSN 0895-4356

Dienstknecht, T.; Schwacha, M. G.; Kang, S. C.; Rue, L. W.; Bland, K. I. & Chaudry, I. H. (2004). Sex steroid-mediated regulation of macrophage/monocyte function in a two-hit model of trauma-hemorrhage and sepsis. *Cytokine,* Vol.25, No.3, pp. 110-118, ISSN 1043-4666

Diodato, M. D.; Knöferl, M. W.; Schwacha, M. G.; Bland, K. I. & Chaudry, I. H. (2001). Gender differences in the inflammatory response and survival following haemorrhage and subsequent sepsis. *Cytokine,* Vol.14, No.3, pp. 162-169, ISSN 1043-4666

Dossett, L. A.; Swenson, B. R.; Evans, H. L.; Bonatti, H.; Sawyer, R. G. & May, A. K. (2008). Serum estradiol concentration as a predictor of death in critically ill and injured adults. *Surgical Infections,* Vol.9, No.1, pp. 41-48, ISSN 1096-2964

Duma, D.; Collins, J. B.; Chou, J. W. & Cidlowski, J. A. (2010). Sexually dimorphic actions of glucocorticoids provide a link to inflammatory diseases with gender differences in prevalence. *Science Signaling,* Vol.3, No.143, pp. 74, ISSN 1937-9145

Dyson, A. & Singer, M. (2009). Animal models of sepsis: why does preclinical efficacy fail to translate to the clinical setting? *Critical Care Medicine,* Vol.37, No.1 Suppl, pp. S30-37, ISSN 1530-0293

Esper, A. M.; Moss, M.; Lewis, C. A.; Nisbet, R.; Mannino, D. M. & Martin, G. S. (2006). The role of infection and comorbidity: Factors that influence disparities in sepsis. *Critical Care Medicine,* Vol.34, No.10, pp. 2576-2582, ISSN 0090-3493

Fish, E. N. (2008). The X-files in immunity: sex-based differences predispose immune responses. *Nature Reviews. Immunology,* Vol.8, No.9, pp. 737-744, ISSN 1474-1733

Fourrier, F.; Jallot, A.; Leclerc, L.; Jourdain, M.; Racadot, A.; Chagnon, J. L.; Rime, A. & Chopin, C. (1994). Sex steroid hormones in circulatory shock, sepsis syndrome, and septic shock. *Circulatory Shock,* Vol.43, No.4, pp. 171-178, ISSN 0092-6213

Grimaldi, C. M.; Cleary, J.; Dagtas, A. S.; Moussai, D. & Diamond, B. (2002). Estrogen alters thresholds for B cell apoptosis and activation. *The Journal of Clinical Investigation,* Vol.109, No.12, pp. 1625-1633, ISSN 0021-9738

Guilbault, C., Stotland, P., Lachance, C., Tam, M., Keller, A., Thompson-Snipes, L., Cowley, E.; Hamilton, T. A.; Eidelman, D. H.; Stevenson, M. M. & Radzioch, D. (2002). Influence of gender and interleukin-10 deficiency on the inflammatory response during lung infection with *Pseudomonas aeruginosa* in mice. *Immunology*, Vol.107, No.3, pp. 297-305, ISSN 0019-2805

Houpikian, P. & Raoult, D. (2005). Blood culture-negative endocarditis in a reference center: etiologic diagnosis of 348 cases. *Medicine*, Vol.84, No.3, pp. 162-173, ISSN 0025-7974

Kahlke, V.; Dohm, C.; Brötzmann, K.; Schreiber, S. & Schröder, J. (2000). Gender-related therapy: early IL-10 administration after hemorrhage restores immune function in males but not in females. *Shock* , Vol.14, No.3, pp. 354-359, ISSN 1073-2322

Kato, K.; Chen, Y.; Nakane, A.; Minagawa, T.; Fujieda, K.; Kimura, T. & Yamamoto, K. (1988). Suppression of delayed-type hypersensitivity in mice pretreated with diethylstilbesterol: involvement of sex hormones in immunomodulation. *Journal of Leukocyte Biology*, Vol.43, No.6, pp. 530-538, ISSN 0741-5400

Kita, E.; Yagyu, Y.; Nishikawa, F.; Hamuro, A.; Oku, D.; Emoto, M.; Katsui, N. & Kashiba, S. (1989). Alterations of host resistance to mouse typhoid infection by sex hormones. *Journal of Leukocyte Biology*, Vol.46, No.6, pp. 538-546, ISSN 0741-5400

Knöferl, M. W.; Angele, M. K.; Diodato, M. D.; Schwacha, M. G.; Ayala, A.; Cioffi, W. G.; Bland, K. I. & Chaudry, I. H. (2002). Female sex hormones regulate macrophage function after trauma-hemorrhage and prevent increased death rate from subsequent sepsis. *Annals of Surgery*, Vol.235, No.1, pp. 105-112, ISSN 0003-4932

Kramer, P. R.; Kramer, S. F. & Guan, G. (2004). 17 beta-estradiol regulates cytokine release through modulation of CD16 expression in monocytes and monocyte-derived macrophages. *Arthritis and Rheumatism*, Vol.50, No.6, pp. 1967-1975, ISSN 0004-3591

Lappen, J. R.; Keene, M.; Lore, M.; Grobman, W. A. & Gossett, D. R. (2010). Existing models fail to predict sepsis in an obstetric population with intrauterine infection. *American Journal of Obstetrics and Gynecology*, Vol.203, No.6, pp. 573-578, ISSN 1097-6868

Laubach, V. E.; Foley, P. L.; Shockey, K. S.; Tribble, C. G. & Kron, I. L. (1998). Protective roles of nitric oxide and testosterone in endotoxemia: evidence from NOS-2-deficient mice. *The American Journal of Physiology*, Vol.275, No.6, pp. H2211-2218, ISSN 0002-9513

Laupland, K. B.; Gregson, D. B.; Zygun, D. A.; Doig, C. J.; Mortis, G. & Church, D. L. (2004). Severe bloodstream infections: a population-based assessment. *Critical Care Medicine*, Vol.32, No.4, pp. 992-997, ISSN 0090-3493

Leone, M. ; Garcin, F. ; Bouvenot, J. ; Boyadjev, I.; Visintini, P.; Albanèse, J. & Martin, C. (2007). Ventilator-associated pneumonia: breaking the vicious circle of antibiotic overuse. *Critical Care Medicine*, Vol.35, No.2, pp. 379-385, ISSN 0090-3493

Leone, M.; Honstettre, A.; Lepidi, H.; Capo, C.; Bayard; F., Raoult, D. & Mege, J.-L. (2004). Effect of sex on *Coxiella burnetii* infection: protective role of 17beta-estradiol. *The Journal of Infectious Diseases*, Vol.189, No.2, pp. 339-345, ISSN 0022-1899

Lopes, J. A.; Fernandes, P.; Jorge, S.; Resina, C.; Santos, C.; Pereira, A.; Neves, J.; Antunes, F. & Gomes da Costa, A. (2010). Long-term risk of mortality after acute kidney injury in patients with sepsis: a contemporary analysis. *BMC Nephrology*, Vol.11, pp. 9, ISSN 1471-2369

Lorber, B. (1997). Listeriosis. *Clinical Infectious Diseases: An Official Publication of the Infectious Diseases Society of America*, Vol.24, No.1, pp. 1-9; quiz 10-11, ISSN 1058-4838

Majetschak, M.; Christensen, B.; Obertacke, U.; Waydhas, C.; Schindler, A. E.; Nast-Kolb, D. & Schade, F. U. (2000). Sex differences in posttraumatic cytokine release of endotoxin-stimulated whole blood: relationship to the development of severe sepsis. *The Journal of Trauma*, Vol.48, No.5, pp. 832-839, ISSN 0022-5282

Maltezou, H. C. & Raoult, D. (2002). Q fever in children. *The Lancet Infectious Diseases*, Vol.2, No.11, pp. 686-691, ISSN 1473-3099

Mandel, T. E. & Cheers, C. (1980). Resistance and susceptibility of mice to bacterial infection: histopathology of listeriosis in resistant and susceptible strains. *Infection and Immunity*, Vol.30, No.3, pp. 851-861, ISSN 0019-9567

Martin, G. S.; Mannino, D. M.; Eaton, S. & Moss, M. (2003). The epidemiology of sepsis in the United States from 1979 through 2000. *The New England Journal of Medicine*, Vol.348, No.16, pp. 1546-1554, ISSN 1533-4406

May, A. K.; Dossett, L. A.; Norris, P. R.; Hansen, E. N.; Dorsett, R. C.; Popovsky, K. A. & Sawyer, R. G. (2008). Estradiol is associated with mortality in critically ill trauma and surgical patients. *Critical Care Medicine*, Vol.36, No.1, pp. 62-68, ISSN 1530-0293

McCombe, P. A.; Greer, J. M. & Mackay, I. R. (2009). Sexual dimorphism in autoimmune disease. *Current Molecular Medicine*, Vol.9, No.9, pp. 1058-1079, ISSN 1875-5666

Melamed, A. & Sorvillo, F. J. (2009). The burden of sepsis-associated mortality in the United States from 1999 to 2005: an analysis of multiple-cause-of-death data. *Critical Care*, Vol.13, No.1, pp. R28, ISSN 1466-609X

Micheli, A.; Ciampichini, R.; Oberaigner, W.; Ciccolallo, L.; de Vries, E.; Izarzugaza, I.; Zambon, P.; Gatta, G. & De Angelis, R. (2009). The advantage of women in cancer survival: an analysis of EUROCARE-4 data. *European Journal of Cancer*, Vol.45, No.6, pp. 1017-1027, ISSN 1879-0852

Morales-Montor, J.; Chavarria, A.; De León, M. A.; Del Castillo, L. I.; Escobedo, E. G.; Sánchez, E. N.; Vargas, J. A.; Hernández-Flores, M.; Romo-González, T. & Larralde, C. (2004). Host gender in parasitic infections of mammals: an evaluation of the female host supremacy paradigm. *The Journal of Parasitology*, Vol.90, No.3, pp. 531-546, ISSN 0022-3395

Moss, M. (2005). Epidemiology of sepsis: race, sex, and chronic alcohol abuse. *Clinical Infectious Diseases: An Official Publication of the Infectious Diseases Society of America*, Vol.41 No.Suppl 7, pp. S490-497, ISSN 1537-6591

Munoz-Suano, A.; Hamilton, A. B. & Betz, A. G. (2011). Gimme shelter: the immune system during pregnancy. *Immunological Reviews*, Vol.241, No.1, pp. 20-38, ISSN 1600-065X

Nachtigall, I.; Tafelski, S.; Rothbart, A.; Kaufner, L.; Schmidt, M.; Tamarkin, A.; Kartachov, M.; Zebedies, D.; Trefzer, T.; Wernecke, K.-D. & Spies, C. (2011). Gender related outcome difference is related to course of sepsis on mixed ICUs - a prospective, observational clinical study. *Critical Care*, Vol.15, No.3, pp. R151, ISSN 1466-609X

Odetola, F. O.; Gebremariam, A. & Freed, G. L. (2007). Patient and hospital correlates of clinical outcomes and resource utilization in severe pediatric sepsis. *Pediatrics*, Vol.119, No.3, pp. 487-494, ISSN 1098-4275

Olubuyide, I. O. (1992). Factors that may contribute to death from typhoid infection among Nigerians. *West African Journal of Medicine*, Vol.11, No.2, pp. 112-115, ISSN 0189-160X

Osborn, T. M.; Tracy, J. K.; Dunne, J. R.; Pasquale, M. & Napolitano, L. M. (2004). Epidemiology of sepsis in patients with traumatic injury. *Critical Care Medicine*, Vol.32, No.11, pp. 2234-2240, ISSN 0090-3493

Pejcic-Karapetrovic, B.; Gurnani, K.; Russell, M. S.; Finlay, B. B.; Sad, S. & Krishnan, L. (2007). Pregnancy impairs the innate immune resistance to *Salmonella typhimurium* leading to rapid fatal infection. *Journal of Immunology*, Vol.179, No.9, pp. 6088-6096, ISSN 0022-1767

Pietropaoli, A. P.; Glance, L. G.; Oakes, D. & Fisher, S. G. (2010). Gender differences in mortality in patients with severe sepsis or septic shock. *Gender Medicine*, Vol.7, No.5, pp. 422-437, ISSN 1878-7398

Pinkhasov, R. M.; Shteynshlyuger, A.; Hakimian, P.; Lindsay, G. K.; Samadi, D. B. & Shabsigh, R. (2010). Are men shortchanged on health? Perspective on life expectancy, morbidity, and mortality in men and women in the United States. *International Journal of Clinical Practice*, Vol.64, No.4, pp. 465-474, ISSN 1742-1241

Pung, O. J.; Luster, M. I.; Hayes, H. T. & Rader, J. (1984). Influence of steroidal and nonsteroidal sex hormones on host resistance in mice: increased susceptibility to *Listeria monocytogenes* after exposure to estrogenic hormones. *Infection and Immunity*, Vol.46, No.2, pp. 301-307, ISSN 0019-9567

Raoult, D. ; Tissot-Dupont, H. ; Foucault, C. ; Gouvernet, J. ; Fournier, P. E. ; Bernit, E. ; Stein, A. ; Nesri, M. ; Harle, J. R. & Weiller, P. J. (2000). Q fever 1985-1998. Clinical and epidemiologic features of 1,383 infections. *Medicine*, Vol.79, No.2, pp. 109-123, ISSN 0025-7974

Rettew, J. A.; Huet-Hudson, Y. M. & Marriott, I. (2008). Testosterone reduces macrophage expression in the mouse of toll-like receptor 4, a trigger for inflammation and innate immunity. *Biology of Reproduction*, Vol.78, No.3, pp. 432-437, ISSN 0006-3363

Rettew, J. A.; Huet, Y. M. & Marriott, I. (2009). Estrogens augment cell surface TLR4 expression on murine macrophages and regulate sepsis susceptibility in vivo. *Endocrinology*, Vol.150, No.8, pp. 3877-3884, ISSN 1945-7170

Rey, A. D.; Mahuad, C. V.; Bozza, V. V.; Bogue, C.; Farroni, M. A.; Bay, M. L.; Bottasso, O. A. & Besedovsky, H. O. (2007). Endocrine and cytokine responses in humans with pulmonary tuberculosis. *Brain, Behavior, and Immunity*, Vol.21, No.2, pp. 171-179, ISSN 0889-1591

Rose, A. M.; Watson, J. M.; Graham, C.; Nunn, A. J.; Drobniewski, F.; Ormerod, L. P.; Darbyshire, J. H. & Leese, J. (2001). Tuberculosis at the end of the 20th century in England and Wales: results of a national survey in 1998. *Thorax*, Vol.56, No.3, pp. 173-179, ISSN 0040-6376

Salem, M. L.; Matsuzaki, G.; Madkour, G. A. & Nomoto, K. (1999). Beta-estradiol-induced decrease in IL-12 and TNF-alpha expression suppresses macrophage functions in the course of *Listeria monocytogenes* infection in mice. *International Journal of Immunopharmacology*, Vol.21, No.8, pp. 481-497, ISSN 0192-0561

Snider, H.; Lezama-Davila, C.; Alexander, J. & Satoskar, A. R. (2009). Sex hormones and modulation of immunity against leishmaniasis. *Neuroimmunomodulation*, Vol.16, No.2, pp. 106-113, ISSN 1423-0216

Soucy, G.; Boivin, G.; Labrie, F. & Rivest, S. (2005). Estradiol is required for a proper immune response to bacterial and viral pathogens in the female brain. *Journal of Immunology*, Vol.174, No.10, pp. 6391-6398, ISSN 0022-1767

Spinedi, E.; Suescun, M. O.; Hadid, R.; Daneva, T. & Gaillard, R. C. (1992). Effects of gonadectomy and sex hormone therapy on the endotoxin-stimulated hypothalamo-pituitary-adrenal axis: evidence for a neuroendocrine-immunological sexual dimorphism. *Endocrinology*, Vol.131, No.5, pp. 2430-2436, ISSN 0013-7227

Stein, A.; Lepidi, H.; Mege, J. L.; Marrie, T. J. & Raoult, D. (2000). Repeated pregnancies in BALB/c mice infected with *Coxiella burnetii* cause disseminated infection, resulting in stillbirth and endocarditis. *The Journal of Infectious Diseases*, Vol.181, No.1, pp. 188-194, ISSN 0022-1899

Suzuki, T.; Shimizu, T.; Yu, H.-P.; Hsieh, Y.-C.; Choudhry, M. A.; Schwacha, M. G. & Chaudry, I. H. (2007). Tissue compartment-specific role of estrogen receptor subtypes in immune cell cytokine production following trauma-hemorrhage. *Journal of Applied Physiology*, Vol.102, No.1, pp. 163-168, ISSN 8750-7587

Textoris, J.; Ban, L. H.; Capo, C.; Raoult, D.; Leone, M. & Mege, J.-L. (2010). Sex-related differences in gene expression following *Coxiella burnetii* infection in mice: potential role of circadian rhythm. *PloS One*, Vol.5, No.8, pp. e12190, ISSN 1932-6203

Theobald, S.; Tolhurst, R. & Squire, S. B. (2006). Gender, equity: new approaches for effective management of communicable diseases. *Transactions of the Royal Society of Tropical Medicine and Hygiene*, Vol.100, No.4, pp. 299-304, ISSN 0035-9203

Tissot-Dupont, H.; Vaillant, V.; Rey, S. & Raoult, D. (2007). Role of sex, age, previous valve lesion, and pregnancy in the clinical expression and outcome of Q fever after a large outbreak. *Clinical Infectious Diseases: An Official Publication of the Infectious Diseases Society of America*, Vol.44, No.2, pp. 232-237, ISSN 1537-6591

Tissot Dupont, H.; Raoult, D.; Brouqui, P.; Janbon, F.; Peyramond, D.; Weiller, P. J.; Chicheportiche, C.; Nezri, M. & Poirier, R. (1992). Epidemiologic features and clinical presentation of acute Q fever in hospitalized patients: 323 French cases. *The American Journal of Medicine*, Vol.93, No.4, pp. 427-434, ISSN 0002-9343

Torres, M. B.; Trentzsch, H.; Stewart, D.; Mooney, M. L.; Fuentes, J. M.; Saad, D. F.; Reeves, R. H. & De Maio, A. (2005). Protection from lethal endotoxic shock after testosterone depletion is linked to chromosome X. *Shock*, Vol.24, No.4, pp. 318-323, ISSN 1073-2322

Trentzsch, H.; Stewart, D. & De Maio, A. (2003). Genetic background conditions the effect of sex steroids on the inflammatory response during endotoxic shock. *Critical Care Medicine*, Vol.31, No.1, pp. 232-236, ISSN 0090-3493

Tsuyuguchi, K.; Suzuki, K.; Matsumoto, H.; Tanaka, E.; Amitani, R. & Kuze, F. (2001). Effect of oestrogen on *Mycobacterium avium* complex pulmonary infection in mice. *Clinical and Experimental Immunology*, Vol.123, No.3, pp. 428-434, ISSN 0009-9104

van Eijk, L. T.; Dorresteijn, M. J.; Smits, P.; van der Hoeven, J. G.; Netea, M. G. & Pickkers, P. (2007). Gender differences in the innate immune response and vascular reactivity following the administration of endotoxin to human volunteers. *Critical Care Medicine*, Vol.35, No.6, pp. 1464-1469, ISSN 0090-3493

Verthelyi, D. (2001). Sex hormones as immunomodulators in health and disease. *International Immunopharmacology*, Vol.1, No.6, pp. 983-993, ISSN 1567-5769

Wafaisade, A.; Lefering, R.; Bouillon, B.; Sakka, S. G.; Thamm, O. C.; Paffrath, T.; Neugebauer, E. & Maegele, M. (2011). Epidemiology and risk factors of sepsis after multiple trauma: an analysis of 29,829 patients from the Trauma Registry of the

German Society for Trauma Surgery. *Critical Care Medicine*, Vol.39, No.4, pp. 621-628, ISSN 1530-0293

Wang, Y. ; Cela, E. ; Gagnon, S. & Sweezey, N. B. (2010). Estrogen aggravates inflammation in *Pseudomonas aeruginosa* pneumonia in cystic fibrosis mice. *Respiratory Research*, Vol.11, 166, ISSN 1465-993X

Yamamoto, Y.; Saito, H.; Setogawa, T. & Tomioka, H. (1991). Sex differences in host resistance to *Mycobacterium marinum* infection in mice. *Infection and Immunity*, Vol.59, No.11, pp. 4089-4096, ISSN 0019-9567

11

The Special Implication of Sex Hormones on Dendritic Cells During Pregnancy

Sabine E. Segerer and Ulrike Kämmerer
University of Würzburg, Department of Obstetrics and Gynaecology, Würzburg, Germany

1. Introduction

Pregnancy bears a great challenge to the immune system: simultaneously, immune cells have to protect the reproductive tract against imminent infections, while the developing conceptus has to be tolerated. To face this problem, a distinct composition of immune cells has to be present in the decidualized endometrium (Gomez-Lopez, Guilbert *et al.*, 2010). The predominant subsets amongst those represent uterine natural killer cells (uNK cells) and cells of the monocyte/macrophage lineage like monocytes, macrophages and dendritic cells (DC) (Loke and King, 1995). Among the latter ones, DC as antigen-presenting cells (APC) are forming an important subgroup (Steinman, 2003).

DC represent a highly adaptive cell type, which can either be transformed into an immunostimulatory phenotype after exposure to inflammatory or infectious signals or into a tolerogenic phenotype preventing T cell activation when located in an adequate anti-inflammatory microenvironment. Establishing contact with invading microorganisms or cells, DC acquire their antigens and process them into antigenic peptides in the context of MHC class I and class II molecules as ligands for antigen-specific T cell receptors. This action is accompanied by migration of DC to secondary lymphoid organs. Here, the processed antigens are presented together with co-stimulatory molecules like CD40, CD80 and CD86 as well as CD83 and MHC molecules (Inaba, Metlay *et al.*, 1990;Steinman, 2003) to select and activate naive T cells (Sallusto and Lanzavecchia, 1999).

Apart from antigens, DC differentiation and maturation is considerably influenced by cytokines, hormones and other soluble factors. Lacking infectious/danger- signals or localiezed in a distinct anti-inflammatory micromilieu (e.g. TGF beta, IL-10), a specific phenotype of DC is generated which prevents T cell activation and which is supposed to protect the semi-allogenic fetus (Rutella, Bonanno *et al.*, 2006).

In human endometrium only a small number of fully matured DC are detected (Rieger, Honig *et al.*, 2004). Thereby, the amount of mature, CD83+ DC is generally low in both pregnant and non-pregnant endometrium with a slight peak in late secretory phase endometrium. During pregnancy, a distinct DC subtype expressing CD14, CD68, HLA-DR and DC-SIGN is found in increased levels in decidua (Bonifaz, Bonnyay *et al.*, 2002;Kammerer, Eggert *et al.*, 2003). These DC, presumably an intertype between immature DC (iDC) and macrophages, are supposed to represent a "pro-fetal" tolerogenic population which is able to induce a TH2 pre-dominant state (Miyazaki, Tsuda *et al.*, 2003) and to suppress the activation of T cells (Kammerer, Eggert *et al.*, 2003).

There is evidence that female sex hormones contribute to the modulation of decidual immune cells into tolerogenic subtypes (for review see: (Kyurkchiev, Ivanova-Todorova *et al.*, 2010) and especially can impact on DC (Segerer, Muller *et al.*, 2009). Thereby, the "micromilieu" determines if the captured antigens are presented in a tolerogenic or immune activating way resulting also in different phenotypes of DC. In the following, we will highlight the impact of the characteristic pregnancy hormones on DC and their potent implication on the development of a tolerogenic subtype of DC.

2. hCG

Human chorionic gonadotropin (hCG) is a heterodimeric hormone of the glycoprotein hormone family and is composed by two subunits linked in a non-covalent way. While the alpha subunit does not differ from the other glycoprotein hormones, the beta subunit of hCG represents the biggest one of the glycoprotein hormones holding a large glycosylated domain which refers to its high stability. hCG represents the very early hormonal factor of pregnancy already produced by the trophoblast layer of the blastocyst before implantation (Bonduelle, Dodd *et al.*, 1988;Lopata and Hay, 1989) and after implantation by the syncytiotrophoblast in increasing amounts (Hoshina, Boothby *et al.*, 1985). The production of hCG reaches a peak between the 10th and 11th week of gestation and thereafter declines to a lower but constant level throughout pregnancy. Preventing luteolysis of the corpus luteum and stimulating the production of progesterone (Keay, Vatish *et al.*, 2004), hCG represents the essential factor to protect and to promote early pregnancy. Despite of these direct effects, hCG can also act as a paracrine factor modulating the proliferation of myometrial smooth muscle cells (Horiuchi, Nikaido *et al.*, 2000;Kornyei, Lei *et al.*, 1993) and increasing endometrial angiogenesis (Berndt, Blacher *et al.*, 2009).

There is also evidence that hCG contributes to maternal tolerance of the developing conceptus by influencing the surrounding immune cells. Thus, experiments on uNK cells revealed that hCG acts as a regulator of uNK cell proliferation (Kane, Kelly *et al.*, 2009). Despite of this direct effect on uNK cell proliferation, hCG can facilitate the adequate establishment and maintenance of pregnancy by inducing the secretion factors which promote angiogeneis by uNK cells and thus could even support placentation (Lash, Schiessl *et al.*, 2006).

Investigations on DC demonstrated hCG receptors to be constitutively expressed by these cells which allows a direct activation of DC via hCG (Yoshimura, Inaba *et al.*, 2003). Experiments on mouse DC revealed that hCG acts in an immunregulatory way by increasing the production of immunosuppressive factors like Interleukin-10 (IL-10) by DC and by reducing antigen-specific T-cell proliferation (Wan, Versnel *et al.*, 2008). In humans, hCG was also able to significantly decrease T-cell stimulatory capacity of DC (Huck, Steck *et al.*, 2005). In contrast, the phenotype of hCG-treated DC ressembeled that of matured DC expressing co-stimulatory molecules like CD 40, CD83 and CD 86 (Segerer, Muller *et al.*, 2009). Thus, hCG seems to be able to induce a tolerogenic subtype of DC even though co-stimulatory molecules of the mature subtype were expressed.

3. Estrogen

Estrogen receptors (ER) alpha and beta (ER α/β) are widely expressed in human endometrium but also in most immune cells (Lindzey, Wetsel *et al.*, 1998). Thereby, they are localized in different cellular compartments. The cytoplasmatic and membrane associated receptors confer to specific intracellular signaling pathways promoting genomic and non-genomic effects. Gene transcription and regulation is also mediated by nuclear ER acting as transcription factors and thus regulating long-term effects (Tamrazi, Carlson *et al.*, 2002;Biswas, Singh *et al.*, 2005). Recently, another estrogen receptor, GPR30, which represents an intracellular transmembrane G protein-coupled receptor was detected (Revankar, Cimino *et al.*, 2005). This receptor is proposed to initiate rapid non-genomic signaling effects and was found to be expressed in human endometrium throughout menstrual cycle and in early pregnancy decidua (Kolkova, Noskova *et al.*, 2010).

B and T lymphocytes were detected to be specific targets of estradiol (Peeva and Zouali, 2005;Nalbandian, Paharkova-Vatchkova *et al.*, 2005;Nalbandian and Kovats, 2005;Smithson, Couse *et al.*, 1998). Thereby, estrogen was able to modulate B lymphopoiesis and the production of immunoglobulins (Ig) where effects were mediated via ERα (Erlandsson, Jonsson *et al.*, 2003). T cell function was found to be modulated by estradiol changing the cytokine profile (Karpuzoglu and Zouali, 2011;Pernis, 2007;Salem, 2004).

Regarding DC, estradiol effects were mediated via ERα and β, both of which are expressed in DC. So far, the intracellular G-protein receptor GPR 30 has not been described in DC. Even though estradiol promotes the differentiation of DC (Paharkova-Vatchkova, Maldonado *et al.*, 2004;Segerer, Muller *et al.*, 2009) towards an immunostimulatory phenotype, expressing co-stimulatory molecules like CD40, CD83 and CD86, T-cell priming was significantly impaired in the presence of estradiol (Segerer, Muller *et al.*, 2009). In addition, investigations of the effects of E2 on murine spleen CD11c-positive dendritic cells revealed an increased stimulatory capacity of DCs and an elevated expression of the anti-inflammatory cytokines like IL-10 (Yang, Hu *et al.*, 2006).

In autoimmune diseases, estrogens seem to have conflicting effects on immune cells. While a reduction of disease activity was seen during pregnancy in multiple sclerosis, it was reported that systemic lupus erythematodes (SLE) could frequently flare up during pregnancy and remit with menopause (Petri, Howard *et al.*, 1991).

It could be speculated, that the effect of estrogen on DC participates in the flare up of SLE during pregnancy: DC generated from monocytes which were isolated from patients suffering from SLE exhibited a matured, pro-inflammatory phenotype, expressing co-stimulatory molecules. In addition, these SLE-DC were very effective in activating T-cells (Ding, Mehta *et al.*, 2006). Perhaps, estrogen could even accelerate the maturation-process of SLE-DC and thus promote disease during ongoing pregnancy.

4. Progesterone

During the menstrual cycle, progesterone is produced by granulosa cells and the corpus luteum (Bachelot and Binart, 2005). In pregnancy, the corpus luteum is rescued 4-5 weeks after implantation. At that time, placental progesterone production becames sufficient to maintain pregnancy (Csapo and Pulkkinen, 1978). Several studies revealed that progesterone acts in an immunosuppressive way (Stites and Siiteri, 1983;Miyaura and Iwata, 2002b). Analysing the effects of progesterone on T lymphocytes, a direct and indirect inhibition of TH1 cell development was detected (Miyaura and Iwata, 2002a). DC cultured under the influence of progesterone changed their phenotype into an immunostimulatory maturated phenotype expressing co-stimulatory molecules (Ivanova, Kyurkchiev *et al.*, 2005;Segerer, Muller *et al.*, 2009). In contrast to effects seen for hCG and estradiol, the capacity of DC to stimulate T-cell proliferation was not significantly altered (Segerer, Muller *et al.*, 2009). However, progesterone had profound effects on rat mDC by suppressing the production of pro-inflammatory cytokines like tumor necrosis factor alpha (TNFα) and interleukin 1beta (IL-1β) as well as by inhibiting the DC-stimulated proliferation of T-cells (Butts, Shukair *et al.*, 2007). Thus, even though the expression of co-stimulatory molecules and T-cell stimulatory capacity was not affected progesterone seems to modulate immune responses by changing the cytokine secretion prolife.

5. Activin A and inhibin A

Activin A represents a distinct growth factor and member of the TGF beta superfamily (Chang, Brown *et al.*, 2002) which is composed by two activin β_A subunits. Its counterpart inhibin A is formed by a dimer consisting of an activin β subunit and a structurally different α subunit (Phillips, Jones *et al.*, 2005). Initially, the function of these glycoprotein hormones was defined as feedback factors regulating the release of the follicle-stimulating hormone (FSH) (Tong, Wallace *et al.*, 2003). Later, it was observed that activin A and inhibin A are endowed by diverse functions acting as cytokines in an autocrine or paracrine manner, too. Thus, activin A was detected to be involved in inflammatory responses (Jones, de Kretser *et al.*, 2004) and acting as a chemoattractant for monocytes (Eramaa, Hurme *et al.*, 1992;Shao, Frigon, Jr. *et al.*, 1992).

During pregnancy, activin A and inhibin A are locally produced by human placenta, decidua and fetal membranes resulting in serum levels in the low ng/ml range peaking at 10 weeks of gestation (Lockwood, Ledger *et al.*, 1997). Both glycoprotein hormones seem to have some impact on implantation and early embryo development (Birdsall, Ledger *et al.*, 1997;Muttukrishna, Jauniaux *et al.*, 2004;Jones, Salamonsen *et al.*, 2002). Furthermore, they have been found to be useful diagnostic markers for pregnancy success. While decreasing activin A levels indicated both an ongoing miscarriage or ectopic pregnancy (Florio, Severi *et al.*, 2007), decreasing inhibin A levels were used as a specific marker to reveal preclinical abortions (Muttukrishna, Jauniaux *et al.*, 2004;Prakash, Laird *et al.*, 2005).

Previous studies revealed that activin A is able to modulate immune responses via type I and II activin receptors on DC (Robson, Phillips *et al.*, 2008). Even though the expression of co-stimulatory molecules was not significantly affected neither by activin A nor inhibin A, both glycoprotein hormones were able to decrease the T-cell stimulatory capacity of DC. Thus, we propose that activin A and inhibin A are distinct modulating factors that could promote the generation of tolerance-inducing DC by affecting their T-cell stimulatory capacity (Segerer, Muller *et al.*, 2008) .

	DC phenotype	**T-cell stimulatory capacity**	**cytokines**
hCG	immunostimulatory (CD40 ↑, CD83 ↑, CD86 ↑)	↓	IL-10 ↑
estrogen	immunostimulatory (CD40 ↑, CD83 ↑, CD86 ↑)	↓	IL-10 ↑
progesterone	immunostimulatory (CD40 ↑, CD83 ↑, CD86 ↑)	↓ (in rats) → (in humans)	TNF-α ↓, IL-1 β ↓ (in rats)
activin A and inhibin A	immunostimulatory (CD40 ↑, CD83 ↑, CD86 ↑)	↓	no significant effects

Table 1.

6. Summary

During pregnancy, the levels of the glycoprotein hormones activin A and inhibin A as well as female sex hormones (hCG, estradiol, progesterone) are substantially elevated in parallel with increased occurrence of cells of the monocyte/macrophage lineage like DC in the decidua. In vitro experiments revealed that all of them can induce a tolerogenic subtype of DC even though effects were found on different levels (reduction of the expression of co-stimulatory molecules, reduction of T-cell stimulation, tolerogenic cytokine-profile). Thus, this distinct mixture of hormonal factors seems to be indispensable to support the development of tolerance-inducing DC which could play a key role in the acceptance of the fetus.

7. References

[1] Bachelot A and Binart N (2005) Corpus luteum development: lessons from genetic models in mice. Curr Top Dev Biol, 68, 49-84.
[2] Berndt S, Blacher S, Perrier dS, Thiry M, Tsampalas M, Cruz A, Pequeux C, Lorquet S, Munaut C, Noel A et al (2009) Chorionic gonadotropin stimulation of angiogenesis and pericyte recruitment. J Clin Endocrinol Metab, 94, 4567-4574.
[3] Birdsall M, Ledger W, Groome N, Abdalla H, and Muttukrishna S (1997) Inhibin A and activin A in the first trimester of human pregnancy. J Clin Endocrinol Metab, 82, 1557-1560.
[4] Biswas DK, Singh S, Shi Q, Pardee AB, and Iglehart JD (2005) Crossroads of estrogen receptor and NF-kappaB signaling. Sci STKE, 2005, e27.
[5] Bonduelle ML, Dodd R, Liebaers I, Van SA, Williamson R, and Akhurst R (1988) Chorionic gonadotrophin-beta mRNA, a trophoblast marker, is expressed in human 8-cell embryos derived from tripronucleate zygotes. Hum Reprod, 3, 909-914.
[6] Bonifaz L, Bonnyay D, Mahnke K, Rivera M, Nussenzweig MC, and Steinman RM (2002) Efficient targeting of protein antigen to the dendritic cell receptor DEC-205 in the steady state leads to antigen presentation on major histocompatibility complex class I products and peripheral CD8+ T cell tolerance. J Exp Med, 196, 1627-1638.
[7] Butts CL, Shukair SA, Duncan KM, Bowers E, Horn C, Belyavskaya E, Tonelli L, and Sternberg EM (2007) Progesterone inhibits mature rat dendritic cells in a receptor-mediated fashion. Int Immunol, 19, 287-296.
[8] Chang H, Brown CW, and Matzuk MM (2002) Genetic analysis of the mammalian transforming growth factor-beta superfamily. Endocr Rev, 23, 787-823.
[9] Csapo AI and Pulkkinen M (1978) Indispensability of the human corpus luteum in the maintenance of early pregnancy. Luteectomy evidence. Obstet Gynecol Surv, 33, 69-81.
[10] Ding D, Mehta H, McCune WJ, and Kaplan MJ (2006) Aberrant phenotype and function of myeloid dendritic cells in systemic lupus erythematosus. J Immunol, 177, 5878-5889.
[11] Eramaa M, Hurme M, Stenman UH, and Ritvos O (1992) Activin A/erythroid differentiation factor is induced during human monocyte activation. J Exp Med, 176, 1449-1452.
[12] Erlandsson MC, Jonsson CA, Islander U, Ohlsson C, and Carlsten H (2003) Oestrogen receptor specificity in oestradiol-mediated effects on B lymphopoiesis and immunoglobulin production in male mice. Immunology, 108, 346-351.

[13] Florio P, Severi FM, Bocchi C, Luisi S, Mazzini M, Danero S, Torricelli M, and Petraglia F (2007) Single serum activin a testing to predict ectopic pregnancy. J Clin Endocrinol Metab, 92, 1748-1753.
[14] Gomez-Lopez N, Guilbert LJ, and Olson DM (2010) Invasion of the leukocytes into the fetal-maternal interface during pregnancy. J Leukoc Biol, 88, 625-633.
[15] Horiuchi A, Nikaido T, Yoshizawa T, Itoh K, Kobayashi Y, Toki T, Konishi I, and Fujii S (2000) HCG promotes proliferation of uterine leiomyomal cells more strongly than that of myometrial smooth muscle cells in vitro. Mol Hum Reprod, 6, 523-528.
[16] 16. Hoshina M, Boothby M, Hussa R, Pattillo R, Camel HM, and Boime I (1985) Linkage of human chorionic gonadotrophin and placental lactogen biosynthesis to trophoblast differentiation and tumorigenesis. Placenta, 6, 163-172.
[17] Huck B, Steck T, Habersack M, Dietl J, and Kammerer U (2005) Pregnancy associated hormones modulate the cytokine production but not the phenotype of PBMC-derived human dendritic cells. Eur J Obstet Gynecol Reprod Biol, 122, 85-94.
[18] Inaba K, Metlay JP, Crowley MT, Witmer-Pack M, and Steinman RM (1990) Dendritic cells as antigen presenting cells in vivo. Int Rev Immunol, 6, 197-206.
[19] Ivanova E, Kyurkchiev D, Altankova I, Dimitrov J, Binakova E, and Kyurkchiev S (2005) CD83 monocyte-derived dendritic cells are present in human decidua and progesterone induces their differentiation in vitro. Am J Reprod Immunol, 53, 199-205.
[20] Jones KL, de Kretser DM, Patella S, and Phillips DJ (2004) Activin A and follistatin in systemic inflammation. Mol Cell Endocrinol, 225, 119-125.
[21] Jones RL, Salamonsen LA, and Findlay JK (2002) Potential roles for endometrial inhibins, activins and follistatin during human embryo implantation and early pregnancy. Trends Endocrinol Metab, 13, 144-150.
[22] Kammerer U, Eggert AO, Kapp M, McLellan AD, Geijtenbeek TB, Dietl J, van Kooyk Y, and Kampgen E (2003) Unique appearance of proliferating antigen-presenting cells expressing DC-SIGN (CD209) in the decidua of early human pregnancy. Am J Pathol, 162, 887-896.
[23] Kane N, Kelly R, Saunders PT, and Critchley HO (2009) Proliferation of uterine natural killer cells is induced by human chorionic gonadotropin and mediated via the mannose receptor. Endocrinology, 150, 2882-2888.
[24] Karpuzoglu E and Zouali M (2011) The multi-faceted influences of estrogen on lymphocytes: toward novel immuno-interventions strategies for autoimmunity management. Clin Rev Allergy Immunol, 40, 16-26.
[25] Keay SD, Vatish M, Karteris E, Hillhouse EW, and Randeva HS (2004) The role of hCG in reproductive medicine. BJOG, 111, 1218-1228.
[26] Kolkova Z, Noskova V, Ehinger A, Hansson S, Casslén B (2010) G protein-coupled estrogen receptor 1 (GPER, GPR 30) in normal human endometrium and early pregnancy decidua. Mol Hum Reprod, 16(10):743-51.
[27] Kornyei JL, Lei ZM, and Rao CV (1993) Human myometrial smooth muscle cells are novel targets of direct regulation by human chorionic gonadotropin. Biol Reprod, 49, 1149-1157.
[28] Kyurkchiev D, Ivanova-Todorova E, and Kyurkchiev SD (2010) New target cells of the immunomodulatory effects of progesterone. Reprod Biomed Online, 21, 304-311.

[29] Lash GE, Schiessl B, Kirkley M, Innes BA, Cooper A, Searle RF, Robson SC, and Bulmer JN (2006) Expression of angiogenic growth factors by uterine natural killer cells during early pregnancy. J Leukoc Biol, 80, 572-580.

[30] Lindzey J, Wetsel WC, Couse JF, Stoker T, Cooper R, and Korach KS (1998) Effects of castration and chronic steroid treatments on hypothalamic gonadotropin-releasing hormone content and pituitary gonadotropins in male wild-type and estrogen receptor-alpha knockout mice. Endocrinology, 139, 4092-4101.

[31] Lockwood GM, Ledger WL, Barlow DH, Groome NP, and Muttukrishna S (1997) Measurement of inhibin and activin in early human pregnancy: demonstration of fetoplacental origin and role in prediction of early-pregnancy outcome. Biol Reprod, 57, 1490-1494.

[32] Loke YW and King A (1995) Human Implantation. Cell Biology and Immunology., Cambridge University Press.

[33] Lopata A and Hay DL (1989) The potential of early human embryos to form blastocysts, hatch from their zona and secrete HCG in culture. Hum Reprod, 4, 87-94.

[34] Miyaura H and Iwata M (2002) Direct and indirect inhibition of Th1 development by progesterone and glucocorticoids. J Immunol, 168, 1087-1094.

[35] Miyazaki S, Tsuda H, Sakai M, Hori S, Sasaki Y, Futatani T, Miyawaki T, and Saito S (2003) Predominance of Th2-promoting dendritic cells in early human pregnancy decidua. J Leukoc Biol, 74, 514-522.

[36] Muttukrishna S, Jauniaux E, McGarrigle H, Groome N, and Rodeck CH (2004) In-vivo concentrations of inhibins, activin A and follistatin in human early pregnancy. Reprod Biomed Online, 8, 712-719.

[37] Nalbandian G and Kovats S (2005) Understanding sex biases in immunity: effects of estrogen on the differentiation and function of antigen-presenting cells. Immunol Res, 31, 91-106.

[38] Nalbandian G, Paharkova-Vatchkova V, Mao A, Nale S, and Kovats S (2005) The selective estrogen receptor modulators, tamoxifen and raloxifene, impair dendritic cell differentiation and activation. J Immunol, 175, 2666-2675.

[39] Paharkova-Vatchkova V, Maldonado R, and Kovats S (2004) Estrogen preferentially promotes the differentiation of CD11c+ CD11b(intermediate) dendritic cells from bone marrow precursors. J Immunol, 172, 1426-1436.

[40] Peeva E and Zouali M (2005) Spotlight on the role of hormonal factors in the emergence of autoreactive B-lymphocytes. Immunol Lett, 101, 123-143.

[41] Pernis AB (2007) Estrogen and CD4+ T cells. Curr Opin Rheumatol, 19, 414-420.

[42] Petri M, Howard D, and Repke J (1991) Frequency of lupus flare in pregnancy. The Hopkins Lupus Pregnancy Center experience. Arthritis Rheum, 34, 1538-1545.

[43] Phillips DJ, Jones KL, Clarke IJ, Scheerlinck JP, and de Kretser DM (2005) Activin A: from sometime reproductive factor to genuine cytokine. Vet Immunol Immunopathol, 108, 23-27.

[44] Prakash A, Laird S, Tuckerman E, Li TC, and Ledger WL (2005) Inhibin A and activin A may be used to predict pregnancy outcome in women with recurrent miscarriage. Fertil Steril, 83, 1758-1763.

[45] Revankar CM, Cimino DF, Sklar LA, Arterburn JB, Prossnitz ER (2005) A transmembrane intracellular estrogen receptor mediates rapid cell signaling. Science, 307(5715):1625-30.

[46] Rieger L, Honig A, Sutterlin M, Kapp M, Dietl J, Ruck P, and Kammerer U (2004) Antigen-presenting cells in human endometrium during the menstrual cycle compared to early pregnancy. J Soc Gynecol Investig, 11, 488-493.

[47] Robson NC, Phillips DJ, McAlpine T, Shin A, Svobodova S, Toy T, Pillay V, Kirkpatrick N, Zanker D, Wilson K et al (2008) Activin-A: a novel dendritic cell-derived cytokine that potently attenuates CD40 ligand-specific cytokine and chemokine production. Blood, 111, 2733-2743.

[48] Rutella S, Bonanno G, Procoli A, Mariotti A, de Ritis DG, Curti A, Danese S, Pessina G, Pandolfi S, Natoni F et al (2006) Hepatocyte growth factor favors monocyte differentiation into regulatory interleukin (IL)-10++IL-12low/neg accessory cells with dendritic-cell features. Blood, 108, 218-227.

[49] Salem ML (2004) Estrogen, a double-edged sword: modulation of TH1- and TH2-mediated inflammations by differential regulation of TH1/TH2 cytokine production. Curr Drug Targets Inflamm Allergy, 3, 97-104.

[50] Sallusto F and Lanzavecchia A (1999) Mobilizing dendritic cells for tolerance, priming, and chronic inflammation. J Exp Med, 189, 611-614.

[51] Segerer SE, Muller N, Brandt J, Kapp M, Dietl J, Reichardt HM, Rieger L, and Kammerer U (2008) The glycoprotein-hormones activin A and inhibin A interfere with dendritic cell maturation. Reprod Biol Endocrinol, 6, 17.

[52] Segerer SE, Muller N, van den BJ, Kapp M, Dietl J, Reichardt HM, Rieger L, and Kammerer U (2009) Impact of female sex hormones on the maturation and function of human dendritic cells. Am J Reprod Immunol, 62, 165-173.

[53] Shao L, Frigon NL, Jr., Young AL, Yu AL, Mathews LS, Vaughan J, Vale W, and Yu J (1992) Effect of activin A on globin gene expression in purified human erythroid progenitors. Blood, 79, 773-781.

[54] Smithson G, Couse JF, Lubahn DB, Korach KS, and Kincade PW (1998) The role of estrogen receptors and androgen receptors in sex steroid regulation of B lymphopoiesis. J Immunol, 161, 27-34.

[55] Steinman RM (2003) Some interfaces of dendritic cell biology. APMIS, 111, 675-697.

[56] Stites DP and Siiteri PK (1983) Steroids as immunosuppressants in pregnancy. Immunol Rev, 75, 117-138.

[57] Tamrazi A, Carlson KE, Daniels JR, Hurth KM, and Katzenellenbogen JA (2002) Estrogen receptor dimerization: ligand binding regulates dimer affinity and dimer dissociation rate. Mol Endocrinol, 16, 2706-2719.

[58] Tong S, Wallace EM, and Burger HG (2003) Inhibins and activins: clinical advances in reproductive medicine. Clin Endocrinol (Oxf), 58, 115-127.

[59] Wan H, Versnel MA, Leijten LM, van Helden-Meeuwsen CG, Fekkes D, Leenen PJ, Khan NA, Benner R, and Kiekens RC (2008) Chorionic gonadotropin induces dendritic cells to express a tolerogenic phenotype. J Leukoc Biol, 83, 894-901.

[60] Yang L, Hu Y, and Hou Y (2006) Effects of 17beta-estradiol on the maturation, nuclear factor kappa B p65 and functions of murine spleen CD11c-positive dendritic cells. Mol Immunol, 43, 357-366.

[61] Yoshimura T, Inaba M, Sugiura K, Nakajima T, Ito T, Nakamura K, Kanzaki H, and Ikehara S (2003) Analyses of dendritic cell subsets in pregnancy. Am J Reprod Immunol, 50, 137-145.

12

Sex Hormones and Neuromuscular Control System

Rose Fouladi
Tehran University, Tehran, Iran

1. Introduction

There is evidence that females sustain more exercise- related musculoskeletal injuries than males. Sex differences in injury rates are apparent in some connective tissues such as ligaments. Although girls and boys have an equal chance of ligament injuries prior to adolescence, girls have a higher rate immediately after maturation (Tursz et al., 1986). Female athletes participating in cutting, jumping and pivoting sports have a 4-6 times greater chance of ACL tearing than their male counterparts (Arendt et al., 1999).

Ligament, tendon, bone and endometrium contain estrogen receptors responsive to female sex hormones. Estrogen has direct effect on soft tissue strength, muscle function and collagen metabolism and behavior. It is demonstrated the influence of female endocrinology on knee joint behavior, as male and females differ substantially in the type, level and periodic exposure of circulating sex hormones after puberty. While hormone levels remain fairly constant in males, females are exposed to rhythmic fluctuations in endogenous hormones during the course of menstrual cycle. The absolute levels of estrogen and progesterone varying considerably during the course of a female's menstrual cycle and there are some variations in the hormonal levels. At the beginning of the menstrual cycle, estrogen (E) and progesterone (P) remain close to their minimum levels. Toward the middle of the cycle, estrogen level rises and in the middle of the luteal phase both E and P levels increase.

Also, estrogen indirectly influences the female neuromuscular system. Neuromuscular patterns in males and females differ during maturation. Males demonstrate power, strength and coordination increasing correlate with their age and maturational stage, whereas girls show little change throughout maturation (Kellis et al., 1999; Beunen et al., 1988). In females, quadriceps strength increases and you know it can increase the tibia anterior translation and subsequently the rate of ACL injury. The reliance of males on a more hamstring dominant strategy may be more protective of the ACL because the hamstring and ACL are agonist to prevent anterior displacement of the tibia on the femur. Also, females have shown more impaired proprioception assessing knee motion into extension than males (Rozzi et al., 1999). Significant slowing of muscle relaxation also occurs during the ovulation (estrogen surge) of the menstrual cycle. Serum estrogen concentrations fluctuate radically throughout the cycle and estrogen has measurable effects on muscle function and tendon and ligament strength.

Moreover Estrogen has effects on the central nervous system. It has demonstrated differences in skill performance in females during different phases of the menstrual cycle, also a decrease in motor skills in the premenstrual phase at the late luteal. These data indicate that estrogen can be effective on neuromuscular function which may facilitate the potential for neuromuscular imbalances to develop in female athletes. There is also evidence that estrogen influences electrical activity of neurons both centrally and peripherally (Lee et al., 2002; Papka et al., 2001; Rozzi et al., 1999). Furthermore, postural control impairments have been demonstrated in females with premenstrual symptoms in the mid-luteal phase (Friden et al., 2003). These findings support the hypothesis that lower extremity neuromuscular performance may be influenced by circulating sex hormones.

Because of existing estrogen and progesterone receptors on the human ACL fibroblasts, females' sex hormones may directly influence the structure and composition of the ACL. Some researchers have indicated different cycle phases for increased incidence of ACL injury. Some of them found that females have a greater risk of ACL injury during the ovulatory phase of the menstrual cycle in which estrogen surge is present (Wojtys et al., 1998). However, the others implicated a significant greater number of ACL injuries occurred onset of the cycle (days 1 and 2) (Slauterbeck et al., 2002). They believed cyclic changes in estrogen and progesterone may change expression of genes encoding tissue-remodeling enzymes and proteins, which in turn could favor either net tissue degradation or repair at specific times during the menstrual cycle.

In some studies, researchers have suggested that the large number of non-contact ACL injuries in female athletes may be related to knee laxity, which might be influenced by hormones. In normal menstruating females, significant increases in knee laxity have been noted in the pre - ovulatory and mid luteal phases of the menstrual cycle compared to menses. This is believed to coincide with elevated levels of estrogen, and estrogen and progesterone respectively. Although hormonal changes might result in increased injury risk for female athletes, the effects of hormonal level on occurrence of injury in these athletes are not fully understood.

In addition to sex hormones receptors, there are mechanoreceptors in human ACL. These mechanoreceptors are referred to as Ruffini receptors, Pacini receptors, Golgy tendon organ-like receptors and free nerve endings that they may have a proprioceptive function (Adachi et al., 2002). Proprioception is an important part of neuromuscular performance, and can be defined as the individual's awareness of his or her extremities' position and motion in space. It involves sensory activities of the tendons, ligaments, capsules and muscles, and can be internal peripheral areas of the body that contribute to postural control, joint stability and conscious sensation of movement. Position sense at the knee joint is influenced by central and peripheral mechanisms, such as muscles, tendons, articulate, cutaneous and ACL receptors (Shultz et al., 2005). The ACL have two complementary functions: mechanical and sensory (proprioception) (Ekenros et al., 2010). It has been implicated that sensory information from the ACL assists in providing functional stability to the knee joint by contributing to neuromuscular control (Riemann et al., 2002).

Since the relationship between ACL injury and female hormone concentration and also, the relationship between ACL injury and neuromuscular control (proprioception) deficit is supported by recent studies. This chapter is going to investigate the relationship between female hormonal level and proprioception, by measuring the knee joint position sense (JPS) and serum estrogen and progesterone concentrations throughout the menstrual cycle.

2. Neuromuscular control and proprioception

Neuromuscular control of the knee is defined as the unconscious response to an afferent signal concerning dynamic knee joint stability. These afferent signals are produced by

Proprioception which refers specially to conscious and unconscious appreciation of joint position, kinesthesia (the sensation of joint motion or acceleration) and the perception of force (an ability to estimate joint loads). These signals are transmitted to the spinal cord via afferent (sensory) pathways. Conscious awareness of joint motion, position and force is essential for motor learning and the anticipation of movements in sport, while unconscious proprioception modulates muscle function and initiates reflex joint stabilization. The efferent (motor) response to sensory information is termed neuromuscular control (Prentice 2011). The deficit of neuromuscular control of the knee joint may be responsible for the high rate of knee injury in female athletes (Hewett et al., 1996; Huston et al., 1996).

The central nervous system (CNS) is the primary mediator for the perception and execution of musculoskeletal control and movement. Perception and sensation of joint movement are monitored by tree main subsystems: 1) the somatosensory system, 2) the vestibular system, and 3) the visual system. The somatosensory system often referred to as proprioception, receives input from peripheral articular and musculotendinous receptors concerning changes in muscle length and tension, in addition to information regarding joint position and motion.

The vestibular system receives information from the vestibules and semicircular canals of the ear, which aid in keeping the body in balance, while the visual system provides the body with visual cues, contributing to balance by providing reference points for orientation.

Information gathered by the somatosensory system, in addition to that from vestibular and visual systems, is processed at three distinct levels of motor control: the spinal level, the brain stem and the higher centers such as the motor cortex, basal ganglia, and cerebellum.

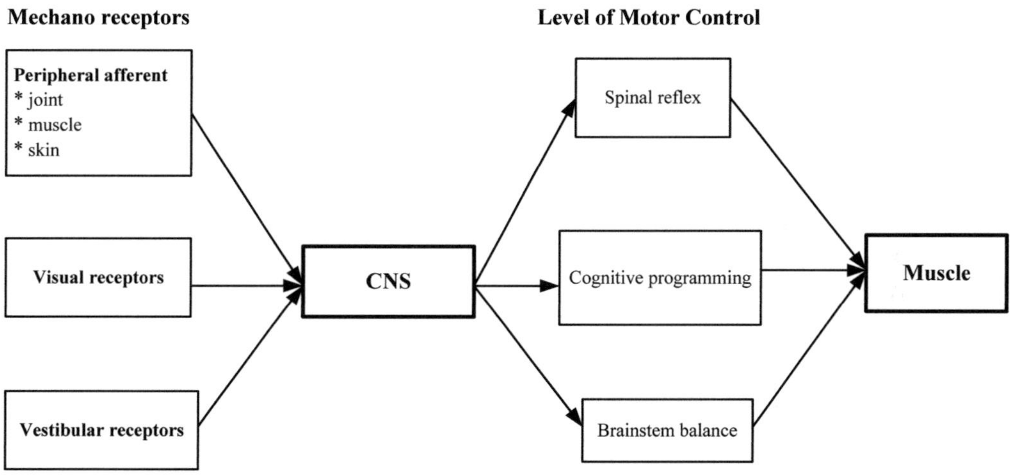

Fig. 1. Neuromuscular control pathway (reproduced from Lephart 1998)

Proprioception and neuromuscular control may be assessed clinically through evaluation of the afferent and efferent neuromuscular pathways. The afferent pathway is qualified through the examination of joint kinesthesia and joint position sensibility, which provide the researcher with a measurement of conscious appreciation of joint motion and position sensibility. Joint kinesthesia is determined clinically by establishing the threshold to detection of passive motion, an assessment of the ability to detect relatively slow passive joint motion. Testing joint position sense, another method of assessing the afferent pathway, determines the ability of the subject to comprehend a presented joint angle and then once removed; actively or passively reproduce the joint angle. Assessment of the efferent pathway is conducted through measurements of balance and muscle activity, which provide a direct determination of the efferent response to afferent stimulation. (Lephart 2000)

3. Hormonal effects on ACL

Sex hormone fluctuations have been associated with tissue alterations and an increased incidence of non-contact ACL injuries among female athletes (Wojtys et al., 2002). Estrogen and progesterone receptors have been detected within the ACL (Liu et al., 1996). Several researchers have suggested the relationship between estrogen peak levels and increased ACL laxity (Shultz et al., 2004; Slauterbeck et al., 2001). This associated change in tissue tolerance may predispose the ACL to failure at lower tensile loads and/or alter the protective muscle reflex actions associated with ACL tissue receptor stimulation (Raunest et al., 1996).

4. Hormonal effects on tissue

Estrogen receptors alpha and beta have been reported in skeletal muscle thereby providing a plausible tissue-based mechanism for influencing neuromuscular control and force transmission pathways (Huijing et al 2005; Wilk et al., 2005). In addition, research has not completely described the influence of sex hormone receptors in skeletal muscles on tissue mechanisms that can alter neuromuscular control (Dedrick et al., 2008).

5. Neuromuscular control mechanisms between sexes

Similar neuromuscular control strategies have been reported between Men and women during landing up until puberty. There is a link between hormonal fluctuations and changes in neuromuscular control, since alterations in hormonal levels constitute a primary change in development after puberty. Neuromuscular control strategies incorporated during a landing sequence appear to change in adult females, where increased knee valgus alignment places the ACL at greater risk of injury (Hewett et al., 2004).

6. Hormonal effects on neuromuscular control

Neuromuscular control patterns, such as fine motor activity and reaction time performance have been reported to fluctuate over the course of the menstrual cycle (Posthuma et al., 1987), with more consistent performance in women using oral contraceptive (OC). It was discovered that there is an increase in postural sway during single limb stance and threshold for detection of passive knee motion in the mid-luteal phase of the cycle (Friden et al., 2003, 2005). Improved neuromuscular coordination may occur in women taking OC with a reduced number of premenstrual symptoms. However, the relationship between fluctuations in ovarian sex hormone levels and neuromuscular strategies has not been fully described (Dedrick et al., 2006).

Neuromuscular patterns in males and females change substantially during maturation. Males demonstrate improve in power, straight and coordination with age that correlate with their maturational stage, whereas, girls show little change throughout maturation.

For example, in study by kelis et al vertical jump height demonstrated by boys increased steadily during maturation, but in girls it did not (Kellis et al., 1999; Beunen et al., 1988).

Neuromuscular control of the knee can be defined as the unconscious to an afferent signal concerning dynamic knee joint stability. The absents of neuromuscular control of the knee joint may be responsible for the increased rate of knee injury in females, but it is not normally measured with the 3 dimensional kinematic system described below and were recorded during the same laboratory evaluation (Lephart et al., 2000).

Changes in neuromuscular control of the knee in adolescent athletes are documented. Several studies have documented a substantial increase in neuromuscular strength and coordination following the growth spurt in adolescent boys but not in the average adolescent girls.

7. Normal menstrual cycle

Normal menstrual cycle in women includes fluctuation of sex hormones' levels in a regular duration that usually takes 21-35 days. Ovarian cycle of the normal menstrual cycle has 2 phases, follicular and luteal. Follicular phase is started by menstruation with 2-4 days bleeding.

Estrogen and progesterone levels are in the lowest level at menses but little by little estrogen increases and it goes up to its highest level just before the ovulation, at the middle of the cycle. Duration of the estrogen surge is so limit and it just takes 24 to 48 hours. After ovulation, both estrogen and progesterone levels go up slowly and they are in their highest level at the middle of luteal phas (Berek et al., 2002).

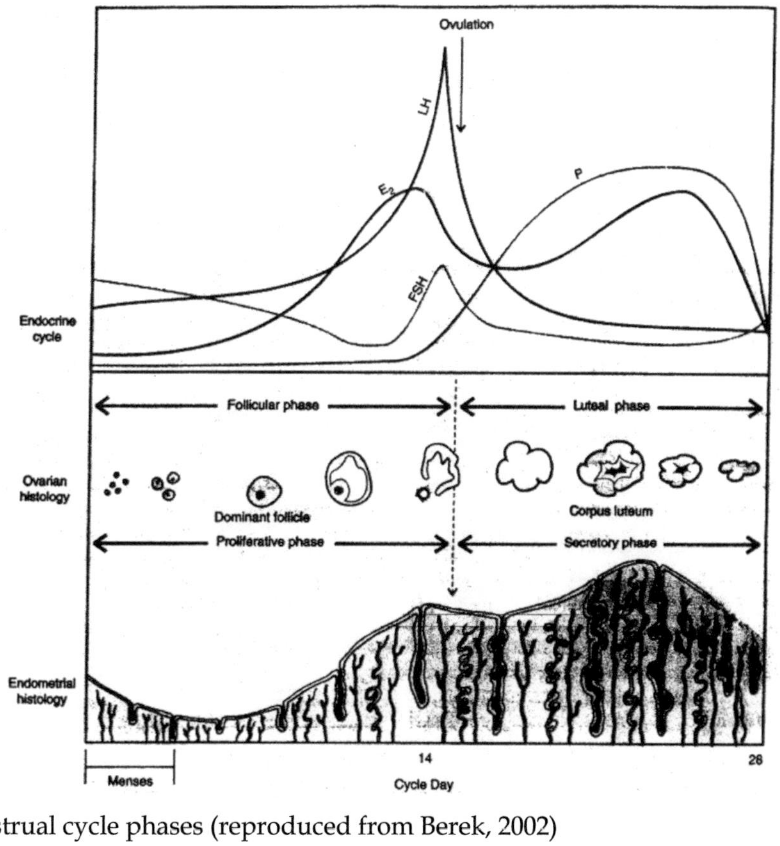

Fig. 2. Menstrual cycle phases (reproduced from Berek, 2002)

8. Procedure

Although, joint proprioception includes some parts, most of the studies have measured JPS as an important part of it. There are different methods for knee JPS evaluation. Some researchers have measured JPS with isokinetic dynamometer- Biodex in non weight bearing position (Aydog et al., 2005; Hertel et al., 2006). In the other studies, JPS was measured by reproduction of the target angle in standing position by using a system comprised of skin markers and digital photography (Stillman BC et al., 2001;Shultz et al., 2003; Shultz et al., 2005; Mir et al., 2008).

In our study the JPS was measured 3 times a month with different level of sex hormones. It was evaluated by reproduction of the target angle (30° flexion) in standing position and absolute angular error (AAE) was considered as a dependent variable.

Testing procedure was completed in an isolated room; the participants were asked to wear loose-fitting shorts. Since previous studies had shown there is no significant difference between the bilateral knee joints' position sense (Herington 2005), we chose the right leg as the tested limb. In all tests, visual cues were eliminated by a blindfold. Each participant was asked to lie down in supine position on the treatment plinth and four circular markers (4 cm in diameter) were attached to their leg at three locations: (1) proximal to a quarter of the distance along a line joining the greater trochanter to the lateral knee joint line, (2) over the fibular neck, (3) over the proximal part of the lateral malleolus. Then each subject asked to sit down (with hip and knee 90° flex), and the fourth marker was attached over the illiotibial tract adjacent to the superior border of the patella. The choice of marker locations was based on previous studies (Deie et al., 2002; Lamoreux et al., 1996). The participant then stood with their feet-shoulder width apart. The left foot was lifted from the floor. The right hand was placed over the chest, and the subject was allowed to use minimum contact of the fingertips in the left hand for balance. One goniometer was adhered onto the wall, out of sight of subject, at angle of 30° as an indicator.

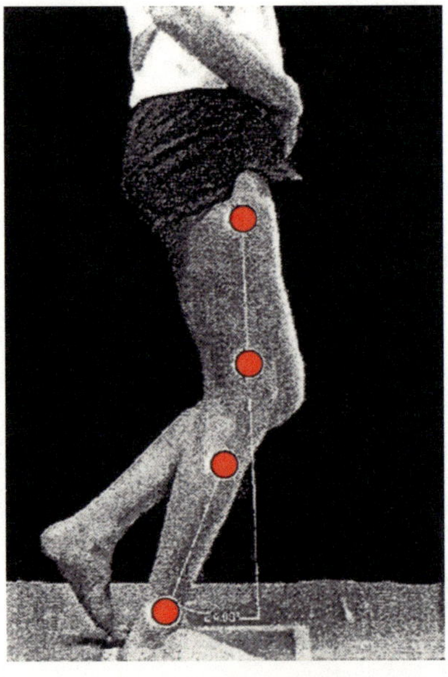

Fig. 3. Measuring the knee joint angle in weight bearing position

9. Joint position sense (JPS) measurement

The movement capture system comprised of digital photography, skin markers and AutoCAD software was utilized for measuring joint angles during the joint position sense test. A digital video camera was located 185cm away from the subject and elevated 65cm from the ground. Photos were taken during movement and holding moments of the leg, respectively. After completing the procedure, the test and replicated angles were measured using the AutoCAD software.

To measure JPS in the knee joint, participants moved their limbs into flexion. Before the tests, each subject watched a video tape showing the squatting movement demonstrated by a trained person performing the movement at a controlled velocity and the subjects were asked to squat as shown in the film. We tried to control velocity approximately, because the JPS accuracy could be influenced by high or low velocity (Stillman et al., 2001). The starting position was knee straightening (0°). The subject stood with eyes closed, and was instructed to: (1) lift the unexamined foot (left limb) from the floor; (2) slowly flex the weight bearing (WB) limb (right limb) until told to stop (~30°); (3) identify the knee position while isometrically holding the test position for about 5 seconds; (4) return to the erect bilateral WB stance (for 7 seconds); and (5) reproduce the previous unilateral flexed position, concentrating on the knee. The holding times used in this study were based on previous studies (Hopper et al., 2003; Marks et al., 1994; Marks et al., 1993). Measurement of knee JPS was repeated three times and the average of the three measurements were calculated in each phase.

In some previous studies JPS was measured in NWB position that is not functional. For example, Aydog et al (2005) evaluated knee JPS throughout the three different phases of the menstrual cycle but they used Biodex System 3 dynamometer to measure knee JPS in a semi-horizontal position. Their method also stimulated cutaneous mechanoreceptors which have an important role on the knee JPS that may change the test accuracy.

In our study, JPS of the knee joint was evaluated in WB position, as it potentially provides more functional information.

10. Blood sampling

At the end of each session, venous blood samples (5 ml) were taken from a superficial forearm vein. The blood sample was allowed to clot at room temperature and then the serum was separated and stored to be analyzed. Serum estrogen and progesterone concentrations were measured with Elisa method by Elisa Reader (SLT model) in Endocrine Research Center lab.

Data was collected throughout the 3 phases of menstrual cycle i.e. early follicular phase (onset of menses), mid-follicular phase (the 7th to 9th days of the cycle) and mid-luteal phase (20th to 23th days of the cycle).

11. Results

11.1 Hormones

Estrogen concentration was found 22.81 (16.75) pg/ml at menses, 125.65 (84.82) at mid-follicular and 179.5 (94.35) at mid-luteal phase. Fig. 4 depicts estrogen concentrations across the menstrual cycle phases. Serum estrogen concentration was significantly higher during the mid-follicular and mid-luteal phases as compared with the early-follicular (menses) phase (P=0.0001). There was no significant difference between peak estrogen concentrations in the mid-follicular versus the mid-luteal phase.

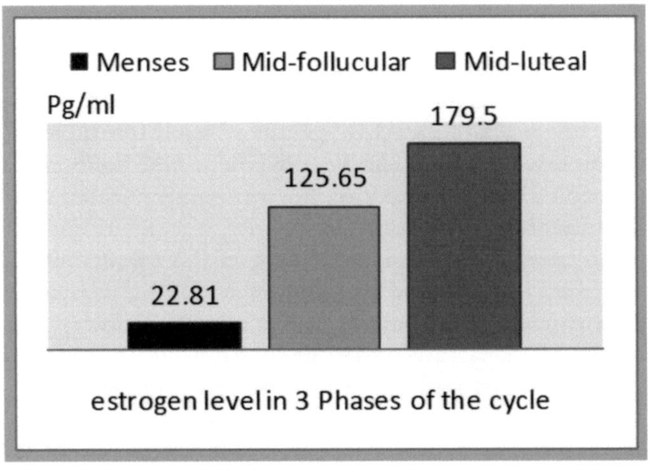

Fig. 4. Estrogen concentrations across three phases of the menstrual cycle

Serum progesterone concentration was found 0.58 (0.62) at menses, 0.51(0.71) at mid-follicular and 7.35(5.87) at mid-luteal phase. These results show that serum progesterone concentration was significantly higher during the mid-luteal phase as compared with the menses and mid-follicular phases (P=0.0001). However there was no significant difference between peak progesterone concentrations in the menses versus mid-follicular phase. Fig. 5 depicts progesterone concentrations across the menstrual cycle phases.

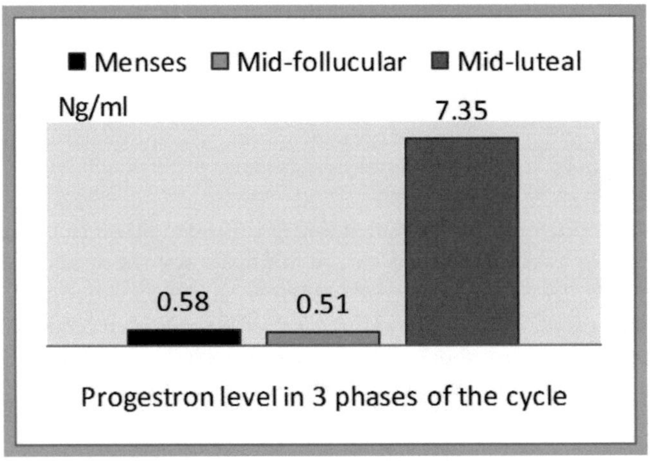

Fig. 5. Progestrone concentrations across the menstrual cycle

12. Joint Position Sense (absolute error of repositioning)

We found females' knee JPS accuracy changes in different phases of menstrual cycle. The greatest amount of mean (SD) value of absolute error was at menses and the least amount of it, was at mid-luteal phase. This finding is also in agreement with previous study that indicated the active knee JPS was significantly reduced during menstruation (Aydog et al., 2005).

	menses	Mid-follicular	Mid-luteal
AAE means	4.18 (2.13)	3.65 (2.78)	2.51 (1.66)

Table 1. The value of absolute angular error across the menstrual cycle

Pearson correlation test showed a negative correlation between AAE and estrogen level with no significant relationship (r= -0.275, p= .058). But, spearman correlation test indicated a negative correlation between AAE and progesterone level with a significant relationship (r= -0.370, p= 0.010). Therefore, the highest level of JPS error was related to the lowest level of estrogen and progesterone. Also, the lowest level of JPS error was related to the highest level of sex hormones. While hormones' levels increase, the knee JPS error decreases. Because of the significant relationship between progesterone and AAE, it seems this hormone has the main effect on the knee JPS accuracy.

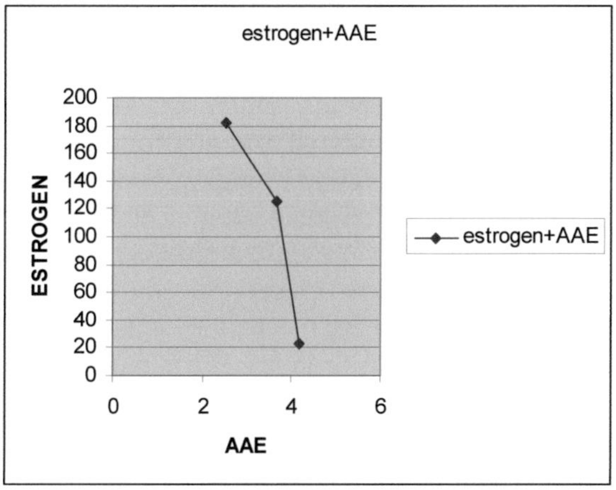

Fig. 6. The linear correlation between estrogen and absolute angular error

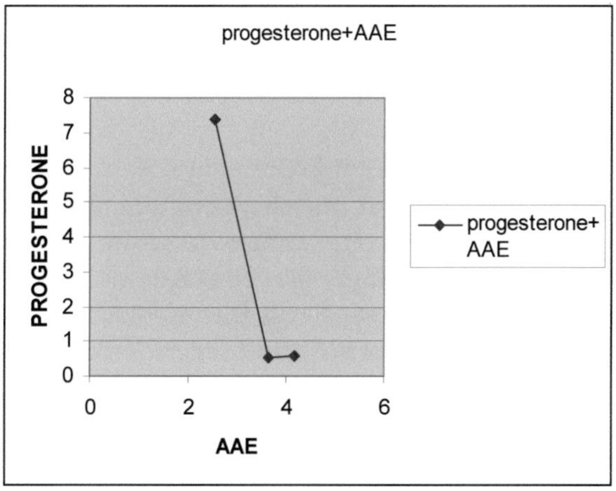

Fig. 7. The linear correlation between progesterone and absolute angular error

13. Discussion

Previous authors report different results regarding changes in knee joint proprioception across the menstrual cycle. The main observation of our study was that higher value of reposition error was found in the menses and the participants made less error in reproduction of joint position sense in two other phases and they were more accurate during the luteal phase. While sex hormones' levels increase, the knee JPS error decreases. The significant relationship was between progesterone and absolute angular error and it seems this hormone has the main effect on the knee JPS accuracy.

These results are due to measurable effects of estrogen on muscle, tendon and ligament strength and function (Sarwer et al., 1996). Estrogen also has influence on the central nervous system and females have different skill performances during different phases of the menstrual cycle (Lebrun et al., 1994). Some researchers demonstrated a decrease in motor skills around the menstruation and this showed that estrogen may influence on neuromuscular function (Posthuma et al., 1987). It is indicated that ACL injuries happened most frequently on day 1 and 2 of menses and it isn't random but occurs usually around the time of menses, when circulating sex- hormones levels decrease and after both estrogen and progesterone elevation (Slauterbeck et al., 2002). In addition, it is believed that proprioception can be influenced by emotional and environmental conditions and because of females' behavioral and emotional character changing in early menstruation increasing in error of knee JPS in menses can be described. Aydog et al (2005) also indicated the active knee JPS was significantly reduced in the menstruation compared to follicular and early luteal phases. They believed that changes in proprioception might be a consequence of changes in distal latency or excitability of the mechanoreceptors.

On the other hand, it is observed that knee laxity exists more in mid-follicular and luteal phases of the females' menstrual cycle. Females with increased knee laxity are less sensitive to joint displacement or loading, and are more reliant on active control of the gastrocnemius and biceps femoris muscles to potentially compensate for reduced passive instability (Shultz et al., 2004; Park et al., 2007).

In another study, some researchers demonstrated increased knee laxity was observed during ovulation (after estrogen serge) but no significant changes in knee mechanics corresponding to menstrual phases were found. They also found knee laxity correlates positively with knee joint loads. They suggested that increased knee joint laxity during menstrual cycle leads to greater knee joint loads in selected high risk movements in healthy young females (Park et al., 2009).

Although, some researchers said knee joint laxity may not explain the higher incidence of females' ACL injury, they suggested that muscle strength and dynamic stability are more important (Bowerman et al., 2006). Some others measured knee JPS with isokinetic dynamometer in sitting position with high skin stimulations and suggested passive joint position sense and joint laxity don't change across the menstrual cycle (Hertel et al., 2006). It is also indicated that ligament laxity does not affect the proprioceptive function of the knee, and it may compensate with muscle contraction (Adachi et al., 2002). These findings are consistent with Johanson's Final Common Input Theory. Based on this theory, due to the joint-tendon-muscle relationship, muscle spindles act with joint afferent information and then send final common signal. As the highest knee joint laxity has been observed in the luteal phase, in the current study the most JPS accuracy can be described.

However, some other researchers didn't find the highest level of laxity in luteal phase, and suggested antagonistic role for progesterone and estrogen. But they found no significant difference of laxity between mid-follicular and luteal phases (Park et al., 2007).
Therefore, according to progesterone effect on knee laxity in the mentioned studies and our finding about its influence on JPS, we suggest progesterone and estrogen are synergies in knee JPS accuracy. Hence we suppose that elevation of both these hormones in luteal phase is the reason of knee joint absolute angular error decreasing and knee JPS accuracy increasing.
The findings of our study are strengthened by controlling many confounding variables such as age, menstrual regularity, previous injuries and length of daytime because of its influence on females' sex hormones (Speroff et al., 2005). We collected all our sampling in one season with almost the same day length during the study. Moreover, we started our study with every participant being in their follicular phase (the menses) and we used the same sequence for all the participants. None of our subjects wasn't pregnant and didn't use oral contraceptive in their 3 recent months because of its effects on their knee joint performance (Lebrun et al., 1994) and it could influence on their postural control (Ekenros et al., 2010). We used skin marker to reduce the skin stimulation and we also used AutoCAD software to measure the knee angles as it has high test-retest reliability. Therefore our JPS test can be considered highly accurate. In the current study, JPS of the knee joint was evaluated in WB position which potentially provides more functional information (Baker et al., 2002).

14. Conclusion

It is concluded that sex hormones, especially progesterone can influence on accuracy of the knee JPS in healthy female athletes. Their reduction at menstruation can reduce the knee JPS accuracy and increase the knee joint injury probability. Knee JPS accuracy decreases in menses, when circulating sex- hormones levels are low and after a time when both were elevated.
As such, Female athletes are at risk of ACL tearing during menstruation. Further studies are needed to investigate the effect of some devices or some ways to protect the knee joint during this high risk time.

15. References

[1] Adachi N, Ochi M, Uchio Y et al (2002) Mechanoreceptors in the anterior cruciate ligament contribute to the joint position sense. Acta Orthop Scand 73:330-334
[2] Arendt EA, Agel J, Dick RW(1999) Anterior cruciate ligament injury patterns among collegiate men and women. J Athl Train 34:86-92
[3] Arendt E, Dick R (1999) Knee injury patterns among men and women in collegiate basketball and soccer. NCAA data and review of literature. Am J Sports Med 23,694-701
[4] Aydog ST, Hascelik Z, Demirel HA, Tetik O, Aydog E, Doral MN (2005). The effects of menstrual cycle on the knee joint position sense:preliminary study. Knee Surg Sports Troumatol Arthrosc 13:649-653.
[5] Baker V, Bannel K, Stillman B, et al (2002) Abnormal knee joint position sense in individuals with patello femoral pain syndrome. J Orthop Res 20:208-14

[6] Berek J S (2002) Berek and Novak's Gynecology. Lippincott Williams & Wilkins, Philadelphia
[7] Beunen G, Malina RM (1988). Growth and physical performance relative to the timing of the adolescent spurt. Exerc Sport Sci Rev 16:503-40
[8] Boden B, Dean G, Feagin J et al (2002) Mechanisms of anterior cruciate ligament injury. Orthop 23, 573-578
[9] Bowerman SJ, Smith DR, Carlson M et al (2006) Comparison of factors influencing ACL injury in male and female athletes and non-athletes. Phys Ther Sport 7:14-152
[10] Cappozzo A, Catani F, Leardini A et al (1996) Position and orientation in space of bones during movement: Experiment of artifacts. Clin Biomech 11:90-100
[11] Dedrick GS, Sizer PhS, Merkle JN et al (2008) Effect of sex hormones on neuromuscular control patterns during landing. J Electromyography Kinesiology 18:68-78
[12] Deie M, Sakamaki Y, Sumen Y et al (2002) Anterior knee laxity in young women varies with their menstrual cycle. Int Orthop 26: 154-156
[13] Ekenros L, Hirschberg AL, Backstrom T, Friden C (2010). Postural control in women with premenstrual symptoms during oral contraceptive treatment. Nordic Federation of Societies of Obstrics and Gynecology 90:97-102.
[14] Frank CB, Jackson DW (1997) The science of reconstruction of the anterior cruciate ligament. J Bone Joint Surg 79A:1556-1576
[15] Friden C, Hirschberg AL et al (2003) The influence of premenstrual symptoms on postural balance and kinesthesia during the menstrual cycle. Gynecol Endocrinol 17:433-40
[16] Friden C, Ramsey DK, Backstrom T et al (2005) Altered postural control during the luteal phase in women with premenstrual symptoms. Neuroendocrinology 81:150-7
[17] Hamlet WP, Liu SH, Panossian V et al (1997) Primary immuno-localization of androgen target cells in the human ACL ligament. Orthop Res 15:657-63
[18] Heitz NA (1999) Hormonal changes throughout the menstrual cycle and increased anterior cruciate ligament laxity in females. J Athl Train 343:144-149
[19] Herrington L (2005) Knee joint position sense: The relationship between open and closed kinetic chain tests. J Sport Rehabil 14:356-362
[20] Hertel J, Williams NI, Olmsted-Kramer LC, Leidy HJ, Putukian M (2006). Neuromuscular performance and knee laxity do not change across the menstrual cycle in female athletes. Knee Surge Sports Traumatol Arthrosc 14:817-822
[21] Hewett T, Stroupe AL, Nance TA, Noyes FR (1996) Plyometric training in female athletes. Decreased impact forces and increased hamstring torques. Am J Sports Med 24:765-73
[22] Hewett T, Myer GD, Ford KR (2004). Decrease in neuromuscular control about the knee with maturation in female athletes. J Bone and Joint Surgery 1601-1608
[23] Hopper DM, Creagh MJ, Formby PA et al (2003) Functional measurement of knee joint position sense after anterior cruciate ligament reconstruction. Arch Phys Med Rehabil 84:868-872
[24] Huijing PA, Jaspers RT (2005) Adaptation of muscle size and myofascial force transmission: a review of some new experimental results. Scand J Med Sci Sports 15:349-80

[25] Huston LJ, Wojtys EM (1996) Neuromuscular performance characteristics in elite female athletes. Am J Sports Med 24:427-36

[26] Kellis SE, Tsitskaris GK, Nikopoulou MD, Mousikou KC (1999). The evaluation of jumping ability of male and female basketball players according to their chronological age and major leagues. J S trength Cond Res 13: 40-6

[27] Lamoreux LW (1996) Coping with soft tissue movement in human motion analysis. In: Harris GF, Smith PA (eds) Human motion analysis: Current applications and future directions, 1st edn. Institute of Electrical and Electrical Engineering, New York, pp 43-47

[28] Lebrun CM (1994) The effect of the phase of the menstrual cycle and the birth control pill in athletic performance. Clin Sports Med 13:419-441

[29] Lee DY, Chai YG, Lee EB, Kim KW et al (2002). Beta-estradiol inhibits high-voltage-activated calcium channel currents in rat sensory neurons via a non-genomic mechanism. Life Sci 70:2047-59

[30] Lephart SM, Pincivero DM, Giraldo Jl et al (1997) The role of proprioception in the management and rehabilitation of athletic injuries. Am J Sports Med 25:130-7

[31] Lephart SM, Pincivero DM, Rozzi SL (1998) . Proprioception of the ankle and knee. Sport Med 25: 149-55.

[32] Liu S H, Al-Shaikh RA, Panossian V et al (1996) Primary immunolocalization of estrogen and progesterone target cells in the human anterior cruciate ligament. Orthop Res Soc 14, 526-533

[33] Marks R (1994) The reliability of knee position sense measurements in healthy women. Physiother Can 46:37-41

[34] Marks R, Quinney HA, Wessel J (1993) Proprioceptive sensibility in women with normal and osteoarthritic knee joints. Clin Rheumatol 12:170-175.

[35] Mir SM, Hadian MR, Talebian S, Naseri N (2008) Functional assessment of knee joint position sense following anterior cruciate ligament reconstruction. Br J Sports Med 300-3

[36] Moller-Neilsen J, Hammar M (1989) Women's soccer injury in relation to the menstrual cycle and oral contraceptive use. Med Sci Sports Exerc 21:126-129

[37] Myklebust G, Maehlum S, Holm I et al (1998) A prospective cohort study of anterior cruciate ligament injuries in elite Norwegian team handball. Scand J Med Sci Sports 8:149-153

[38] Papka RE, Storey-Workley M et al (2001) Estrogen recetor-α and Β-immunoreactivity and mRNA in neurons of sensory and autonomic ganglia and spinal cord. Cell Tissue Res 304:193-214

[39] Park SK, Stefanyshyn DJ, Hart DA et al (2007) Influence of hormones on knee joint laxity and joint mechanics in healthy females. J Biomech 40(52)

[40] Park SK, Stefanyshyn DJ, Ramage B (2009) Relationship between knee joint laxity and knee joint mechanics during the menstrual cycle. Br J Sports Med 43:174-179.

[41] Park SK, Stefanyshyn DJ, Ramage B, Hart DA, Ronsky JL (2009) Alterations in knee joint laxity during the menstrual cycle in healthy women leads to increases in joint loads during selected athletic movements. Am J Sports Med 37:1169

[42] Posthuma BW, Bass MJ, Bull SB et al (1987) Detecting changes in functional ability in women with premenstrual syndrome. Am J Obstet Gynecol159:275-278

[43] Prentice WE (2011) Rehabilitation techniques: For sports medicine and athletic training. 5th edn. The McGraw-Hill companies, New York, pp: 122-139.

[44] Raunest J, Sager M, Burgener E (1996) Proprioceptive mechanisms in the cruciate ligaments: and electromugraphic study on reflex activity in the thigh muscles. J Trauma 41:488-93

[45] Riemann BL, Lephart SM (2002) The sensory system. Part II: The role of proprioception in motor control and functional joint stability. J Athl Train 37:80-84

[46] Rozzi SL, Lephart SM, Fu FH (1999) Effects of muscular fatigue on knee joint laxity and neuromuscular characteristics of male and female athletes. J Athl Train 34,106-114

[47] Rozzi SL, Lephart SM, Gear WS (1999) Knee joint laxity and neuromuscular characteristics of male and female soccer and basketball players. Am J Sports Med 27:312-319

[48] Sarwer R, Beltran NB, Rutherford OM (1996) Changes in muscle strength, relaxation rate and fatiguability during the human menstrual cycle. J Physiol 493:267-272

[49] Sciore P, Smith S, Frank CB (1997) Detection of receptors for estrogen and progesterone in human ligaments and rabbit ligaments and tendons by RT-PCR. Trans Orthop Res Soc 22:51

[50] Slauterbeck JR, Fuzie SF, Smith MP et al (2002) The menstrual cycle, sex hormones and anterior cruciate ligament injury. J Athl Train 37:275-280

[51] Shultz SJ, Carcia CR, Perrin DH (2004) Knee joint laxity affects muscle activation patterns in the healthy knee. J Electromyogr Kines14:475-483

[52] Shultz SJ, Sander TC, Kirk SE et al (2005) Sex differences in knee joint laxity change across the female menstrual cycle. J Sports Med Phys Fitness 45:594-603

[53] Shultz SJ, Sander TC, Johnson KM et al (2004) Relationship between sex hormones and anterior knee laxity across the menstrual cycle. Med Sci Sports Exerc 36:1165-1174

[54] Speroff L, Fritz MA 2005 Clinical gynecologic endocrinology and infertility. Lippincott W illiams E Wilkins. 7th ed., A wolters kluwer company. pp:187-225

[55] Stillman BC, McMeeken JM (2001) The role of weight bearing in the clinical assessment of knee joint position sense. Aust J Physiother 47(4):247-53

[56] Tursz A, Crost M (1986) Sports-related injuries in children. A study of their characteristics, frequency and severity, with comparision to other type of accidental injuries. Am J sports Med 14:294-299

[57] Wilk A, Gustafsson T, Esbjornsson M et al (2005) Expression of oestrogen receptor α and β is higher in skeletal muscle of highly endurance-trained than of moderately active men. Acta Physiol Scand 184:105-12

[58] Wojtys EM, Huston LJ, Lindenfeld TN et al (1998) Association between the menstrual cycle and anterior cruciate ligament injuries in female athletes. Am J Sports Med 26:614-9

[59] Wojtys EM, Huston LJ, Boynton MD et al (2002) The effect of the menstrual cycle on anterior cruciate ligament injuries in women as determined by hormone levels. Am J Sports Med 30:182-8

[60] Yu WD, Hatch JD, Panossian V et al (1999) Effect of estrogen on cellular growth and collagen synthesis of human ACL. Clin Orthop Rel Res 366:229-238

13

Acute and Chronic Testosterone Responses to Physical Exercise and Training

Eduardo Lusa Cadore and Luiz Fernando Martins Kruel
Exercise Laboratory Research, Physical Education School,
Federal University of Rio Grande do Sul
Brazil

1. Introduction

High-intensity physical training is a powerful stimulus to acute increases in blood steroid hormone levels (Ahtiainen et al., 2005; Cadore et al., 2008a, 2008b, 2009a; Häkkinen & Pakarinen, 1994a, 1995; Staron et al., 1994). Moreover, strength training (ST) has been shown to stimulate greater increases in testosterone levels when compared to aerobic training (Copeland, et al., 2002; Tremblay et al., 2003), which can be explained by the powerful influence of the anaerobic glycolytic pathway in stimulating acute hormonal increases in response to exercise (Kraemer & Ratamess, 2005). This stimulus features control mechanisms independent from luteinising hormone (LH) stimulation (Fahrner & Hackney, 1998; Lu et al., 1997), and some factors related to the training session are directly associated with this response (Cadore et al., 2008c; Häkkinen et al., 1988; Häkkinen & Pakarinen, 1995, Kraemer et al., 1993; Smilios et al., 2003, 2006).

Despite the well-known acute hormonal response to physical exercise (Kraemer et al., 1990; Hansen et al., 2001; Cadore et al., 2009c), data on resting concentrations remain controversial. Some studies demonstrate increased resting testosterone levels following ST (Ahtiainen et al., 2003; Häkkinen et al., 1998; Izquierdo et al., 2006; Kraemer et al., 1993; Kraemer et al., 1999; Marx et al., 2001; Staron et al., 1994), leading authors to suggest this type of training as a form of intervention for maintaining testosterone levels during ageing (Kraemer et al., 1999). However, increases in resting testosterone levels were not observed in middle-aged (Cadore et al. 2008a) or elderly people (Häkkinen et al., 2000, 2001a; Kraemer et al., 1999). Chronic adaptations to ST apparently occur at the level of cellular androgen receptors (ARs), given that ARs present on muscle cells seem to increase in number in response to this type of training (Inoue et al., 1994; Willoughby & Taylor, 2004), and this adaptation may result in improved hormone-receptor interaction (Bamman et al., 2001; Willoughby & Taylor, 2004).

Conversely, reductions in testosterone levels associated with increases in cortisol levels have been observed in response to aerobic training in athletes subjected to high-volume training (Maïmoun et al., 2003). These alterations may be associated with the overtraining process and consequent suppression of the hypothalamic-pituitary-gonadal and adrenocortical axis (Bell et al., 2001; Hu et al., 1999; Kraemer et al., 1995). Nevertheless, reductions in testosterone levels may occur without overtraining. This alteration may be transient, reflecting the variation in volume and training intensity, and it may be explained by changes in plasma volume (Hu et al., 1999; Kraemer & Ratamess, 2005; Maïmoun et al., 2003).

It has been suggested that the neuromuscular adaptations observed during ST (Häkkinen et al., 2000, 2001b; Tsolakiis et al., 2004) are partly mediated by acute responses to circulating testosterone levels resulting from the training session (Kraemer & Ratamess, 2005) as well as modifications in the cellular receptors present on muscle cells (Ahtiainen et al., 2011; Kadi et al., 2000). Besides the known effects exerted by these hormones on muscle metabolism (Bhasin et al., 2001), the magnitude of increase in muscular strength in individuals subjected to strength training has been associated with testosterone concentration and other hormone-related parameters (i.e., the testosterone:cortisol ratio and testosterone:sex hormone-binding globulin (SHBG)) (Cadore et al., 2010; Häkkinen et al., 1988, 2000; Häkkinen & Pakarinen, 1993a, 1993b; Izquierdo et al., 2001). The figure 1 shows a Schematic diagram of the mechanism of training adaptations: anabolic process as adaptation to strength training and chronic catabolic process resulting from excessive volume of both strength and aerobic training.

Due to the possible importance of acute hormone responses, as well as chronic adaptation of androgen receptors due to strength training, it may be important to determine which aspects of training influence these responses to establish an optimum anabolic environment during a training session or period. Therefore, the objective of this chapter is to review existing data on the influence of testosterone levels on physical training and to determine which factors related to the training session are associated with the acute and chronic hormone responses the endocrine system to exercise.

2. Testosterone and strength trainability

Testosterone is a powerful stimulator of protein synthesis, specifically in the context of muscle metabolism (Griggs et al., 1989). Its effects are exerted through the interaction between the hormone and its specific receptor located on the muscle cell (Bamman et al., 2001). The main mechanism through which testosterone induces protein synthesis is the activation and induction of the proliferation of satellite cells, which subsequently incorporate into muscle fibres, resulting in an increase in myonuclear number (Kadi et al., 2000). Moreover, this hormone is capable of influencing strength production by stimulating the transition of type II fibres to a more glycolytic profile (Ramos et al., 1998), increasing the secretion of insulin-like growth factor I (IGF-I), mediated by its influence on the amplitude of growth hormone (GH) pulses (Bross et al., 1999) as well as its influence on the production of neurotransmitters that are important for muscle contraction (Kraemer et al., 1999).

Several studies demonstrate that among individuals subjected to the same volume and intensity of ST, those presenting higher testosterone levels achieve greater muscular strength and/or power following training (Ahtiainen et al., 2003; Cadore et al., 2010; Häkkinen et al., 1988; Häkkinen & Pakarinen, 1993a). This suggests that the trainability of individuals is related to testosterone and hormonal parameters associated with this hormone, such as the testosterone:sex hormone-binding globulin (SHBG) ratio and the testosterone:cortisol ratio, as demonstrated by results obtained in published studies (Ahtiainen et al., 2003; Cadore et al., 2010; Häkkinen et al., 1988; Häkkinen & Pakarinen, 1993a). Furthermore, in transversal studies that investigated middle-aged and elderly individuals, strength production was correlated to serum testosterone levels (Häkkinen & Pakarinen, 1993a; Cadore et al., 2008a).

Häkkinen et al. (1988) investigated male weightlifting athletes (22.3 ± 2.1 years) and observed a correlation between testosterone:cortisol and testosterone:SHBG ratios and the variations in maximum strength and rate of force development (RFD), respectively, as a result of ST (r =

0.77 and r = 0.84, P < 0.05). In an investigation of the relationship between the endocrine system and strength production, Häkkinen & Pakarinen (1993a) observed a correlation between maximum strength and testosterone levels as well as testosterone:SHBG ratio (r = 0.62 and 0.68, respectively, P < 0.01). A study by Izquierdo et al. (2001) revealed that individuals with greater increases in isometric strength following ST also showed higher total (r = 0.78, P < 0.01) and free (r = 0.71, P < 0.05) testosterone levels. The same trend was observed in data obtained by Ahtiainen et al. (2003) when evaluating highly trained men subjected to a 21-week ST program, where positive correlations were observed between the changes in isometric strength and total testosterone (r = 0.84, P < 0.01), the testosterone:cortisol ratio (r = 0.88, P < 0.01) and the isometric strength development and free testosterone (pre-training values: r = 0.78, P < 0.05 and post-training values: r = 0.82, P < 0.05). A study conducted in our laboratory by Cadore et al. (2008a) showed significant correlations between testosterone:SHBG ratios and DHEA concentrations as well as strength production in bench press, leg press and squat exercises (r = 0.55 to 0.82, P < 0.05 to P < 0.001) in trained and untrained middle-aged men. In another study, Cadore et al. (2010) showed significant correlations between increases in the strength of knee extensors and average basal total testosterone levels throughout the training period (3 measurements in 12 weeks of training) (r = 0.94, P < 0.01) and the average total testosterone:cortisol ratio (r = 0.93, P < 0.01). Table 1 shows the results obtained from studies where correlations between hormonal parameters and variables related to muscle strength were identified. One aspect that must be emphasised is that other structural factors, such as pennation angle and fibre type composition, may interfere with strength production (Ramos et al., 1998), just as the volume and intensity of ST largely influence the increase in strength resulting from training (Marx et al., 2001).

Author	Strength performance vs. sex hormonal parameters
Ahtianinen *et al.*, 2003	↑ MVC after ST with TT and TT:COR ratio (r=0.84 and 0.88, P<0.01), and MVC after ST with FT post training (r=0.82, p<0.05)
Cadore *et al.*, 2008a	Squat 1 RM values with TT:SHBG and DHEA before (r=0.71 and 0.65, respectively) and after ST bout (r=0.76 and 0.82, respectively) (p<0.01 to 0.05).
Cadore et al., 2010	↑ knee extension 1 RM values after ST with TT and TT:COR ratio (r=0.94 and 0.93, respectively, p<0.01)
Häkkinen & Pakarinen, 1993a	TT and TT:SHBG with MVC and RFD (r = 0.66 to 0.69, p<0.01)
Häkkinen & Pakarinen, 1993b	↑ MVC after ST with TT and TT:COR (r=0.57 and 0.61, respectively, p<0.05)
Häkkinen *et al.*, 1988	Annual average of TT:COR ratio and MVC (r=0.77, p<0.05); and, annual average of TT:SHBG ratio and ↑ RFD after ST (r=0.84, p<0.05)
Häkkinen *et al.*, 2000	↑ 1 RM values after ST with FT and TT (r=0.55 and 0.43, respectively, p<0.05)
Izquierdo *et al.*, 2001	↑ MVC after ST with TT and FT (r = 0.78 and 0.71, respectively, p<0.01).

Table 1. Relatioship between sex hormonal parameters and strength performance. TT: total testosterone; FT: free testosterone; COR: cortisol; DHEA, dehidroepiandrosterone; SHBG: sex hormone binding globuline; ↑: increases; MVC: maximal voluntary contraction (maximal isometric strength); and, 1 RM: one-maximum repetition (maximal dynamic strength); ST: strength training.

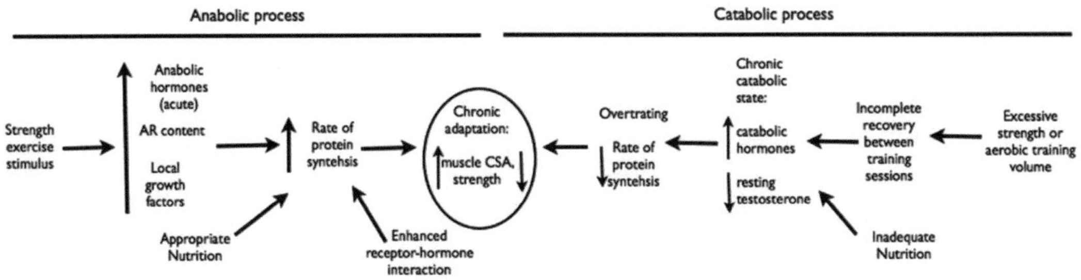

Fig. 1. Schematic diagram of the mechanism of training adaptations: anabolic process as adaptation to strength training and chronic catabolic process resulting from excessive volume of both strength and aerobic training. AR, androgen receptor; CSA, cross-sectional area.

3. Acute testosterone responses to physical exercise

Acute testosterone responses to ST exhibit plasticity, and their pattern depends on factors related to the training session, such as volume, intensity, method (i.e., single or multiple sets) (Cadore et al., 2009a; Häkkinen & Pakarinen, 1993a; McCaulley et al., 2009), type of muscle contraction (Durand et al., 2003; Kraemer et al., 2006) and muscle mass involved (Häkkinen et al., 1998), as well as factors such as age (Kraemer et al., 1999; Cadore et al., 2009a) and the individual's level of training (Ahtiainen et al., 2003; Cadore et al., 2008a, 2009; Kraemer et al., 1999). The response of testosterone levels to ST may expose the skeletal musculature to an elevated peripheral hormonal concentration, which may improve the interaction between the hormone and its cellular receptors (Hoffman et al., 2003, Willoughby & Taylor, 2004). Regarding aerobic training, even though the importance of the anabolic hormone response remains unclear, it seems that testosterone is more responsive to higher intensity exercises (Enea et al., 2009) and a longer duration of exercises (Harris et al., 1989; Trembley et al., 2005).

3.1 Possibles physiological mechanisms for the stimulus

The response of testosterone levels to exercise sessions may reflect certain regulatory mechanisms in addition to the processes that regulate the secretion of this hormone at rest (Fahrner and Hackney, 1998; Lu et al., 1997). A study conducted by Lu et al. (1997) demonstrated that exercise-induced increase in testosterone levels in male rats correlated with an increase in blood lactate levels. Following this observation, the authors proceeded to conduct an *in vitro* study where lactate was infused into the rats' testes, and a dose-dependent increase in testosterone was observed. Methods of ST aimed at achieving muscle hypertrophy or resistance have been shown to cause high lactate production (McCaulley et al., 2009; Smilios et al., 2003), suggesting a strong relationship between the mechanism of testosterone increase and lactate stimulation in the testes (Lu et al., 1997).

Other mechanisms may be responsible for the exercise-induced increase in testosterone levels, among which are increased sympathetic activity in response to exercise (Fahrner and Hackney, 1998) and blood flow and vasodilation related to the release of nitric oxide, which increases hormone secretion (Meskaitis et al., 1997). Even though various studies have used different strength training exercise protocols, Kraemer et al. (1999) and Ahtiainen et al.

(2003) suggest that these mechanisms may also be mediators of testosterone increase in response to this type of training.

3.2 The influence of strength training variables on testosterone responses

It may be stated that the hormonal response to exercise is connected to certain characteristics inherent to the training session, such as the number of sets and repetitions, the relative intensity (percentage of 1 maximum repetition - 1 RM) and time intervals (McCaulley et al., 2009). The amount of work done during ST may be a determining factor in the acute hormone response, leading to an optimum combination of anabolic and catabolic hormone stimulation. This, in turn, may result in a more favourable environment for neuromuscular adaptations to training, resulting in increases in muscle strength and mass (Smilios et al., 2003).

The preponderant influence of volume on the hormonal response to different training methods was observed by Häkkinen and Pakarinen (1993b), who compared the hormonal response to a session involving 20 sets of 1 RM with a session composed by 10 sets of 10 repetitions at 70% of 1 RM; both ST bout were conducted with 3-minute intervals between sets. The authors observed a significant increase ($P<0.05$) in total (22%) and free (23%) testosterone in response to the high-volume training and no increase in the training session that included a higher load and fewer repetitions. Smilios et al. (2003) showed that the hormone response observed in young men increased as the number of sets in each session increased, approaching maximum strength, muscle hypertrophy and resistance. These authors observed that when the number of sets was increased from 4 to 6, the anabolic hormone levels stabilised, while cortisol levels continued to increase. Their results suggest that modifying the volume of a ST session causes alterations in the balance between anabolic and catabolic hormones. When considering different training methods, McCaulley et al. (2009) observed a higher total testosterone response to muscle hypertrophy protocols when compared to protocols that aimed at developing maximum strength and power, despite equalisation of the total work load for each session (load x sets x repetitions). When investigating the influence of the total muscle mass involved in training, Häkkinen et al. (1998b) demonstrated a greater testosterone response in young and elderly men using protocols involving simultaneous use of the lower and upper limbs (27%). However, an increase in hormone levels was also observed for protocols that involved the upper and lower limbs separately ($P<0.01$), indicating that the greater the amount of muscle mass involved, the greater the acute total testosterone response.

Regarding the influence of resting intervals on the acute hormone response, the smaller the interval between sets, the greater the stimulus (Kraemer et al., 1990). Nevertheless, when the sets are performed with maximum repetitions, the interval appears to have no influence within a certain intensity range, as demonstrated by Ahtiainen et al. (2005), who showed that there was no difference in acute hormone response between two protocols of 10 RM with 2- and 5-minute intervals. Notwithstanding, sessions with moderate to high intensity that involve multiple sets and short time intervals, during which energy is derived mainly from glycolytic lactate metabolism, appear to be the greatest stimulus for the steroid hormone response to ST.

Little is known about the influence of combined aerobic and strength training (i.e., concurrent training) on the acute testosterone response. A study by Goto et al. (2005) demonstrated that the GH response to strength training was found to be suppressed by prior aerobic training. However, no differences were observed in strength training-induced testosterone concentrations, with or without prior aerobic training, possibly due to the low-volume protocol used in the study. However, unpublished data from our laboratory show that the manipulation of the order of modalities (strength and aerobic) may, in fact, influence the testosterone response produced by concurrent training sessions. A significant increase was observed in both protocols following the first modality, though levels remained high only at the end of the training session when the protocol involved aerobic training followed by strength training; the same response was not observed when strength training was performed before aerobic training. When comparing acute testosterone responses to strength and aerobic training, some studies show that strength training appears to stimulate greater increases in testosterone levels when compared to aerobic training (Copeland et al., 2002, Tremblay et al., 2003). In a previous study (Cadore et al., 2009a), we showed significantly higher salivary free testosterone responses to water-based resistance exercise compared with water-based aerobic exercise in both young and elderly healthy men. These results can be explained by the powerful influence of the anaerobic glycolytic pathway on acute hormonal increases in response to exercise (Kraemer & Ratamess, 2005).

3.3 The Influence of age and training status

The profile of the population subjected to training sessions is one of the factors that influence hormone response to ST. Studies aimed at investigating this response in different age groups have mainly observed lower responses in elderly individuals as demonstrated by Kraemer et al. (1999). For instance, when comparing acute total and free testosterone responses in groups of men aged 30 ± 5 and 62 ± 3 years, Kraemer et al. (1999) demonstrated that even though both groups showed an increase in free testosterone, a lower testosterone response was observed in the elderly group. According to these authors, the reduced response is associated with andropause, which is characterised by a smaller number and decreased secretory capacity of Leydig cells due to ageing. Similar results were observed by Cadore et al. (2009a), where elderly individuals showed significantly lower free-testosterone responses to water-based resistance exercise than young men.

The individual's training status may also influence the response of the endocrine system to ST (Cadore et al., 2008a, 2009b; Kraemer et al., 1992), given that different anabolic responses may occur before and after a period of ST. Kraemer et al. (1992) investigated weightlifting male athletes aged 17 ± 2 years and observed that individuals with more than 2 years of training presented higher acute testosterone responses. A study by Cadore et al. (2008a) observed different patterns of hormone response in trained and untrained middle-aged men (40 ± 4 years) after a ST protocol. Significant increases in free testosterone (27%) were observed in members of the trained group, whereas significant increases in both total (28%) and free (22%) testosterone as well as DHEA (127%) were observed in the untrained group ($P<0.05$). These results may suggest a higher capacity for testosterone dissociation from carrier proteins, increasing the bioactivity of the hormone without the need for an increase in production. A study by Kraemer et al. (1999) showed higher free testosterone responses in young and elderly individuals following 10 weeks of periodic strength training. Some results suggest the existence of specific responses to certain types of training, as demonstrated in a study developed by Tremblay et al. (2003). The study showed greater increases in anabolic hormone levels in response to strength training in strength-trained subjects when compared to aerobically trained individuals, whereas aerobically trained subjects produced higher hormonal responses to aerobic exercise when compared to strength-trained individuals.

However, the influence of the training status on the testosterone response to ST was not found in many studies. When submitting untrained and previously strength-trained individuals to a 21-week strength training protocol, Ahtiainen et al. (2003) observed similar alterations in total and free testosterone for both groups before and after training. This discrepancy may be due to factors such as sample profile, exercise protocol or potential changes in plasma volume. Moreover, testosterone responses to this type of exercise may be influenced by the relationship of the hormone with its cellular receptors, given that this interaction appears to be greater in trained individuals and that they thus may not require the same magnitude of an acute response in order to obtain an optimum hormone-receptor interaction (Ahtiainen et al., 2011; Willoughby & Taylor, 2004).

4. Chronic endocrine adaptations to physical training

4.1 Basal testosterone adaptations induced by strength training

While some studies demonstrate an increase in the resting levels of testosterone as an adjustment to ST (Izquierdo et al., 2006; Kraemer et al., 1995; Nicklas et al., 1995; Raastad et al., 2003; Tsolakis et al., 2004), other studies have observed no significant differences in this parameter (Ahtiainen et al., 2003; Hansen et al., 2001; Hickson et al., 1994). So far, available data indicate that only young individuals are capable of altering their resting hormone concentrations (Häkkinen et al., 1988; Staron et al., 1994; Tsolakis et al., 2004), whereas middle-aged and elderly individuals show no significant changes in such parameters (Häkkinen & Pakarinen, 1994; Häkkinen et al., 2000; 2001a; Izquierdo et al., 2006; Ryan et al., 1994). Increases in resting levels of testosterone seem to occur during periods of high-volume (Kramer et al., 1995; Marx et al., 2001) and high-intensity training (Staron et al., 1994; Kraemer et al., 1998; Raastad et al., 2003). These changes may occur in men (Häkkinen et al., 1988) and women (Marx et al., 2001) in response to long (Häkkinen et al., 1988; Marx et al., 2001) or short training periods (Staron et al., 1994; Kraemer et al., 1998).

The influence of training volume on chronic adaptations of basal testosterone was described in a study by Marx et al. (2001), which 34 women (22 ± 5 years) were evaluated before and after performing a 24-week ST protocol. In this study, resting levels of testosterone were measured in order to compare groups of ST performing single vs. multiple sets. The results showed an increase in testosterone in both training groups, and the first adaptations took place after 12 weeks of training. However, after 24 weeks of training, only the multiple sets group had further increases in their resting testosterone levels, which was higher in this point than after 12 weeks, and higher than the single set ST group. Even though the performance of high-volume ST sessions may induce higher acute increases in catabolic hormones (Smilios et al., 2003), the study developed by Marx et al. (2001) demonstrated that high-volume and high-intensity ST may lead to higher chronic increases in anabolic hormones compared to low-volume ST. This may contribute to the greater strength production observed in individuals who trained with multiple sets when compared to those who trained with simple sets (Kemmler et al., 2004).

The Table 2 shows subjects characteristics, training protocol and results from some of the studies that have investigated resting hormone adaptations to ST. Nevertheless, modifications in resting concentrations appear to be transient, resulting from the increase or decrease in intensity and, mainly, in volume (Ahtiainen et al., 2003). However, the precise role of resting testosterone concentrations in neuromuscular adaptation to training is yet to be determined.

Author	Subjects	Training protocol	Results
Ahtiainen *et al.*, 2003	Young previously trained and untrained men	21 weeks, 2 times/week, 8-10 RM	↑ FT in trained after 14 weeks; no modifications after 21 weeks
Cadore *et al.*, 2008a	Middle-aged long-term trained and untrained men	10 ± 5 years of strength training, 4 times a week, 8-12 RM	No difference at rest, different responses to exercise
Häkkinen *et al.*, 2001a	Elderly men	21 weeks, 40-80% of 1 RM	No modifications
Häkkinen *et al.*, 1988	Elite powerlifters young men	Two years, 5 times/week	↑ TT
Staron et al., 1994	Young men and women	8 weeks, 3 times/week, 6-12 RM	↑ TT in men
Häkkinen & Pakarinen, 1994	Middle-aged and elderly men and women	12 weeks, 3 times/week, 40-80% of 1 RM	No modifications
Izquierdo *et al., 2001*	Young men and women	16 weeks, 3 times/week, 50-80% of 1 RM	No modifications
Kraemer *et al.*, 1995	Military young men	12 weeks, 4 times/week, 3-10 RM, strength vs. concurrent training	↑ TT after concurrent training
Kraemer *et al.*, 1999	Young and elderly men	10 weeks, 3 times/week, 3-15 RM	↑ FT jovens
Marx *et al.*, 2001	Young women	24 weeks, 3-15 RM, single vs. 3 sets per exercise	↑ TT in both groups after 12 weeks, higher after 3 sets training group
Nicklas *et al.*, 1995	Middle-aged and elderly men	16 weeks, 3 times/week, 5-15 RM	No modifications
Ryan *et al.*, 1994	Elderly men	16 weeks, 3 times/week, 5-15 RM	No modifications

Table 2. Testosterone modifications at rest after strength training: TT: total testosterone; FT: free testosterone; ↑: increases; RM: maximal repetitions.

4.2 Changes in circulating testosterone in response to aerobic training

With regards to aerobic training, studies have demonstrated that endurance athletes have lower testosterone levels when compared to sedentary individuals (Strüder et al., 1998; Maïmoun et al., 2003). However, Strüder et al. (1998) showed that although testosterone levels were indeed lower in elderly male runners compared to age-matched sedentary subjects, the same was not true for previously sedentary subjects who performed aerobic training for 20 weeks 3 times per week with an intensity of 50 to 65% of aerobic power. A previous study conducted in our laboratory (Cadore et al., 2010) demonstrated a significant reduction in free testosterone in elderly men following 12 weeks of aerobic training on a cycle ergometer 3 times per week with intensity varying between 55 and 85% of aerobic power (9.7 ± 2.8 vs. 7.9 ± 3.0 pg/mL, P < 0.01). Possible discrepancies between the results of different studies may reflect the different intensities and volumes used, given that the intensity used by Strüder et al. (1999), for instance, was lower than the intensity used in our study (Cadore et al., 2010). However, in animal models, Hu et al. (1999) observed a significant reduction in testosterone levels in rats submitted to continuous swimming for 3 weeks. Levels were restored to normal following 6 weeks of training, suggesting an adjustment to training on LH secretion in the endocrine system that was associated with negative feedback. Even though testosterone reduction during aerobic training has not been clearly demonstrated, it is possible that a certain amount of time is necessary for the endocrine system to adapt to the volume and intensity of training when these factors exceed a certain stimulus threshold (Calbet et al., 1993; Kraemer & Ratamess, 2005; Maïmoun et al., 2003).

Though high-volume physical training may result in the suppression of testosterone via direct inhibition due to the effect of cortisol on the testes (Brownlee et al., 2005), this does not completely explain the occurrence of testosterone reduction with aerobic training, given that increases in basal cortisol levels and the consequent testicular suppression are most commonly related to overtraining. In fact, testosterone levels have been shown to be reduced in endurance athletes with no alterations in cortisol levels (Maïmoun et al., 2003) as well as in non-athletes subjected to aerobic training (Cadore et al. 2010). Furthermore, other mechanisms, such as hypervolemia, increased utilisation of the hormone by muscle tissue and increased hepatic degradation of the hormone, may be responsible for the decrease in testosterone levels that result from endurance training (Izquierdo et al., 2004).

4.3 Changes in muscle cell androgen receptors

Evidence shows that cell adjustments may be key factors for training-induced hypertrophy (Ahtiainen et al., 2011; Deschenes et al., 1994; Inoue et al., 1993, 1994; Kadi et al., 2000; Bamman et al., 2001; Willoughby & Taylor, 2004; Ratamess et al., 2005). Some of these adjustments correspond to an increase in the number of androgen receptors (AR) in the muscle, and they are apparently dependent on the pattern of acute testosterone response to exercise (Willoughby & Taylor, 2004). A greater number of ARs and an increased sensitivity of these receptors to the hormone may improve the trophic effects of testosterone on target cells (Kadi et al., 2000). Inoue et al. (1993) subjected male rats to training using electrical stimulation and demonstrated that muscle hypertrophy occurred in parallel with a significant increase in cellular ARs. In a different study, Inoue et al. (1994) observed that the suppression of androgen receptors by receptor antagonists reduced the increase in muscle mass obtained with electrical stimulation.

Kadi et al. (2000) measured the number of ARs per area of muscle fibre in the superior trapezius and the *vastus lateralis* muscle of high-performance weightlifting men. The sample was composed of trained individuals with (31 ± 3 years) and without (28 ± 8 years) the use of exogenous anabolic steroids as well as untrained individuals (23 ± 3 years). Results showed higher numbers of ARs per area of muscle fibre in the superior trapezius of individuals from both trained groups when compared with untrained individuals. Moreover, individuals using exogenous anabolic steroids presented higher values than those that were only training (P<0.05). Surprisingly, these differences were observed only in the superior trapezius. The proportion between the different types of muscle fibres present in each of the evaluated muscle groups (i.e., type I and type II) may have influenced the different behaviours of the androgen receptors in response to training. In fact, while studying rats subjected to strength training, Deschenes et al. (1994) were only able to observe an increase in the number of ARs in muscles with a predominance of fast glycolytic fibres, whereas muscles with a predominance of slow oxidative fibres showed decreased numbers of ARs.

Willoughby & Taylor (2004) conducted a study where 18 young men were subjected to 3 sessions of ST with 3 sets of 8 to 10 RM. Results showed a significant increase in protein synthesis, AR expression and AR messenger RNA following the training sessions, where values increased up to 202% 48 hours after the third session. Furthermore, the study revealed a correlation between testosterone increase (significant following all sessions) and an increase in the number of receptors ($r = 0.89$, $P < 0.05$). These results suggest that the hormone-receptor complex constitutes an important element in the mechanism responsible for mediating the adjustments to strength training, such as an increase in muscle strength and exercise-induced hypertrophy (Inoue et al., 1993; Kadi et al., 2000; Willoughby & Taylor 2004).

5. Conclusion

As noted in the studies presented in this chapter, there is a connection between the trainability of individuals subjected to ST and their levels of circulating testosterone. However, factors related to the training sessions and population profile seem to influence acute and chronic hormone responses, which result in a plasticity in the pattern of testosterone response to physical exercise, particularly strength training. Among the types of strength training sessions, high-volume protocols with moderate to high intensity (70-85% 1 RM), which are typically used to achieve muscle hypertrophy and predominantly rely on the glycolytic lactate metabolic pathway, appear to stimulate greater responses. Moreover, the increase in the number of ARs appears to have a key role in muscle hypertrophy observed with ST. However, determining which factors might be related to the hormone response to ST may be of great importance for the prescription of a training session and determination of the optimum period that will optimise the anabolic environment determined by testosterone and thus maximise the neuromuscular adaptations resulting from strength training.

6. Acknowledgements

We thank specially to CAPES and CNPq government associations for their support to this project.

7. References

Ahtiainen J.P.; Pakarinen, A.; Alen, M.; Kraemer, W.J. & Häkkinen, K. (2003). Muscle hypertrophy, hormonal adaptations and strength development during strength training in strength-trained and untrained men. *European Journal of Applied Physiology*, Vol. 89, No. 6 (Aug 2003) pp. 555-63, ISSN 1419-6339

Ahtiainen J.P.; Pakarinen, A.; Alen, M.; Kraemer, W.J.; & Häkkinen, K. (2005). Short vs. long rest period between the sets in hypertrophic resistance training: influence on muscle strength, size, and hormonal adaptations in trained men. *Journal of Strength and Conditioning Research*, Vol 19, No. 3, pp. 572-582, ISSN 1064-8011

Ahtiainen J.P.; Hulme, J.J.; Kraemer, W.J.; Lehti, M.; Nyman, K.; Selanne, H.; Alen, M.; Pakarinen, A.; Komulainen, J.; Kovanen, V.; Mero, A.A. & Häkkinen, K. (2011). Heavy resistance exercise training and skeletal muscle androgen receptor expression in younger and older men. Steroids, Vol. 76, No. 1-2 (Jan 2011), pp. 183-192, ISSN 0039-128X

Bamman, M.M.; Ship, J.R.; Jiang, J.; Gower, B.A.; Hunter, G.R.; Goodman, A.; McLafferty, J.R. & Urban, R.J. (2001). Mechanical load increases muscle IGF-I and androgen receptor mRNA concentration in humans. *American Journal of Physiology: Endocrinology and Metabolism,* Vol. 280, No. 3 (Mar 2001), pp. 383-90, ISSN 0193-1849

Bell, G.J.; Syrotuik, D.; Martin, T.P.; Burnham, R. & Quinney, H.A. (2000). Effect of concurrent strength and endurance training on skeletal muscle properties and hormone concentrations in humans. *European Journal of Applied Physiology,* Vol. 81, No. 5 (mar 2000), pp. 418-427, ISSN 1419-6339

Bhasin, S.W.; Woodhouse, L.;, Casaburi, R.; Singh, A.B.; Bhasin, D.; Berman, N., Chen, X.; Yarasheske, K.E.; Magliano, L.; Dzekov, C.; Dzekov, J.; Bros, R.; Philips, J.; Sinha-Hikim, I.; Shen, R. & Storer, T.W. (2001). Testosterone dose-response relationships in healthy young men. *American Journal of Physiology: Endocrinology Metabolism,* Vol. 281, No. 6, (Dec 2001), pp. 1172-1181, ISSN 0193-1849

Bross, R.; Javanbakht, M. & Bhasin, S. (1999). Anabolic intervention for aging-associated sarcopenia. *The Journal of Clinical Endocrinology and Metabolism,* Vol. 84, No. 10, pp. 3420-3430, ISSN 0021-972X

Brownlee, K.K.; Moore, A.W. & Hackney, A.C. (2005). Relationship between circulating cortisol and testosterone: influence of physical exercise. *Journal of Sports Science and Medicine,* Vol. 4, pp. 76-83, ISSN 1303-2968

Cadore, E.L.; Lhullier, F.L.R.; Brentano, M.A.; Silva, E.M.; Ambrosini, M.B.; Spinelli, R.; Silva, R.F. & Kruel, L.F.M. (2008a). Hormonal responses to resistance exercise in long-term trained and untrained middle-aged men. *Journal of Strength and Conditioning Research,* Vol. 22, No. 5 (Sep 2008) pp. 1617-1624, ISSN 1064-8011

Cadore, E.; Lhullier, F.; Brentano, A.; Silva, E.; Ambrosini, M., Spinelli, R., Silva, R.F. & Kruel, L.F.M. (2008b). Correlations between serum and salivary hormonal concentrations in response to resistance exercise. *Journal of Sports Sciences,* Vol. 26, No. 10 (Aug 2008) pp. 1067-1072, ISSN 0264-0414

Cadore, E.L.; Brentano, M.A.; Lhullier, F.L.R. & Kruel, L.F.M. (2008c). Factors concerned with the testosterone and cortisol response to strength training. *Revista Brasileira de Medicina do Esporte,* Vol. 14, No. 1, (Jan/Fev 2008), pp. 74-78, ISSN 1517-8692

Cadore, E.L.; Lhullier, F.L.; Alberton, C.L.; Almeida, A.P.; Sapata, K.B.; Korzenowski, A.L.; & Kruel, L.F. (2009a). Salivary hormonal responses to different water-based exercise protocols in young and elderly men. *Journal of Strength and Conditioning Research,* Vol. 23, No. 9, (Dec 2009), pp. 2695-2701, ISSN 1064-8011

Cadore E.L.; Lhullier, F.; Arias Brentano, A.; Marczwski da Silva, E.; Bueno Ambrosini, M.,;Spinelli, R.; Ferrari Silva, R.; Martins Kruel, L.F. (2009b). *Journal of Sports Medicine and Physical Fitness,* 49, No. 3 (Sep 2009), pp. 301-307, ISSN 0022-4707

Cadore, E.L.; Pinto, R.S.; Lhullier, F.L.R.; Correa, C.S.; Alberton, C.L.; Pinto, S.S.; Almeida, A.P.V.; Tartaruga, M.P.; Silva, E.M. & Kruel, L.F.M. (2010). Physiological effects of concurrent training in elderly men. *International Journal of Sports Medicine,* 31, No. 10 (Oct 2010), pp. 689-697. ISSN 0172-4622

Calbet, J.A.L.; Navarro, M.A.; Barbany, J.R.; Manso, J.G.; Bonnin, M.R. & Valero, J. (1993). Salivary steroid changes and physical performance in highly trained cyclists. *International Journal of Sports Medicine,* Vol. 14, No. 3, (Apr 1993), pp. 111-117, ISSN 0172-4622

Copeland, J.L.; Consitt, L.A. & Tremblay, M.S. (2002). Hormonal Responses to endurance and resistance exercise in females aged 19-69 years. *The Journal of Gerontology,* Vol. 57, No. 4 , (Apr 2002), pp. B158-B165) ISSN 0022-1422

Deschenes, M.R.; Maresh, C.M.; Armstrong, L.E.; Covault, J.; Kraemer, W.J.; Crivello, J.F. (1994). Endurance and resistance exercise induce muscle fiber type specific responses in androgen binding capacity. *Journal of Steroid Biochemistry and Molecular Biology* Vol. 50, No 3-4, (Aug 1994), pp. 175-179, ISSN 0960-0760

Durand, J.R.; Castracane, V.D.; Hollander, D.B.; Trynieck, J.L.; Bamman, M.M.; O'neal, S.; Hebert, E.P. & Kraemer, R.R. (2003). Hormonal responses from concentric and eccentric muscle contractions. *Medicine and Science in Sports and Exercise* 2003, Vol. 35, No. 6, (Jun 2003), pp. 937-943, ISSN 0195-9131

Enea, C.; Boisseau, N.; Mulliez, J.; Millet, C.; Ingrand, I.; Diaz, V. & Dugué, B. (2009). Effects of menstrual cycle, oral contraception, and training on exercise-induced changes in circulating DHEA-sulphate and testosterone in young women. *European Journal of Applied Physiology,* Vol. 106, No. 3, (Jun 2009), pp. 365-373, ISSN 1419-6339

Fahrner, C.L. & Hackney, A.C. (1998). Effects of endurance exercise on free testosterone concentration and binding affinity of sex hormone binding globulin (SHBG). *International Journal of Sports Medicine,* Vol. 19, No. 1, (Jan 1998), pp. 2-15, ISSN 0172-4622

Goto, K.; Higashiyama, M.; Ishii, N. & Takamatsu, K. (2005). Prior endurance exercise attenuates growth hormone responses to subsequent resistance exercise. *European Journal of Applied Physiology,* Vol. 94, No. 3, (Jun 2005), pp. 333-338, ISSN 1419-6339

Griggs, R.C.; Kingston, W.; Jozefowcz, R.F.; Herr, B.E.; Forbes, G. & Halliday, D. (1989) Effects of testosterone on muscle mass and muscle protein synthesis. *Journal of Applied Physiology,* Vol. 66, No 1, (Jan 1989), pp. 498-503, ISSN 8750-7587

Häkkinen, K. & Pakarinen, A. (1993a). Acute hormonal responses to two different fatiguing heavy-resistance protocols in male athletes. *Journal of Applied Physiology,* Vol. 74, No. 2, (Feb 1993), pp. 882-887, ISSN 8750-7587

Häkkinen K, Pakarinen A. (1993b). Muscle strength and serum testosterone, cortisol and SHBG concentrations in middle-aged and elderly men and women. *Acta Physiologica Scandinavica,* Vol. 148, No. 2 (Jun 1993), pp. 199-207, ISSN 0001-6772

Häkkinen, K. & Pakarinen, A. (1994) Serum hormones and strength development during strength training in middle-aged and elderly males and females. *Acta Physiologica Scandinavica,*Vol. 150, No. 2 (Feb 1994), pp. 211-219, ISSN 0001-6772

Häkkinen, K. & Pakarinen, A. (1995). Acute hormonal responses to heavy resistance exercise in men and women at different ages. *International Journal of Sports Medicine,* Vol. 16, No. 8, (Aug 1995), pp. 507-513, ISSN 0172-4622

Häkkinen K.; Pakarinen, A.; Alen, M.; Kauhanen, H.; Komi, P.V. (1988). Neuromuscular and hormonal adaptations in athletes to strength training in two years. *Journal of Applied Physiology,* Vol. 65, No. 6, (Dec 1988), pp. 2406-2412, ISSN 8750-7587

Häkkinen, K.; Pakarinen, A.; Newton, R.U.; Kraemer, W.J. (1998). Acute hormonal responses to heavy resistance lower and upper extremity exercise in young versus old men.

European Journal of Applied Physiology Vol. 77, No. 4, (Mar 1998), pp. 312-19 ISSN 1419-6339

Häkkinen, K.; Pakarinen, A.; Kraemer, W.J.; Newton, R.U. & Alen, M. (2000). Basal concentrations and acute responses of serum hormones and strength development during heavy resistance training in middle-aged and elderly men and women. *Journal of Gerontology: Biological Sciences*, Vol. 55, No. 2, (Feb 2000), pp. B95-B105, ISSN 0022-1422

Häkkinen, K.; Pakarinen, A.; Kraemer, W.J.; Häkkinen, A.; Valkeinen, H. & Alen, M. (2001a). Selective muscle hypertrophy, changes in EMG and force, and serum hormones during strength training in older women. *Journal of Applied Physiology*, Vol. 91, No. 2, (Aug 2001), pp. 569-80, ISSN 8750-7587

Häkkinen, K.; Kraemer, W.J.; Newton, R.U. & Alen, M. (2001b). Changes in electromyographic activity, muscle fibre and force production characteristics during heavy resistance/power strength training in middle-aged and older men and women. *Acta Physiologica Scandinavica*, Vol .171, No 1, (Jan 2001), pp. 51-62, ISSN 0001-6772

Hansen, S.; Kvorning, T.; Kjaer, M. & Sjogaard, G. (2001). The effect of short-term strength training on human skeletal muscle: the importance of physiologically elevated hormone levels. *Scandinavian Journal of Medicine and Science in Sports*, Vol. 11, No. 6, (Dec 2001), pp. 347-54. ISSN 0905-7188

Harris, B.; Cook, N.J.; Walker, R.F.; Read, G.F.; Riad-Fahmy, D. (1989). Salivary steroids and psychometric parameters in male marathon runners. *British Journal of Sports Medicine*; 23 (2): 89-93. ISSN 0306-3674

Hickson, R.C.; Hidaka, K.; Foster, C.; Falduto, M.T. & Chatterton Jr, R.T. (1994). Successive time courses of strength development and steroid hormone responses to heavy-resistance training. *Journal of Applied Physiology*, Vol. 76 No. 2, (Feb 1994), 663-670, ISSN 8750-7587

Hoffman, J.R.; Im, J.; Rundell, K.W.; Kang, J.; Nioka, S.; Speiring, B.A.; Kime, R. & Chance, B. (2003). Effects of muscle oxygenation during resistance exercise on anabolic hormone response. *Medicine and Science in Sports and Exercise* Vol. 35, No. 11, (Nov 2003), pp. 1929-34. ISSN 0195-9131

Hu, Y.; Asano, K.; Mizuno, K.; Usuki, S.; Kawamura, Y. (1999). Serum testosterone responses to continuous and intermittent exercise training in male rats. *International Journal of Sports Medicine*, Vol. 20, No. 1 (Jan 1999), pp. 12-16, ISSN 0172-4622

Inoue, K.; Yamasaki, T.; Fushiki, T.; Kano, T.; Moritani, T.; Itoh, K. & Sugimoto E. (1993). Rapid increase in the number of androgen receptors following electrical stimulation of the rat muscle. *European Journal of Applied Physiology*, Vol. 66, No. 2 (Feb. 1993), pp. 134-40, ISSN 1419-6339

Inoue, K.; Yamasaki, T.; Fushiki, T, Okada, Y. & Sugimoto, E. (1994). Androgen receptor antagonist suppresses exercise-induced hypertrophy of skeletal muscle. *European Journal of Applied Physiology*, Vol. 69, No. 1, (Jan 1994), pp. 88-91, ISSN 1419-6339

Izquierdo, M.; Häkkinen, K.; Ibañez, J.; Garrues, M.; Antón, A.; Zúniga, A.; Larrión, J.L. & Gorostiaga, E.M. (2001). Effects of strength training on muscle power and serum hormones in middle-aged and older men. *Journal of Applied Physiology*, Vol. 90, No. 4, (Apr 2001), pp. 1497-1507, ISSN 8750-7587

Izquierdo, M.; Ibañez, J.; Häkkinen, K.; Kraemer, W.J.; Ruesta, M. & Gorostiaga, E.M. (2004). Maximal strength and power, muscle mass, endurance and serum hormones in weightlifters and road cyclists. Journal of Sports Sciences, Vol. 22, No. 5, (May 2004), pp. 465-478, ISSN 0264-0414

Izquierdo, M.; Ibañez, J.; González-Badillo, J.J.; Häkkinen, K.; Ratamess, N.A.; Kraemer, W.J.; French, D.N.; Eslava, J.; Altadill, A.; Asiain, X. & Gorostiaga, E.M. (2006). Differential effects of strength training leading to failure versus not to failure on hormonal responses, strength or power gains. *Journal of Applied Physiology* Vol. 100, No. 5, (May 2006), pp. 1646-1656, ISSN 8750-7587

Kadi, F.; Bonnrud, P.; Eriksson, A. & Thornell, L.E. (2000). The expression of androgen receptors in human neck and limb muscles: effects of training and self-administration of androgenic steroids. *Histochemistry and Cell Biology*, Vol. 113, No 1, (Jan 2000), pp. 25-29, ISSN 0948-6143

Kemmler, W.K.; Lauber, D.; Engelke, K. & Weineck, J. (2004). Effects of single- vs. multiple-set resistance training on maximun strength and body composition in trained postmenopausal women. *Journal of Strength and Conditioning Research*, Vol. 18, No. 4, (Nov 2004), pp. 689–694, ISSN 1064-8011

Kraemer, R.R.; Hollander, D.B.; Reeves, G.V.; Francois, M.; Ramadan, Z.G.; Meeker, B.; Tryniecki, J.L.; Hebert, E.P. & Castracane, V.D. (2006). Similar hormonal responses to concentric and eccentric muscle actions using relative loading. *European Journal of Applied Physiology* Vol. 96, No. 5, (Mar 2006), pp. 551-557, ISSN 1419-6339

Kraemer, W.J.; Marchitelli, L.J.; Gordon, S.E.; Harman, E.; Dziados, J.E,.; Mello, R.; Frykman, P.; McCurry, D. & Fleck, S.J. (1990). Hormonal and growth factor responses to heavy resistance exercise protocols. *Journal of Applied Physiology*, Vol. 69, No. 4, (Oct 1990), pp. 1442-1450, ISSN 8750-7587

Kraemer, W.J.; Fry, A.C.; Warren, B.J.; Stone, M.H.; Fleck, S.J.; Kearney, J.T.; Conroy, B.P.; Maresh, C.M.; Weseman, C.A.; Triplett, N.T. & Gordon, S.E. (1992).Acute hormonal responses in elite junior weightlifters. *International Journal of Sports Medicine*, Vol. 13, No. 2, (Feb 1992), pp. 103-109, ISSN 0172-4622

Kraemer, W.J.; Fleck, S.J.; Dziados, J.E.; Harman, E.A.; Marchitelli, L.J.; Gordon, S.E.; Mello, R.; Frykman, P.N.; Koziris, L.P. & Triplett, N.T. (1993). Changes in hormonal concentrations after different heavy-resistance exercise protocols in women. *Journal of Applied Physiology*, Vol. 75, No. 2 (Aug 1993), pp. 494-504, ISSN 8750-7587

Kraemer, W.J.; Patton, J.F.; Gordon, S.E.; Harman, E.A.; Deschenes, M.R.; Reynolds, K.; Newton, R.U.; Triplett, N.T. & Dziados, J.E. (1995). Compatibility of high-intensity strength and endurance training on hormonal and skeletal muscle adaptations. *Journal of Applied Physiology* Vol. 78, No 3, (Mar 1995), pp. 976-989, ISSN 8750-7587

Kraemer, W.J.; Staron, R.S.; Hagerman, F.C.; Hikida, R.S.; Fry, A.C.; Gordon, S.E.; Nindl, B.C.; Gothshalk, L.A.; Volek, J.S.; Marx, J.O.; Newton, R.U. & Häkkinen, K. (1998). The effects of short-term resistance training on endocrine function in men women. *European Journal of Applied Physiology* 1998;Vol. 78, No. 1, (Jun 1998), pp. 69-76, ISSN 1419-6339

Kraemer, W.J.; Häkkinen, K.; Newton, R.U.; Nindl, B.C.; Volek, J.S.; McCormick, M.; Gothshalk, L.A.; Gordon, S.E.; Fleck, S.J.; Campbell, W.W.; Putukian, M. & Evans, W.J. (1999). Effects of resistance training on hormonal response patterns in younger vs. older men. *Journal of Applied Physiology* Vol. 87, No. 3, (Sep 1999), pp. 982-992, ISSN 8750-7587

Kraemer, W.J. & Ratamess, N.A. (2005). Hormonal responses and adaptation to resistance exercise and training *Sports Medicine,* Vol. 35, No. 4, pp. 339-361, ISSN 0193-1849

Lu, S.; Lau, C.; Tung, Y.; Huang, S.; Chen,Y.; Shih, H., Tsai, S.C.; Lu, C.C.; Wang, S.W.; Chen, J.J.; Chien, E.J.; Chien, C.H. & Wang, P.S. (1997). Lactate and the effects of exercise on testosterone secretion: evidence for the involvement of cAMP-mediated mechanism. *Medicine and Science in Sports and Exercise,* Vol. 29, No. 8, (Aug 1997), pp. 1048-1054, ISSN 0195-9131

Maïmoun, L.; Lumbroso, S.; Manetta, J.; Paris, F.; Leroux, J.L. & Sultan, C. (2003). Testosterone is significantly reduced in endurance athletes without impact on bone mineral density. *Hormone Research* Vol. 59, No. 6, pp. 285-292, ISSN 0301-0163

Marx, J.O.; Ratamess, N.A.; Nindl, B.C.; Gotshalk, L.A.; Volek, J.S.; Dohi, K.; Bush, J.A.; Gómez, A.L.; Mazzetti, S.A.; Fleck, S.J.; Newton, R.U. & Häkkinen, K. (2001). Low-volume circuit versus high-volume periodized resistance training in women. *Medicine and Science in Sports and Exercise,* Vol. 33, No. 4, (Apr 2001), pp. 635-643, ISSN 0195-9131

McCaulley, G.O.; McBride, J.M.; Cormie, P.; Hudson, M.B.; Nuzzo, J.L.; Quindry, J.C.; & Triplett, N.T. (2009). Acute hormonal and neuromuscular to hypertrophy, strength and power type resistance exercise. *European Journal of Applied Physiology,* Vol. 105, No. 5, (Mar 2009), pp. 695-704, ISSN 1419-6339

Meskaitis, V.J.; Harman, F.S.; Volek, J.S.; Nindl, B.C.; Kraemer, W.J.; Weinstok, D. & Deaver, D.R. (1997) Effects of exercise on testosterone and nitric oxide production in the rats testis. *The Journal of Andrology Supplement* 1997; p. 31, ISSN 0196-3635

Nicklas, B.J.; Ryan, A.S.; Treuth, M.M.; Harman, S.M.; Blackman, M.R.; Hurley, B.F. & Rogers, M.A. (1995). Testosterone, growth hormone and IGF-I responses to acute and chronic resistive exercise in men aged 55-70 years. *International Journal of Sports Medicine,* Vol.16, No. 7, (Oct 1995), pp. 445-450, ISSN 0172-4622

Raastad, T.; Glomsheler, T.; Bjoro, T. & Hallen, J. (2003). Recovery of skeletal muscle contractility and hormonal responses to strength exercise alter two weeks of high-volume strength training. *Scandinavian Journal of Medicine and Science in Sports,* Vol. 13, No. 3 (Jun 2003), pp.159-168, ISSN 0905-7188

Ramos, E.; Frontera, W.R.; Llopart, A. & Feliciano, D. (1998). Muscle strength and hormonal levels in adolescents: gender related differences. *International Journal of Sports Medicine* 1998;Vol. 19, No 8, (Nov 1998), pp. 526-531, ISSN 0172-4622

Ratamess, N.A.; Kraemer, W.J.; Volek, J.S.; Maresh, C.M.; Vanheest, J.L.; Sharman, M.J.; Rubin, M.R.; French, D.N.; Vescovi, J.D.; Silvestre, R.; Hatfield, D.L.; Fleck, S.J. & Deschenes, M.R. (2005). Androgen receptor content following heavy resistance exercise in men. *Journal of Steroid Biochemistry and Molecular Biology,* Vol. 93, No. 1, (Jan 2005), pp. 35-42, ISSN 0960-0760

Ryan, A.S.; Treuch, M.S.; Rubin, M.A.; Miller, J.P.; Nicklas, B.J.; Landis, D.M.; Pratley, R.E.; Libanati, C.R.; Gundberg, C.M. & Hurley, B.F. (1994) Effects of strength training on bone mineral density: hormonal and bone turnover relationships. *Journal of Applied Physiology,* Vol. 77, No. 4, (Oct 1994), pp.1678-1684, ISSN 8750-7587

Smilios, I.; Pilianidis, T.; Karamouzis, M.; Parlavantzas, A. & Tokmakidis SP. (2007). Hormonal responses after strength endurance resistance exercise protocol in young and elderly males. *International Journal of Sports Medicine,* Vol. 28, No. 5, (May 2007), pp. 401-406, ISSN 0172-4622

Smilios, I.; Pilianidis, T.; Karamouzis, M. & Tokmakidis, S. Hormonal responses after various resistance exercise protocols. *Medicine and Science in Sports and Exercise,* Vol 35, No. 4, (Apr 2003), pp. 644-654, ISSN 0195-9131

Staron, R.S.; Karapondo, D.L.; Kraemer, W.J.; Fry, A.C.; Gordon, S.E.; Falkel, J.E.; Hagerman, F.C. & Hikida, R.S. (1994). Skeletal muscle adaptations during early phase of heavy-resistance training in men and women. *Journal of Applied Physiology,* Vol. 76, No. 3, (Mar 1994), pp. 1247-1255, ISSN 8750-7587

Strüder, H.K.; Hollmann, W.; Platen, P.; Rost, R.; Wiecker, H.; Kirchhof, O. & Weber, K. (1999). Neuroendocrine system and mental function in sedentary and endurance-trained elderly males. *International Journal of Sports Medicine,* Vol. 20, No. 3 (Apr 1999), pp. 159-166, ISSN 0172-4622

Tremblay, M.S.; Copeland, J.L. & Van Helder, W. (2004). Effect of training status and exercise mode on endogenous steroid hormones in men. *Journal of Applied Physiology,* Vol. 96, No. 2, (Feb 2004), pp. 531-539, ISSN 8750-7587

Tremblay, M.S.; Copeland, J.L. & Van Helder, W. (2005). Influence of exercise duration on post-exercise steroid hormone responses in trained males. *European Journal of Applied Physiology,* Vol.94, No. 5-6, (Aug 2005), pp. 505-513, ISSN 1419-6339

Tsolakis, C.K.; Vagenas, G.K. & Dessypris, A.G. (2004). Strength adaptations and hormonal responses to resistance training and detraining in preadolescent males. *Journal of Strength and Conditioning Research,* Vol. 18, No. 3, (Aug 2004), pp.625–629, ISSN 1064-8011

Willoughby, D.S. & Taylor, L. (2004). Effects of sequential bouts of resistance exercise on androgen receptor expression *Medicine and Science in Sports and Exercise,* Vol. 36, No. 9, (Sep 2004), pp.1499-1506, ISSN 0195-9131

14

Hand Grip Strength in Relation to Morphological Measures of Masculinity, Fluctuating Asymmetry and Sexual Behaviour in Males And Females

Stefan Van Dongen and Ellen Sprengers
Antwerp University
Belgium

1. Introduction

Human evolutionary history is, as that of any other species, characterized by phenotypic and genetic changes as a result of natural and/or sexual selection. In spite of the fact that we live in relatively unnatural environments (especially in our Western culture), signals of this evolutionary history are tractable and allow gaining insights in ancestral processes of selection. One important aspect that has received a lot of attention is the process of mate selection and attractiveness (e.g., Thornhill & Gangestad, 1999). The central working hypothesis is that particular morphological features correlate with 'genetic' quality or mate value. Selection would then favour preferences for these features (i.e., evaluated to be attractive) such that choosing a mate baring these features would increase reproductive success. This has driven research in evolutionary psychology, and the main focus has been on attractiveness, secondary sex characteristics as hormone markers, hormone levels and fluctuating asymmetry (e.g., Thornhill & Gangestad, 1999).

Overall, there is growing evidence that (especially) women evaluate sex-typical characteristics of the face, body and voice in men and that their preference may vary across the menstrual cycle. Also in women, typically feminine characteristics are judged to be more attractive. Although the adaptive value of these preferences is much more difficult to study, it appears reasonable to assume that more masculine characteristics in males correlate with increased circulating testosterone levels which in turn positively associate with dominance and physical performance while feminine characteristics reflect oestrogen levels which associate with increased fertility. Thus, there is evidence that these hormone-mediated characteristics bare information that, at least ancestrally, are important for mate selection and expected fitness. An interesting and open question then is why the sexual dimorphism in humans has not evolved to be more extreme. Most likely, some cost is associated to develop more masculine for males and/or more feminine for females. Alternatively, there is some evidence of an intra locus sexual conflict affecting fitness of siblings (Garver-Apgar et al., 2011). Most attention in the literature has been devoted to the association between masculinity and other measures of health, like fluctuating asymmetry (FA). Three possible outcomes have been proposed. More masculine or feminine features are (assumed to be) associated to higher testosterone or oestrogen levels, respectively, which, in turn, may act as an immunosuppressant (Little et al., 2008). It has, therefore, often been argued that larger secondary sexual characteristics should be related to a healthier immune system because only healthy individuals can afford the high sex hormone handicap (Little et al., 2008). On the other hand, Getty (2002) and Kokko et al. (2002) have noted that, because of trade-offs between investment in reproductive traits and somatic investment (e.g., immune defences), high quality individuals may, under intense sexual selection, be 'forced' to invest in reproduction to such a large degree that they actually have worse health and poorer survival prospects than individuals of low quality. Thus, if both symmetry and masculinity/femininity signal quality, both should be positively correlated where high quality males can grow symmetric and masculine and high quality females can grow symmetric and feminine (e.g., Little et al., 2008). However, if sexual selection drives high quality individuals to display extreme masculine/feminine features, these may come at the expense of health. Under such a scenario, high quality individuals preferred for mating, with high circulating sex hormones (testosterone or estrogens) and/or associated morphological expression of masculinity/femininity would develop a less symmetric body relative to individuals with lower circulating hormones and less extreme morphological expression of masculinity/femininity. Recently, Puts (2010) argued that androgen-dependent masculine traits may be produced in proportion to inherited immunocompetence, so that good-gene males end up little healthier than average. The regulation of androgen levels and the response to them may thus have evolved as a means of producing sexually selected traits in proportion to a male's ability to safely bare them. If so, little or no relationship between sexual dimorphism and FA is expected, as individuals would trade inherited immunocompetence for sexual competitiveness (masculinity in males, femininity in females). A recent review found little evidence for an association between FA and sexual dimorphism, supporting Puts (2010) view, but further research was clearly recommended (Van Dongen submitted manuscript). Clearly, there is a need for an integrative approach studying associations between masculinity/femininity, health and sexual behaviour simultaneously. Furthermore, the associations between different measures of masculinity/femininity are not well understood.

Indeed, measures of masculinity and femininity can be obtained in many different ways. Body masculinity is often measured objectively by the shoulder-to-hip ratio (SHR), while femininity is reflected by the well known waist-to-hip ratio (WHR). Facial masculinity/femininity can be expressed by facial shape (Little et al., 2008) and recently one study suggested that the eye-mouth-eye (EME) angle would also reliably reflect masculinity/femininity (Danel & Pawlowski, 2007). Next to these objective measurements, masculinity/femininity is often studied through ratings of pictures by the opposite sex. To evaluate the fitness-relevance of variation in masculinity/femininity, some have studied associations with sexual behaviour, like age of first sexual contact and number of sexual partners (or promiscuity). Others have studies associations with dominance. More recently, associations with physical stress have been of interest and more specifically, hand-grip strength (HGS) appears to be very relevant in this context. Physical strength, and its closely related HGS, may play an important role in male-male competition, and also appears to be, albeit weakly, related to survival (e.g., Gallup et al., 2008). Results from several recent studies are summarized in Table 1, and suggest that HSG is a promising measure of masculinity, yet, also shows some heterogeneity. In addition, there seems to be a lack of studies investigating associations between HGS and other objective measures of masculinity/femininity.

In this study we present data on relationships between HGS and i) objective measures of facial masculinity/femininity; ii) fluctuating asymmetry; iii) attractiveness and vi) sexual behaviour in a population of young males and females. The dataset presented here was not very large (total sample size of 100). Therefore, it cannot provide strong conclusions. Although the study of associations with HGS in this context is relatively new, quite some estimates have been published. It is therefore timely to review these results and combine them with the newly presented data here to come to more robust conclusions and suggestions for further research. We therefore also present a meta-analysis of all available data.

Hypothesis tested	gender	N	Reference
HGS related significantly to 2D:4D in two samples	m	88+52	Fink et al 2006
HGS related positively to rated masculinity, dominance and attractiveness	m	32	Fink et al 2007
HGS related to SHR, aggressive behavior, age at first sexual intercourse and promiscuity	m	82	Gallup et al 2007
HGS did not relate to 2D:4D	m	82	
HGS did not relate to any of the above	f	61	
HGS related to facial attractiveness and SHR, but not to number of partners and age at first sexual intercourse	m	38	Shoup & Gallup, 2008
HGS related to perception of dance ability	m	40	Hugill et al. 2009
HGS related to victimization, popularity but not aggression	m/f	255	Gallup et al., 2010
HGS related to perceived aggressiveness, dominance and health, but not with attractiveness	m	69	
HGS did not relate to perceived aggressiveness, attractiveness, dominance and health	f	93	

Table 1. Overview of results of relationships between hand-grip strength (HGS) and measures of masculinity and sexual behavior in previous studies.

2. Materials and methods

2.1 Study design

We measured bilateral asymmetry and masculinity/femininity from scans (HP scanjet G4050, 4800*9600 DPI) of hands and photographs (Nikon D70, 6 megapixel) of faces of 52 men and 48 women with an average age of 22.6 (SD = 2.66) and 22.3 (SD = 1.87) years respectively. The degree of handedness was also self-evaluated on a scale of 0 (extreme left-handed) to 10 (extreme right-handed). Hand-grip strength (HGS) was determined using a Biometrics precision dynamometer. For each participant, the strength was determined twice on each side and the maximum value was obtained as HGS. All participants also completed a questionnaire asking for their age of first sexual contact and their total lifetime number of sexual partners. Each photograph was rated for its attractiveness by 10 to 30 opposite sex raters. As the repeatability of these ratings was about 30%, reliable estimates of attractiveness were obtained.

For each participant the length of the left and right 2nd (D2), 3rd (D3), 4th (D4) and 5th digit (D5) as well as the width of the palm of the hand (P) were independently measured 3 times and averaged (Fig.1). On each photograph, initially 7 landmarks were placed on each side of the face to obtain measures of facial asymmetry: i.e.; the width of the eye (EW), the distance between the pupil of the eye and the widest point at the side of the nostrils (EN), and the distance between the cheek bone and the corner of the mouth (CM) (Fig.1). Landmarks were placed in 3 independent sessions (i.e., on three separate days) and distances were averaged across sessions to reduce measurement error. In addition, since traits within hands and face showed correlations in the signed FA, traits were averaged within hands and faces to obtain two composite estimates (handFA and faceFA1, see Van Dongen et al., 2009 for details). The relative lengths of the second to fourth digit (2D:4D ratio) was also calculated (see also Van Dongen, 2009).

In addition, 19 landmarks were placed (Fig. 1) and based on these landmarks, a procrustes analysis was performed in MorphoJ (available at: http://www.flywings.org.uk/MorphoJ_page.htm; Klingenberg, 2011) to extract an overall measure of facial FA (faceFA2). In addition, facial masculinity was obtained as outlined in Little et al. (2008) and the EME angle was also calculated (Daniel & Pawlowski, 2007). Masculinity was also obtained from the procrustes analysis in MorphoJ by performing a canonical variate analysis for sexual dimorphism. This will allow to visualize the sexual dimorphism and to correlate the canonical variate with the measure obtained following Little et al (2008) and as outlined in Fig.1. An average measure of facial masculinity was obtained from the four individual measures after standardisation. All measurements were performed in ImageJ, freely available at http://rsb.info.nih.gov/ij/. First we tested if measures of masculinity differed between males and females using t-tests. The correlations among the masculinity measures (facial, EME angle, HGS, 2D:4D) were also graphically explored using a biplot from a principal component analysis. Next, correlations with FA, sexual behaviour and attractiveness were also investigated.

2.2 Literature search and meta-analysis

Studies investigating associations between HGS, attractiveness, FA, other forms of masculinity/femininity, sexual behaviour and dominance were obtained from Web of Science and PubMed. Six papers were found of which results are summarized in Table 1. Effect sizes (Pearson's correlations) from these studies as well as the results presented here were grouped in 5 different categories: masculinity measures (objective measurements on body or face); digit ratios; ratings (of masculinity, dominance, popularity); sexual behaviour (age of first contact, promiscuity) and attractiveness. Effect sizes in these categories and for males and females were presented in a funnel plot (i.e., in relation with sample size) to explore problems of publication bias. Effect sizes were then compared among the 5 categories and between males and females by a mixed model ANOVA with reference as random effect.

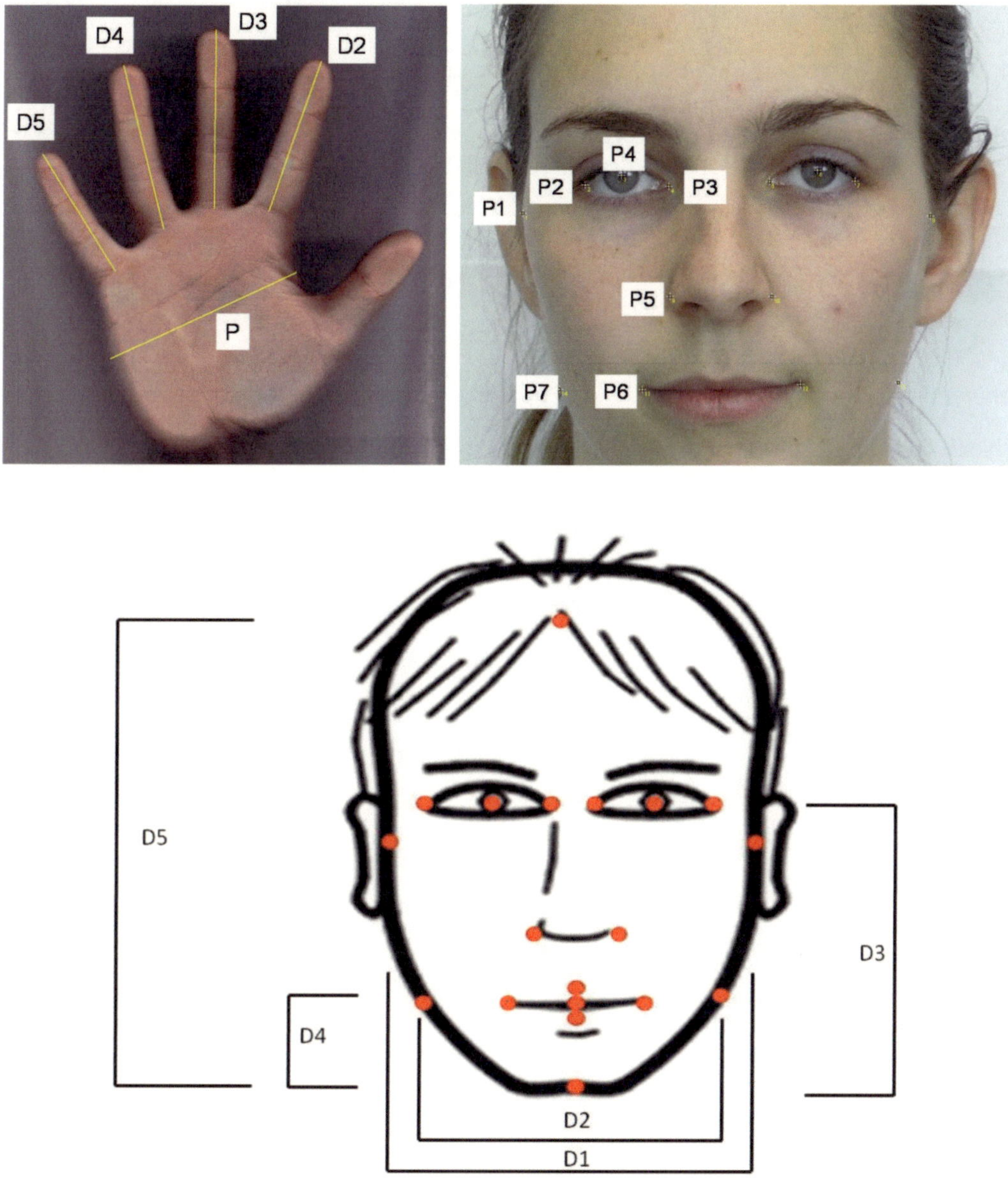

Fig. 1. Top: Scan of right hand with indication of four digit lengths (D2 to D5) and width of hand palm (P) (left) and Landmarks located at both sides of facial photographs, and linear distances derived: eye width (EW: P2-P3), distance from cheekbone to corner of mouth (CM: P1- P6), distance between pupil and most lateral side of nostril (PN: P4-P5) (right). Bottom: Position of landmarks placed on pictures of all faces (see also Little et al., 2008). Sexual dimorphism was calculated by four measures: Cheekbone prominence (D1/D2); Face width/lower face height (D1/D3); Jaw height / lower face height (D4/D3) and Lower face height / Face height (D3/D5).

3. Results

3.1 Measures of masculinity/femininity and sexual dimorphism

Each of the four measures of masculinity (based on the landmarks in Fig. 1) showed a statistically significant sexual dimorphism (Table 2). Therefore, an average measure was obtained after standardisation (further called facial masculinity or masc_face).

	males	females	t-statistic	p-value
Cheekbone prominence	1.13	1.17	t_{97}=4.25	<0.0001
Face width / lower face height	1.17	1.23	t_{97}=4.50	<0.0001
Jaw height / lower face height	0.42	0.41	t_{97}=-2.72	0.008
Lower face height / face height	0.59	0.57	t_{97}=-3.14	0.002

Table 2. Tests of facial sexual dimorphism in the four individual measures (Fig. 1).

Facial shape also differed significantly between males and females based on the geometric morphometrics approach (p<0.0001). The shape differences are given in Figure 2.

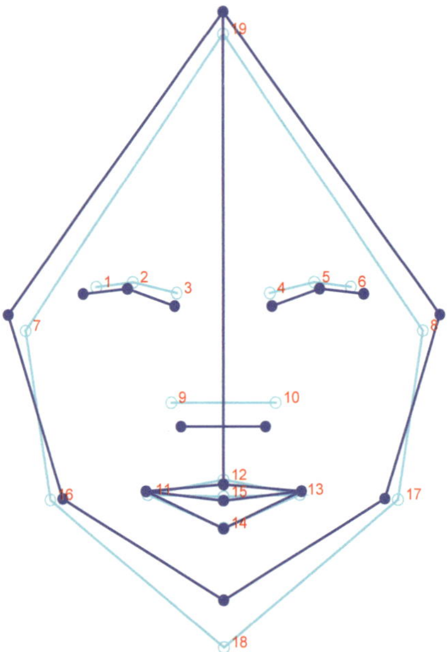

Fig. 2. Shape differences between males (light blue) and females (dark blue) from the canonical covariate analysis on the procrustes coordinates.

The canonical variate of the shape difference between males and females correlated strongly with facial masculinity as calculated above (see Table 2 for details). Thus, facial masculinity as measured by the relative proportions of different distances in the face (Table 2; Little et al., 2008) closely reflects the sexual dimorphism present in the landmarks used. We, therefore, used facial masculinity based on the relative proportions of the distances in Figure 1 for comparability with other studies.

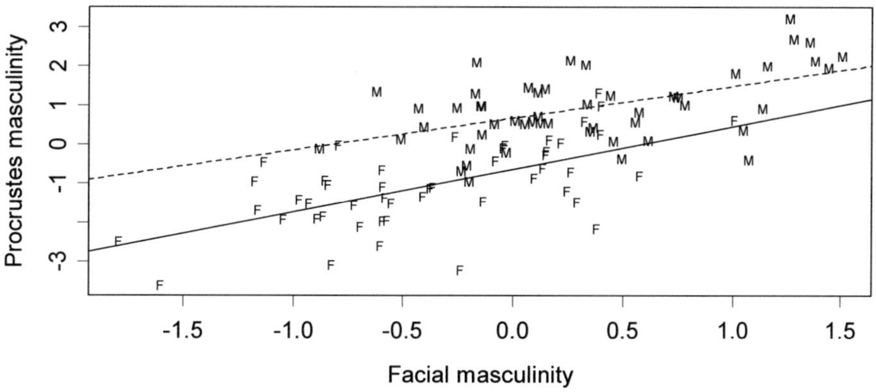

Fig. 3. Association between facial masculinity as obtained following Little et al. (2008) (facial masculinity) and the canonical variate obtained from the geometrics morphometrics approach (procrustes masculinity).

Across males and females:										
	FAhand	FAface1	FAface2	2D:4D	masc_face	HGS	angle	#partners	AFC	attract
FAhand					-	-	-	-	-	-
FAface1	0.05	-	-	-	-	-	-	-	-	-
FAface2	0.08	**0.42*****	-	-	-	-	-	-	-	-
2D:4D	-0.08	0.14	0.13	-	-	-	-	-	-	-
masc_face	-0.06	0.13	0.08	0.07	-	-	-	-	-	-
HGS	0.05	-0.01	-0.16	-0.05	**0.42*****	-	-	-	-	-
angle	-0.12	-0.15	**-0.22***	0.02	-0.16	-0.06	-	-	-	-
#partners	**-0.28****	**-0.22***	-0.01	-0.06	-0.07	-0.05	0.12	-	-	-
AFC	0.17	**0.31****	**0.20**	0.02	-0.02	0.08	-0.04	-0.64***	-	-
attract.	-0.04	**0.21***	0.02	0.03	-0.08	**-0.25***	0.06	0.06	-0.14	-
By sex (males above diagonal/females below diagonal)										
	FAhand	FAface1	FAface2	2D:4D	masc_face	HGS	angle	#partners	AFC	attract
FAhand	-	-0.13	-0.10	-0.10	-0.20	0.07	-0.04	-0.21	**0.29***	0.01
FAface1	0.26	-	**0.40****	0.08	0.21	-0.03	0.12	-0.23	**0.33***	-0.13
FAface2	**0.35**	**0.46****	-	0.19	0.27	-0.11	-0.08	**-0.32***	0.20	0.08
2D:4D	-0.01	0.24	0.00	-	0.27	0.04	0.10	-0.14	0.02	0.09
masc_face	0.04	0.04	0.01	0.06	-	0.12	0.09	0.04	-0.17	0.26
HGS	-0.08	-0.13	-0.24	0.17	0.25	-	-0.03	0.09	-0.04	0.04
angle	-0.27	**-0.33***	**-0.40****	-0.11	**-0.34***	0.11	-	0.17	0.01	0.06
#partners	**-0.36***	-0.21	0.03	0.00	-0.02	0.05	0.04	-	**-0.65*****	-0.04
AFC	-0.04	**0.29**	**0.24***	-0.10	-0.05	-0.09	-0.08	**-0.62*****	-	-0.07
attract	-0.07	-0.26	-0.07	--0.11	-0.04	-0.18	0.01	0.04	-0.16	-

Table 3. Correlation coefficients and statistical significance (*: p<0.05; **: p<0.01; ***: p<0.001, indicated in bold) of associations among fluctuating asymmetry (FA) values (hand and face), measures of masculinity (face, hand grip strength (HGS), eye-mouth-eye angle and digit ratio (2D:4D)), sexual behavior (number of partners and age of first sexual contact (AFC)) and attractiveness. Correlations are given across both sexes (top table) and for males and females separately (bottom table).

Next to the facial masculinity studied here (which was significantly dimorphic: $t_{97}=5.69$, $p<0.0001$), only one other measure of masculinity/femininity also showed a significant sexual dimorphism in our sample. Males showed significantly higher HGS ($t_{97}=10.1$, $p<0.0001$), but no differences were observed for 2D:4D ($t_{94}=1.54$, $p=0.12$) and the EME angle ($t_{97}=0.92$, $p=0.36$) (see also Fig. 4). Across males and females, only HGS and facial masculinity showed a significant positive correlation (Table 3), a pattern that appeared consistent among both sexes (Fig.5), albeit not significantly so within sexes (Table 3). In woman, the EME angle and facial masculinity were negatively correlated, yet, unexpectedly, slightly positively in males (Table 3, Fig. 5). A principal component analysis of the

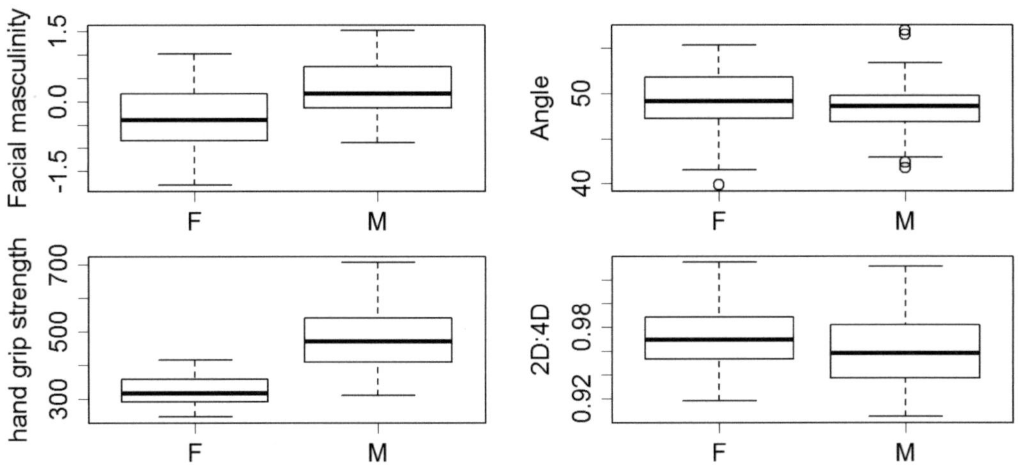

Fig. 4. Boxplots of the differences in measures of potentially sexually dimorphic traits: from top left to bottom right: facial masculinity based on the 19 landmarks, eye-mouth-eye angle, handgrip strength and digit ratio)

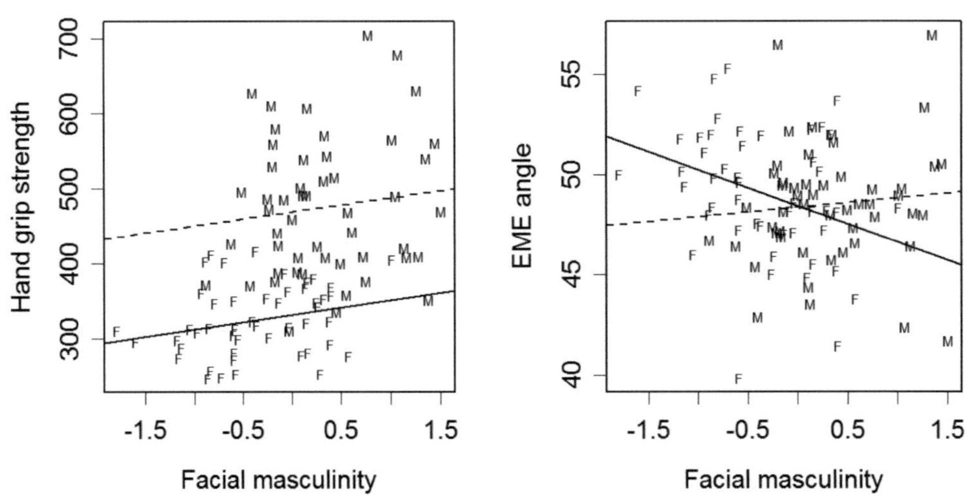

Fig. 5. Associations between measures of masculinity that were statistically significant (Table 3).

masculinity traits confirmed the lack of strong correlations. The first principal component explained 37% of the total variation and was determined by HGS and facial masculinity. The second and third each explained about 25% of the total variation and each reflected one other variable, 2D:4D and EME angle respectively (Fig.6). Thus, in order to capture a large amount of the variation, three components were required, one of which only combined variation across two variables.

3.2 Asymmetry measurements

The degree of measurement error (ME) of FA (i.e., the percentage of variance due to ME relative to the total variance (FA+ME)) due to scanning and placing landmarks, were the following: D2: 16%; D3: 20%; D4: 18%; D5: 13%. None of the hand measurements showed significant directional asymmetry (all $p > 0.05$). After standardization, asymmetries of hand-traits were averaged into a single measure of asymmetry per individual (FAhand). Both handedness and asymmetry in power between right and left hand were significantly correlated with the signed asymmetry of the hand (handedness: $r = 0.33$, $p = 0.001$; power: $r = 0.30$, $p = 0.001$) (see also Van Dongen et al., 2009). For the three facial characteristics measurements were less accurate (EW: 57%; EN: 14%; CM: 73%). Facial FA showed significant directional asymmetry (all $p > 0.05$), two facial traits (EW: $t_{99} = 3.2$, $p = 0.002$ and PN: $t_{99} = 1.98$, $p = 0.05$) showed larger values on the right side, on average.

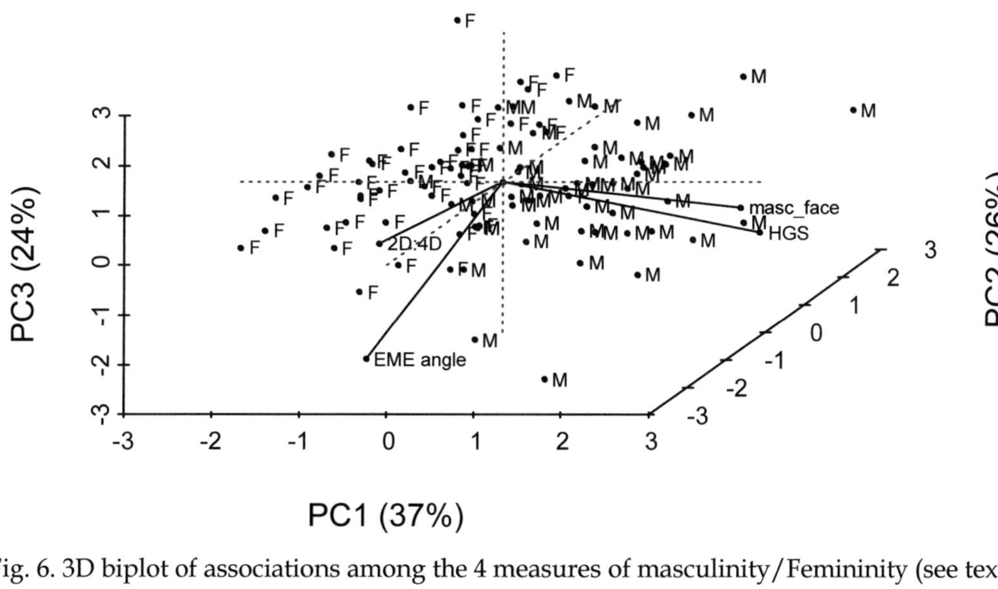

Fig. 6. 3D biplot of associations among the 4 measures of masculinity/Femininity (see text for details).

Because the three measurements of facial FA did not show high accuracy (though did show associations with sexual behavior, see Van Dongen et al., 2009 and below) we decided to take additional measurement on the face in the form of 19 landmarks. Procrustes ANOVA showed significant directional asymmetry ($F_{31,1798}=2.42$, $p<0.0001$) and significant FA ($F_{1798,1426}=2.28$, $p<0.0001$).

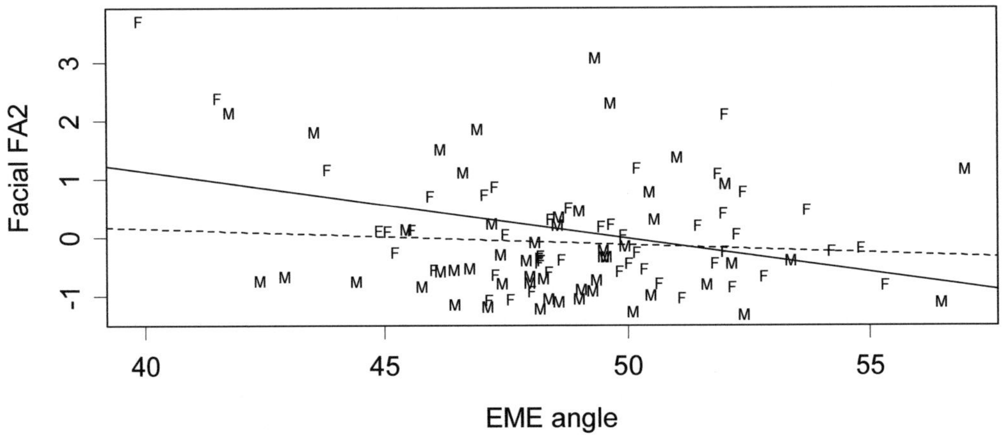

Fig. 7. Associations between eye-mouth-eye angle and facial asymmetry in males (dashed line) and females (solid line).

3.3 Correlations among FA, masculinity and sexual behaviour

All correlations, across both sexes and for males and females separately, are provided in Table 3. It is important to realize that many tests are being performed and some of them are significant at the 5% level just by chance. It is, therefore, only relevant to interpret correlations significant at the 5%/135=0.04% level (after Bonferonni correction). The only correlations which are significant at this level are situated between FA and sexual behaviour, between the number of partners and age of first sexual contact, between the two measures of facial FA, and between facial masculinity and HGS (Table 3). One correlation that is worth mentioning (albeit not significant after Bonferonni correction) is the negative association between EME angle and facial FA in woman (Table 3) indicating a wider (more feminine) EME angle to be associated with higher facial FA (Fig.7).

3.4 Meta-analysis

A funnel graph of all available effect sizes is provided in figure 8. There does not appear to be a problem of publication bias (correlation between sample size and effect size = -0.11, d.f.=81, p=0.29). 16 out of 83 estimates were statistically significant (20%) and 64 out of 83 estimates were in the expected direction (i.e., a positive effect size) (77%), a proportion that is significantly higher than 50% ($p<0.0001$). The average weighted effect size across all estimates equalled 0.19 (0.05), which was significantly different from zero (t_7=4.00, p=0.007). Thus, on average there appears to be a robust correlation. However, average effect sizes were only half as high in females (difference=-0.10 (0.03), $F_{1,74}$=11.3, p=0.001), and differed significantly among the broad categories of masculinity and sexual behaviour ($F_{1,66}$=3.06, p=0.015). Although most two-by-two comparisons were not statistically significant, averaged across males and females, the highest effect sizes that were significant at the 0.01 level were found for objective measurements of bodily and facial masculinity (average effect size: 0.24 (0.05)) and ratings of dominance and attractiveness of opposite sex raters (average effect size: 0.22 (0.05)). Lower effect sizes, albeit still significant at the 0.05 level, were observed for 2D:4D (average effect size: 0.13 (0.05)) and measures of sexual behaviour (average effect size: 0.14 (0.05)). The remaining two were even somewhat lower, no longer statistically significant but still in the expected direction: attractiveness (average effect size:

0.12 (0.08)) and self rated dominance, aggression and popularity (average effect size: 0.09 (0.05)). These differences appeared comparable between males and females as there was no significant interaction ($F_{5,68}$=2.00, p=0.09), but the power to detect an interaction was probably small. Therefore, we also present average effect sizes by sex (Table 4).

Category	sex	effect size (SE)	p-value
2D:4D	males	**0.15 (0.06)**	0.02
	females	**0.11 (0.06)**	0.10
Attractiveness*	males	**0.24 (0.09)**	0.01
	females	-0.07 (0.12)	0.57
Masculinity	males	**0.24 (0.06)**	<0.001
	females	**0.24 (0.06)**	<0.001
Ratings*	males	**0.29 (0.05)**	<0.001
	females	0.10 (0.08)	0.24
self ratings	males	**0.12 (0.05)**	0.04
	females	0.06 (0.05)	0.30
sexual behavior*	males	**0.24 (0.06)**	<0.001
	females	0.04 (0.06)	0.52

Table 4. Average weighted effect sizes of the associations between hand grip strength and other measures of masculinity (masculinity: objective measurements; ratings: ratings of masculinity and dominance by opposite sex raters; self ratings: own evaluations of masculinity, dominance, popularity; digit ratios (2D:4D), attractiveness and sexual behavior) for males and females. Categories where males have a significantly higher effect size are indicated by a * (although the interaction was not statistically significant, see text for details).

4. Discussion

4.1 Associations between masculinity, attractiveness, fluctuating asymmetry and sexual behaviour

This study, albeit small in terms of new data added to the existing literature, did not provide strong evidence that measures of masculinity would be related to sexual behaviour, attractiveness or fluctuating asymmetry. Clearly, sample sizes were relatively small, yet, it did allow to detect robust associations between FA and measures of sexual behaviour (see Van Dongen et al., 2009 for further discussion), but not attractiveness (this study). Thus, this suggests that sample sizes were sufficiently large for some aspects (i.e., associations with FA), and that asymmetry may be more closely related to sexual behaviour and promiscuity that masculinity. Nevertheless, many others have shown associations between masculinity and both attractiveness and sexual behaviour, such that this small study clearly cannot cast any doubt on the relevance of masculinity and hormone levels in human sexual behaviour and attractiveness. However, there is some doubt about the associations among different measures of masculinity and their association with sex-hormone levels (e.g., Koehler et al., 2004; Campbell et al., 2010). In this study, associations among the four objective measures were weak, with the exception of the association between facial masculinity and hand grip strength. HGS also showed a clear sexual dimorphism, as did facial masculinity. However, eye-mouth-eye angle and 2D:4D did not show correlations with facial masculinity or HGS and were not sexually dimorphic. Results for 2D:4D are discussed elsewhere (Van Dongen 2009). For EME angle, one study of similar size as this one did show a sexual dimorphism and associations with attractiveness (Danel & Pawlowski, 2007). The results presented here thus question the generality of the usefulness of EME angle as a measure of masculinity and calls for further research. In spite of the fact that EME angle did not show a sexual dimorphism in this study and did not relate to masculinity (except perhaps weakly in woman), sexual behaviour or attractiveness, there was some suggestion that it correlated with facial FA. This certainly warrants further study since associations between FA and measures of masculinity are at best very weak and results vary among studies (Van Dongen submitted manuscript).

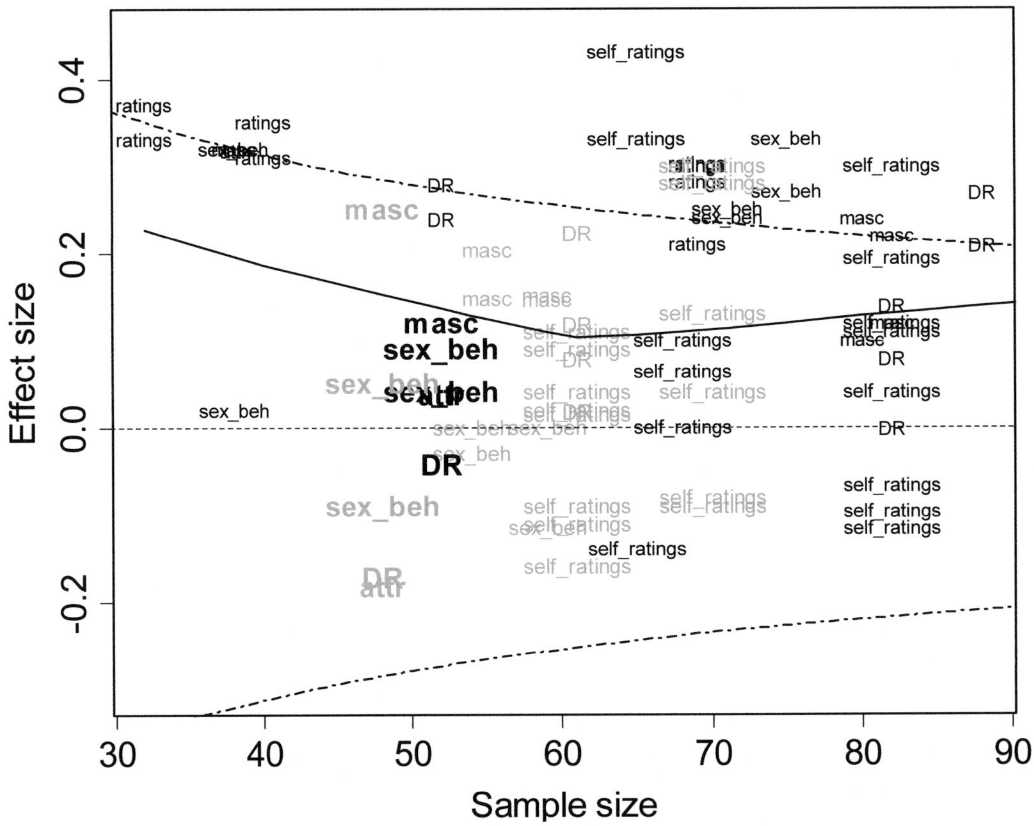

Fig. 8. Funnel graph (effect sizes vs. sample size) of the associations between hand grip strength and other measures of masculinity (masc: objective measurements; ratings: ratings of masculinity and dominance by opposite sex raters), self ratings (own evaluations of masculinity, dominance, popularity, …), digit ratios (DR: 2D:4D), attractiveness (attr) and sexual behavior (sex_beh). Dash-dotted lines represent critical values for the effect sizes, where more extreme values are statistically significant at the 0.05 level. The solid line the lowess curve of the association (or rather the lack of it in this case). effect sizes for males are given in black, those of females in grey, and estimates from this study are provided in a larger bold font.

4.2 Handgrip strength as a measure of masculinity

Our results show that HGS relates to facial masculinity (but not 2D:4D) in both males and females. HGS has only recently been put forward as a useful measure of masculinity (Table 1), and we here present an overview of the current literature. There appears to be a highly significant and robust average weighted effect size of about 0.2, of correlations between HGS and different correlates of masculinity/femininity. There also appears to be some variation in the effect sizes. On the average, effect sizes were smaller in females and lowest for sexual behaviour and self rated dominance, aggression and popularity. Although there was no significant interaction between sex and type of masculinity measure, the p value was only 0.09, suggesting that the difference between may not have been similar for the different categories. Although we should interpret these test with caution (and await further study), the differences in effect sizes between males and females were strongest for attractiveness, sexual behaviour and rated masculinity. In each of these, relatively strong average effect sizes were observed for males, and nearly zero for females (Table 4). Thus, HGS appears to be related to objectively measured masculinity in both males and females (Table 4 and data from this study), and to a lesser extent with 2D:4D (Table 4). For all other categories, no significant associations were found for females (Table 4). Although it may be to preliminary at this point to make any firm conclusions, our results and the combined analysis of the data from the literature suggests that HGS relates to morphological measures of masculinity alone in females, but also to attractiveness, rated and self-rated masculinity and dominance and sexual behaviour in males.

5. Conclusion

In this paper we study associations between objective morphological measures of masculinity/femininity and physical strength (handgrip strength) in relation to developmental instability (as measured by fluctuating asymmetry, FA), attractiveness and sexual behaviour. In spite of the relatively small sample sizes, we were able to detect associations between FA and sexual behaviour (further discussed in Van Dongen et al., 2009), yet not with our measures of masculinity. We next focussed on a relatively recently studied measure of masculinity/femininity, namely physical strength expressed as handgrip strength (HGS). We reviewed results from the recent literature and demonstrated a robust association between HGS and other measures of masculinity/femininity. In addition, we were able to detect some sources of variation. On the one hand, HGS related to morphological features of bodily masculinity (and to a lesser extent but still significantly so to 2D:4D ratios) equally strong in both males and females. However, associations between HGS and either attractiveness, (self-)ratings of dominance, masculinity and popularity and sexual behaviour were weaker or absent in females compared to males. Thus, based on the available literature we conclude that physical strength is determined by circulating hormones affecting morphologically dimorphic structures, yet affects behaviour and the physical expression of it in males only. Physical strength and masculinity is thus likely to play a role in male-male competition and as a signal of mate value in sexual selection.

6. References

Campbell, B.C., Dreber, A., Apicella, C.L., Eisenberg, D.T.A, Gray, P.B., Little, A.C., Garcia, J.R., Zamore, R.S. & Lum, J.K. 2010. Testosterone exposure, dopaminergic reward, and sensation seeking in young men. Physiology and behavior 99: 451-456.

Danel, D. & Pawlowski, B. 2007. Eye-mouth-eye angle as a good indicator of face masculinization, asymmetry, and attractiveness (Homo sapiens). Journal of comparative Psychology 121: 221-225.

Fink, B., Neave, N. & Seydel, H. 2007. Male facial appearance signals physical strength to women. American Journal of Human Biology 19: 82-87.

Gallup, A.C., White, D.D. & Gallup G.G. 2007. Handgrip strength predicts sexual behavior, body morphology, and aggression in male college students. Evolution and human behavior. 28: 423-429.

Gallup, A.C., O'Brien, D.T., White, D.D. & Wilson, D.S. 2010. Handgrip strength and socially dominant behavior in male adolescents. Evolutionary Psychology 8: 229-243.

Garver-Apgar, C.E., Eaton, M.A., Tybur, J.M. & Thompson, M.E. 2011. Evidence of intralocus sexual conflict: physically and hormonally masculine individuals have more attractive brothers relative to sisters. Evolution and human behavior in press.

Getty, T. (2002). Signaling health versus parasites. *American Naturalist, 159,* 363-371.

Klingenberg, C. P. 2011. MorphoJ: an integrated software package for geometric morphometrics. *Molecular Ecology Resources* 11: 353-357

Koehler, N., Simmons, L.W., & Rhodes, G. 2004. How well does second-to-fourth-digit ratio in hands correlate with other indications of masculinity in males? Proc R Soc. Lond B (suppl.) 271: S296-S298.

Kokko, H., Brooks, R., McNamara, J.M. & Houston, A.I. (2002). The sexual selection continuum. *Proceedings of the Royal Society of London* B, 269,1331-1340.

Little, A. C., Jones, B. C., Waitt, C., Tiddeman, B. P., Feinberg, D. R., Perrett, D. I. Apicella, C. L. & Marlowe, F. W. (2008). Symmetry is related to sexual dimorphism in faces: Data across culture and species. *PLoS One, 3,* e2106.

Puts, D. A. 2010. Beauty and the beast: Mechanisms of sexual selection in humans. *Evolution and Human Behavior, 31,*157-175.

Shoup, M.L. & Gallup, G.G. 2008. Men's faces convey information about their bodies and their behavior: what you see is what you get. Evolutionary psychology 6: 469-479.

Thornhill, R. & Gangestad, S.W. 1999. Facial attractiveness. trends in Cognitive Sciences. 3: 452-460

Van Dongen Stefan. (2009). A critical re-evaluation of the association between 2D:4D ratios and fluctuating asymmetry in humans. *Annals of human biology, 36,* 186-198.

Van Dongen, S., Cornille, R. & Lens, L. 2009. Sex and asymmetry in humans: What is the role of developmental instability. *Journal of Evolutionary Biology*, 22, 612-622

15

Sex Differences in the Developmental Programming of Adult Disease

Jeffrey S. Gilbert and Christopher T. Banek
Department of Human Physiology, University of Oregon
USA

1. Introduction

A significant body of knowledge has established that stressors in early life have long-term health consequences on the adult organism. This has given rise to the Developmental Origins of Health and Adult Disease (DOHAD) hypothesis. Among the several broad themes that have emerged from the clinical and experimental investigations into the DOHAD hypothesis; perhaps none is as intriguing as the role of biological sex and sex hormones in the progression and development of adult diseases. Despite the significant progress in recent years, many uncertainties remain with respect to the roles of biological sex and gonadal steroids in the progression of human diseases in general, and in the mechanisms underlying sex differences in developmental programming in particular.

While sexual dimorphism is widely recognized in the progression of many diseases (e.g. cardiovascular), it appears that the primary pathways leading to these differences exert distinct influences during fetal and adult life. The mechanisms by which biological sex contributes to these processes is a rapidly expanding area of investigation drawing upon studies interrogating systems at the molecular, cellular and whole organism physiological levels. From these investigations several intriguing hypotheses have been proposed. These include developmental programming due to: 1) endocrine disruption resulting from exogenous sex steroids and/or analogs or nutritional stress during development; 2) chromosomal regulation of sex dimorphism in the transcriptome of mammalian tissues; and 3) sex specific responses to stressors during fetal life. The goal of this chapter is to place into perspective the current body of knowledge in the rapidly growing area of sex differences in developmental programming with a primary focus on cardiovascular diseases.

2. Periods of susceptibility to developmental programming

Developmental programming can be defined as the response by the developing organism to specific stimuli during critical periods of organogenesis that results in persistent effects on the adult phenotype. It is now recognized as an important determinant of adult health. Acceptance and understanding of this concept derives from human epidemiological studies suggesting that many metabolic diseases such as cardiovascular disease (Barker, 1993), chronic kidney disease (Li *et al.*, 2007), type II diabetes mellitus (Hovi *et al.*, 2007;Hofman *et al.*, 1997), and hypertension (Roseboom *et al.*, 2001) are associated with low birth weight. Since developing organisms pass more physiological benchmarks prior to birth than during any other time in life, it is not surprising that deviations in the timing or nature of these developmental steps have functional consequences in later life. Hence, it is vitally important to understand early life gene-environment interactions that can increase predisposition to adult disease. Figure 1 provides an overview of the timing of the susceptibilities for various organs systems and processes in developmental programming.

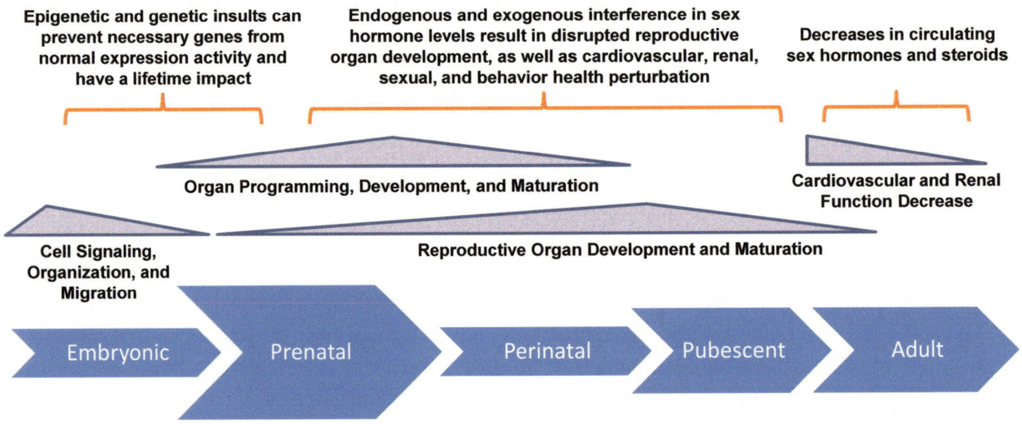

Fig. 1. *Organogenesis and Maturation Disruption.* Timeline depicts separate stages of mammalian organ development and maturation and the relative sensitivity to various programming stimuli. Listed above are necessary processes during this period for normal growth and the activity (light blue). At the top are the perturbations that can interfere with proper development.

2.1 Embryonic development

Susceptibility to programming events begins very early in life and surprisingly sex differences are already present. The transcriptome of male and female pre-implantation embryos differ such that several genes located on the X chromosome are more expressed in bovine and human female versus male embryos (Gutierrez-Adan *et al.*, 2000;Taylor *et al.*, 2001;Wrenzycki *et al.*, 2002;Peippo *et al.*, 2002) while autosomal genes expressed in trophoblast cells, such as those for interferon-γ (Larson *et al.*, 2001), human choriogonadotropic hormone (Haning, Jr. *et al.*, 1989), and numerous other imprinted genes (Paldi *et al.*, 1995;Kovtun *et al.*, 2000;Durcova-Hills *et al.*, 2004) are also not expressed or methylated the same across the sexes. Morphological differences exist as well; male and female embryos differ in rates of development as early as the first few days post-fertilization. Bovine (Avery *et al.*, 1992;Yadav *et al.*, 1993), murine (Valdivia *et al.*, 1993) and ovine embryos (Bernardi & Delouis, 1996) produced *in vitro* often fall into fast-cleaving and slow-cleaving groups that are predominantly male and female, respectively. Interestingly, Sood *et al.* reported a sex dichotomy in the genes expressed in male and female placentas (Sood *et al.*, 2006) using microarray analysis and identified genes in villous samples such as JAK1, IL2RB, Clusterin, LTBP, CXCL1, and IL1RL1 that were expressed at higher levels in female placentas.

2.2 Fetal development

The fetal period is a critical time for organogenesis. As gestation progresses and the embryo becomes a fetus, the sex dimorphism of early development re-appears around mid-gestation as male fetuses become larger than age-matched females (Hindmarsh *et al.*, 2002;Crawford *et al.*, 1987;Parker *et al.*, 1984). From clinical and experimental studies we know that this size difference persists to term (Hindmarsh *et al.*, 2002;Parker *et al.*, 1984;Gilbert *et al.*, 2007a;Gilbert *et al.*, 2006a). Underlying these morphological differences are specific sex related differences in endocrinology and metabolism. While androgens are recognized for their role in male maturation, they are also essential to development of the female fetus. Production of androgens in both the ovaries and the adrenal cortex in females is essential to folliculogenesis and mammary development. Levels below the required amount for normal development have been shown to diminish the development of the tissues aforementioned. Exposure of female fetuses to androgens may not necessarily disrupt normal development of the ovaries, but may result in altered expression of steroidogenic proteins (Hogg *et al.*, 2011). Increased androgens are also associated with female fetuses developing male-like sexual behavior, increased aggression, delayed vaginal opening (Meisel & Ward, 1981).

Sex differences at the molecular level also persist from embryonic into fetal life. Baserga *et al.* have reported that gestation in the rat cyclooxygenase-2 (COX-2) levels were higher in the female than the male kidney at day of gestation (DG) 8, although not significantly increased at DG 21. In contrast, 11β-Hydroxysteroid Dehydrogenase 2 (11β-HSD2) levels were higher in the male control kidney at DG 21. Both of these gene products play important roles in renal function and alterations in either could have developmental and/or functional effects in the kidney (Baserga *et al.*, 2007b). Similarly, sex differences have also been reported in the ontogeny of gene expression in the renal RAS (Gilbert *et al.*, 2007a).

Similar to the kidney, the mammary gland undergoes discrete phases of development. However, in contrast to the kidney, the mammary has important developmental phases that extend into adulthood. In early pregnancy, the processes of fetal mammary development are thought to occur independently of influences from systemic hormones (Hennighausen & Robinson, 2001). After mid-gestation, placental hormones enter fetal circulation and initiate canalization of the early ductal system. It is during this period that exposure to endocrine mimetics may exert an influence on subsequent risk of breast cancer in the offspring (Xue & Michels, 2007). While the origin and the purpose of these sex differences in fetal development remain unclear, it may simply reflect different trajectories of fetal development between the sexes; however, this may also underlie sex differences in developmental programming.

2.3 Post-natal

It has long been observed that growth restricted fetuses which develop metabolic syndrome often experience "catch-up growth" and surpass normal birth weight controls (Hales & Ozanne, 2003). While it is clear that catch-up growth plays a role in the manifestations of developmental programming it has been difficult to identify the specific peri-natal *vs.* post-natal influences involved. Disordered vascular function is thought to contribute to programming of cardiovascular health but the cause and effect relationships remain uncertain (Martin *et al.*, 2000;Leeson *et al.*, 2001;Goodfellow *et al.*, 1998). There are recognized sex differences in arterial pressure and the progression of renal disease, both of which are thought to involve interactions of the renin angiotensin system and sex steroids (Sandberg & Ji, 2003;Silva-Antonialli *et al.*, 2004). Most current evidence points to sex steroids as the most important factor influencing sex differences in post-natal cardiovascular function.

In contrast to organs such as the kidney that complete development *in utero*, several reproductive organs such as the mammary undergo significant developmental changes during post-natal life and sometimes well into adulthood. A significant portion of mammary development begins at puberty and continues throughout an individual's reproductive years (Hinck & Silberstein, 2005) and renders this particular organ to more critical periods susceptible to programming influences. Aberrant signaling during these phases may initiate abnormal growth of the ductal epithelium, possibly resulting in alterations in risk for subsequently developing mammary cancer.

Interestingly, Wlodek, *et al.* found that uteroplacental insufficiency, via uterine restriction in rats, resulted in reduced alveolar proliferation (Wlodek *et al.*, 2009). We have reported that growth restricted female rats from hypertensive mothers have a much higher incidence of mammary tumors when exposed to N-nitroso-N-methylurea than normal birthweight control rats (Gingery *et al.*, 2011). Thus, differentiation events of the mammary epithelium occurring mid- to late-gestation may provide a substrate sensitive to sub-optimal intrauterine conditions or environmental exposures that could set the stage for subsequent development of cancer.

The transcriptome continues to display sex differences in adulthood, such as in differences in expression of mRNA for osmoregulatory, drug and steroid metabolizing proteins in the murine kidney and liver (Rinn *et al.*, 2004). It is therefore not unreasonable to hypothesize sex differences exist within a molecular framework and that there are many potential avenues, from embryonic life on into adulthood, through which sex differences may interact with developmental programming stimuli to result in sex specific alterations.

3. Endocrine disruption

It has become nearly axiomatic that endocrine signaling by gonadal steroids like estradiol and testosterone are important contributors to the development and maintenance of long-term health and/or disease. Endocrine disruption generally occurs as a consequence of one or more of four main characteristics of the compound under study: agonist, antagonist, modification, and/or altering synthesis (Derfoul *et al.*, 2003). Some compounds can have a pleiotropic effect in which at least two signaling pathways known to be independent from each other are impacted. Moreover, endogenous sexual hormones and mimetics include: estrone, estriol, estradiol, human chorionic gonadotropin, testosterone, progesterone, prostaglandins, and several other estrogens and androgens. While endocrine disruptors are traditionally considered to be environmental pollutants, there are numerous physiological stressors that may generate disturbances of endocrine signaling pathways. Further, in Table 1 we highlight the main classes of steroidogenic endocrine disruptors and the manners in which they become accessible to organisms. To this end, we have considered a variety of physiological models under the general theme of endocrine disruption.

3.1 Endogenous hormones/mimetics

Females on average are at lesser of a risk for cardiovascular disease during the premenopausal state, but significantly are at increased risk for cardiovascular and renal disease after menopause, nearing comparable rates to male disease development (Gilbert & Nijland, 2008;Sakemi *et al.*, 1995). In adult growth-restricted females, an ovariectomy can lead to an increase in renal-induced hypertension, compared to subjects with the ovaries still intact(Ojeda *et al.*, 2007a). These observations allude to the idea that estrogens have a cardiac

Sex Hormone Disruption	Reported Mimetics	Reported Conduits of Exposure
Estrogens	Polychlorinated (PCB) and polybrominated (PBB) biphenyls, dichlorodiphenyltrichloroethane (DDT), Dichlordiphenyldichloro-ethylene (DDE), methoxychlor, diethylstilbestrol (DES), alkylphenols, cadmium, bisphenyl-A (BPA).	Dielectric fluids and electronics; hard plastics; pesticides; insecticides; synthetic estrogens; sewage degradation, batteries and television screens; plastics and dental sealants
Androgens	Kepone , procymidone, dichlorodiphenyldichloroethylene (DDE), vinclosolin, 2,3,7,8-tetrachlorodibenzodioxin (TCDD)	Insecticides; pesticides; fungicides; herbicides
Prostaglandins	Phthalates, COX inhibiting pharmaceuticals	Soft plastics, paints, inks; prescription pharmaceuticals

Table 1. *Overview of exogenous steroid mimetics.* Exogenous endocrine mimetics have been reported to have agonistic and/or antagonistic behavior in mammals. Exposures to these compounds occur through various types of materials in a variety of settings.

and renal protective component that is attenuated during post-menopausal state (Rubinow & Girdler, 2011;Ojeda *et al.*, 2007a). But, estrogen differences between the sexes cannot alone explain the disease development differences because androgens have been observed to have cardioprotective properties as well (Manolakou *et al.*, 2009).

Androgens are important in fetal development regardless of sex. During the first trimester of development, the male fetus maturation is dictated by the presence of androgens, which if disrupted can lead to several conditions such as testicular cancer, lower sperm count and motility, and cryptorchidism (Manikkam *et al.*, 2004;Bormann *et al.*, 2011;Recabarren *et al.*, 2008). With below-normal levels of testosterone, the male fetus fails to properly develop the testes, known as testicular dysgenesis. In contrast, excess testosterone is linked to altered development of the seminiferous tubules and lower sperm count and motility. Taken together these studies show proper control of androgen levels in males is essential to normal reproductive development (Manikkam *et al.*, 2004;Bormann *et al.*, 2011).

In growth restricted males, increased testosterone levels have been shown to lead to an increase in angiotensin II sensitivity and this in turn may lead to increased susceptibility to hypertension (Ojeda *et al.*, 2010). Recently, Ojeda et al. showed high incidence of hypertension coinciding with growth restriction is dependent on circulating testosterone levels. The castration of adult growth restricted males resulted in mitigation of the hypertension, which contrasted the observations of no blood pressure change after castration of normal growth, hypertensive male rats (Ojeda *et al.*, 2007a).

The concept of endocrine disruption leading to developmental programming can be extended to the fetal renin-angiotensin system (RAS) as well. Interestingly, this system is responsive not only to pharmacological manipulation but also to nutritional stress as well. Indeed, work from several laboratories has provided insights regarding the role of the RAS in cardiac development (Beinlich *et al.*, 1991;Beinlich & Morgan, 1993;Beinlich *et al.*, 1995;Samyn *et al.*, 1998;Segar *et al.*, 1997;Segar *et al.*, 2001;Sundgren *et al.*, 2003). In particular, Sundgren *et al.* demonstrated that Ang II promotes hyperplastic growth during early gestation, whereas Beinlich *et al.* have reported neonatal hypertrophic growth in the pig

(Beinlich *et al.*, 1995;Sundgren *et al.*, 2003). The intra-cardiac RAS also appears to be sensitive to nutritional stress as demonstrated recently by Gilbert et al. in a study that shows decreased immunoreactive AT1 and AT2 in the mid-gestation left ventricle of fetal sheep gestated in ewes that were subjected to 50% global nutrient restriction (Gilbert *et al.*, 2005b).

3.2 Exogenous hormones/mimetics/antagonists

Exposure to a variety of environmental factors may generate exogenous interference with endocrine systems through mimetic or antagonistic activity. This is a rapidly growing area of research with implications for both environmental and public health. Several known exogenous estrogen antagonists include polychlorinated (PCB) and polybrominated (PBB) biphenyls, dichlorodiphenyltrichloroethane (DDT), methoxychlor, diethylstilbestrol, 17β-estradiol, alkylphenols sewage degradation, cadmium, and the infamous bisphenyl-A (BPA) (Sonnenschein & Soto, 1998;Derfoul *et al.*, 2003). Xenoestrogens may exist in the system at levels that do not elicit strong or detectable estrogenic effects individually, but it has been shown that these have additive effects and several xenoestrogens in the system can act together to induce estrogenic activity. (Sonnenschein & Soto, 1998) This additive effect brings rise to the idea that some materials we are exposed to may pass inspection individually for tolerable levels of these endocrine disrupting compounds, but in concert with low levels of the xenoestrogens may have phenotypic effects *in utero*. Since estrogen is mainly required in maturation and growth, it is common to not see congenital endocrine complications until adolescence or even as late as adulthood (Derfoul *et al.*, 2003). Overexposure of estrogens to the fetus has been suggested to stunt growth and alter bone development (Derfoul *et al.*, 2003;Sonnenschein & Soto, 1998). In contrast to the large number of estrogen disruptors, only several androgen antagonists have been identified and studied. These are insecticide ingredients such as kepone and procymidone, dichlorodiphenyldichloroethyle (DDE), vinclosolin, and 2,3,7,8-tetrachlorodibenzodioxin (TCDD) (Sonnenschein & Soto, 1998). While very little to no androgen agonists have been discovered (Sonnenschein & Soto, 1998) it has been reported that exposure to androgen antagonists like DDE is linked to development of recurrent respiratory tract infection (Carey *et al.*, 2007).

Prostaglandins are important to many sexual processes in both men and women, but little has been done on that research to describe endocrine disruption targeting prostaglandins. Interference in prostaglandin pathways has been associated with the development of several types of cancer and cardiovascular disorders. The alteration of synthesis of prostaglandins from arachadonic acid through the COX enzyme has been shown disrupt endocrine processes. Several phthalates that are similar to pharmaceutical COX inhibitors, were found to disrupt the levels of prostaglandin synthesis (Kristensen *et al.*, 2011). Chronic inhibition of COX activity is known to have deleterious effects on renal and cardiovascular function, resulting in mild to moderate hypertension and even renal failure. Developmental sex differences in this system have been reported and show that renal COX-2 expression is higher in female fetuses at gestational day 21 than age matched male fetuses (Baserga *et al.*, 2007a). Prostaglandin synthesis pathways are relatively understudied but may provide important insights into the development of sex differences in adult disease.

4. Sex differences in developmental programming

Numerous studies have documented sex-differences in the incidence and severity of cardiovascular diseases such as coronary artery disease, heart failure, cardiac hypertrophy, and sudden cardiac death (Gilbert *et al.*, 2006b;Ojeda *et al.*, 2008;Grigore *et al.*, 2008). These differences in the expression of cardiovascular disease may be related in part to intrinsic sex-differences in myocardial function. Many recent studies have provided evidence that indicates a sex dichotomy also exists in the physiological responses to developmental challenges as they relate to the programming of subsequent cardio-renal function. These studies have largely been interpreted in one of two ways: 1) that male and female fetuses adapt differently to developmental stressors; or 2) that male and female sex steroids have a profound influence on the development and progression of developmentally programmed disease states. Moreover, since sex differences are apparent quite early in embryonic development and are independent of sex hormones; developing a third line of reasoning to suggest innate differences between the sexes play a role in the response of the developing organism to stressors may yield useful insights. Viewed in concert several primary remaining questions emerge: Do innate sex differences originating in fetal life predispose organisms to adult diseases in general and developmentally programmed outcomes in particular? Do post-natal sex differences drive specific fetal adaptations to *in utero* stressors that generate differential outcomes? Or perhaps it is a combination of these scenarios?

4.1 Human studies

A small number of clinical studies have investigated sex differences in renal function as it relates to developmentally programmed hypertension. The larger body of work in this area has detailed differences in cardiovascular parameters and stress responses. Nevertheless, several interesting findings have been reported that confirm the idea that women are "reno-protected" during early adulthood. A recent report from the Nord Trøndelag Health Study (1995-1997) in Norway found intrauterine growth restriction (IUGR), high blood pressure and low normal renal function were associated in 20-30 year olds (Hallan *et al.*, 2008). Although the degree of impaired renal function was small in these young adults, it was significant and more consistent in men than women (Hallan *et al.*, 2008). Similarly, Kistner *et al.* reported women born pre-term had increased blood pressure but no signs of adverse renal function as young adults (Kistner *et al.*, 2000).

Other studies have evaluated cardiovascular responses between male and female subjects that were growth restricted *in utero*. In one such study, Ward and colleagues reported women born small were far more susceptible to stress-induced increases in systolic blood pressure (Ward *et al.*, 2004). A recent study by Jones *et al.* has shown that there are marked sex differences in the way size at birth is associated with alterations in cardiovascular physiology established in childhood (Jones *et al.*, 2008). Further evidence that markers of impaired fetal growth are related to autonomic cardiovascular control involving modulation of both sympathetic and parasympathetic function but in a sex-specific manner has also been provided in an adult Australian cohort by the same group (Jones *et al.*, 2007). The authors reported women, but not men, who were small at birth demonstrated increased low-frequency blood pressure variability at rest and during stress, reduced levels of high-frequency heart period variability and a reduction in baroreflex sensitivity.

4.2 Animal studies

Studies utilizing animal models have employed a range of stressors in a variety of species to induce fetal growth restriction and test hypotheses regarding the developmental origins of disease (summarized in Table 2). Perhaps the most common model to date has focused on maternal nutrient restriction (MNR), either as a decrease in total caloric intake or an isocaloric decrease in protein content; studies to understand the consequences of maternal obesity from the DOHAD perspective are gaining (Grigore *et al.*, 2008;Mcmillen & Robinson, 2005;Gallou-Kabani *et al.*, 2007;Khan *et al.*, 2005;Khan *et al.*, 2003;Taylor *et al.*, 2004).

Programming Insult	Species	Adult outcomes reported in the literature
Maternal overnutrition	Rat, mouse, sheep	Hypertension (females), reduced vascular compliance, Endothelial dysfunction, aortic hypoplasia, decreased renal Na^{+}, K^{+} ATPase activity, decreased locomotor activity (female>male)
Maternal undernutrition	Rat, sheep, baboon	Hypertension (male>female), growth restriction, altered expression of renin-angiotensin system
Placental insufficiency	Rat	Hypertension (male>female), growth restriction, glucose intolerance
Maternal renal insufficiency	Rat, rabbit	Hypertension (female>male)
Ang II receptor inhibition	Rat	Hypertension, decreased nephron number, glomerulosclerosis (male>female), interstitial fibrosis (male>female)
Glucocorticoid excess	Rat, sheep	Hypertension (sex and age dependent), glomerulosclerosis
Androgen excess	Rat, mouse, sheep, human	Hypertension (male>female), decreased endothelial function, ovarian dysgenesis, increased ANG-2 sensitivity (GR males), increased male-like sexual behavior (female), growth retardation, delayed vaginal opening, increased aggression
Estrogen deficiency	Rat, mouse, sheep, human	Hypertension (postmenopausal women), infertility, abnormal mammary growth

Table 2. *Summary of developmental programming studies and outcomes.* A variety of developmental insults lead to long-term health consequences for the offspring. (References found in Sections 2 and 3.)

4.2.1 Models of nutrient restriction

Others have shown that considerable sex differences are observed in the response to MNR between male and female baboon fetuses near term (Cox *et al.*, 2008). Evidence from MNR studies suggest female progeny are less affected than their male siblings (Ozaki *et al.*, 2001;Woods *et al.*, 2005;McMullen & Langley-Evans, 2005b;McMullen & Langley-Evans, 2005a) although these observations may depend on the extent of the nutrient restriction (Hoppe *et al.*, 2007). These studies generally show decreased nephron endowment and altered expression of components of the intra-renal renin-angiotensin system (Ozaki *et al.*, 2001;Woods *et al.*, 2005;McMullen & Langley-Evans, 2005b;McMullen & Langley-Evans, 2005a;Hoppe *et al.*, 2007). Hemmings *et al.* have reported impairment of the myogenic response in the mesenteric vascular bed of pregnant adult females exposed to MNR during development (Hemmings *et al.*, 2005). MNR during the pre-implantation period in the rat resulted in elevated BP in male offspring only (Kwong *et al.*, 2000). Restriction of specific nutrients other than protein has also been evaluated. A maternal low-sodium diet in rats has recently been associated with increased maternal plasma renin activity and correlated with IUGR, increased blood pressure, and reduced creatinine clearance in female offspring but not in males (Battista *et al.*, 2002).

Similar to the results observed in many small animal models, not all large animal models show clear effects of MNR on the offspring. In addition, only a subset of these studies has been evaluated for sex differences. Previous work has shown male sheep and baboon fetuses are more susceptible to the effects of poor maternal nutrition (Gilbert *et al.*, 2005a;Gilbert *et al.*, 2006a;Gilbert *et al.*, 2007a). Studies in sheep have shown global caloric restriction impairs nephrogenesis and alters intrarenal immunoreactive AT_1, AT_2 and renin expression in gestational age and gender specific ways (Gilbert *et al.*, 2007a). Further, only male offspring of these NR ewes are hypertensive (Gilbert *et al.*, 2005a). While the mechanisms by which NR alters gene expression remains unclear in our model, data from Lillycrop *et al.* and Burdge *et al.*, both employing protein restriction in the rat suggests deficiency of methyl donors may alter gene methylation patterns and in turn effect changes in gene expression (Lillycrop *et al.*, 2005;Burdge *et al.*, 2007;Lillycrop *et al.*, 2007;Lillycrop *et al.*, 2008). It remains unclear whether the increased risk to the males is a result of gene-environment interactions originating during or after gestation. Further studies are needed to thoroughly investigate these possibilities.

4.2.2 Models of utero-placental and renal insufficiency

Models of utero-placental insufficiency are quite intriguing as they are relevant to multiple maternal health issues as well as to the developmental programming of hypertension. Alexander *et al.* have shown that reduced uterine perfusion pressure during the last trimester of pregnancy in the rat programs hypertension in the offspring and in a sex specific manner (Grigore *et al.*, 2007;Alexander, 2003). Further, in this model both the RAS and sex steroids have been implicated in the observed sex differences in hypertension (Ojeda *et al.*, 2007b;Ojeda *et al.*, 2007a;Grigore *et al.*, 2007). In contrast, the two kidney-one wrapped kidney (2K,1W) model of hypertension resulted in hypertension in 30 week old female offspring only (Denton *et al.*, 2003). Interestingly, plasma renin activity was significantly lower in the female offspring of hypertensive mothers at 10 weeks of age ($P<0.05$), suggesting that development of the renin-angiotensin system was altered. The differences in the factors elaborated by the ischemic placenta and poorly perfused kidney illustrate the complexity of the interactions between the maternal endocrine milieu and fetal development. Whereas reduced renal perfusion primarily activates the RAS, the ischemic placenta produces a variety of humoral and locally acting factors such as sFlt-1 (soluble fms-like tyrosine kinase-1) and tumor necrosis factor (TNF)-α that have far reaching effects.

Recent studies in the rat and baboon have shown chronic reductions of utero-placental blood flow elevates levels of sFlt-1 in the placenta, amniotic fluid and maternal plasma (Gilbert *et al.*, 2007b;Makris *et al.*, 2007). In the rat, this has been associated with decreased fetal growth and subsequent hypertension that is sex dependent (Alexander, 2003;Ojeda *et al.*, 2007a). Recent studies in rodents have shown elevated sFlt-1 levels alone results in fetal growth restriction (Lu *et al.*, 2007b;Bridges *et al.*, 2008). Furthermore, Lu *et al.* have followed the mouse offspring of these pregnancies and reported sex specific effects regarding the development of hypertension as only male mice have higher blood pressure in this model (Lu *et al.*, 2007a). Viewed together, these studies strongly suggest that in addition to the immediate well being of the mother, a long term outlook with regards to the well being of the fetus must also be considered during complicated and/or high risk pregnancies.

4.2.3 Maternal obesity

Maternal obesity is associated with a variety of conditions including maternal hypertension, hypertriglyceridemia, hyperglycemia and insulin resistance (Wilson & Grundy, 2003), that are independently correlated with a suboptimal *in utero* environment and consequently linked to DOHAD. Several human studies have described a positive correlation between maternal weight and/or adiposity and blood pressure of teenage children (Lawlor *et al.*, 2004;Cho *et al.*, 2000;Laor *et al.*, 1997), leading Boney *et al* to conclude from their examination of large for gestational age babies and the incidence of childhood metabolic syndrome, that "given the increased obesity prevalence in children exposed to either maternal diabetes or maternal obesity, there are implications for perpetuating the cycle of obesity, insulin resistance, and their consequences in subsequent generations." Few, if any, of the studies in humans include offspring sex as a co-variable (Boney *et al.*, 2005).

Important information with regard to maternal nutrient excess and sex-associated difference comes largely from animal models. Studies show hypertension in male rat offspring after exposure to a maternal diet high in saturated fat (or low in linoleic acid) that is not present in females (Langley-Evans, 1996). In contrast, Elahi *et al.* reported mice fed high fat diets long before the onset of gestation are hypercholesterolemic, hypertensive and produce hypertensive, hypercholesterolemic female offspring (Elahi *et al.*, 2008). Moreover, treatment of the dams with pravastatin lowered blood pressure and cholesterol levels in those offspring (Elahi *et al.*, 2008). Because the numerous pleiotropic effects of statins the mechanisms for these effects remain unclear, nevertheless these observations provide insights for further studies.

In a model more resembling high fat food consumption in humans, Armitage *et al.* demonstrated that a diet rich in fat fed to pregnant rats results in male offspring gaining more body weight and presenting with decreased renal renin activity when compared to females (Armitage *et al.*, 2005). Offspring from this model are reportedly hypertensive, exhibit increased aortic stiffness, decreased aortic smooth muscle cell number, endothelial dysfunction and decreased renal Na+, K+-ATPase activity. The bulk of these changes were independent of sex except for increased blood pressure where female offspring were hypertensive while the males were not (Khan *et al.*, 2003;Samuelsson *et al.*, 2008). Further, Khan et al. reported female offspring have reduced locomotor activity at 180 days of age compared to male offspring of pregnant rats fed a high fat diet during pregnancy (Khan *et al.*, 2003). In addition, this research group used cross-fostering techniques after birth to show that the hypertension in females is attained whether exposure to maternal high fat diet occurs before and during pregnancy or during the suckling period (Khan *et al.*, 2005). While the mechanisms responsible for programming due to high fat diets remain unclear, the report that statin treatment has beneficial effects on the offspring highlights at least one potential mechanism, alterations in lipid metabolism (Elahi *et al.*, 2008). In addition, it has been suggested that high levels of butyric acid that may result from a high fat diet could lead to changes in chromatin structure and result in epigenetic alterations (Junien, 2006). Taken together these observations highlight an important role for nutrition and intermediate metabolites in developmental programming.

4.2.4 Endocrine disruption

The importance of environmental exposures to endocrine disruptors during pregnancy has long been noted. Factors derived from *Pinus ponderosa* needles (e.g. isocupressic acid) and leaves from *Veratrum californicum* have long been observed to have profound impacts on the pregnancies of livestock (Short *et al.*, 1995;Panter *et al.*, 1992;Wu *et al.*, 2002). Moreover, the observations that ingestion of *Veratrum californicum* by sheep at specific times of gestation resulted in fetal malformations and prolonged gestation laid the foundation for experimental evidence that supports a crucial role for glucocorticoids and the fetal hypothalamic pituitary axis in the onset of parturition (Liggins, 1994;Challis *et al.*, 2000). Similarly, carbenoxolone, an active ingredient of licorice may also inhibit production of cortisol and disrupt normal HPA signaling between the mother and fetus. These findings point to a role for maternal and fetal stressors that alter glucocorticoid levels during pregnancy as important mediators of developmental programming. One such physiological stressor is exercise during pregnancy which has been reported to have a variety of effects on the offspring in hypertensive rats (Gilbert *et al.*, 2008). Whereas moderate exercise lowered blood pressure in female offspring and increased body density in both male and female progeny, a high volume of exercise resulted in post-natal growth failure followed by catch-up growth but only females suffered exacerbated hypertension (Gilbert *et al.*, 2002). Using a dexamethazone injection model, O'Reagan *et al.* showed similar effects on BP in males and females but the magnitude of hypertension and a greater stress-induced hypertension was observed in males. In another study, prenatal dexamethasone (DEX) treatment significantly enhanced the arterial pressure response to acute stress only in female Wistar rats, while DEX augmented the elevation in heart rate during stress only in male rats (Bechtold *et al.*, 2008).
Ortiz *et al.* have shown antenatal DEX elevates blood pressure in female offspring at three weeks of age while only male offspring had increased blood pressure at six months of age (Ortiz *et al.*, 2003). Interestingly, despite the observation only male DEX-treated rats were hypertensive at six months of age, both male and female offspring showed signs of glomerulosclerosis when compared to control rats (Ortiz *et al.*, 2003). Similar work has shown that a postnatal diet rich in ω-3 (n-3) fatty acids attenuates the effects of DEX on blood pressure in the offspring (Wyrwoll *et al.*, 2006) in a sex independent manner. With the wide ranging effects reported in the glucocorticoid models, continued studies are required to tease out the mechanisms of sex-specific responsivity in this programming model.

Another intriguing area of investigation garnering attention involves the role of the maternal RAS during pregnancy and/or lactation in pregnancy outcome and offspring health. These approaches may be in the form of administration of RAS inhibitors (Salazar *et al.*, 2008) or altered sodium diet as described above (Battista *et al.*, 2002). RAS inhibition at the level of the AT_1 receptor is reported to have several sex specific effects that manifest post-partum (Loria *et al.*, 2007b;Saez *et al.*, 2007;Salazar *et al.*, 2008). Saez *et al.* found that AT_1 inhibition reduces nephron number similarly in male and female rats, but the subsequent glomerulosclerosis and interstitial fibrosis are greater in males than in females. Further, the male rats are also reported to have a significant papillary atrophy (Saez *et al.*, 2007). Functional differences include impaired urinary-concentrating ability during a prolonged dehydration in the male offspring (Loria *et al.*, 2007b) and impaired excretory capacity following acute volume expansion (Loria *et al.*, 2007a).

Although the present data clearly indicate inhibition of the RAS during pregnancy has well defined and deleterious effects on renal development and function in the offspring, current studies are less clear on the effects of more subtle perturbations of the RAS (e.g. via dietary alterations, etc.) on the long term health of the offspring. Further work in these areas will help define the importance of these pathways in the developmental programming of health and disease.

5. Potential mechanisms underlying sex differences in developmental programming

A variety of mechanisms have been postulated with regard to DOHAD (summarized in Figure 2). While the contribution of sex to the developmental origins of disease is widely recognized, it seems sex may exert distinctly different influences during fetal and adult life. For example, while male fetuses may be more susceptible to *in utero* nutrient privation (Gilbert *et al.*, 2007a), female fetuses may have increased susceptibility to gestational over-nutrition (Khan *et al.*, 2003). The reasons for this remain nebulous; however, one clue may be held in the long observed differences in growth rates exhibited by male and female fetuses *in utero* (Parker *et al.*, 1984). Hence, a faster growing male fetus may experience greater or lesser degrees of these nutritional insults compared to a female counterpart. Differences in the rate at which the male develops compared to the female likely contribute to gender differences in stress responses during pregnancy (Ozaki *et al.*, 2001). It remains unclear whether male fetuses have increased metabolism compared to female fetuses. Hence, the

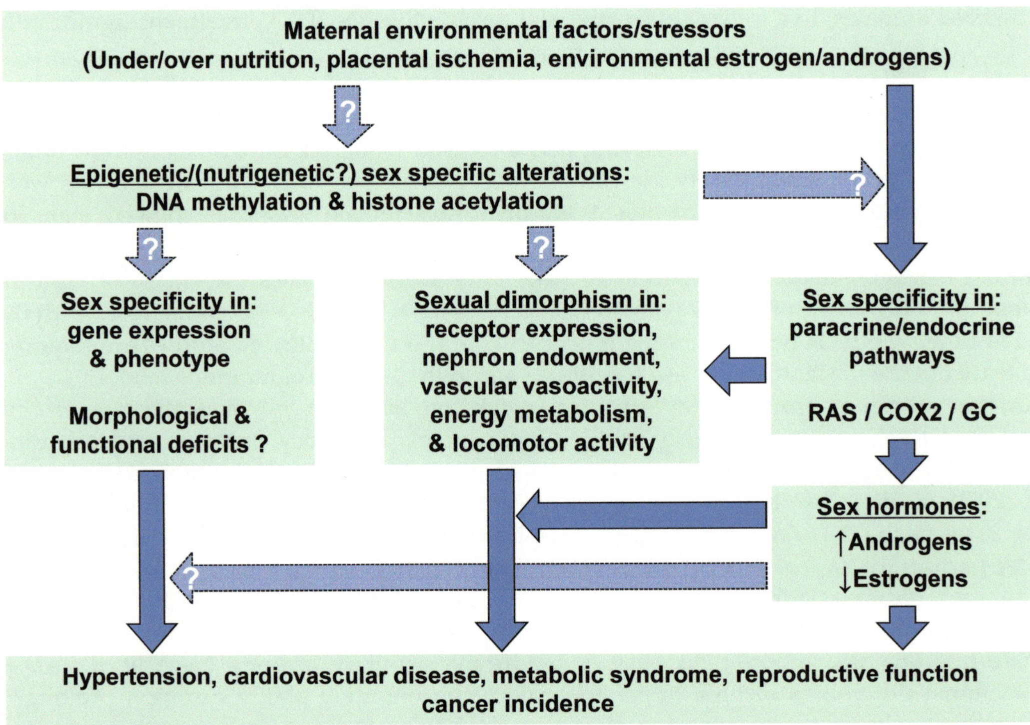

Fig. 2. *Proposed mechanisms of sexual dimorphism in developmental programming.* Research has revealed the dependence on the stimuli that result in normal development, but several connections are yet to be defined. Dark blue arrows with solid outline indicate observed pathways, like blue arrows with dotted outline represent putative connections.

chromosomal complement of the fetus may affect maternal metabolism and as the mother carrying a male fetus endures NR, the male fetus will face greater hardship than a female fetus in an equivalent pregnancy. In contrast, the female fetus in a pregnancy with an over-nourished mother could face similar hardship via different pathways.

5.1 Innate sex differences

While the existence of sexually dimorphic phenotypes is rather obvious, the mechanisms that underlie this process have remained a matter of interest. Using a theoretical model to examine the evolutionary association between X-linkage and sexually dimorphic phenotypes, Rice concluded that "sex chromosomes facilitate the evolution of sexual dimorphism and that X-linked genes have a predominant role in coding for sexually dimorphic traits" (Rice, 1984). In the ensuing twenty-five years support for this thesis has grown to include functional grouping of X chromosome gene content. Genes expressed in brain (Zechner *et al.*, 2001), for example, are particularly abundant on the X chromosome. In contrast, and perhaps of importance to potential paternal contributions to the interactions between fetus and the maternal environment, placentally expressed genes are relatively rare on the X chromosome (Ko *et al.*, 1998).

It has been recognized in humans that blood pressure is higher in men than in women (Burt *et al.*, 1995) and this difference originates during adolescence and persists into adulthood (Yong *et al.*, 1993). Further, males show an enhanced propensity to progress towards renal injury and decreased renal function than do females in several species (Neugarten *et al.*, 2002;Reckelhoff *et al.*, 1998;Sandberg & Ji, 2003). Although the roots of this difference have been linked to the RAS (Miller *et al.*, 1999), a role for an alteration in the ratio of sex steroids has also been proposed. Androgens have been linked with the progression of renal injury (Reckelhoff *et al.*, 1998;Sandberg & Ji, 2003) while estrogens have been proposed as being protective of renal function (Sandberg & Ji, 2003). Moreover, it seems that sex may exert distinctly different influences during fetal and adult life. Whereas male fetuses may be more susceptible to *in utero* nutrient privation (Gilbert *et al.*, 2007a), female fetuses appear to have increased susceptibility to gestational over-nutrition (Khan *et al.*, 2003). The reasons for this are not clear; however, one clue may be held in the long observed differences in growth rates exhibited by male and female fetuses *in utero* (Parker *et al.*, 1984). Despite findings that seem to clearly identify sex hormones as a likely culprit, recent efforts have raised many further questions and much remains unclear regarding the role of innate sex *vs.* sex steroids in developmental programming.

5.2 Epigenetic mechanisms

Epigenetic phenomena appear to be central to the induction of persistent and heritable changes in gene expression that occur without alteration of DNA sequence (Akintola *et al.*, 2008;Bird, 1986;Holliday & Ho, 2002;Wyrwoll *et al.*, 2007). While most cells in an organism contain the same DNA, gene expression varies widely across various tissues. Epigenetic mechanisms underlie this tissue- and cell-type-specific gene expression (Waterland & Michels, 2007) and include CpG methylation, histone modification (acetylation) and the activity of autoregulatory DNA-binding proteins (Kelly & Trasler, 2004). Moreover, since DNA methylation and histone acetylation are implicated in the silencing of gene expression, X-inactivation and X-linked dosage differences (Chow *et al.*, 2005), one might argue that sex-bias in differential gene expression linked to DOHAD also has its roots in methylation. Indeed, these processes appear to have many sex specific features.

Because moderate folate depletion can induce genome-wide DNA methylation (Jacob *et al.*, 1998), genomic methylation may be useful as an integrative biomarker of methyl donor nutritional status (Mason, 2003). While considerable work has been initiated in this area with regards to developmental programming, little work has focused specifically on sex differences. Interestingly, sheep exposed to a methyl deficient diet during pregnancy produce hypertensive male offspring compared to females of similar rearing, as well as to male and female controls (Sinclair *et al.*, 2007). The authors then evaluated 1400 CpG sites (primarily gene promoter associated) in fetal liver at 90 days of gestation (term=150d) and reported that more than half of the affected loci were specific to males. These observations suggest male-specific demethylation that could provide a mechanistic basis for the phenotypic sex differences observed in that study (Sinclair *et al.*, 2007). In addition, the emerging fields of nutrigenetics and metabolomics (Mutch *et al.*, 2005;Goodacre, 2007) seem poised to shed further light on these operational characteristics of these mechanisms.

Alternatively, it has also been hypothesized that when genes are expressed in multiple tissues or serve several functions they should show less sex bias than genes that are more specialized (Ellegren & Parsch, 2007). The genes such as those involved in the RAS are certainly expressed in multiple tissues, yet these genes are also closely associated with sex differences in the developmental origins of cardio-renal diseases. Clearly there is a tremendous gap in our understanding of these complex topics and further studies are needed to clarify these matters particularly in the light of the differences reported regarding fetal gender and the developmental response to maternal over- and under-nutrition.

5.3 Sex steroids

In contrast to the sex-related dichotomy observed in response to nutritional stressors, when faced with a robust stressor such as AT_1 antagonism (Loria *et al.*, 2007a;Loria *et al.*, 2007b;Saez *et al.*, 2007;Salazar *et al.*, 2008), severe protein restriction (Woods *et al.*, 2001), or chronic reductions uterine perfusion pressure (Ojeda *et al.*, 2007a;Alexander, 2003) both male and female fetuses are affected similarly *in utero.* Nonetheless a dichotomy emerges later in life with females being less impacted by their suboptimal *in utero* experience (Loria *et al.*, 2007a;Loria *et al.*, 2007b;Saez *et al.*, 2007;Salazar *et al.*, 2008). The apparent benefit of being female in scenarios such as this are supported by recent work that suggested estrogens confer a protective effect on intrauterine growth restricted females that prevents the development of programmed hypertension (Ojeda *et al.*, 2007a). Moreover, the observation that ovariectomy leads to a significant increase in blood pressure in growth-restricted females with no significant effect in controls makes a strong case for the post-developmental involvement of estrogens. Indeed, estrogen replacement reversed the effect of ovariectomy on blood pressure in growth-restricted offspring as did renin angiotensin system blockade (Ojeda *et al.*, 2007a).

Studies on the role of sex hormones in expression of components of renal renin angiotensin in healthy Sprague Dawley rats, have suggested that an estrogen-mediated attenuation of renal AT_1 binding is a potential mechanism by which estrogen exerts protection from vascular and renal disease in females (Rogers *et al.*, 2007). When this inhibition is lifted following ovariectomy in their model, or in diabetes or menopause, the resulting increased angiotensin II signaling increases both the degree of susceptibility to vascular and renal disease and the rate of existing disease progression (Rogers *et al.*, 2007).

Testosterone has also been implicated in the progression of hypertension in male growth restricted offspring (Ojeda *et al.*, 2007b). The potential underlying mechanisms have been

studied by Sullivan (Sullivan *et al.*, 2007) who has described a relationship between androgens and the development of albuminuria, and the renal protection afforded by estrogen, in spontaneously hypertensive rats. There is some evidence to suggest that both over activity of the renin angiotensin system and oxidative stress likely contributing to sex differences in the progression to renal injury. Treatment with either an AT_1 blocker and/or an ACE inhibitor blunts the occurrence of renal injury in males (Lazaro *et al.*, 2005). Male spontaneously hypertensive rats (SHR), which exhibit some signs of a programming model such as smaller size at birth when compared to Wistar-Kyoto control rats, exhibit androgen-dependent increases in blood pressure and albuminuria that are independent of renal cortical angiotensin II levels and oxidative stress (Sullivan *et al.*, 2007). In contrast, a female specific form of hypertension during pregnancy, preeclampsia, is reportedly not to be influenced by the levels of circulating testosterone levels during pregnancy (Tuutti *et al.*, 2011).
Interestingly, the cardio-renal protective effects of estrogens has not been a universal finding (Salazar *et al.*, 2008). Considering the differences between the models employed by different laboratories, one possibility could be the magnitude of the insult to the kidney during development has an influence on the extent of protection that may be afforded by female sex hormones in later life. It is widely recognized that differences in sex hormones contribute to considerable sexual dimorphism in the transcriptome of a variety of mammalian tissues and organs (Rinn & Snyder, 2005); however, it has only recently been recognized that androgen/estrogen independent mechanisms may operate at the transcriptional level to regulate sex differences (Tullis *et al.*, 2003). This possibility represents an alternate pathway that may be at work contributing to the observations that the relationship between sex hormones and blood pressure is far more complex than simply the balance of estrogen *vs.* testosterone (Ojeda *et al.*, 2007a). Taken together, it appears that the influence of sex on the developmental origins of disease may reach far beyond the widely recognized role of sex hormones. Alternatively, recent work implicates growth hormone (GH) in sex dependent differences in renal expression of glomerular AT_1 during hypertrophy following uninephrectomy; male rat kidneys show increased glomerular AT_1 expression, whereas females do not (Mok *et al.*, 2003). Because there is sexual dimorphism in GH release these observations may hold implications for both normal and pathological growth and development of the kidney.

6. Concluding remarks

From a clinical perspective it is hoped that increased understanding and awareness of developmental programming will lead to better diagnostic, preventative and therapeutic measures. The persistence of programmed effects is likely due to covalent modifications of the genome resulting from changes in promoter methylation and histone acetylation. The emerging fields of metabolomics and nutrigenetics suggest many of these alterations are likely a result of changes in the metabolic flux during critical periods of development. While epigenetic phenomena are central to the induction of persistent and heritable changes in gene expression that occur without alteration of DNA sequence, their contribution to the intensively studied sex differences in developmental programming remains uncertain. While reversal of these molecular changes may be possible and to improve long-term health outcomes if interventions are timed appropriately, loss of function in existing structures may be difficult to overcome if developmental plasticity is no longer present. For example it is difficult to see how any deficit in nephron endowment can be remedied. Nevertheless, continued investigation using hypothesis driven mechanistic studies that incorporate sexual dimorphism into the models rather than attempt to control for sex differences by omitting male and/or female subjects are needed to identify target pathways for possible intervention.

7. Acknowledgements

The authors regret that, because of space limitations, we have been unable to cite all the primary literature in the field. This work is supported by American Heart Association Grant 10SDG2600040.

8. References

Akintola AD, Crislip ZL, Catania JM, Chen G, Zimmer WE, Burghardt RC, & Parrish AR (2008). Promoter methylation is associated with the age-dependent loss of N-cadherin in the rat kidney. *Am J Physiol Renal Physiol* 294, F170-F176.

Alexander BT (2003). Placental Insufficiency Leads to Development of Hypertension in Growth-Restricted Offspring. *Hypertension* 41, 457-462.

Armitage JA, Lakasing L, Taylor PD, Balachandran AA, Jensen RI, Dekou V, Ashton N, Nyengaard JR, & Poston L (2005). Developmental programming of aortic and renal structure in offspring of rats fed fat-rich diets in pregnancy. *J Physiol (Lond)* 565, 171-184.

Avery B, Jorgensen CB, Madison V, & Greve T (1992). Morphological development and sex of bovine in vitro-fertilized embryos. *Mol Reprod Dev* 32, 265-270.

Barker DJ (1993). Fetal origins of coronary heart disease. *Br Heart J* 69, 195-196.

Baserga M, Hale MA, Wang ZM, Yu X, Callaway CW, McKnight RA, & Lane RH (2007a). Uteroplacental insufficiency alters nephrogenesis and downregulates cyclooxygenase-2 expression in a model of IUGR with adult-onset hypertension. *Am J Physiol Regul Integr Comp Physiol* 292, R1943-R1955.

Baserga M, Hale MA, Wang ZM, Yu X, Callaway CW, McKnight RA, & Lane RH (2007b). Uteroplacental insufficiency alters nephrogenesis and downregulates cyclooxygenase-2 expression in a model of IUGR with adult-onset hypertension. *Am J Physiol Regul Integr Comp Physiol* 292, R1943-R1955.

Battista MC, Oligny LL, St Louis J, & Brochu M (2002). Intrauterine growth restriction in rats is associated with hypertension and renal dysfunction in adulthood. *Am J Physiol Endocrinol Metab* 283, E124-E131.

Bechtold AG, Vernon K, Hines T, & Scheuer DA (2008). Genetic predisposition to hypertension sensitizes borderline hypertensive rats to the hypertensive effects of prenatal glucocorticoid exposure. *J Physiol (Lond)* 586, 673-684.

Beinlich CJ & Morgan HE (1993). Control of growth in neonatal pig hearts. *Mol Cell Biochem* 119, 3-9.

Beinlich CJ, Rissinger CJ, & Morgan HE (1995). Mechanisms of rapid growth in the neonatal pig heart. *J Mol Cell Cardiol* 27, 273-281.

Beinlich CJ, White GJ, Baker KM, & Morgan HE (1991). Angiotensin II and left ventricular growth in newborn pig heart. *J Mol Cell Cardiol* 23, 1031-1038.

Bernardi ML & Delouis C (1996). Sex-related differences in the developmental rate of in-vitro matured/in-vitro fertilized ovine embryos. *Hum Reprod* 11, 621-626.

Bird AP (1986). CpG-rich islands and the function of DNA methylation. *Nature* 321, 209-213.

Boney CM, Verma A, Tucker R, & Vohr BR (2005). Metabolic Syndrome in Childhood: Association With Birth Weight, Maternal Obesity, and Gestational Diabetes Mellitus. *Pediatrics* 115, e290-e296.

Bormann CL, Smith GD, Padmanabhan V, & Lee TM (2011). Prenatal testosterone and dihydrotestosterone exposure disrupts ovine testes development. *Reproduction.*

Bridges JP, Gilbert JS, Colson D, Dukes M, Babcock SA, Ryan MJ, & Granger JP (2008). Soluble Flt-1 induces hypertension and vascular dysfunction in pregnant rats. *The FASEB Journal* 22, 969.

Burdge GC, Slater-Jefferies J, Torrens C, Phillips ES, Hanson MA, & Lillycrop KA (2007). Dietary protein restriction of pregnant rats in the F0 generation induces altered methylation of hepatic gene promoters in the adult male offspring in the F1 and F2 generations. *Br J Nutr* 97, 435-439.

Burt VL, Whelton P, Roccella EJ, Brown C, Cutler JA, Higgins M, Horan MJ, & Labarthe D (1995). Prevalence of Hypertension in the US Adult Population : Results From the Third National Health and Nutrition Examination Survey, 1988-1991. *Hypertension* 25, 305-313.

Carey MA, Card JW, Voltz JW, Germolec DR, Korach KS, & Zeldin DC (2007). The impact of sex and sex hormones on lung physiology and disease: lessons from animal studies. *Am J Physiol Lung Cell Mol Physiol* 293, L272-L278.

Challis JRG, Matthews SG, Gibb W, & Lye SJ (2000). Endocrine and Paracrine Regulation of Birth at Term and Preterm. *Endocr Rev* 21, 514-550.

Cho NH, Silverman BL, Rizzo TA, & Metzger BE (2000). Correlations between the intrauterine metabolic environment and blood pressure in adolescent offspring of diabetic mothers. *The Journal of Pediatrics* 136, 587-592.

Chow JC, Yen Z, Ziesche SM, & Brown CJ (2005). Silencing of the mammalian X chromosome. *Annu Rev Genomics Hum Genet* 6, 69-92.

Cox LA, Glenn J, Schiabritz-Loutsevitch NE, Nathanielsz PW, & Nijland MJ (2008). Sex effects of maternal nutrient restriction (MNR) on renal transcriptome expression in the 0.9 gestation (G) fetal baboon. *Reproductive Sciences* 15, 120A.

Crawford MA, Doyle W, & Meadows N (1987). Gender differences at birth and differences in fetal growth. *Hum Reprod* 2, 517-520.

Denton KM, Flower RL, Stevenson KM, & Anderson WP (2003). Adult Rabbit Offspring of Mothers With Secondary Hypertension Have Increased Blood Pressure. *Hypertension* 41, 634-639.

Derfoul A, Lin FJ, Awumey EM, Kolodzeski T, Hall DJ, & Tuan RS (2003). Estrogenic endocrine disruptive components interfere with calcium handling and differentiation of human trophoblast cells. *J Cell Biochem* 89, 755-770.

Durcova-Hills G, Burgoyne P, & McLaren A (2004). Analysis of sex differences in EGC imprinting. *Developmental Biology* 268, 105-110.

Elahi MM, Cagampang FR, ANTHONY FW, Curzen N, Ohri SK, & Hanson MA (2008). Statin Treatment in Hypercholesterolemic Pregnant Mice Reduces Cardiovascular Risk Factors in Their Offspring. *Hypertension* 51, 939-944.

Ellegren H & Parsch J (2007). The evolution of sex-biased genes and sex-biased gene expression. *Nat Rev Genet* 8, 689-698.

Gallou-Kabani C, Vige A, Gross MS, Boileau C, Rabes JP, Fruchart-Najib J, Jais JP, & Junien C (2007). Resistance to high-fat diet in the female progeny of obese mice fed a control diet during the periconceptual, gestation, and lactation periods. *Am J Physiol Endocrinol Metab* 292, E1095-E1100.

Gilbert JS, Cox L, Babcock SA, Shade R, Nathanielsz PW, & Nijland MJ (2006a). Gender specific effects of moderate maternal nutrient restriction (NR) in the first half of pregnancy on fetal renal renin-angiotensin system (RAS). *Journal of the Society for Gynecologic Investigation* 13, 207A.

Gilbert JS, Cox LA, Mitchell G, & Nijland MJ (2006b). Nutrient-restricted fetus and the cardio-renal connection in hypertensive offspring. *Expert Rev Cardiovasc Ther* 4, 227-237.

Gilbert JS, Ford SP, Lang AL, Pahl LR, Drumhiller MC, Babcock SA, Nathanielsz PW, & Nijland MJ (2007a). Nutrient restriction impairs nephrogenesis in a gender-specific manner in the ovine fetus. *Pediatr Res* 61, 42-47.

Gilbert JS, Knoblich PR, & Steck S (2002). Effects of regular, voluntary gestational exercise on the development of hypertension in offspring. *Faseb Journal* 16, A1141.

Gilbert JS, Lang AL, Grant AR, & Nijland MJ (2005a). Maternal nutrient restriction in sheep: hypertension and decreased nephron number in offspring at 9 months of age. *J Physiol* 565, 137-147.

Gilbert JS, Lang AL, & Nijland MJ (2005b). Maternal nutrient restriction and the fetal left ventricle: Decreased angiotensin receptor expression. *Reprod Biol Endocrinol* 3, 27.

Gilbert JS & Nijland MJ (2008). Sex differences in the developmental origins of hypertension and cardiorenal disease. *Am J Physiol Regul Integr Comp Physiol* 295, R1941-R1952.

Gilbert JS, Babcock SA, & Granger JP (2007b). Hypertension Produced by Reduced Uterine Perfusion in Pregnant Rats Is Associated With Increased Soluble Fms-Like Tyrosine Kinase-1 Expression. *Hypertension* 50, 1142-1147.

Gilbert JS, Nijland MJ, & Knoblich P (2008). Placental ischemia and cardiovascular dysfunction in preeclampsia and beyond: making the connections. *Expert Review of Cardiovascular Therapy* 6, 1367-1377.

Gingery A, Johnson BK, & Gilbert JS (2011). Fetal Growth Restriction Results in Increased Mammary Tumor Development. *The FASEB Journal* 25, 851.

Goodacre R (2007). Metabolomics of a Superorganism. *Journal of Nutrition* 137, 259S-266.

Goodfellow J, Bellamy MF, Gorman ST, Brownlee M, Ramsey MW, Lewis MJ, Davies DP, & Henderson AH (1998). Endothelial function is impaired in fit young adults of low birth weight. *Cardiovascular Research* 40, 600-606.

Grigore D, Ojeda NB, & Alexander BT (2008). Sex differences in the fetal programming of hypertension. *Gend Med* 5 Suppl A, S121-S132.

Grigore D, Ojeda NB, Robertson EB, Dawson AS, Huffman CA, Bourassa EA, Speth RC, Brosnihan KB, & Alexander BT (2007). Placental insufficiency results in temporal alterations in the renin angiotensin system in male hypertensive growth restricted offspring. *Am J Physiol Regul Integr Comp Physiol* 293, R804-R811.

Gutierrez-Adan A, Oter M, Martinez-Madrid B, Pintado B, & De La FJ (2000). Differential expression of two genes located on the X chromosome between male and female in vitro-produced bovine embryos at the blastocyst stage. *Mol Reprod Dev* 55, 146-151.

Hales CN & Ozanne SE (2003). The dangerous road of catch-up growth. *J Physiol* 547, 5-10.

Hallan S, Euser AM, Irgens LM, Finken MJ, Holmen J, & Dekker FW (2008). Effect of intrauterine growth restriction on kidney function at young adult age: the Nord Trondelag Health (HUNT 2) Study. *Am J Kidney Dis* 51, 10-20.

Haning RV, Jr., Curet LB, Poole WK, Boehnlein LM, Kuzma DL, & Meier SM (1989). Effects of fetal sex and dexamethasone on preterm maternal serum concentrations of human chorionic gonadotropin, progesterone, estrone, estradiol, and estriol. *Am J Obstet Gynecol* 161, 1549-1553.

Hemmings DG, Veerareddy S, Baker PN, & Davidge ST (2005). Increased Myogenic Responses in Uterine but not Mesenteric Arteries from Pregnant Offspring of Diet-Restricted Rat Dams. *Biol Reprod* 72, 997-1003.

Hennighausen L & Robinson GW (2001). Signaling Pathways in Mammary Gland Development. *Developmental Cell* 1, 467-475.

Hinck L & Silberstein GB (2005). Key stages in mammary gland development: the mammary end bud as a motile organ. *Breast Cancer Res* 7, 245-251.

Hindmarsh P, Geary M, Rodeck C, Kingdom JC, & Cole T (2002). Intrauterine Growth and its Relationship to Size and Shape at Birth. *Pediatric Research* 52, 263-268.

Hofman PL, Cutfield WS, Robinson EM, Bergman RN, Menon RK, Sperling MA, & Gluckman PD (1997). Insulin resistance in short children with intrauterine growth retardation. *J Clin Endocrinol Metab* 82, 402-406.

Hogg K, McNeilly AS, & Duncan WC (2011). Prenatal androgen exposure leads to alterations in gene and protein expression in the ovine fetal ovary. *Endocrinology* 152, 2048-2059.

Holliday R & Ho T (2002). DNA methylation and epigenetic inheritance. *Methods* 27, 179-183.

Hoppe CC, Evans RG, Bertram JF, & Moritz KM (2007). Effects of dietary protein restriction on nephron number in the mouse. *Am J Physiol Regul Integr Comp Physiol* 292, R1768-R1774.

Hovi P, Andersson S, Eriksson JG, Jarvenpaa AL, Strang-Karlsson S, Makitie O, & Kajantie E (2007). Glucose Regulation in Young Adults with Very Low Birth Weight. *The New England Journal of Medicine* 356, 2053-2063.

Jacob RA, Gretz DM, Taylor PC, James SJ, Pogribny IP, Miller BJ, Henning SM, & Swendseid ME (1998). Moderate Folate Depletion Increases Plasma Homocysteine and Decreases Lymphocyte DNA Methylation in Postmenopausal Women. *Journal of Nutrition* 128, 1204-1212.

Jones A, Beda A, Osmond C, Godfrey KM, Simpson DM, & Phillips DIW (2008). Sex-specific programming of cardiovascular physiology in children. *Eur Heart J* ehn292.

Jones A, Beda A, Ward AMV, Osmond C, Phillips DIW, Moore VM, & Simpson DM (2007). Size at Birth and Autonomic Function During Psychological Stress. *Hypertension* 49, 548-555.

Junien C (2006). Impact of diets and nutrients/drugs on early epigenetic programming. *J Inherit Metab Dis* 29, 359-365.

Kelly TL & Trasler JM (2004). Reproductive epigenetics. *Clin Genet* 65, 247-260.

Khan IY, Dekou V, Douglas G, Jensen R, Hanson MA, Poston L, & Taylor PD (2005). A high-fat diet during rat pregnancy or suckling induces cardiovascular dysfunction in adult offspring. *Am J Physiol Regul Integr Comp Physiol* 288, R127-R133.

Khan IY, Taylor PD, Dekou V, Seed PT, Lakasing L, Graham D, Dominiczak AF, Hanson MA, & Poston L (2003). Gender-Linked Hypertension in Offspring of Lard-Fed Pregnant Rats. *Hypertension* 41, 168-175.

Kistner A, Celsi G, Vanpee M, & Jacobson SH (2000). Increased blood pressure but normal renal function in adult women born preterm. *Pediatric Nephrology* 15, 215.

Ko MS, Threat TA, Wang X, Horton JH, Cui Y, Wang X, Pryor E, Paris J, Wells-Smith J, Kitchen JR, Rowe LB, Eppig J, Satoh T, Brant L, Fujiwara H, Yotsumoto S, & Nakashima H (1998). Genome-wide mapping of unselected transcripts from extraembryonic tissue of 7.5-day mouse embryos reveals enrichment in the t-complex and under-representation on the X chromosome. *Hum Mol Genet* 7, 1967-1978.

Kovtun IV, Therneau TM, & McMurray CT (2000). Gender of the embryo contributes to CAG instability in transgenic mice containing a Huntington's disease gene. *Human Molecular Genetics* 9, 2767-2775.

Kristensen DM, Skalkam ML, Audouze K, Lesne L, Desdoits-Lethimonier C, Frederiksen H, Brunak S, Skakkebaek NE, Jegou B, Hansen JB, Junker S, & Leffers H (2011). Many putative endocrine disruptors inhibit prostaglandin synthesis. *Environ Health Perspect* 119, 534-541.

Kwong WY, Wild AE, Roberts P, Willis AC, & Fleming TP (2000). Maternal undernutrition during the preimplantation period of rat development causes blastocyst abnormalities and programming of postnatal hypertension. *Development* 127, 4195-4202.

Langley-Evans SC (1996). Intrauterine programming of hypertension in the rat: nutrient interactions. *Comp Biochem Physiol A Physiol* 114, 327-333.

Laor A, Stevenson DK, Shemer J, Gale R, & Seidman DS (1997). Size at birth, maternal nutritional status in pregnancy, and blood pressure at age 17: population based analysis. *BMJ* 315, 449-453.

Larson MA, Kimura K, Kubisch HM, & Roberts RM (2001). Sexual dimorphism among bovine embryos in their ability to make the transition to expanded blastocyst and in the expression of the signaling molecule IFN--ä. *Proceedings of the National Academy of Sciences of the United States of America* 98, 9677-9682.

Lawlor DA, Najman JM, Sterne J, Williams GM, Ebrahim S, & Smith GD (2004). Associations of Parental, Birth, and Early Life Characteristics With Systolic Blood Pressure at 5 Years of Age: Findings From the Mater-University Study of Pregnancy and Its Outcomes. *Circulation* 110, 2417-2423.

Lazaro A, Gallego-Delgado J, Justo P, Esteban V, Osende J, Mezzano S, Ortiz A, & Egido J (2005). Long-term blood pressure control prevents oxidative renal injury. *Antioxid Redox Signal* 7, 1285-1293.

Leeson CPM, Kattenhorn M, Morley R, Lucas A, & Deanfield JE (2001). Impact of Low Birth Weight and Cardiovascular Risk Factors on Endothelial Function in Early Adult Life. *Circulation* 103, 1264-1268.

Li S, Chen SC, Shlipak M, Bakris G, McCullough PA, Sowers J, Stevens L, Jurkovitz C, McFarlane S, Norris K, Vassalotti J, Klag MJ, Brown WW, Narva A, Calhoun D, Johnson B, Obialo C, Whaley-Connell A, Becker B, & Collins AJ (2007). Low birth weight is associated with chronic kidney disease only in men. *Kidney Int* 73, 637-642.

Liggins GC (1994). The role of cortisol in preparing the fetus for birth. *Reprod Fertil Dev* 6, 141-150.

Lillycrop KA, Phillips ES, Torrens C, Hanson MA, Jackson AA, & Burdge GC (2008). Feeding pregnant rats a protein-restricted diet persistently alters the methylation of specific cytosines in the hepatic PPAR alpha promoter of the offspring. *Br J Nutr* 100, 278-282.

Lillycrop KA, Slater-Jefferies JL, Hanson MA, Godfrey KM, Jackson AA, & Burdge GC (2007). Induction of altered epigenetic regulation of the hepatic glucocorticoid receptor in the offspring of rats fed a protein-restricted diet during pregnancy suggests that reduced DNA methyltransferase-1 expression is involved in impaired DNA methylation and changes in histone modifications. *Br J Nutr* 97, 1064-1073.

Lillycrop KA, Phillips ES, Jackson AA, Hanson MA, & Burdge GC (2005). Dietary Protein Restriction of Pregnant Rats Induces and Folic Acid Supplementation Prevents Epigenetic Modification of Hepatic Gene Expression in the Offspring. *Journal of Nutrition* 135, 1382-1386.

Loria A, Reverte V, Salazar F, Saez F, Llinas MT, & Salazar FJ (2007a). Changes in renal hemodynamics and excretory function induced by a reduction of ANG II effects during renal development. *Am J Physiol Regul Integr Comp Physiol* 293, R695-R700.

Loria A, Reverte V, Salazar F, Saez F, Llinas MT, & Salazar FJ (2007b). Sex and age differences of renal function in rats with reduced ANG II activity during the nephrogenic period. *Am J Physiol Renal Physiol* 293, F506-F510.

Lu F, Bytautiene E, Tamayo E, Gamble P, Anderson GD, Hankins GD, Longo M, & Saade GR (2007a). Gender-specific effect of overexpression of sFlt-1 in pregnant mice on fetal programming of blood pressure in the offspring later in life. *Am J Obstet Gynecol* 197, 418-5.

Lu F, Longo M, Tamayo E, Maner W, Al-Hendy A, Anderson GD, Hankins GDV, & Saade GR (2007b). The effect of over-expression of sFlt-1 on blood pressure and the occurrence of other manifestations of preeclampsia in unrestrained conscious pregnant mice. *American Journal of Obstetrics and Gynecology* 196, 396.

Makris A, Thornton C, Thompson J, Thomson S, Martin R, Ogle R, Waugh R, McKenzie P, Kirwan P, & Hennessy A (2007). Uteroplacental ischemia results in proteinuric hypertension and elevated sFLT-1. *Kidney Int* 71, 977-984.

Manikkam M, Crespi EJ, Doop DD, Herkimer C, Lee JS, Yu S, Brown MB, Foster DL, & Padmanabhan V (2004). Fetal programming: prenatal testosterone excess leads to fetal growth retardation and postnatal catch-up growth in sheep. *Endocrinology* 145, 790-798.

Manolakou P, Angelopoulou R, Bakoyiannis C, & Bastounis E (2009). The effects of endogenous and exogenous androgens on cardiovascular disease risk factors and progression. *Reprod Biol Endocrinol* 7, 44.

Martin H, Hu J, Gennser G, & Norman M (2000). Impaired Endothelial Function and Increased Carotid Stiffness in 9-Year-Old Children With Low Birthweight. *Circulation* 102, 2739-2744.

Mason JB (2003). Biomarkers of Nutrient Exposure and Status in One-Carbon (Methyl) Metabolism. *Journal of Nutrition* 133, 941S-9947.

Mcmillen IC & Robinson JS (2005). Developmental Origins of the Metabolic Syndrome: Prediction, Plasticity, and Programming. *Physiol Rev* 85, 571-633.

McMullen S & Langley-Evans SC (2005a). Maternal low-protein diet in rat pregnancy programs blood pressure through sex-specific mechanisms. *Am J Physiol Regul Integr Comp Physiol* 288, R85-R90.

McMullen S & Langley-Evans SC (2005b). Sex-Specific Effects of Prenatal Low-Protein and Carbenoxolone Exposure on Renal Angiotensin Receptor Expression in Rats. *Hypertension* 01.

Meisel RL & Ward IL (1981). Fetal female rats are masculinized by male littermates located caudally in the uterus. *Science* 213, 239-242.

Miller JA, Anacta LA, & Cattran DC (1999). Impact of gender on the renal response to angiotensin II. *Kidney Int* 55, 278-285.

Mok KY, Sandberg K, Sweeny JM, Zheng W, Lee S, & Mulroney SE (2003). Growth hormone regulation of glomerular AT1 angiotensin receptors in adult uninephrectomized male rats. *Am J Physiol Renal Physiol* 285, F1085-F1091.

Mutch DM, Wahli W, & Williamson G (2005). Nutrigenomics and nutrigenetics: the emerging faces of nutrition. *The FASEB Journal* 19, 1602-1616.

Neugarten J, Kasiske B, Silbiger SR, & Nyengaard JR (2002). Effects of sex on renal structure. *Nephron* 90, 139-144.

Ojeda NB, Grigore D, & Alexander BT (2008). Intrauterine growth restriction: fetal programming of hypertension and kidney disease. *Adv Chronic Kidney Dis* 15, 101-106.

Ojeda NB, Royals TP, Black JT, Dasinger JH, Johnson JM, & Alexander BT (2010). Enhanced sensitivity to acute angiotensin II is testosterone dependent in adult male growth-restricted offspring. *Am J Physiol Regul Integr Comp Physiol* 298, R1421-R1427.

Ojeda NB, Grigore D, Robertson EB, & Alexander BT (2007a). Estrogen Protects Against Increased Blood Pressure in Postpubertal Female Growth Restricted Offspring. *Hypertension* 50, 679-685.

Ojeda NB, Grigore D, Yanes LL, Iliescu R, Robertson EB, Zhang H, & Alexander BT (2007b). Testosterone contributes to marked elevations in mean arterial pressure in adult male intrauterine growth restricted offspring. *Am J Physiol Regul Integr Comp Physiol* 292, R758-R763.

Ortiz LA, Quan A, Zarzar F, Weinberg A, & Baum M (2003). Prenatal dexamethasone programs hypertension and renal injury in the rat. *Hypertension* 41, 328-334.

Ozaki T, Nishina H, Hanson MA, & Poston L (2001). Dietary restriction in pregnant rats causes gender-related hypertension and vascular dysfunction in offspring. *J Physiol* 530, 141-152.

Paldi A, Gyapay G, & Jami J (1995). Imprinted chromosomal regions of the human genome display sex-specific meiotic recombination frequencies. *Curr Biol* 5, 1030-1035.

Panter KE, James LF, & Molyneux RJ (1992). Ponderosa pine needle-induced parturition in cattle. *J Anim Sci* 70, 1604-1608.

Parker AJ, Davies P, Mayho AM, & Newton JR (1984). The ultrasound estimation of sex-related variations of intrauterine growth. *Am J Obstet Gynecol* 149, 665-669.

Peippo J, Farazmand A, Kurkilahti M, Markkula M, Basrur PK, & King WA (2002). Sex-chromosome linked gene expression in in-vitro produced bovine embryos. *Molecular Human Reproduction* 8, 923-929.

Recabarren SE, Rojas-Garcia PP, Recabarren MP, Alfaro VH, Smith R, Padmanabhan V, & Sir-Petermann T (2008). Prenatal testosterone excess reduces sperm count and motility. *Endocrinology* 149, 6444-6448.

Reckelhoff JF, Zhang H, & Granger JP (1998). Testosterone exacerbates hypertension and reduces pressure-natriuresis in male spontaneously hypertensive rats. *Hypertension* 31, 435-439.

Rice WR (1984). Sex chromosomes and the evolution of sexual dimorphism. *Evolution* 38, 735-742.

Rinn JL, Rozowsky JS, Laurenzi IJ, Petersen PH, Zou K, Zhong W, Gerstein M, & Snyder M (2004). Major molecular differences between mammalian sexes are involved in drug metabolism and renal function. *Dev Cell* 6, 791-800.

Rinn JL & Snyder M (2005). Sexual dimorphism in mammalian gene expression. *Trends Genet* 21, 298-305.

Rogers JL, Mitchell AR, Maric C, Sandberg K, Myers A, & Mulroney SE (2007). Effect of sex hormones on renal estrogen and angiotensin type 1 receptors in female and male rats. *Am J Physiol Regul Integr Comp Physiol* 292, R794-R799.

Roseboom TJ, van der Meulen JH, van Montfrans GA, Ravelli AC, Osmond C, Barker DJ, & Bleker OP (2001). Maternal nutrition during gestation and blood pressure in later life. *J Hypertens* 19, 29-34.

Rubinow DR & Girdler SS (2011). Hormones, heart disease, and health: individualized medicine versus throwing the baby out with the bathwater. *Depress Anxiety* 28, E1-E15.

Saez F, Castells MT, Zuasti A, Salazar F, Reverte V, Loria A, & Salazar FJ (2007). Sex Differences in the Renal Changes Elicited by Angiotensin II Blockade During the Nephrogenic Period. *Hypertension* 49, 1429-1435.

Sakemi T, Toyoshima H, Shouno Y, & Morito F (1995). Estrogen attenuates progressive glomerular injury in hypercholesterolemic male Imai rats. *Nephron* 69, 159-165.

Salazar F, Reverte V, Saez F, Loria A, Llinas MT, & Salazar FJ (2008). Age-sodium sensistive hypertension and sex-dependent renal changes in rats with a reduced nephron number. *Hypertension* 51, 1184-1189.

Samuelsson AM, Matthews PA, Argenton M, Christie MR, McConnell JM, Jansen EHJ, Piersma AH, Ozanne SE, Twinn DF, Remacle C, Rowlerson A, Poston L, & Taylor PD (2008). Diet-Induced Obesity in Female Mice Leads to Offspring Hyperphagia, Adiposity, Hypertension, and Insulin Resistance: A Novel Murine Model of Developmental Programming. *Hypertension* 51, 383-392.

Samyn ME, Petershack JA, Bedell KA, Mathews MS, & Segar JL (1998). Ontogeny and regulation of cardiac angiotensin types 1 and 2 receptors during fetal life in sheep. *Pediatr Res* 44, 323-329.

Sandberg K & Ji H (2003). Sex and the renin angiotensin system: implications for gender differences in the progression of kidney disease. *Adv Ren Replace Ther* 10, 15-23.

Segar JL, Dalshaug GB, Bedell KA, Smith OM, & Scholz TD (2001). Angiotensin II in cardiac pressure-overload hypertrophy in fetal sheep. *Am J Physiol Regul Integr Comp Physiol* 281, R2037-R2047.

Segar JL, Scholz TD, Bedell KA, Smith OM, Huss DJ, & Guillery EN (1997). Angiotensin AT1 receptor blockade fails to attenuate pressure-overload cardiac hypertrophy in fetal sheep. *Am J Physiol* 273, R1501-R1508.

Short RE, Ford SP, Grings EE, & Kronberg SL (1995). Abortifacient response and plasma vasoconstrictive activity after feeding needles from ponderosa pine trees to cattle and sheep. *J Anim Sci* 73, 2102-2104.

Silva-Antonialli MM, Tostes RCA, Fernandes L, Fior-Chadi DR, Akamine EH, Carvalho MH, Fortes ZB, & Nigro D (2004). A lower ratio of AT1/AT2 receptors of angiotensin II is found in female than in male spontaneously hypertensive rats. *Cardiovascular Research* 62, 587-593.

Sinclair KD, Allegrucci C, Singh R, Gardner DS, Sebastian S, Bispham J, Thurston A, Huntley JF, Rees WD, Maloney CA, Lea RG, Craigon J, McEvoy TG, & Young LE (2007). DNA methylation, insulin resistance, and blood pressure in offspring determined by maternal periconceptional B vitamin and methionine status. *Proceedings of the National Academy of Sciences* 104, 19351-19356.

Sonnenschein C & Soto AM (1998). An updated review of environmental estrogen and androgen mimics and antagonists. *J Steroid Biochem Mol Biol* 65, 143-150.

Sood R, Zehnder JL, Druzin ML, & Brown PO (2006). Gene expression patterns in human placenta. 103, 5478-5483.

Sullivan JC, Semprun-Prieto L, Boesen EI, Pollock DM, & Pollock JS (2007). Sex and sex hormones influence the development of albuminuria and renal macrophage infiltration in spontaneously hypertensive rats. *Am J Physiol Regul Integr Comp Physiol* 293, R1573-R1579.

Sundgren NC, Giraud GD, Stork PJ, Maylie JG, & Thornburg KL (2003). Angiotensin II stimulates hyperplasia but not hypertrophy in immature ovine cardiomyocytes. *J Physiol* 548, 881-891.

Taylor DM, Handyside AH, Ray PF, Dibb NJ, Winston RML, & Ao A (2001). Quantitative measurement of transcript levels throughout human preimplantation development: analysis of hypoxanthine phosphoribosyl transferase. *Molecular Human Reproduction* 7, 147-154.

Taylor PD, Khan IY, Hanson MA, & Poston L (2004). Impaired EDHF-mediated vasodilatation in adult offspring of rats exposed to a fat-rich diet in pregnancy. *J Physiol (Lond)* 558, 943-951.

Tullis KM, Krebs CJ, Leung JYM, & Robins DM (2003). The Regulator of Sex-Limitation Gene, Rsl, Enforces Male-Specific Liver Gene Expression by Negative Regulation. *Endocrinology* 144, 1854-1860.

Tuutti EK, Hamalainen EK, Sainio SM, Hiilesmaa VK, Turpeinen UL, Alfthan HV, & Stenman UH (2011). Serum testosterone levels during early pregnancy in patients developing preeclampsia. *Scand J Clin Lab Invest.*

Valdivia RP, Kunieda T, Azuma S, & Toyoda Y (1993). PCR sexing and developmental rate differences in preimplantation mouse embryos fertilized and cultured in vitro. *Mol Reprod Dev* 35, 121-126.

Ward AM, Moore VM, Steptoe A, Cockington RA, Robinson JS, & Phillips DI (2004). Size at birth and cardiovascular responses to psychological stressors: evidence for prenatal programming in women. *J Hypertens* 22, 2295-2301.

Waterland RA & Michels KB (2007). Epigenetic Epidemiology of the Developmental Origins Hypothesis. *Annual Review of Nutrition* 27, 363-388.

Wilson PWF & Grundy SM (2003). The Metabolic Syndrome: Practical Guide to Origins and Treatment: Part I. *Circulation* 108, 1422-1424.

Wlodek M, Ceranic V, O'Dowd R, Westcott K, & Siebel A (2009). Maternal Progesterone Treatment Rescues the Mammary Impairment Following Uteroplacental Insufficiency and Improves Postnatal Pup Growth in the Rat. *Reprod Sci.*

Woods LL, Ingelfinger JR, Nyengaard JR, & Rasch R (2001). Maternal protein restriction suppresses the newborn renin-angiotensin system and programs adult hypertension in rats. *Pediatr Res* 49, 460-467.

Woods LL, Ingelfinger JR, & Rasch R (2005). Modest maternal protein restriction fails to program adult hypertension in female rats. *Am J Physiol Regul Integr Comp Physiol* 289, R1131-R1136.

Wrenzycki C, Lucas-Hahn A, Herrmann D, Lemme E, Korsawe K, & Niemann H (2002). In Vitro Production and Nuclear Transfer Affect Dosage Compensation of the X-Linked Gene Transcripts G6PD, PGK, and Xist in Preimplantation Bovine Embryos. *Biol Reprod* 66, 127-134.

Wu LS, Chen JC, Sheu SY, Huang CC, Kuo YH, Chiu CH, Lian WX, Yang CJ, Kaphle K, & Lin JH (2002). Isocupressic acid blocks progesterone production from bovine luteal cells. *Am J Chin Med* 30, 533-541.

Wyrwoll CS, Mark PJ, & Waddell BJ (2007). Developmental programming of renal glucocorticoid sensitivity and the renin-angiotensin system. *Hypertension* 50, 579-584.

Wyrwoll CS, Mark PJ, Mori TA, Puddey IB, & Waddell BJ (2006). Prevention of Programmed Hyperleptinemia and Hypertension by Postnatal Dietary {omega}-3 Fatty Acids. *Endocrinology* 147, 599-606.

Xue F & Michels KB (2007). Intrauterine factors and risk of breast cancer: a systematic review and meta-analysis of current evidence. *The Lancet Oncology* 8, 1088-1100.

Yadav BR, King WA, & Betteridge KJ (1993). Relationships between the completion of first cleavage and the chromosomal complement, sex, and developmental rates of bovine embryos generated in vitro. *Mol Reprod Dev* 36, 434-439.

Yong LC, Kuller LH, Rutan G, & Bunker C (1993). Longitudinal Study of Blood Pressure: Changes and Determinants from Adolescence to Middle Age. The Dormont High School Follow-up Study, 1957-1963 to 1989-1990. *American Journal of Epidemiology* 138, 973-983.

Zechner U, Wilda M, Kehrer-Sawatzki H, Vogel W, Fundele R, & Hameister H (2001). A high density of X-linked genes for general cognitive ability: a run-away process shaping human evolution? *Trends Genet* 17, 697-701.

16

WW Domain-Containing Oxidoreductase is a Potential Receptor for Sex Steroid Hormones

Won-Pei Su[1], Shu-Hui Chen[2], Szu-Jung Chen[1],
Pei-Yi Chou[1], Chun-Cheng Huang[1] and Nan-Shan Chang[1,3,4]
[1]*Institute of Molecular Medicine, National Cheng Kung University, Tainan, Taiwan,*
[2]*Department of Chemistry, National Cheng Kung University, Tainan, Taiwan,*
[3]*Department of Neuroscience and Physiology, SUNY Upstate Medical University, Syracuse, NY,*
[4]*Department of Neurochemistry, NYS Institute of Basic Research in Developmental Disabilities, Staten Island, NY,*
[1,2]*ROC*
[3,4]*USA*

1. Introduction

1.1 Biosynthesis and metabolism of estrogens

Estrogen is a steroid hormone that comprises a group of compounds, including estrone (E1), estradiol (E2) and estriol (E3). E2 is an ovarian hormone necessary for the development of secondary sexual characteristics and function of the reproductive system in females. It also plays important roles in non-reproductive organs by multiple pathways. Estrogens are produced primarily by developing follicles in the ovaries, the corpus luteum, and the placenta. Some estrogens are also produced in smaller amounts by other tissues such as the liver, adrenal glands, and the breasts. E2 is converted from testosterone and E1 from rostenedione; both conversions are regulated by a dehydrogenase enzyme, aromatase. Estrogens are eliminated from the body by metabolic conversion to hormonally inactive and water-soluble metabolites that are excreted in the urine and/or feces. The metabolic disposition of estrogens includes oxidative metabolism (Martucci et al., 1993) and conjugative metabolism by glucuronidation (Zhu, et al., 1996), sulfonation (Hernandez et al., 1992) and/or *O*-methylation (Ball & Knuppen, 1980). Hydroxylation at the C-2 and C-4 position of E2 (17β-Estradiol) yields the catecholestrogens (CEs), 2-hydroxyestrone (2-OHE1) and 2-hydroxyestradiol (2-OHE2), 4-hydroxyestrone (4-OHE1) and 4-hydroxyestradiol (4-OHE2) while hydroxylation at the C-16 α position yields 16 α-hydroxyestrone (16 α-OHE1), which is subsequently converted to estriol (E3) (Ball & Knuppen, 1980; Zhu & Conney, 1998). The hydroxylated products exert very different biological properties: the 16 α-hydroxy and 4-hydroxy metabolites are active estrogens, whereas the 2-hydroxy metabolites are not as active (Fishman & Martucci, 1980; Swaneck & Fishman, 1988). However, the binding and redox cycling activities of CEs can be blocked via *O*-methylation by catechol-O-methyltransferase (COMT), which converts 2-OHE1/E2 and 4-OHE1/E2 to their methoxy derivatives 2-MeOHE1, 2-MeOHE2, 4-MeOHE1, and 4-MeOHE2, respectively (Albin et al., 1993; Cheng et al., 1998; Falany & Falany, 1996). Although liver is the major organ of the estrogen metabolism, some estrogen hydroxylation enzymes are selectively expressed in other tissues. Our recent data indicated that trace amounts (<0.9 fg/cell) of estrogens are produced in the endogenous breast cancer cells (MCF-7) (Huang et al., 2011). Moreover, E2 treatment substantially induced E1 and estrogen metabolites in MCF-7 cells, indicating the expression of estrogen metabolizing enzymes in breast cancer cells as well.

1.2 Estrogen receptors

E2 is most known to act by binding to and activating two estrogen receptors (ERs), ERα and ERβ (Mosselman et al., 1996), which belongs to the super-family of nuclear receptors (McDonnel & Norris, 2002). Like many nuclear receptors, ERs are consisted of hypervariable *N*-termini that contribute to the transaction function; namely, a highly conserved DNA binding domain responsible for DNA binding and dimerization and *C*-terminal domain, which is involved in ligand binding, nuclear localization, and ligand-dependent transaction function. It is well established that E2 can activate ERα and promote cancer formation in experimental animals, which is associated with cell proliferation. In contrast, the activated ERβ suppresses cell proliferation and colon cancer xenograft growth, probably as a consequence of ERβ-mediated inhibition of cell-cycle pathways (Hartman et al., 2009). E2 action involves ligand-mediated activation of ERα and ERβ, which binds directly with estrogen response element (ERE) in the promoters of target genes and recruits various coactivators to mediate transcriptional regulation. There is a general consensus that hormonally active compounds may directly or indirectly activate transcription factors through ER binding and promote gene transcription and cell proliferation, in particular in cells responding to the hormones by growth. Many anti-cancer drugs for estrogen-dependent breast tumor have been developed based on their antagonistic effect on E2 binding so as to affect protein expression.

1.3 Non-classical estrogen actions

E2, however, could also induce estrogenic effects in ER-negative systems through signaling pathways more commonly associated with growth factor activation of cell surface receptors such as G-protein-coupled receptor (GPCR) GPR30 to transactivate epidermal growth factor receptor (EGFR) and activate the MAPK cascade *via* the release of surface-associated heparin binding epidermal growth factor (Filardo et al., 2002). E2 may also trigger the transcription of non-estrogen responsive genes through kinase activation. It has been demonstrated that this GPR30-dependent estrogen induction of MAPK is transient and under the control of a cAMP-dependent negative feedback loop. Whereas, our phosphoproteomics data (Wu et al., 2011) suggested that the growth factor-mediated pathways also occur in ER-dependent cells. Furthermore, accumulating evidence reveals that many unexpected non-classical responses such as estrogen-derived reactive oxidative stress (ROS) may also be induced (Yeh et al., 2005; Miro et al., 2011). The interaction between estrogen-derived ROS and proliferation machinery has not been elucidated yet.

1.4 Non-classical estrogen receptors

Based on a review of data scattered in the literature, we suggest that some of the effects exerted by active estrogen may be mediated by specific intracellular receptors or effectors, which are different from the classical estrogen receptor. It is most likely that additional isoforms of the classical ERs or putative receptors with the ligand binding domain are potential candidates of E2 receptors. Moreover, active estrogen metabolites such as catechol estrogens are not merely to simplify the secretion of estrogen, but may have their own biological roles (Zhu & Conney, 1998). Receptors of estrogen metabolites are distinct and different from classical ERs (Markides & Liehr, 2005). A locally formed estrogen metabolite may exert a biological effect important for the action of the parent hormone. Cytochrome P450 family are the major enzymes catalyzing nicotinamide adenine dinucleotide phosphate (reduced form) (NADPH*)-dependent oxidative metabolism of estrogens to multiple hydroxylated metabolites. The estrogen biosynthesis enzyme, aromatase, whose function is to aromatize androgens in order to produce estrogens, is a member of the cytochrome P450 superfamily. Since estrogen and estrogen metabolites are substrates of specific reductases or oxidases, we suspect that cellular proteins, which possess an oxidoreductase domain, are candidates of novel estrogen receptors. These novel receptors may possess important and unique biological functions that are not directly associated with the classical estrogen action.

2. Oxidoreductases and sex steroid hormones

2.1 17β-hydroxysteroid dehydrogenases

Biologically active sex steroid hormones are metabolically converted in normal and cancerous tissues and organs. Estrogen provides a proliferative effect in majority of ER-positive breast cancer cells. Enzymes responsible for metabolizing steroid hormones are aromatase, estrone sulfatases, and 17β-hydroxysteroid dehydrogenases (17β-HSDs) (Jansson, 2009; Aka et al., 2009). These enzymes are present in breast cancer tissues (Miki et al., 2009). There are reductive and oxidative 17β-HSDs. The reductive 17β-HSDs are responsible for manufacturing active androgens and estrogens by catalyzing the formation of the hydroxy group at position 17β of the steroid backbone. The oxidative 17β-HSD transforms the hydroxy group into keto and inactivates the steroids. The type 3 17β-HSD (17β-HSD3) is reductive, structurally similar to 17β-HSD12, and present in the testis. 17β-HSD3 recognizes androgen by catalyzing the transformation of 4-androstenedione into testosterone (Geissler et al., 1994). 17β-HSD12 catalyzes the transformation of both androgens and estrogens (Blanchard & Luu-The, 2007; Liu et al., 2007). *Caenorhabditis elegans* LET-767 is known to metabolize androgens and estrogens, and the gene appears to share a common ancestor with human types 17β-HSD3 and HSD12 (Desnoyers et al., 2007). High levels of expression of 17β-HSD1 have been shown to be associated with poor prognosis in breast cancer and late relapse among patients with ER-positive breast tumors (Sasaki et al., 2010; Jansson et al., 2009). In contrast, significant downregulation of 17β-HSD2 is also correlated with decreased survival in ER-positive breast cancer (Sasaki et al., 2010; Jansson et al., 2009). Similarly, significantly reduced expression of 17β-HSD14 mRNA in breast cancer is also associated with decreased survival (Jansson et al., 2009). Overall, there are 14 different types of 17β-HSDs (Marchais-Oberwinkler et al., 2011). These oxidoreductases are central to the estrogen and androgen steroid metabolism by catalyzing final steps of the steroid biosynthesis. Indeed, 17β-HSDs act like receptor molecules. While these proteins are involved in many diseases such as breast cancer, prostate cancer, endometriosis, osteoporosis, and brain cancer, 17β-HSDs are of considerable interest in therapeutic targeting.

2.2 Estrogen metabolites and biological effects

Despite the wealthy knowledge of estrogen/ER in signaling, metabolism and diseases (Tam et al., 2011; Okoh et al., 2011; Nilsen, 2008; Mueck & Seeger, 2007; Straub, 2007), the signal pathways underlying the biological effects of estrogen metabolites are largely unknown. Estrogen metabolites could provide growth signal for cancer cells, and yet they may become toxic to normal cells (Obi et al., 2011; Sepkovic & Bradlow, 2009; Chen at al., 2008). The metabolites may invoke inflammatory lung diseases such as asthma, cystic fibrosis, and chronic obstructive pulmonary disease in women (Tam et al., 2011). Estrogen metabolite 16α-hydroxyestrone exerts estrogenic activity through covalent ER binding, whereas 2-hydroxyestrone would have anti-estrogenic capabilities (Obi et al., 2011). The ratios of these metabolites appear to be critical in controlling breast cancer cell growth. 2-Hydroxyestradiol and 4-hydroxyestradiol are implicated in tumorigenesis via increasing cell proliferation and the formation of reactive oxygen species for possibly generating deoxyribonucleic acid mutations (Joubert et al., 2009). The E2 metabolite 2-methoxyestradiol exerts apoptosis in many cancer cell types (Verenich & Gerk, 2010).

2.3 Short chain alcohol dehydrogenase/reductase (SDR)

Long-term exposure to estrogen and metabolites influences the development of breast cancer in women. The underlying mechanisms appear to be mainly involved in 1) estradiol/ERα signaling for stimulation of cell proliferation, and 2) formation of genotoxic metabolites of estradiol for binding to DNA and causing depurination and mutations (Santen et al., 2009). We suspect that naturally occurring dehydrogenases/reductases (including 17β-HSDs), which possess binding sites for sex steroid hormones, may act as receptors and play an alternative role in breast cancer progression. For example, short-chain dehydrogenases/reductases (SDRs) are composed of a large family of NAD(P)(H)-dependent oxidoreductases, sharing sequence motifs with similar functions (Kavanagh et al., 2008; Jörnvall et al., 2010). SDR enzymes play critical roles in metabolism for lipid, amino acid, carbohydrate, cofactor, and hormones, as well as in redox sensor mechanisms (Kavanagh et al., 2008). The SDR enzymes are normally 250–300 amino acid residues in length, which possesses a catalytic tetrad of Asn-Ser-Tyr-Lys (N-S-Y-K), and provides a platform for enzymatic activities encompassing several EC classes, including oxidoreductases, epimerases and lyases (Kavanagh et al., 2008).

3. WW domain-containing Oxidoreductase

3.1 Tumor suppressor WWOX/FOR/WOX1 – a protein possessing WW and SDR domains

WW domain-containing oxidoreductase, designated WWOX, FOR, or WOX1, is a protein possessing both WW domains and an SDR domain. The human and mouse *WWOX/Wwox* gene was first isolated independently by 3 laboratories in year 2000 (Smith et al., 2007; Del Mare et al., 2009; Chang et al., 2007, 2010; reviews). Human *WWOX* gene possesses approximately 1 million bases with 9 exons and codes for a 46-kDa protein containing 414 amino acids. Due to frequent genetic alterations, *WWOX* gene is generally considered as a tumor suppressor. The reason for the genetic alterations is probably associated with its localization on a common fragile site *FRA16D* on chromosome ch16q23.3-24.1. The *WWOX* gene encodes the WWOX/WOX1 protein. Substantial evidence reveals that this protein possesses a tumor suppressor function (Chang et al., 2007; Smith et al., 2007; Del

Mare et al., 2009; Chang et al., 2010; Chang et al., 2001). It is documented that there is a relative high percentage of loss of heterozygosity (LOH) from 30 to 50% in human *WWOX* gene in many types of cancer cells (Chang et al., 2007; Smith et al., 2007; Del Mare et al., 2009; Chang et al., 2010).

The WWOX/WOX1 protein is composed of a nuclear localization sequence (NLS), two *N*-terminal WW domains (containing conserved tryptophan residues), a *C*-terminal short-chain alcohol dehydrogenase/reductase (SDR) domain, and probably a functional *C*-terminal tail named D3 (Hong et al., 2007; Hsu et al., 2008; Lin et al., 2011) (Figure 1). The putative tertiary structures of the first WW domain and the C-terminal SDR domain are shown. The solution structure of the second WW domain has been documented (Wang et al., 2007).

The *N*-terminal conserved first WW domain, which has been categorized as a group I WW domain, binds many proteins containing a PPXY motif(s), where P is proline, Y is tyrosine and X is any amino acid (Chang et al., 2007; Smith et al., 2007; Del Mare et al., 2009; Chang et al., 2010). Among these WWOX/WOX1-binding protein targets are p73, activator protein 2γ (AP-2, ErbB4, Ezrin, small integral membrane protein of the lysosome/late endosome (SIMPLE), c-Jun, and runt-related transcription factor 2 (RUNX2) (Chang et al., 2007; Del Mare et al., 2009; Chang et al., 2010). While most of the observations were from ectopic expression to enhance the binding, physiological consequences of the binding interactions are largely unknown.

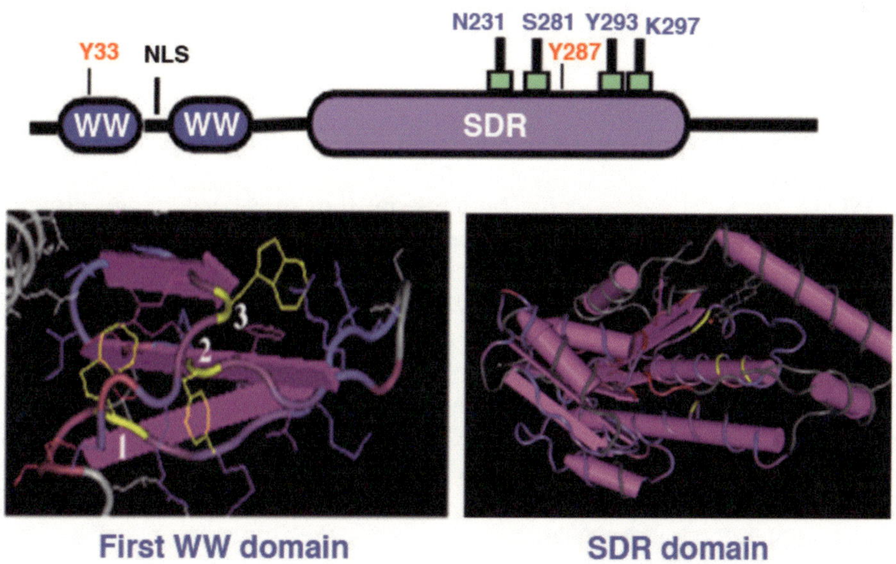

Fig. 1. WWOX and simulated tertiary structures. The predicted amino acid sequence of WW domain-containing oxidoreductase, designated WWOX, FOR, or WOX1, possesses two *N*-terminal WW domains, a nuclear localization signal sequence (NLS), and a *C*-terminal short-chain alcohol dehydrogenase/reductase (SDR) domain, where Tyr33 and Tyr287 are the hosphorylation sites, and NSYK is the binding motif for sex steroid hormones. Simulated structures of the first WW domain and the SDR domain are shown (1= 1st tryptophan; 2= Try33 phosphorylation site; 3= 2nd tryptophan; see yellow). Also, NSYK residues are marked in yellow.

When WWOX/WOX1 becomes activated by stress stimuli such as UV light and tumor necrosis factor, Tyr33 is phosphorylated in the first WW domain (Chang, 2002; Chang et al., 2003a, 2003b, 2005a, 2007; Lai et al., 2005; Lo et al., 2008). Tyrosine kinase Src is known to phosphorylate Tyr33 in WWOX/WOX1 (Aqeilan et al., 2004a). The activated WWOX/WOX1 interacts with a large spectrum of proteins without possessing a PPXY motif(s), including proteins in the stress signaling and apoptotic response, as well as transcription factors (Chang et al., 2007, 2010; Del Mare et al., 2009). These proteins are p53 (Lo et al., 2008; Chang et al., 2001, 2003a, 2005a, 2005b; Lai et al., 2005), JNK1 (Lo et al., 2008; Chang et al., 2003a), MDM2 (Chang et al., 2005a), Zfra (Hong et al., 2007; Hsu et al., 2008), and Hyal-2 (Hsu et al., 2009).

The *C*-terminal SDR domain in WOX1/WWOX has been shown to bind Tau, a microtubule-binding protein involved in neurodegeneration (Sze et al., 2004). Functional consequence of this binding is also unknown. It is postulated that WOX1/WWOX binds Tau to prevent hyperphosphorylation by enzymes such as ERK, Cdk5, GSK-3β and JNK, thereby preventing tau aggregation as found in the hippocampi of patients with Alzheimer's disease (Sze et al., 2004). WOX1/WWOX physically interacts with MEK1 in T leukemia cells, and PMA (phorbol myristate acetate) modulates the binding interactions (Lin et al., 2011). PMA-induced dissociation of the WOX1/MEK1 interactions leads to apoptosis of Jurkat T cells, suggesting there is a critical switch in cell death for T cell leukemia upon the dissociation of WOX1/MEK1 (Lin et al., 2011). MEK1 has been shown to bind to both the WW and SDR domain of WOX1 with differential affinities. How this differential binding strength affects cell growth and death and correlates with biological activities is unknown and remains to be established.

3.2 WWOX/WOX1 activation and its role in multiple signaling networks *in vitro* and *in vivo*

WWOX/WOX1 interacts with many proteins in the stress signaling, growth, gene transcription, and apoptosis regulations, suggesting it is involved in multiple signal networks. For example, WWOX/WOX1 controls the activation of transcription factors, including p53 (Lo et al., 2008; Chang et al., 2001, 2003a, 2003b, 2005a, 2005b; Lai et al., 2005), p73 (Aqeilan et al., 2004a), AP2γ (Aqeilan et al., 2004b), c-Jun (Gaudio et al., 2006; Li et al., 2009), and CREB (Li et al., 2009). By immunoelectron microscopy, FRET (Förster resonance energy transfer) and co-immunoprecipitation, we have revealed the complex formation of the Tyr33-phosphorylated or activated WOX1 with p-CREB and p-c-Jun *in vivo* (Li et al., 2009). Interestingly, WOX1 blocks the prosurvival CREB-, CRE-, and AP-1-mediated promoter activation *in vitro*. In contrast, WOX1 enhances promoter activation regulated by c-Jun, Elk-1 and NF-κB (Li et al., 2009).

Tyr33-phosphorylated WOX1 is central to the stability and function of tumor suppressor p53. The activated WOX1 binds and stabilizes p53 with Ser46 phosphorylation, which is necessary for the apoptotic function of p53 (Chang et al., 2005a).

Numerous factors are known to induce Tyr33 phosphorylation in WWOX/WOX1, including sex steroid hormones (Chang et al., 2005b), transforming growth factor beta (Hsu et al., 2009), complement C1q (Hong et al., 2009), UV light, and anisomycin (Chang et al., 2001, 2003a, 2005a). Stress stimuli induce relocation of WWOX/WOX1 to the mitochondria and nuclei both *in vitro* and *in vivo*. When neurons are subjected to injury by axotomy, neurotoxin and long-term exposure to constant light in rats, WOX1 becomes activated via

Tyr33 phosphorylation and accumulation in the mitochondria and nuclei (Chen et al., 2005; Lo et al., 2008; Li et al., 2009). Tyr287 in WWOX/WOX1 can undergo phosphorylation by activated tyrosine kinase 1 (Ack1) for polyubiquitination and protein degradation in prostate cancer cells (Mahajan et al., 2005).

3.3 Alteration of human *WWOX* gene in cancer

Cumulative reports have shown deletion or epigenetic alteration of human *WWOX* gene induces loss of protein expression in malignant cancer (Del Mare et al., 2009; Chang et al., 2007, 2010). For example, as demonstrated in most recent reports, both tumor suppressor genes *FHIT* and *WWOX* are deleted in primary effusion lymphoma (PEL) cell lines (Roy et al., 2011). Loss of WWOX occurs during the progression and development of gastric cancer (Maeda et al., 2010). *Helicobacter pylori / H. pylori* infection induces methylation of *WWOX* gene in human gastric cancer, suggestive of the role of epigenetic modification by H. pylori in causing cancer (Yan et al., 2011). Interestingly, polymorphism Pro-282-Ala in *WWOX* gene may have a risk factor for differentiated thyroid carcinoma (Cancemi et al., 2011). Also, hypermethylation of *WWOX* gene promoter region and mutations in the gene, encoding the SDR domain, appears to contribute to lung carcinogenesis (Baykara et al., 2010). Overall, it is not surprising to observe complete loss of *WWOX* gene and protein in invasive or metastatic cancer cells.

In most cases, cancer specimens from patients cannot represent the very early stages of cancer development. In this regard, our knowledge concerning how and when *WWOX* gene is altered is still lacking. We have examined the time-related *Wwox* gene alteration in hairless mice during the initiation and progression of cutaneous squamous cell carcinoma (SCC) (Lai et al., 2005). During the acute phase of UVB exposure in hairless mice, WOX1 protein was significantly upregulated and became activated in epidermal cells in 24 hours. After the inflammatory phase, the mice developed cutaneous SCC in 3 months, with significant reduction of WOX1 protein and its Tyr33 phosphorylation, but without down-regulation of *Wwox* mRNA. In normal human and mouse skin, keratinocyte differentiation involves upregulation of human WWOX/WOX1, isoform WOX2, and Tyr33 phosphorylation prior to cornification and death (Lai et al., 2005). However, there are significant reductions in WOX1 and WOX2 proteins and their Tyr33 phosphorylation in non-metastatic and metastatic cutaneous SCC, but without down-regulation of *WWOX* mRNA. These observations suggest an additional mechanism for the inactivation of *WWOX* mRNA and a translational blockade of *WWOX* mRNA to protein.

By immunohistochemistry, it was reported that WWOX protein levels are not decreased but rather elevated in gastric and breast carcinoma (Watanabe et al., 2003), challenging the notion of WWOX as a classical tumor suppressor. Nonetheless, the stages of cancer cells are unknown. We have examined the hyperplasia stage of prostate cancer development and shown the increased expression levels of WWOX/WOX1 protein and isoforms (Chang et al., 2005b)

3.4 WWOX/WOX1 localization and signaling

Normal cells of the epithelial origin express WWOX/WOX1. These cells include skin keratinocytes and sebaceous gland cells, lung epithelial cells, epithelial cells of the digestive system, Leydig cells, follicular cells, prostate epithelial cells, and mammary gland cells.

Many of these cells are responsive to stimulation by sex steroid hormones. During terminal differentiation of kerationcytes, WWOX/WOX1 expression is increased steadily prior to cornification. Whether this also reflects an increased oxidoreductase activity of WWOX/WOX1 in the keratinocytes is unknown. WWOX/WOX1 is accumulated in the nuclei during the terminal differentiation of keratinocytes (Lai et al., 2005). Substantial evidence shows that accumulation of WWOX/WOX1 in the nuclei may induce death of cancer cells in culture (Chang et al., 2007, 2010). Also, during axotomy, WWOX/WOX1, along with CREB, NF-κB and many transcription factors, relocates to the nuclei, and this appears to contribute to the eventual death of neurons (Li et al., 2009). Similar observations for the accumulation of WWOX/WOX1 in the nuclei have been shown in animal models using neurotoxin MPP+ and long-term constant light exposure to cause neuronal death (Lo et al., 2008; Chen at al., 2005).

3.4.1 WWOX/Ezrin interactions

WWOX/WOX1 is known to be associated in part with the cell membrane/cytoskeleton area, and thereby serves as a sensor of environmental cues (Chang et al., 2010). WWOX/WOX1 receives and integrates signals from cell surface by undergoing Tyr33-phosphorylation and relocation to the nuclei *in vitro* and *in vivo* (Chang et al., 2010; review). Nuclear WWOX may either enhance or inhibit the promoter activities regulated by SMAD, NF-κB, c-JUN, CREB and other transcription factors (Gaudio et al., 2006; Li et al., 2009; Chang et al., 2010). By immunoelectron microscopy, WWOX/WOX1 can exist alone at the membrane/cytosleleton (Hsu et al., 2009), or it can be in binding with Ezrin (Jin el al., 2006), Hyal-2 (Hsu et al., 2009), or other cytoskeletal proteins (Cheng et al., unpublished). PKA-mediated phosphorylation of ezrin is central to the apical localization of WWOX protein in parietal cells, and that disruption of ezrin-WWOX interaction reduces the apical localization of WWOX (Jin et al., 2006). Ezrin directly binds to the first WW domain of WWOX via its C-terminal tyrosine-containing polyproline sequence (470)PPPPPPVY(477) (Jin et al., 2006).

3.4.2 TGF-β/Hyal-2/WWOX/Smad4 signal pathway

We have recently demonstrated that transforming growth factor beta (TGF-β) induces relocation of WWOX/WOX1 to the nuclei in response to TGF-β1 in many types of cells, except in certain breast cancer cells (Hsu et al., 2009). Under physiological conditions, TGF-β1 binds membrane TβRII as a cognate receptor for recruiting TβRI, followed by phosphorylating Smad2 and 3, recruiting Smad4, and the Smad2/3/4 complex binding to responsive elements in the nucleus. In TβRII-deficient HCT116 cells, we showed that membrane hyaluronidase Hyal-2 acts as a cognate receptor for TGF-β1 (Hsu et al., 2009). TGF-β1 binds to a surface-exposed segment in the catalytic domain of Hyal-2 in the microvilli, followed by rapidly recruiting WWOX. The WWOX/Hyal-2 complex appears to recruit Smad4 for enhancing SMAD-responsive promoter activation. Hyaluronan is also a ligand for Hyal-2, suggesting that both hyaluronan and TGF-β1 may compete for the binding with membrane Hyal-2. Thus, we propose an alternative scenario that hyaluronan enhances the binding of TGF-β1 with Hyal-2 without transmitting the signal. Presumably, TGF-β1 is trapped on the cell surface by hyaluronan and Hyal-2. Upon hyaluronan degradation, the signal event may start. Two reports showed that hyaluronan blocks TGF-β signaling by inducing trafficking of TGF-β receptors to lipid raft-associated pools, which facilitates increased receptor turnover (Ito et al., 2004; Webber et al., 2009).

3.4.3 Complement protein C1q as an activator of WWOX/WOX1

Purified serum C1q is able to rapidly induce the activation of WWOX/WOX1 (Hong et al., 2009). Complement C1q induces apoptosis of cancer cells overexpressing WWOX/WOX1, and the induced cell death is independent of the complement classical activation pathway. When WWOX/WOX1 is deficient in cells, C1q fails to cause apoptosis, indicating the presence of a novel pathway of programmed cell death. As determined by time-lapse surface plasmon-enhanced two-photon total internal reflection fluorescence (TIRF) microscopy (He et al., 2009, 2010), C1q induces the formation of clusters of microvilli and destabilizes the adherence in WOX1-overexpressing prostate DU145 cancer cells, without causing exposure of phosphatidylserine (PS) on the outer leaflet of the plasma membrane (Hong et al., 2009). Ultimately, these cells undergo shrinkage, membrane blebbing, and death (Hong et al., 2009). The observations suggest a critical role of WWOX/WOX1 in cell adherence and microvillus formation. Indeed, benign prostatic hyperplasia and prostate cancer have a significantly reduced expression of tissue C1q, compared to age-matched normal prostate tissues (Hong et al., 2009), suggesting that they can grow favorably as long as WWOX/WOX1 is also downregulated.

3.5 A role of WWOX/WOX1 in metabolism

3.5.1 WWOX/WOX1 is associated with plasma HDL levels

Low serum HDL-cholesterol (HDL-C) is known to be one of the risk factors for coronary artery disease. Three recent studies demonstrated that *WWOX* gene is associated with the alterations of plasma HDL levels (Lee et al., 2008; Sáez et al., 2010; Leduc et al., 2011). By genotyping of single nucleotide polymorphisms (SNPs), Lee et al. identified one SNP, rs2548861, in the intron 8 of *WWOX* gene with region-wide significance for low HDL-C in dyslipidemic families of Mexican and European descent and in low-HDL-C cases and controls of European descent. They concluded that there is a significant association between HDL-C and a *WWOX* variant with an allele-specific cis-regulatory function. Similar approaches, coupled with mouse genome mapping, were also used to indicate the association of *WWOX* gene with HDL cholesterol and triglyceride levels (Sáez et al., 2010; Leduc et al., 2011).

3.5.2 WWOX/WOX1 plays a role in aerobic metabolism

Genetic knockout models have revealed the functional properties of WWOX. In a *Drosophila* model, Wwox is shown to play a key role in aerobic metabolism probably via functional interactions with CG6439/isocitrate dehydrogenase (*Idh*) and Cu-Zn superoxide dismutase (*Sod*) (O'Keefe et al., 2011). Varied Wwox expression also causes altered levels of endogenous reactive oxygen species. A direct interaction between Wwox and the functional interactors has not been demonstrated.

3.5.3 *Wwox* gene knockout mice models

Targeted ablation of mouse *Wwox* gene at exons 2-4 appears to increase the incidence of spontaneous formation of tumors in heterozygous mice (Aqeilan et al., 2007). Importantly, the effect of *Wwox* gene knockout has a significant effect on bone metabolism defects (Aqeilan et al., 2008). The whole body *Wwox* gene-ablated mice can only survive for approximately one month. The molecular mechanism of this regard is not known. In addition, the knockout mice are also defective in the reproductive system (Ludes-Meyers et al., 2009). Inactivation of *Wwox* gene induces mammary tumorigenesis, and the tumors tend to have loss of estrogen receptor-α (ER) and progesterone receptor (Abdeen et al., 2011).

4. WWOX/WOX1 is a candidate hormone receptor

How breast cancer cells develop estrogen-independent growth is not known. Hormone-independent breast cancer cells are normally ER-negative and highly invasive. Prognosis for patients is poor. WWOX/WOX1 possesses an NSYK motif for hormone binding. Depending upon cell lines, estrogen or androgen may induce WWOX/WOX1 phosphorylation at Tyr33 (Chang et al., 2005b). Activated WWOX/WOX1 relocates to the nucleus to induce apoptosis in certain cells. Conceivably, loss of WWOX/WOX1 in invasive breast cancer allows them to grow independently of hormones. TFAP2C plays a critical role in gene regulation in hormone responsive breast cancer. *WWOX* gene is one of the transcriptional targets of TFAP2C (Woodfield et al., 2010), suggesting a role of WWOX in the hormonal response.

4.1 17β-estradiol (E2) induces WWOX/WOX1 activation

The NSYK motif for binding with estrogen and androgen in WWOX/WOX1 is predicted to be N232, S281, Y293, and K297 (Chang et al., 2003b; review). We have investigated whether androgen and estrogen activate WWOX/WOX1 (Chang et al., 2005b). In COS7 fibroblasts, E2 induces Tyr33 phosphorylation in WWOX/WOX1, and both E2 and WWOX/WOX1 co-translocate to the nuclei (Chang et al., 2005b) (Figure 2). E2 at μM levels induces apoptosis of COS7 cells. It appears that when a sufficient amount of WWOX/WOX1 is accumulated in the nucleus, apoptosis occurs. However, it is not clear whether E2 binds to the NSYK motif. Indeed, E2 stimulates the formation of p53 and WOX1 complex, which is found in the nucleus (Chang et al., 2005b) (Figure 3). In contrast, JNK1 blocks the relocation of p53/WOX1 to the nucleus (Chang et al., 2005b). JNK1 binds and blocks WOX1 and p53 activation *in vivo* (Chang et al., 2003), and that dominant-negative JNK1 spontaneously induces WOX1 nuclear translocation. Whether there is a direct binding interaction between E2 and p53 or JNK1 is unknown.

E2 could not induce accumulation of WWOX/WOX1 in the nuclei of ER-positive breast MCF-7. ER-negative breast MDA-MB-231 and MDA-MB-435S are metastatic and have very low levels of WWOX/WOX1. Reconstitution of WWOX/WOX1 in these cells is expected to restore their sensitivity to estrogen. Interestingly, E2 and androsterone induce WWOX/WOX1 activation in androgen receptor (AR)-negative prostate DU145 cells, indicating that ER and AR are probably not involved in the E2-induced WWOX/WOX1 activation. Taken together, WWOX/WOX1 is a potential receptor for sex steroid hormones (Figure 4). Whether this protein metabolizes estrogen or androgen remains to be determined. Also, whether WWOX/WOX1 possesses an enzymatic activity in oxidation/reduction is still elusive.

4.2 Estrogen-induced apoptosis

Majority of ER-positive breast cancer cells depend upon estrogen for growth. It appears that these cells may become sensitive to estrogen-mediated apoptosis upon long-term deprivation of estrogen, followed by re-introducing estrogen. Whether WWOX/WOX1 is involved in the conferred sensitivity is not known. A recent study showed that AIB1

(Amplified in Breast Cancer-1) is responsible for E2-mediated apoptosis in breast MCF-7: cells (Hu et al., 2011). Computational analysis revealed that AIB1 integrates signals from G-protein-coupled receptors, PI3 kinase, Wnt and Notch signal pathways, which affect cell growth and death. Interestingly, it has been hypothesized that ER conformation affects E2-induced cell death (Maximov et al., 2011).

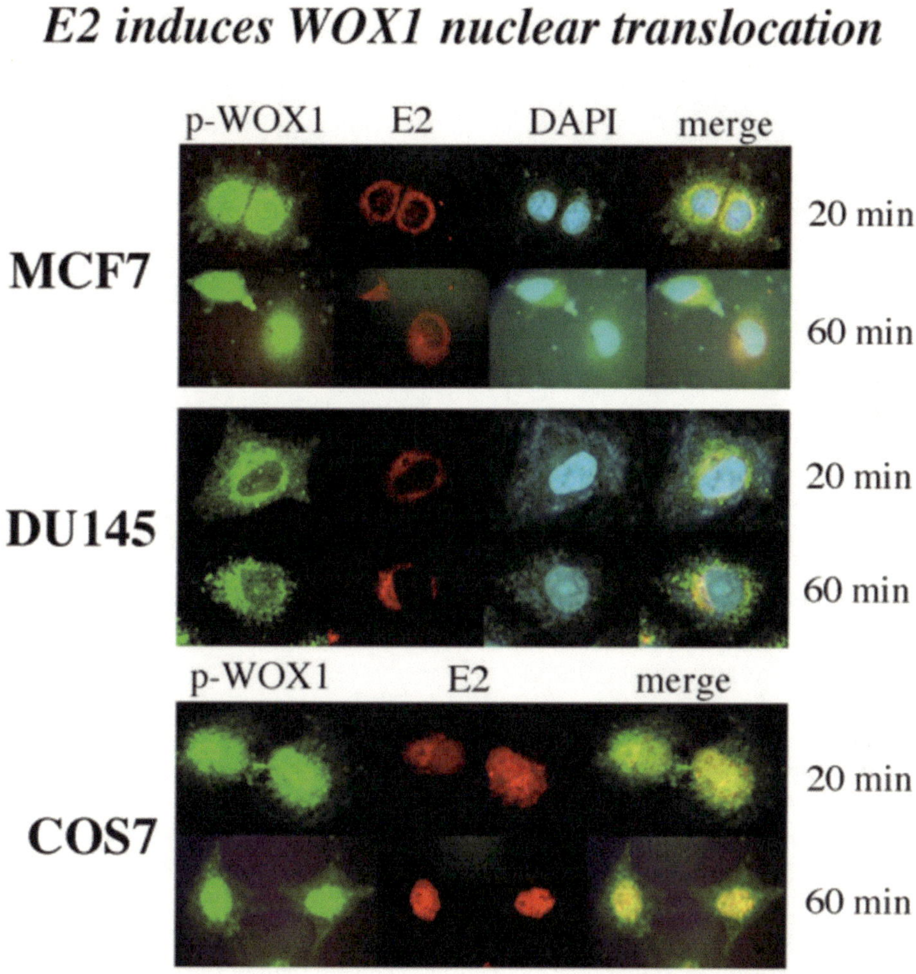

Fig. 2. 17β-estradiol (E_2) stimulates phosphorylation of WWOX/WOX1 at Tyr33, and co-tranalocation of WOX1 with E2 to the nucleus in COS7 fibroblasts. Stimulation of COS7 fibroblasts with E2 (40 nM) for 1 hr resulted in activation of WOX1 via Tyr33 phosphorylation (p-WOX1) and nuclear translocation, along with E2. Both p-WOX1 and E2 were stained with specific antibodies. WOX1 undergoes activation in ER-positive MCF-7 cells, whereas E2 is retained in the cytoplasm. Both WOX1 and E2 are retained in the cytoplasm without undergoing nuclear translocation in AR-negative DU145 cells.

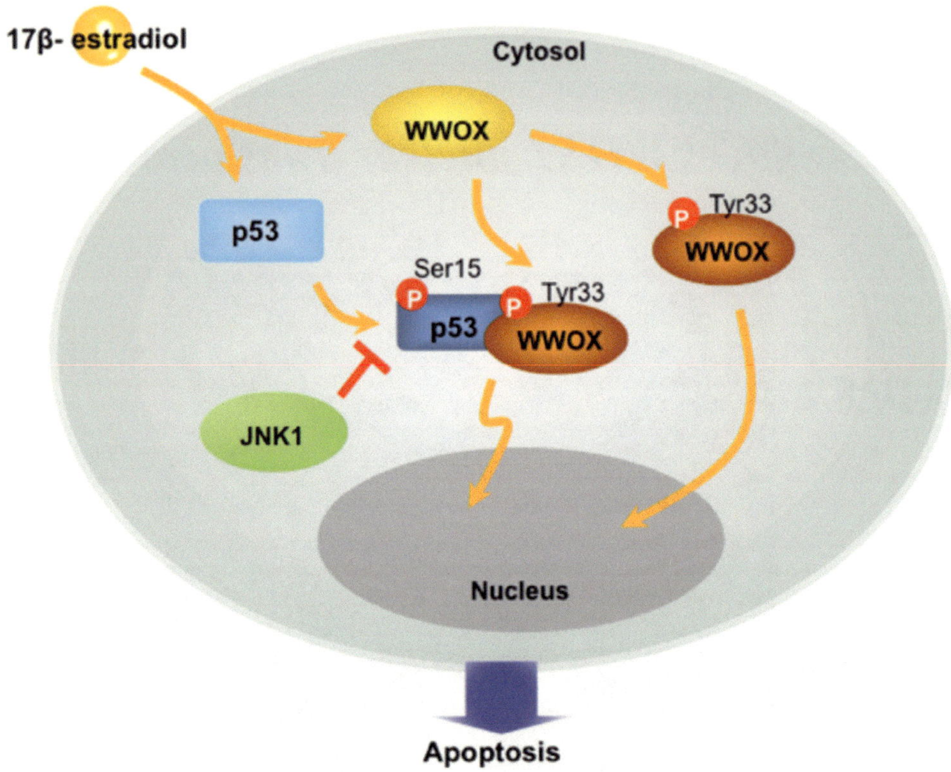

Fig. 3. E2 induces co-translocation of p53 and WWOX/WOX1 to the nuclei of COS7. *In vitro* experiments support the likely scenario that E2 induces the complex formation of Tyr33-phosphorylated WOX1 and Ser15-phosphorylated p53, and the complex relocates to the nuclei (Chang et al., 2005b). JNK1 is also associated with the p53/WOX1 in the cytosol, but fails to undergo nuclear relocation. JNK1 blocks the nuclear accumulation of p53/WOX1.

4.3 Hormone-independence in breast cancer and perspectives

Development of hormone-independence in breast cancer patients involves a complicated event that underlies a network structure rather than individual molecular components. It is critical to probe the "disease systems" from a gene regulatory network to a cell, a tissue, or even an entire organism. Areas of this regard in terms of development independence in breast cancer are largely unknown. Invasive breast cancer cells exhibit a high frequency of loss of heterozygosity of *WWOX* gene. Wild type WWOX/WOX1 is responsive to estrogen-induced activation, via Tyr33 phosphorylation and nuclear translocation, for controlling cell growth. Thus, loss of *WWOX* gene in invasive breast cancer cells is likely to result in hormone resistance.

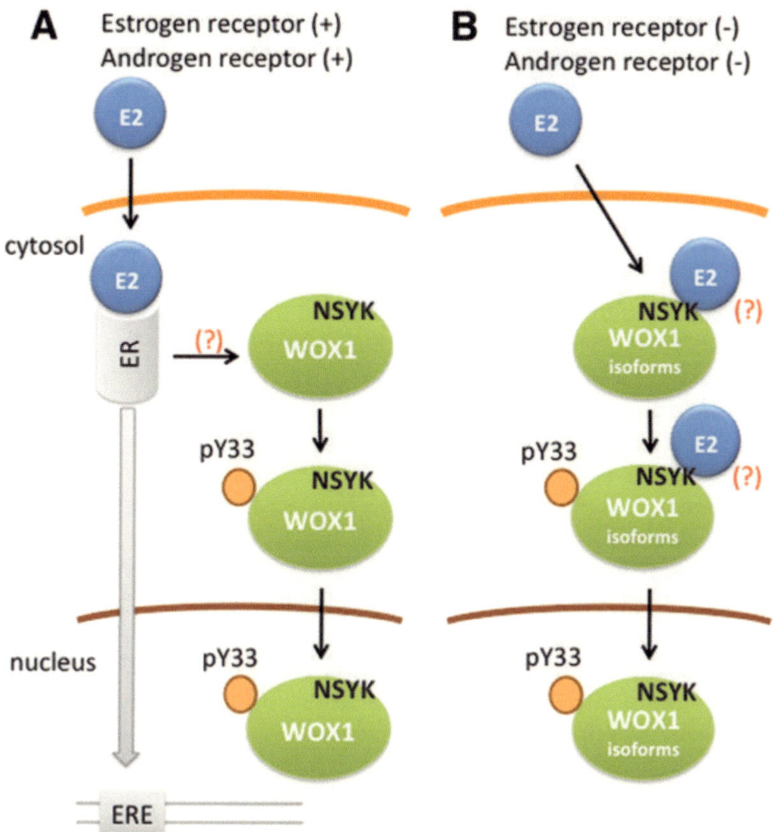

Fig. 4. Schematic illustration of E2/WWOX signaling. (**A**) In ER-positive cells, E2 binds ER and other proteins, and the complex translocates the nucleus to control gene transcription by binding to estrogen responsive elements (EREs) in chromosomal DNA. Alternatively, E2 may co-translocate with WOX1 to the nuclei. (**B**) In ER-negative, metastatic breast cancer cells, the wild type WWOX or WOX1 is deficient, whereas isoforms WOX2 and WOX8 may be present. These proteins provide the NSYK motif for binding with estrogen or androgen for relocating to the nucleus.

5. Acknowledgement

Research was supported, in part, by the Department of Defense, USA (W81XWH-08-1-0682), the National Science Council, Taiwan, ROC (NSC96-2320-B-006-014, 98-2628-B-006-041-MY3, and 98-2628-B-006-045-MY3), the National Health Research Institute, Taiwan, ROC (NHRI-EX99-9705BI), and the National Cheng Kung University Landmark Projects (C0167 & R026) (to NS Chang).

6. References

Abdeen S.K.; Salah Z.; Maly B.; Smith Y.; Tufail R.; Abu-Odeh M.; Zanesi N.; Croce C.M.; Nawaz Z. & Aqeilan R.I. (2011). Wwox inactivation enhances mammary tumorigenesis. *Oncogene*, (Apr 2011), ISSN

Aka J.A.; Mazumdar M. & Lin S.X. (2009). Reductive 17beta-hydroxysteroid dehydrogenases in the sulfatase pathway: critical in the cell proliferation of breast cancer. *Mol. Cell Endocrinol.*, Vol.301, No.1-2, (Mar 2009) pp. 183-190, Review, ISSN

Albin N.L.; Massaad C.; Toussaint M.C.; Mathieu J.; Morizet O.; Parise A.; Gouyette A. & Chabot G.G. (1993). Main Drug-metabolizing Enzyme Systems in Human Breast Tumors and Peritumoral Tissues. *Cancer Res,* Vol.53, No.15, (Aug 1993) pp. 3541-3546, ISSN

Aqeilan R.I.; Hassan M.Q.; de Bruin A.; Hagan J.P.; Volinia S.; Palumbo T.; Hussain S.; Lee S.H.; Gaur T.; Stein G.S.; Lian J.B. & Croce C.M (2008). The WWOX tumor suppressor is essential for postnatal survival and normal bone metabolism. *J. Biol. Chem.* Vol.283, No.31, (Aug 2008) pp. 21629-21639, ISSN

Aqeilan R.I.; Palamarchuk A.; Weigel R.J.; Herrero J.J.; Pekarsky Y. & Croce C.M. (2004b) Physical and functional interactions between the Wwox tumor suppressor protein and the AP-2gamma transcription factor. *Cancer Res*, Vol.64, No.22, (Nov 2004) pp. 8256-61, ISSN

Aqeilan R.I.; Pekarsky Y.; Herrero J.J.; Palamarchuk A.; Letofsky J.; Druck T.; Trapasso F.; Han S.Y.; Melino G.; Huebner K. & Croce C.M. (2004a). Functional association between Wwox tumor suppressor protein and p73, a p53 homolog. *Proc. Natl. Acad. Sci. USA*, Vol.101, No.13, (Mar 2004) pp. 4401-4406, ISSN

Aqeilan R.I.; Trapasso F.; Hussain S.; Costinean S.; Marshall D.; Pekarsky Y.; Hagan J.P.; Zanesi N.; Kaou M.; Stein G.S.; Lian J.B. & Croce C.M. (2007). Targeted deletion of Wwox reveals a tumor suppressor function. *Proc. Natl. Acad. Sci. USA,* Vol.104, No.10, (Mar 2007) pp. 3949-3954, ISSN

Ball P. & Knuppen R. (1980). Catecholoestrogens (2- and 4-hydroxyoestrogens): chemistry, biogenesis, metabolism, occurrence and physiological significance. *Acta Endocrinol.*, Vol.232, (1980) pp. 1–127, ISSN

Baykara O., Demirkaya A., Kaynak K., Tanju S., Toker A., Buyru N. (2010) WWOX gene may contribute to progression of non-small-cell lung cancer (NSCLC). Tumour Biol Vol.31, No.4,(Aug 2010) pp.315-20, ISSN

Baykara O., Demirkaya A., Kaynak K., Tanju S., Toker A., Buyru N. (2010) WWOX gene may contribute to progression of non-small-cell lung cancer (NSCLC). Tumour Biol Vol.31, No.4,(Aug 2010) pp.315-20, ISSN

Blanchard P.G. & Luu-The V. (2007). Differential androgen and estrogen substrates specificity in the mouse and primates type 12 17ß-hydroxysteroid dehydrogenase. *J. Endocrinol.*, Vol.194, No.2, (Aug 2007) pp. 449-455, ISSN

Cancemi L., Romei C., Bertocchi S., Tarrini G., Spitaleri I., Cipollini M., Landi D., Garritano S., Pellegrini G., Cristaudo A., Pinchera A., Barale R., Elisei R., Landi S., Gemignani F. (2011) Evidences that the polymorphism Pro-282-Ala within the tumor suppressor gene WWOX is a new risk factor for differentiated thyroid carcinoma. Int J Cancer Vol.129, No.12,(Dec 2011) pp.2816-24, ISSN

Cancemi L., Romei C., Bertocchi S., Tarrini G., Spitaleri I., Cipollini M., Landi D., Garritano S., Pellegrini G., Cristaudo A., Pinchera A., Barale R., Elisei R., Landi S., Gemignani F. (2011) Evidences that the polymorphism Pro-282-Ala within the tumor suppressor gene WWOX is a new risk factor for differentiated thyroid carcinoma. Int J Cancer Vol.129, No.12,(Dec 2011) pp.2816-24, ISSN

Chang J.Y.; He R.Y.; Lin H.P.; Hsu L.J.; Lai F.J.; Hong Q.; Chen S.J. & Chang N.S. (2010). Signaling from membrane receptors to tumor suppressor WW domain-containing oxidoreductase. *Exp. Biol. Med.* (Maywood), Vol.235, No.7, (Jul 2010) pp. 796-804, ISSN

Chang N.S. (2002). A potential role of p53 and WOX1 in mitochondrial apoptosis (review). *Int. J. Mol. Med.*, Vol.9, No.1, (Jan 2002) pp. 19-24, ISSN

Chang N.S.; Doherty J. & Ensign A. (2003a). JNK1 physically interacts with WW domain-containing oxidoreductase (WOX1) and inhibits WOX1-mediated apoptosis. *J. Biol. Chem. Vol.* 278, No.11, (Mar 2003) pp. 9195-9202, ISSN

Chang N.S.; Doherty J.; Ensign A.; Lewis J.; Heath J.; Schultz L.; Chen S.T. & Oppermann U. (2003b). Molecular mechanisms underlying WOX1 activation during apoptotic and stress responses. *Biochem. Pharmacol.*, Vol.66, No.8, (Oct 2003) pp. 1347-1354, ISSN

Chang N.S.; Doherty J.; Ensign A.; Schultz L.; Hsu L.J. & Hong Q. (2005a). WOX1 is essential for tumor necrosis factor-, UV light-, staurosporine-, and p53-mediated cell death, and its tyrosine 33-phosphorylated form binds and stabilizes serine 46-phosphorylated p53. *J. Biol. Chem.*, Vol.280, No.52, (Dec 2005) pp. 43100-43108, ISSN

Chang N.S.; Hsu L.J.; Lin Y.S.; Lai F.J. & Sheu H.M. (2007). WW domain-containing oxidoreductase: a candidate tumor suppressor. *Trends Mol. Med.*, Vol.13, No.1, (Jan 2007) pp. 12-22, ISSN

Chang N.S.; Pratt N.; Heath J.; Schultz L.; Sleve D.; Carey G.B. & Zevotek N. (2001). Hyaluronidase induction of a WW domain-containing oxidoreductase that enhances tumor necrosis factor cytotoxicity. *J. Biol. Chem.*, Vol.276, No.5, (Feb 2001) pp. 3361-3370, ISSN

Chang N.S.; Schultz L.; Hsu L.J.; Lewis J.; Su M. & Sze C.I. (2005b). 17beta-Estradiol upregulates and activates WOX1/WWOXv1 and WOX2/WWOXv2 in vitro: potential role in cancerous progression of breast and prostate to a premetastatic state in vivo. *Oncogene, Vol.*24, No.4, (Jan 2005) pp. 714-723, ISSN

Chen J.Q.; Brown T.R. & Yager J.D. (2008). Mechanisms of hormone carcinogenesis: evolution of views, role of mitochondria. *Adv. Exp. Med. Biol.*, (2008) 630:1-18, Review, ISSN

Chen S.T.; Chuang J.I.; Cheng C.L.; Hsu L.J. & Chang N.S. (2005). Light-induced retinal damage involves tyrosine 33 phosphorylation, mitochondrial and nuclear translocation of WW domain-containing oxidoreductase in vivo. *Neuroscience*, Vol.130, No.2, (2005) pp. 397-407, ISSN

Cheng Z.; Rios G.R.; King C.D.; Coffman B.L.; Green M.D.; Mojarrabi B.; Mackenzie P.I. & Tephly T.R. (1998). Glucuronidation of catechol estrogens by expressed human UDP-glucuronosyltransferases (UGTs) 1A1, 1A3, and 2B7. *Toxicol Sci.*, Vol.45, No1, (Sep 1998) pp. 52-57, ISSN

Del Mare S.; *Salah* Z. & Aqeilan R.I. (2009). WWOX: its genomics, partners, and functions. *J. Cell Biochem.*, Vol.108, No.4, (Nov 2009) pp. 737-745, ISSN

Desnoyers S.; Blanchard P.G.; St-Laurent J.F.; Gagnon S.N.; Baillie D.L. & Luu-The V. (2007). Caenorhabditis elegans LET-767 is able to metabolize androgens and estrogens and likely shares common ancestor with human types 3 and 12 17beta-hydroxysteroid dehydrogenases. *J. Endocrinol.*, Vol.195, No.2, (Nov 2007) pp.271-279, ISSN

Falany J.L. & Falany C.N. (1996). Expression of Cytosolic Sulfotransferases in Normal Mammary Epithelial Cells and Breast Cancer Cell Lines1. *Cancer Res*, Vol.56, No.7, (Apr 1996) pp. 1551-1555, ISSN

Filardo E.J.; Quinn J.A.; Frackelton A.R. Jr. & Bland K.I. (2002). Estrogen action via the G protein-coupled receptor, GPR30: stimulation of adenylyl cyclase and cAMP-mediated attenuation of the epidermal growth factor receptor-to-MAPK signaling axis. *Mol. Endocrinol,* Vol.16, No.1, (Jan 2002) pp. 70-84, ISSN

Fishman J. & Martucci C. (1980). Biological properties of 16alpha-hydroxyestrone: Implications in estrogen physiology and pathophysiology. *J. Clin. Endocrinol Metab.,* Vol.51, No.3, (Sep 1980) pp. 611-615, ISSN

Gaudio E.; Palamarchuk A.; Palumbo T.; Trapasso F.; Pekarsky Y.; Croce C.M. & Aqeilan R.I. (2006). Physical association with WWOX suppresses c-Jun transcriptional activity. *Cancer Res,* Vol.66, No.24, (Dec 2006) pp. 11585-11589, ISSN

Geissler W.M.; Davis D.L.; Wu L.; Bradshaw K.D.; Patel S.; Mendonca B.B.; Elliston K.O.; Wilson J.D.; Russell D.W. & Andersson S. (1994). Male pseudohermaphroditism caused by mutations of testicular 17 beta-hydroxysteroid dehydrogenase 3. *Nat. Genet.,* Vol.7, No.1, (May 1994) pp. 34-39, ISSN

Hartman J.; Edvardsson K.; Lindberg K.; Zhao C.; Williams C.; Strom A. & Gustafsson J.A. (2009). Tumor repressive functions of estrogen receptor B in SW480 colon cancer cells. *Cancer Res,* Vol.69, No.15, (Aug 2009) pp. 6100-6106, ISSN

He R.Y.; Lin C.Y.; Su Y.D.; Chiu K.C.; Chang N.S.; Wu H.L. & Chen S.J. (2010). Imaging live cell membranes via surface plasmon-enhanced fluorescence and phase microscopy. *Opt. Express,* Vol.18, No.4, (Feb 2010) pp. 3649-3659, ISSN

He R.Y.; Su Y.D.; Cho K.C.; Lin C.Y.; Chang N.S.; Chang C.H. & Chen S.J. (2009). Surface plasmon-enhanced two-photon fluorescence microscopy for live cell membrane imaging. *Opt. Express,* Vol.17, No.8, (Apr 2009) pp. 5987-5997, ISSN

Hernandez, J.S.; Watson R.W.; Wood TC & Weinshilboum R.M. (1992). Sulfation of estrone and 17 β-estradiol in human liver. Catalysis by thermostable phenol sulfotransferase and by dehydroepiandrosterone sulfotransferase. *Drug Metab. Dispos.,* Vol.20, No.3, (May-Jun 1992) pp. 413-422, ISSN

Hong Q.; Hsu L.J.; Schultz L.; Pratt N.; Mattison J. & Chang N.S. (2007). Zfra affects TNF-mediated cell death by interacting with death domain protein TRADD and negatively regulates the activation of NF-kappaB, JNK1, p53 and WOX1 during stress response. *BMC Mol. Biol.,* Vol.8, (Jun 2007) pp. 50, ISSN

Hong Q.; Sze C.I.; Lin S.R.; Lee M.H.; He R.Y.; Schultz L.; Chang J.Y.; Chen S.J.; Boackle R.J.; Hsu L.J. & Chang N.S. (2009). Complement C1q activates tumor suppressor WWOX to induce apoptosis in prostate cancer cells. *PLoS One,* Vol.4, No.6, (Jun 2009) p. e5755, ISSN

Hsu L.J.; Hong Q.; Schultz L.; Kuo E.; Lin S.R.; Lee M.H.; Lin Y.S. & Chang N.S. (2008). Zfra is an inhibitor of Bcl-2 expression and cytochrome c release from the mitochondria. *Cell Signal,* Vol.20, No.7, (Jul 2008) pp. 1303-1312, ISSN

Hsu L.J.; Schultz L.; Hong Q.; Van Moer K.; Heath J.; Li M.Y.; Lai F.J.; Lin S.R.; Lee M.H.; Lo C.P.; Lin Y.S.; Chen S.T. &Chang N.S. (2009). Transforming growth factor beta1 signaling via interaction with cell surface Hyal-2 and recruitment of WWOX/WOX1. *J. Biol. Chem.,* Vol.284, No.23, (Jun 2009) pp. 16049-16059, ISSN

Hu ZZ, Kagan BL, Ariazi EA, Rosenthal DS, Zhang L, Li JV, Huang H, Wu C, Jordan VC, Riegel AT, Wellstein A. (2011) Proteomic analysis of pathways involved in estrogen-induced growth and apoptosis of breast cancer cells. PLoS One Vol. 6. No. 6,(July 27) p.e20410, ISSN

Huang H.J.; Chiang P.H. & Chen S.H. (2011). Quantitative analysis of estrogens and estrogen metabolites in endogenous MCF-7 breast cancer cells by liquid chromatography-tandem mass spectrometry. *J. Chromatogr. B.*, Vol.879, No.20, (Jun 2011) pp. 1748-1756, ISSN

Ito T.; Williams JD.; Fraser DJ. & Phillips AO. (2004). Hyaluronan regulates transforming growth factor-beta1 receptor compartmentalization. *J Biol Chem,* Vol.279, No. 24, (Jun 2004) pp.25326-25332, ISSN

Jansson A. (2009). 17Beta-hydroxysteroid dehydrogenase enzymes and breast cancer. *J. Steroid Biochem. Mol. Biol.*, Vol.114, No.1-2, (Mar 2009) pp. 64-67, Review, ISSN

Jansson A.; Delander L.; Gunnarsson C.; Fornander T.; Skoog L.; Nordenskjöld B. & Stål O. (2009). Ratio of 17HSD1 to 17HSD2 protein expression predicts the outcome of tamoxifen treatment in postmenopausal breast cancer patients. *Clin. Cancer Res,* Vol.15, No.10, (May 2009) pp. 3610-3616, ISSN

Jin C.; Ge L.; Ding X.; Chen Y.; Zhu H.; Ward T.; Wu F.; Cao X.; Wang Q. & Yao X. (2006). PKA-mediated protein phosphorylation regulates ezrin-WWOX interaction. *Biochem. Biophys. Res Commun.*, Vol.341, No.3, (Mar 2006) pp. 784-791, ISSN

Jörnvall H.; Hedlund J.; Bergman T.; Oppermann U. & Persson B. (2010). Superfamilies SDR and MDR: from early ancestry to present forms. Emergence of three lines, a Zn-metalloenzyme, and distinct variabilities. *Biochem. Biophys. Res Commun.*, Vol.396, No.1, (May 2010) pp. 125-130, Review, ISSN

Joubert A.; Van Zyl H.; Laurens J. & Lottering M.L. (2009). C2- and C4-position 17beta-estradiol metabolites and their relation to breast cancer. *Biocell*, Vol.33, No.3, (Dec 2009) pp. 137-140, Review, ISSN

Kavanagh K.L.; Jörnvall H.; Persson B. & Oppermann U. (2008). Medium- and short-chain dehydrogenase/reductase gene and protein families : the SDR superfamily: functional and structural diversity within a family of metabolic and regulatory enzymes. *Cell Mol. Life Sci.*, Vol.65, No.24, (Dec 2008) pp. 3895-3906, Review, ISSN

Lai F.J.; Cheng C.L.; Chen S.T.; Wu C.H.; Hsu L.J.; Lee J.Y.; Chao S.C.; Sheen M.C.; Shen C.L.; Chang N.S. & Sheu H.M. (2005). WOX1 is essential for UVB irradiation-induced apoptosis and down-regulated via translational blockade in UVB-induced cutaneous squamous cell carcinoma in vivo. *Clin. Cancer Res,* Vol.11, No.16, (Aug 2005) pp. 5769-5777, ISSN

Leduc M.S.; Lyons M.; Darvishi K.; Walsh K.; Sheehan S.; Amend S.; Cox A.; Orho-Melander M.; Kathiresan S.; Paigen B. & Korstanje R. (2011). The mouse QTL map helps interpret human genome-wide association studies for HDL cholesterol. *J. Lipid Res,* Vol.52, No.6, (Jun 2011) pp. 1139-1149, ISSN

Lee J.C.; Weissglas-Volkov D.; Kyttälä M.; Dastani Z.; Cantor R.M.; Sobel E.M.; Plaisier C.L.; Engert J.C.; van Greevenbroek M.M.; Kane J.P.; Malloy M.J.; Pullinger C.R.; Huertas-Vazquez A.; Aguilar-Salinas C.A.; Tusie-Luna T.; de Bruin T.W.; Aouizerat B.E.; van der Kallen C.C.; Croce C.M.; Aqeilan R.I.; Marcil M.; Viikari J.S.; Lehtimäki T.; Raitakari O.T.; Kuusisto J.; Laakso M.; Taskinen M.R.; Genest J. & Pajukanta P. (2008). WW-domain-containing oxidoreductase is associated with low plasma HDL-C levels. *Am. J. Hum. Genet*, Vol.83, No.2, (Aug 2008) pp. 180-192, ISSN

Li M.Y.; Lai F.J.; Hsu L.J.; Lo C.P.; Cheng C.L.; Lin S.R.; Lee M.H.; Chang J.Y.; Subhan D.; Tsai M.S.; Sze C.I.; Pugazhenthi S.; Chang N.S. & Chen S.T. (2009). Dramatic co-activation of WWOX/WOX1 with CREB and NF-kappaB in delayed loss of small dorsal root ganglion neurons upon sciatic nerve transection in rats. *PLoS One*, Vol.4, No.11, (Nov 2009) pp. e7820, ISSN

Lin H.P.; Chang J.Y.; LinS.R.; Lee M.H.; Huang S.S.; Hsu L.J. & Chang N.S. (2011). Identification of an *in vivo* MEK/WOX1 complex as a master switch for apoptosis in T cell leukemia. *Genes &Cancer*, in press.

Liu H.; Zheng S.; Bellemare V.; Pelletier G.; Labrie F. & Luu-The V. (2007). Expression and localization of estrogenic type 12 17beta-hydroxysteroid dehydrogenase in the cynomolgus monkey. *B.M.C. Biochem.*, Vol8, (Feb 2007) pp. 2, ISSN

Lo C.P.; Hsu L.J.; Li M.Y.; Hsu S.Y.; Chuang J.I.; Tsai M.S.; Lin S.R.; Chang N.S. & Chen S.T. (2008). MPP+-induced neuronal death in rats involves tyrosine 33 phosphorylation of WW domain-containing oxidoreductase WOX1. *Eur J Neurosci.*, Vol.27, No.7, (Apr 2008) pp. 1634-1646, ISSN

Ludes-Meyers J.H.; Kil H.; Parker-Thornburg J.; Kusewitt D.F.; Bedford M.T. & Aldaz C.M. (2009). Generation and characterization of mice carrying a conditional allele of the Wwox tumor suppressor gene. *PLoS One*, Vol.4, No.11, (Nov 2009) p. e7775, ISSN

Maeda N.; Semba S.; Nakayama S.; Yanagihara K. & Yokozaki H. (2010). Loss of WW domain-containing oxidoreductase expression in the progression and development of gastric carcinoma: clinical and histopathologic correlations. *Virchows Arch*, Vol.457, No.4, (Oct 2010) pp. 423-32, ISSN

Mahajan N.P.; Whang Y.E.; Mohler J.L. & Earp H.S. (2005). Activated tyrosine kinase Ack1 promotes prostate tumorigenesis: role of Ack1 in polyubiquitination of tumor suppressor Wwox. *Cancer Res*, Vol.65, No.22, (Nov 2005) pp. 10514-10523, ISSN

Marchais-Oberwinkler S.; Henn C.; Möller G.; Klein T.; Negri M.; Oster A.; Spadaro A.; Werth R.; Wetzel M.; Xu K.; Frotscher M.; Hartmann R.W. & Adamski J. (2011). 17β-Hydroxysteroid dehydrogenases (17β-HSDs) as therapeutic targets: Protein structures, functions, and recent progress in inhibitor development. *J. Steroid Biochem. Mol. Biol.*, Vol.125, No.1-2, (May 2011) pp. 66-82, ISSN

Markides C.S. & Liehr J.G. (2005). Specific binding of 4-hydroxyestradiol to mouse uterine protein: evidence of a physiological role for 4-hydroxyestradiol. *J. Endocrinol*, Vol.185, No.2, (May 2005) pp. 235-242, ISSN

Martucci, C.P. & Fishman, J. (1993). P450 enzymes of estrogen metabolism. *Pharmacol. Ther.*, Vol.57, No.2-3, (Feb-Mar 1993) pp. 237-257, Review, ISSN

Maximov P., Sengupta S., Lewis-Wambi J.S., Kim H.R., Curpan R.F., Jordan V.C. (2011) The Conformation of the Estrogen Receptor Directs Estrogen-Induced Apoptosis in Breast Cancer: A Hypothesis. Horm Mol Biol Clin Investig Vol.5, No.1,(Mar 2011) pp.27-34, ISSN

McDonnel D.P. & Norris J.D. (2002). Connections and regulation of the human estrogen receptor. *Science, Vol.296, No.5573, (May 2002) pp. 1642-1644, ISSN*

Miki Y.; Suzuki T. & Sasano H. (2009). Intracrinology of sex steroids in ductal carcinoma in situ (DCIS) of human breast: comparison to invasive ductal carcinoma (IDC) and non-neoplastic breast. J. Steroid Biochem. Mol. Biol., Vol.114, No.1-2, (Mar 2009) pp. 68-71, Review, ISSN

Miro A.M.; Sastre-Serra J.; Ponsa D.G.; Vallea A.; Rocaa P. & Oliver J. (2011). 17β-Estradiol regulates oxidative stress in prostate cancer cell lines according to ERalpha/ERbeta ratio. *Journal of Steroid Biochemistry & Molecular Biology,* Vol.123, No.3-5, (Feb 2011) pp. 133-139, ISSN

Mosselman S.; Polman J. & Dijkema R. (1996). ER beta: identification and characterization of a novel human estrogen receptor. *FEBS Lett.*, Vol.392, No.1, (Aug 1996) pp. 49-53, ISSN

Mueck A.O. & Seeger H. (2007). Breast cancer: are estrogen metabolites carcinogenic? *Climacteric.*, Suppl. 2, (Oct 2007) pp. 62-65, Review, ISSN

Nilsen J. (2008). Estradiol and neurodegenerative oxidative stress. (2008). *Front Neuroendocrinol.*, Vol.29, No.4, (Oct 2008) pp. 463-475, Review, ISSN

Obi N.; Vrieling A.; Heinz J. & Chang-Claude J. (2011). Estrogen metabolite ratio: Is the 2-hydroxyestrone to 16α-hydroxyestrone ratio predictive for breast cancer? *Int. J. Womens Health*, Vol.3, (Feb 2011) pp. 37-51, ISSN

O'Keefe L.V.; Colella A.; Dayan S.; Chen Q.; Choo A.; Jacob R.; Price G.; Venter D. & Richards R.I. (2011). Drosophila orthologue of WWOX, the chromosomal fragile site FRA16D tumour suppressor gene, functions in aerobic metabolism and regulates reactive oxygen species. *Hum.Mol.Genet*, Vol.20, No.3, (Feb 2011) pp. 497-509, ISSN

Okoh V.; Deoraj A. & Roy D. (2011). Estrogen-induced reactive oxygen species-mediated signalings contribute to breast cancer. *Biochim. Biophys. Acta.*, Vol.1815, No.1, (Jan 2011) pp. 115-133, Review, ISSN

Roy D.; Sin S.H.; Damania B. & Dittmer D.P. (2011). Tumor suppressor genes FHIT and WWOX are deleted in primary effusion lymphoma (PEL) cell lines. *Blood*, (Jun 2011), ISSN

Sáez M.E.; González-Pérez A.; Martínez-Larrad M.T.; Gayán J.; Real L.M.; Serrano-Ríos M. & Ruiz A. (2010). WWOX gene is associated with HDL cholesterol and triglyceride levels. *B.M.C. Med. Genet*, Vol.11, (Oct 2010) pp.148, ISSN

Santen R.; Cavalieri E.; Rogan E.; Russo J.; Guttenplan J.; Ingle J. & Yue W. (2009). Estrogen mediation of breast tumor formation involves estrogen receptor-dependent, as well as independent, genotoxic effects. *Ann. N. Y. Acad. Sci.*, Vol.1155, (Feb 2009) pp. 132-140, Review, ISSN

Sasaki Y.; Miki Y.; Hirakawa H.; Onodera Y.; Takagi K.; Akahira J.; Honma S.; Ishida T.; Watanabe M.; Sasano H. & Suzuki T. (2010). Immunolocalization of estrogen-producing and metabolizing enzymes in benign breast disease: comparison with normal breast and breast carcinoma. *Cancer Sci.*, Vol.101, No.10, (Oct 2010) pp. 2286-2292, ISSN

Sepkovic D.W. & Bradlow H.L. (2009). Estrogen hydroxylation--the good and the bad. *Ann. N. Y. Acad. Sci.*, Vol.1155, (Feb 2009) pp.57-67, Review, ISSN

Smith D.I.; McAvoy S.; Zhu Y. & Perez D.S. (2007). Large common fragile site genes and cancer. *Semin Cancer Biol.*, Vol.17, No.1, (Feb 2007) pp. 31-41, ISSN

Straub R.H. (2007). The complex role of estrogens in inflammation. *Endocr. Rev.*, Vol.28, No.5, (Aug 2007) pp. 521-574, Review, ISSN

Swaneck G.E. & Fishman J. (1988). Covalent binding of the endogenous estrogen 16 alpha-hydroxyestrone to estradiol receptor in human breast cancer cells: Characterization and intranuclear localization. *Proc. Natl. Acad. Sci. USA*, Vol.85, No21, (Nov 1988) pp. 7831-7835, ISSN

Sze C.I.; Su M.; Pugazhenthi S.; Jambal P.; Hsu L.J.; Heath J.; Schultz L. & Chang N.S. (2004). Down-regulation of WW domain-containing oxidoreductase induces Tau phosphorylation in vitro. A potential role in Alzheimer's disease. *J. Biol. Chem.*, Vol.279, No.29, (Jul 2004) pp. 30498-30506, ISSN

Tam A.; Morrish D.; Wadsworth S.; Dorscheid D.; Man S.P. & Sin D.D. (2011). The role of female hormones on lung function in chronic lung diseases. *B.M.C. Womens Health*, Vol.11, (Jun 2011) pp. 24, ISSN

Verenich S. & Gerk P.M. (2010). Therapeutic promises of 2-methoxyestradiol and its drug disposition challenges. *Mol. Pharm.*, Vol.7, No.6, (Dec 2010) pp. 2030-2039, Review, ISSN

Wang Y.; Addess K.J.; Chen J.; Geer L.Y.; He J.; He S.; Lu S.; Madej T.; Marchler-Bauer A.; Thiessen P.A.; Zhang N. & Bryant S.H. (2007). MMDB: annotating protein sequences with Entrez's 3D-structure database. *Nucleic Acids Res*, (Jan 2007) 35(Database issue):D298-300, ISSN

Watanabe A., Hippo Y., Taniguchi H., Iwanari H., Yashiro M., Hirakawa K., Kodama T., Aburatani H. (2003) An opposing view on WWOX protein function as a tumor suppressor. Cancer Res Vol.63, No.24,(Dec 2003) pp.8629-33, ISSN

Watanabe A., Hippo Y., Taniguchi H., Iwanari H., Yashiro M., Hirakawa K., Kodama T., Aburatani H. (2003) An opposing view on WWOX protein function as a tumor suppressor. Cancer Res Vol.63, No.24,(Dec 2003) pp.8629-33, ISSN

Webber J.; Jenkins RH.; Meran S.; Phillips A. & Steadman R. (2009). Modulation of TGFbeta1-dependent myofibroblast differentiation by hyaluronan. *Am J Pathol*, Vol.175, No.1, (Jul 2009) pp. 148-160, ISSN

Woodfield G.W.; Chen Y.; Bair T.B.; Domann F.E.; Weigel R.J. (2010). Identification of primary gene targets of TFAP2C in hormone responsive breast carcinoma cells. *Genes Chromosomes Cancer*, Vol.49, No.10, (Oct 2010) pp. 948-962, ISSN

Wu C.J.; Chen Y.W.; Tai J.H. & Chen S.H. (2011). Quantitative phosphoproteomics studies using stable isotope dimethyl labeling coupled with IMAC-HILIC-nanoLC-MS/MS for estrogen-induced transcriptional regulation. *J. Proteome Res*, Vol.10, No.3, (Mar 2011) pp. 1088-1097, ISSN

Yan J., Zhang M., Zhang J., Chen X., Zhang X. (2011) Helicobacter pylori infection promotes methylation of WWOX gene in human gastric cancer. Biochem Biophys Res Commun Vol.408, No.1,(Apr 2011) pp.99-102, ISSN

Yan J., Zhang M., Zhang J., Chen X., Zhang X. (2011) Helicobacter pylori infection promotes methylation of WWOX gene in human gastric cancer. Biochem Biophys Res Commun Vol.408, No.1,(Apr 2011) pp.99-102, ISSN

Yeh M.C.S.; Ni J.; Yin Y.; Chang E.; Zang M. & Wen X. (2005). Functions of estrogen receptor in prostate and prostate cancer, in: Basic Mechanisms and Therapeutic Approaches. *W.S. Publishing, New Jersey*, 2005, pp. 293–313

Zhu B.T. & Conney A.H. (1998). Functional role of estrogen metabolism in target cells: review and perspectives. *Carcinogenesis*, Vol.19, No.1, (Jan 1998) pp. 1-27, ISSN

Zhu, B.T.; Suchar, L.S.; Huang, M.-T. & Conney, A.H. (1996). Similarities and differences in the glucuronidation of estradiol and estrone by UDPglucuronosyltransferase in liver microsomes from male and female rats. *Biochem. Pharmacol.*, Vol.51, No.9, (May 1996) pp. 1195-1202, ISSN

17

Sex Steroids in Insects and the Role of the Endosymbiont *Wolbachia*: A New Perspective

Ilaria Negri[1] and Marco Pellecchia[2]
[1]*DIVAPRA - University of Turin*
[2]*Koiné - Consulenze Ambientali S.n.c. Parma*
Italy

1. Introduction

Sex steroids play a pivotal role in sex differentiation and sex reversal in several species of vertebrates, both with genotypic and environmental sex determination systems (Nakamura, 2010; Norris & Carr, 2006). Steroidal sex hormones can be found naturally in both sexes of vertebrates, although the proportions of hormones may differ between males and females. Feminization of males or masculinization of females can be induced by altering the levels of 'female' and 'male' hormones, respectively. Estrogens for example have a feminizing effect on gonadal differentiation in many species of fish, amphibians, reptiles, and birds (Guiguen et al., 2010; Nakamura, 2009, 2010). In humans, androgen receptor defect disorder may lead to gonadal feminization and, in its complete form, the syndrome causes sex reversal of genotypical (XY) males and a female phenotype (Oakes et al., 2008).

Vertebrate-like sex steroids occur in several groups of invertebrates including nematodes, arthropods, echinoderms, but full information on the precise action and function of sex steroids is still missing (Janer & Porte, 2007). Some intriguing data have been provided in mollusks, where an involvement of steroids in gender determination and sexual differentiation of the brain, and even in a "superfeminization syndrome", has been demonstrated (Oehlmann et al., 2006; Wang & Croll, 2004).

In insects the existence of sex hormones is under debate. Indeed sex differentiation is generally thought to be a strictly genetic process, in which each cell decides its own sexual fate autonomously, based on its sex chromosome constitution. Therefore, differentiation of primary and secondary sexual characteristics should be exclusively under the control of the genotype of each single cell (Schütt & Nöthiger, 2000; Steinmann-Zwicky et al., 1989). This hypothesis was born studying insect gynandromorphs, i.e. aberrant specimens with an intermediate feature between female and male (according to the Greek roots gyne = female, aner = male, morphe = form; Fig. 1). In the fruit fly *Drosophila melanogaster*, gynandromorphs may arise when one embryonic nucleus loses an X chromosome and the insects possess a mixture of XX (i.e. female) and X0 (i.e. male) tissues. According to Gilbert (2000), because there are no sex hormones in insects to modulate such events, each cell makes its own sexual "decision".

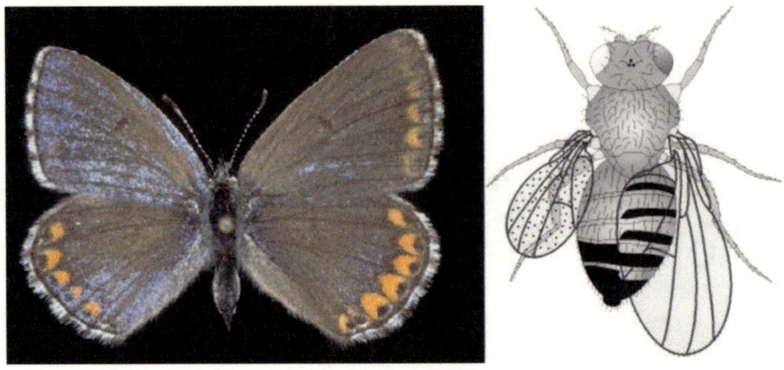

Fig. 1. Gynandromorphs, i.e. aberrant specimens made up of both female and male cells, are common in insects. On the left: *Polyommatus bellargus* (Lepidoptera, Lycaenidae) mosaic gynandromorph in which male (blue) and female (brown) features are mixed (Courtesy of R. Villa, Bologna, Italy). On the right: *D. melanogaster* bilateral gynandromorph in which one side is female and the other male (Modified from Griffiths et al., (2000). *An introduction to genetic analysis*, 7th edition, New York: W. H. Freeman).

However recent data demonstrate that in insects as in vertebrates, non-autonomous (= hormonal) sex determination controls sex dimorphism (DeFalco et al., 2008). In the germ line of the *D. melanogaster* embryo there is evidence for both autonomous and non-autonomous regulation of sexual identity, but non-autonomous signals from the soma are dominant, and germ cells establish their sexual identity as they contact the somatic gonad (Casper & Van Doren, 2009; DeFalco et al., 2008). In fact, XX (i.e. female) and XY or X0 (i.e. male) germ cells are not irrevocably committed to female or male identity, respectively (Waterbury et al., 2000).

According to these results, the presence of signals coordinating the development of a gender-specific phenotype (i.e. sex hormones) is conceivable. In his fine review, De Loof (2006) suggests that the loss of an X chromosome in *Drosophila* embryonic cells possibly makes the mutant cells react differently to a given hormonal environment and/or signals from their neighbours than XX cells.

Finally, it is noteworthy to note that, in addition to gynandromorphs, intersexes specimens do exist in insects. As previously discussed, gynandromorphism is the simultaneous presence within the same organism of genotypically and phenotypically male and female tissues rather than of masculinized or feminized tissues, as is the case with intersexes. Indeed intersexes are characterised by phenotypically male and female regions, but genetically homogeneous pattern (Laugé, 1985; White, 1973). In 1934, for example, Whiting and colleagues described individuals of the hymenopteran *Habrobracon juglandis* which were found to be genetically male but with feminized genitalia.

How can the existence of intersexes be explained, if each cell makes its own sexual decision?

2. Ecdysteroids: A role as sex hormones in insects?

De Loof (2006) proposes that ecdysteroids are the best candidates for a role as sex steroids in insects since, for example, they are involved in the appearance of sex dimorphic structures; are produced by the gonads; and induce different gender-specific physiological effects. Indeed the role of ecdysteroids is not restricted to moulting but they have a much wider effect on the insect biology, both at the larval and adult stages.

Insect moulting is induced by the steroid hormone 20-hydroxyecdysone (20E). Ecdysone pulses in the insects' hemolymph trigger moulting, and the presence or absence of juvenile hormone determines whether moults will lead to another larval stage or, through metamorphosis, to a pupa and an adult form (Gilbert at al., 2002). The 20E precursor is secreted by the prothoracic glands after their stimulation by the brain prothoracicotropic hormone (PTTH) whose release is governed by both intrinsic factors, like the body size, and extrinsic factors, like photoperiod and temperature (Gilbert at al., 2002).

Dietary cholesterol is then converted to 20E thanks to many hydroxylation reactions catalysed by cytochrome P450 enzymes of microsomal and/or mitochondrial origin, the final step being characterised by the action of a P450 monooxygenase that hydroxylates the ecdysone s.s. (E) at carbon 20.

Cytochrome P450s are encoded by the Halloween genes family, first characterised in *D. melanogaster* and then described in lots of insect species (Christiaens et al., 2010; Rewitz et al., 2007).

Once 20E is biosynthesized, it binds the heterodimeric nuclear receptor EcR/USP composed of EcR (Ecdysone Receptor) and USP (Ultraspiracle, homologous to the vertebrate retinoid-X receptor), which shares many commonalities with the human thyroid hormone receptor. Then, the EcR/USP complex activates the transcriptional processes underlying the cellular and morphogenetic moulting cascade events (Gilbert et al., 2002). In *D. melanogaster*, pulses of 20E throughout fly development have proved to regulate cell proliferation, differentiation, and programmed cell death in a highly controlled manner. During metamorphosis, for example, ecdysone is a primary regulator of apoptosis in larval tissues such as salivary glands, midgut and neural tissues which are destroyed or remodelled into an "adult" form (Mottier et al., 2004; Tsuzuki et al., 2001). The activation and execution of ecdysis (i.e. shedding of the old cuticle during embryonic and larval development) are controlled by a series of peptide hormones produced by Inka cells and neuropeptides within the central nervous system, whose expression is again under ecdysteroid control (Zitnan et al., 2007).

In adults the role played by ecdysteroids is much less explored: for example, it has been demonstrated that they control several important aspects of reproduction, including ovarian development and oogenesis (Carney & Bender, 2001; Raikhel et al., 2005; Riddifort, 1993; Swevers & Iatrou, 2003). In many insect species 20E is also directly involved in the regulation of vitellogenin biosynthesis by the female fat body, a metabolic tissue functionally analogous to the vertebrate liver, and it can also induce vitellogenin synthesis in males (Bownes et al., 1983; Bownes et al., 1996; Huybrechts & De Loof, 1977; Zhu et al., 2007). The 20E has also been shown to affect sexual behaviour, having a role in courtship initiation by males, and promoting male-male sexual attraction (Ganter et al., 2007).

De Loof (2006, 2008) suggests that ecdysteroids already served as sex hormones long before they acquired a function in moulting. In particular, 20E secreted by the follicle cells of the insect ovary could be the physiological equivalent of vertebrate estrogens, while E - the precursor of the active moulting hormone 20E - should act as a distinct hormone, being the physiological equivalent of the vertebrate testosterone (De Loof & Huybrechts, 1998; De Loof, 2006). Indeed, by using *Drosophila* larval organ culture Beckstead and colleagues (2007) demonstrate that E can regulate a set of genes that are distinct from those controlled by 20E, thus confirming that it may exert different biological (=hormonal) functions from 20E.

3. Ecdysteroids and *Wolbachia*: Different roles and different manipulations

Wolbachia are members of the order Rickettsiales (α-Proteobacteria), a diverse group of symbionts with parasitic, mutualistic or commensal lifestyle. The genus *Wolbachia* is known to infect exclusively invertebrates, namely nematodes and arthropods, being widely spread in insects where it is estimated to occur in up to 66% of the species (Hilgenboecker et al., 2008; Werren et al., 2008). *Wolbachia* bacteria, and specifically the species *W. pipientis*, are transmitted through the germ line from the mother to the offspring and, occasionally, between individuals of phylogenetically distant species (Stouthamer et al., 1999). The trans-ovarial inheritance of *Wolbachia* in insects seems to be mediated by bacteryocite-like cells (cells specialized for harbouring endosymbionts) in the ovary of the infected mother, which degenerate thus ensuring transmission of bacteria to germ line cells and then to the progeny (Sacchi et al., 2010).

Phylogenetic studies based on 16S ribosomal sequences reveal that *Wolbachia* bacteria are divided into eight different supergroups: two are commonly found in Nematoda (mainly in filarial but also in non filarial species), whereas the other six supergroups are found primarily in Arthropoda, including insects, mites, spiders, scorpions and isopod crustaceans (Werren et al., 2008).

A unique feature shared by Arthropoda and Nematoda is the ability to replace the exoskeleton, a process known as ecdysis. This shared characteristic is thought to reflect a common ancestry, giving rise to the clade Ecdysozoa (Ewer, 2005a). Although the exoskeleton composition varies among ecdysozoans, the process of moulting itself is similar within the clade: the epidermis undergoes cell division producing a larger surface and separates from the exoskeleton. Then the epidermis secretes a new exoskeleton that remains soft until the residues of the old cuticle are shed at ecdysis. The new cuticle then expands and hardens (Ewer, 2005a, 2005b).

As previously discussed, arthropod moulting is induced by the steroid hormone 20E and a role for ecdysteroids in nematode ecdysis has also been observed. In filarial nematodes, moulting seems to be regulated by ecdysteroid-like hormones: in *Dirofilaria immitis*, for example, moulting from the third to the fourth larval stage can be induced in vitro by the 20E of insects (Wabrick et al., 1993), and orthologs of insects nuclear receptors involved in ecdysone response have been found (Crossgrove et al., 2008; Ghedin et al., 2007; Tzertzinis et al., 2010). In *Caenorhabditis elegans* these nuclear receptors are also involved in the regulation of sex determination and reproductive development (Höss & Weltje, 2007; Motola et al., 2006) and, interestingly, ecdysone has also a role in the fertility and microfilaria release in filarial worms (Barker et al., 1991).

In nematodes, *Wolbachia* is an obligate symbiont, as worms depend on bacteria for survival. Antibiotic curing of *Wolbachia* "infection" inhibits nematode fertility and development, suggesting a specific role for the symbiont in host oogenesis, embryogenesis and moulting (Arumugam et al., 2008; Casiraghi et al., 2002; Frank et al., 2010).

In arthropods the bacterium is able to manipulate the host reproduction in order to increase the number of infected females. The effects of the *Wolbachia* infection include cytoplasmic incompatibility, that is an aberrant or considerably reduced offspring production if uninfected females mate with infected males, or if the parents are infected with different *Wolbachia* strains; thelytokous parthenogenesis, in which infected virgin females produce daughters; feminization, in which infected genetic males develop as females; and male-killing, in which infected males die (Stouthamer et al., 1999; Werren et al., 2008).

Such phenotypic variability is thought to be linked to high genome plasticity of insect-borne *Wolbachia*, since all the sequenced genomes of the symbiont contain high number of repetitive sequences, including IS (insertion sequences) elements and prophage-like sequences (Iturbe-Ormaetxe & O'Neill, 2007; Wu et al., 2004).

According to us, except for cytoplasmic incompatibility that is a secondary effect of the infection, the phenotypic effects observed in arthropods might not be so different, but strictly interconnected, and possibly all ascribable to feminization.

Indeed, male killing could be just an unsuccessful "attempt" at feminization by *Wolbachia*. Male-killing is known in several insect species, where males die during embryogenesis or development. Insight into the mechanism of male killing comes from the moths *Ostrinia scapulalis* and *O. furnacalis*, where *Wolbachia* kills genetic males during the larval development. Intriguingly, a partial *Wolbachia* curing leads to the appearance of lepidopteran intersexes having exclusively male genotype (Kageyama & Traut, 2003). Accordingly, a partial feminization of genetic males does occur, while a complete feminization is incompatible with the survival of the male genotype (Kageyama & Traut, 2003; Sakamoto et al., 2007).

Regarding the parthenogenesis induction by *Wolbachia*, this phenomenon has been demonstrated in several haplodiploid species of mites, hymenopterans and thrips, where males naturally develop (parthenogenetically) from unfertilized haploid eggs and females from fertilized diploid eggs (Arakaki et al., 2001; Stouthamer et al., 1990; Weeks & Breeuwer, 2001). In *Wolbachia*-infected species, unfertilized eggs are subjected to a "diploidy" restoration, giving origin to (infected) females. Recently, Giorgini and colleagues (2009) observed that in the (haplodiploid) wasp *Encarsia hispida*, the symbiont *Cardinium* (which belongs to the only bacterial group known to cause similar reproductive manipulations of *Wolbachia*) doesn't induce, as expected, thelytokous parthenogenesis but feminization. In fact antibiotic treatment results in uninfected diploid male offspring, thus demonstrating that diploidy restoration is a necessary condition, but not sufficient, to elicit female development. Therefore, *Cardinium* is responsible for the feminization of the hymenopteran genetic males.

Since in studies concerning the parthenogenesis induction by *Wolbachia* no cytogenetic analyses have been performed on males produced by cured females, the hypothesis that the symbiont actually induces feminization rather than parthenogenesis may be conceivable.

As will be discussed later, feminization deals with sex determination and differentiation much more directly than the other *Wolbachia*-induced phenotypes, thus offering the opportunity to shed light on processes governing arthropod development and reproduction, and on the involvement of the endosymbiont in such processes.

On the whole, the data available in the literature suggest that the phenotypic effects induced by *Wolbachia* may be linked to differences in host physiology, and in particular to endocrine-related processes governing development and reproduction which in insects display high variability.

Interestingly, *Wolbachia* bacteria are known to localize in many hosts' steroidogenic tissues. In different insect species, the endosymbiont has been observed in the cytoplasm of the follicular cells (Gonella et al. 2011; Sacchi et al., 2010) (Fig. 2). In *Drosophila*, *Wolbachia* microinjected into the abdominal cavity has shown a tropism towards somatic stem cells that differentiate in follicular cells (Frydman et al., 2006). In insects the follicular epithelium is one of the major niches deputed to the synthesis of ecdysteroids (Swevers et al., 2005).

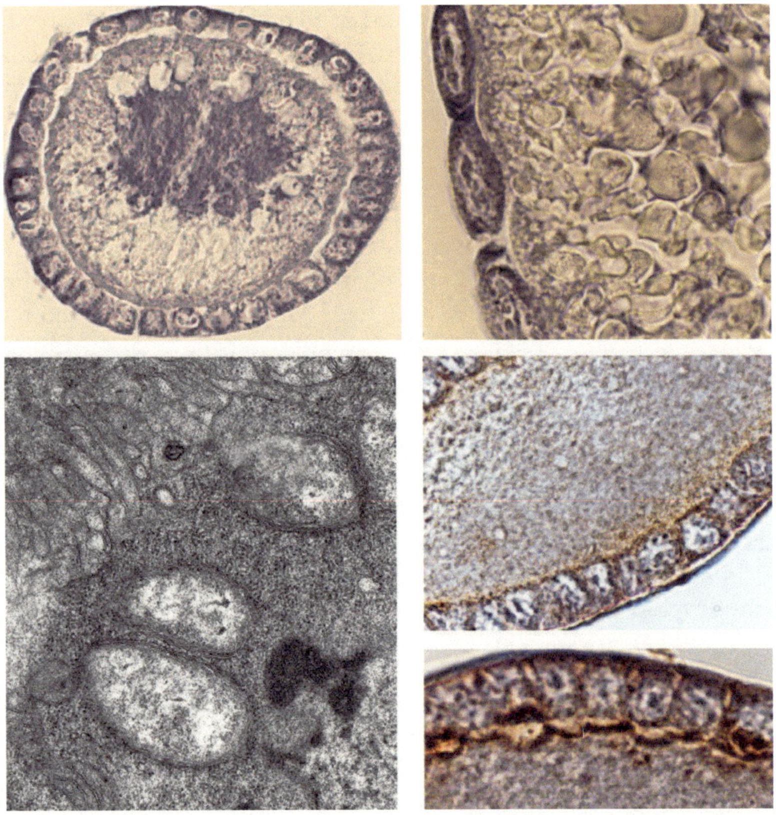

Upper left and right: A *Zyginidia pullula* (Hemiptera, Cicadellidae) oocyte surrounded by a single layer of follicle cells (gallocyanin–chrome alum reaction on leafhopper ovary sections). Lower left: TEM micrograph of a *Wolbachia*-infected *Z. pullula* follicle cell filled with bacteria. Lower right: Immuno-histochemical reactions showing strong positivity (brown) to anti-wsp (*Wolbachia* surface protein) antibody in the leafhopper's follicular epithelium.

Fig. 2. *Wolbachia* localization in the follicular epithelium of the gonad's host.

Moreover, the endosymbiont is frequently associated to host's fat bodies, the other major niche for steroid synthesis (Kamoda et al., 2000; Thummel & Chory, 2002) (Fig. 3).
Therefore, it is conceivable that *Wolbachia* may interfere with insect reproduction and development by modulating host hormonal pathways, as it has already been shown for isopod crustaceans and will be explained in the following section.

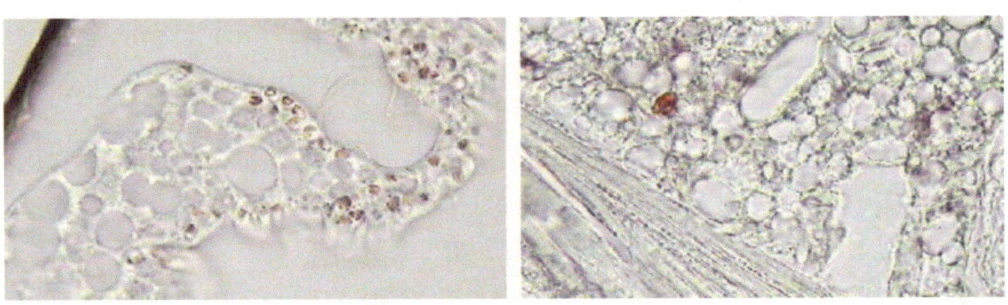

Fig. 3. In-situ hybridization with a specific probe for *Wolbachia* 16S rRNA on *Zyginidia pullula* fat body shows positive staining (red), indicating that the tissue is filled with bacteria.

4. *Wolbachia* and the feminization of the arthropod host

In arthropods, feminization induced by *Wolbachia* was first described in isopod crustaceans (Bouchon et al., 2008; Martin et al., 1973; Rigaud et al., 1999) and, later, the phenomenon was studied in the lepidopteran species *Eurema hecabe*, *Ostrinia scapulalis* and *O. furnacalis*, and the hemipteran species *Zyginidia pullula* (Hiroki et al., 2002; Kageyama & Traut, 2003; Negri et al., 2006; Sakamoto et al., 2007).

In Crustacea, which are phylogenetically close to insects, sex differentiation and development of secondary sexual characteristics are driven by an androgenic hormone (AH), secreted by the androgenic gland (AG), whose action inhibits female differentiation (Legrand et al., 1987; Sagi & Khalaila, 2001). In fact, Crustacea are by default female and the expression of male secondary characteristics is only possible by the production of AH. Indeed, the ablation of the AG results in the degeneration from male to the female form, whereas injection with purified extracts of the AH or implantation of AGs into females results in the development of external male sexual characteristics or the complete sex reversal (Charniaux-Cotton, 1954; Sagi et al., 1997; Suzuki & Yamasaki, 1998). Therefore, it has been suggested that in Crustacea sex reversal is actually due to masculinisation of females or de-masculinisation of males (Ford, 2008).

The feminization effect induced by *Wolbachia* in isopods is thought to be linked to interactions between the bacterium and the AG differentiation process or, more probably, the AH receptors (Bouchon et al., 2008; Rigaud & Juchault, 1998). Indeed, in *Armadillidium vulgare* genetic males, AH mRNA can be detected at the beginning of male gonad differentiation, and AH may thus have an early and local action by inducing male differentiation of embryonic gonads (Negri et al., 2010). *Wolbachia* could then induce feminization (or de-masculinisation?) by targeting AH receptors, thereby inhibiting AG differentiation (Juchault & Legrand, 1985). If *Wolbachia* bacteria are experimentally inoculated in adult males, the AG become hypetrophic, but the host soon develops female genital apertures, probably because the AH receptors are no longer functional due to the infection (Martin et al., 1973; Martin et al., 1999).

In insect species, *Wolbachia* is able to feminize genetical males and, in all these cases, the existence of intersexes linked to *Wolbachia* effects has been described: in the presence of signals coordinating the development of a gender specific phenotype, intersexes might arise from a conflict between male and female sex hormones and/or receptors (Hiroki et al., 2002; Kageyama & Traut, 2003; Negri et al., 2006; Sakamoto et al., 2007).

In *E. hecabe*, feminizing *Wolbachia* acts continuously throughout the larval development to produce the female phenotype (Narita et al., 2007). As a consequence, if the bacteria act on sex differentiation rather than sex determination, sex hormone (i.e. ecdysteroid) pathways should be involved. Some clues are provided by studies on infected *E. hecabe*, where an incomplete *Wolbachia* suppression during host development, i.e. when host sex differentiation is not yet completed, leads to larval/pupal moulting defects (Narita et al., 2007). In particular, some individuals show morphological abnormalities (i.e. curled, folded or asymmetric wings), while a certain number of insects do not pupate: dissection of dead pupae reveals that many of them have actually completed adult morphogenesis but failed to escape from the pupal case (Narita et al., 2007). Interestingly, similar moulting defects may be obtained in knockdown insects using RNA interference techniques on ecdysone receptors. For example, some treated nymphs of the german cockroach *Blattella germanica* do not moult into adults, maintaining both nymphal and adult structures of ectodermal origin duplicated, whereas those nymphs that moulted into adults show characteristic deformations in the wing extension (Cruz et al., 2006). Also *Drosophila* EcR mutants are characterised by pupal lethality: specimens rarely eclose and the pharate adults dissected from the pupal case show abnormalities (Davies et al., 2005).

Moreover, since in some lepidopteran species the ecdysteroid titer has been proven to regulate sex specific wing development (Lobbia et al., 2003), sexually intermediate traits in wing morphology observed in *E. hecabe* specimens subjected to a partial *Wolbachia* curing could also be attributed to the ecdysteroid action.

In the other lepidopteran species *Ostrinia scapulalis* and *O. furnacalis*, *Wolbachia* has the ability to feminize genetic males, but - as discussed above - a complete feminization is fatal, and genetical males die (Kageyama and Traut, 2003; Sakamoto et al., 2007). In these species male-killing occurs during the larval development while the role played by ecdysteroids is crucial. In other insects, the sex-specific killing action by *Wolbachia* occurs during embryogenesis (Dyer& Jaenike, 2004; Fialho & Stevens, 2000; Jiggins et al., 2001; Zeh et al., 2005). Embryogenesis takes place in a steroid hormone-enriched environment where steroid hormones act for the coordination of morphogenetic movements (De Loof, 2006; Kozlova & Thummel, 2003; Gaziova et al., 2004). Thus, if male-killing *Wolbachia* interacts with the host hormonal pathway involving ecdysteroids, this could interfere with the processes required for a normal development of males.

Unfortunately, little information about sex-specific action of ecdysteroids during insect embryogenesis and development is available, and it mainly concerns the effects of endocrine disrupting chemicals. For example, in the housefly *Musca domestica* and in the midge *Chironomus riparius* the sex ratio is affected by the ecdysteroid agonist bisphenol A (Izumi et al., 2008; Lee & Choi, 2007). Another ecdysteroid agonist, tebufenozide, exerts similar effects on *C. riparius* and the moth *Platynota idaeusalis* (Biddinger et al., 2006; Hahn et al., 2001). Female-biased sex ratios are also obtained after a treatment performed on the midge larvae with the ecdysteroid antagonist ethynil estradiol (Hahn et al., 2001; Lee & Choi, 2007).

According to some authors, the observed sex-specific effect could be explained by considering insect steroids as sex hormones. In particular, larval or embryo males die because they are subjected to an unsuitable, i.e. female, hormonal environment (Hahn et al., 2001).

Recent studies on the moth *Ostrinia scapulalis* are providing new data on the molecular bases of the *Wolbachia*-host interaction. Sugimoto and colleagues (2010) analysed the expression of the *doublesex* gene (*dsx*) in *Ostrinia* intersexes (= partially feminized males) generated from antibiotic treated mothers. *Doublesex* is the highly conserved gene at the bottom of the sex determination cascades in insects, and it is known to regulate the somatic sexual differentiation through the sex specific proteins DSXf (female) and DSXm (male). (Burtis & Baker, 1989). In particular, *dsx* resides at the junction of a complex network of regulatory interactions that include homeotic genes, ligand-based signal transduction cascades, and other transcriptional regulators for the differentiation of sexually dimorphic structures (Burtis, 2002; Rideout et al., 2010). In *Drosophila* males, feminization may be induced by modifying dsx expression. The ectopical expression of DSXf with the complete removal of endogenous DSXm may cause external complete feminization (Waterbury et al., 1999); even the XY (male) germ line may be feminized by ectopical expression of DSXf (Waterbury et al., 2000).

As expected, in somatic tissues of *O. scapulalis* males and females, the sex-specific isoform of DSX was found; while in the gonads the opposite sex was also weakly expressed, maybe because reproductive organs comprise also undifferentiated germ cells where both DSXf and DSXm could be expressed (Sugimoto et al., 2010). In intersex individuals originated from

Wolbachia-cured mothers, both female- and male-specific isoforms are present, suggesting that the symbiont may interfere either with the sex-specific splicing of the gene *dsx* itself or (more probably) with another upstream process involved in sex determination/differentiation (Sugimoto et al., 2010).

Male- and female-specific isoforms of DSX share a zinc finger DNA-binding domain (designated as the DM motif), which is widely conserved in the Animal Kingdom, from corals to nematodes, from arthropods to vertebrates, and characterize the *dmrt* family of genes (Erdman & Burtis, 1993; Murphy et al., 2010; Matsuda et al., 2002; Raymond et al., 1998; Smith et al., 2009; Yoshimoto et al., 2008; Zhu et al., 2000).

Despite the attention that *dmrt* factors have received, to date it has not been well elucidated how *dmrts* mediate their activities, and putative downstream targets have yet to be characterized.

In some vertebrates, such as fish, it has been demonstrated that sex steroid hormones affect *dmrt1* expression (Herpin & Schartl, 2011), thus it would be of capital interest to verify changes in *O. scapulalis dsx* expression following steroid treatments, and if feminizing *Wolbachia* may play a role in modulating *dsx* expression by interaction with hormonal pathways.

New insights into the mechanisms underlying the bacterium-host interaction have been provided by studies on the leafhopper *Z. pullula*. In this hemipteran species, *Wolbachia*-infected genetic males develop into intersexes with a female phenotype, which retain secondary male features in the ano-genital zone (Negri et al., 2006) (Fig. 4).

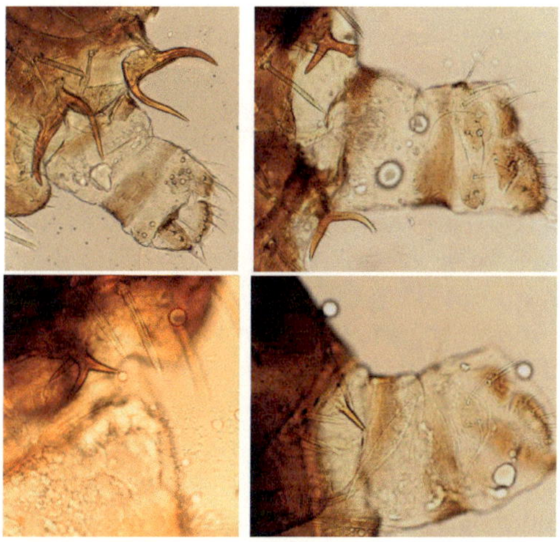

Fig. 4. *Zyginidia pullula* males feminized by *Wolbachia* maintain typical male structures (the so-called upper pygofer appendages) localized in the last abdominal segments. These forked chitinous structures are completely absent in normal females. In feminized males they appear well developed (upper left), or not completely developed but reduced to a stump (lower right).

Leafhopper feminized males are vital and even active reproductively. In laboratory rearing, couplings are often observed (Fig. 5), meaning that these individuals have a feminine 'sex appeal', and progeny is occasionally obtained (Negri et al., 2006). In addition to feminized males with ovaries ("intersex females"), some rare intersexes bear male gonads ("intersex males") (Negri et al., 2009a) (Fig. 5). Interestingly, "intersex males" possess a *Wolbachia* density approximately four orders of magnitude lower than "intersex females" (Negri et al., 2009a).

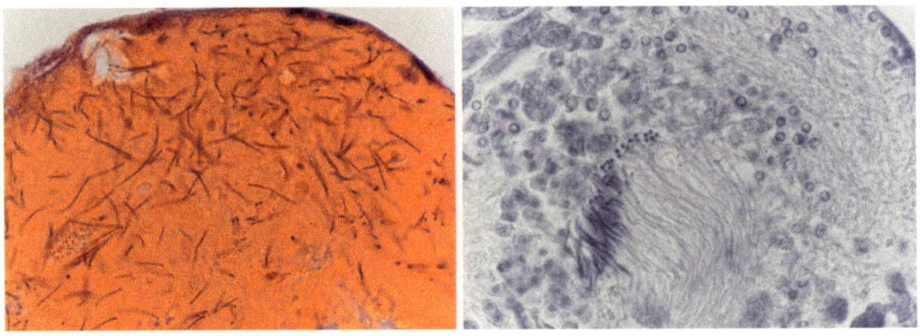

Fig. 5. On the left: a spermatheca of an intersex female of *Zyginidia pullula* full of sperms after after mating (haematoxylin/eosin stain on leafhopper gonad sections). On the right: testis of an intersex male showing different stages of spermatogenesis (gallocyanin-chrome alum reaction on leafhopper gonad sections).

Recent data demonstrate that *Wolbachia* infection is able to modulate the leafhopper's genomic imprinting through cytosine methylation of the host DNA (Negri et al., 2009a, 2009b).

Genomic imprinting is a phenomenon whereby a gene, or a region of a chromosome, is reversibly modified so that it retains a sort of "memory" of its own genetic history. The term imprinting, originally coined referring to a complex behaviour of the X chromosome in the dipteran insect *Sciara coprophila* (Crouse, 1960), indicates a situation in which the activity of the imprinted genes or chromosomes is determined by the sex of the parent that transmits them, and the altered expression is limited to the somatic tissue of the progeny, whereas the germ line is not permanently altered (Surani, 1998). Epigenetic changes are based on molecular mechanisms including methylation of cytosines, remodelling of chromatin structure through histone chemical modifications and RNA interference. These molecular processes can activate, reduce or completely disable the activity of genes.

Methylation of cytosine residues in the DNA is currently one of the most studied epigenetic mechanisms (Bender, 2004). This robust but reversible marking of genomic DNA is catalyzed by a conserved family of enzymes called DNA methyltransferases (DNMTs), which have been extensively studied in mammals, plants and fungi (Goll & Bestor, 2005).

Until now, the genomic imprinting has been found in vertebrates (Martin & McGowan 1995; Sharman 1971; Surani 1998) and invertebrates, including lots of insect species (Rewieved in Lyko & Maleszka, 2011). In particular, in the hymenopteran wasp *Nasonia vitripennis* and in the coccid *Planococcus citri* imprinting is related to sex determination (Beukeboom et al. 2007; Field et al. 2004); in *P. citri* it has been clearly assessed that DNA methylation is deeply involved in the establishment of the differential sex-specific genomic imprinting.

At a molecular level, in the hemipteran *Z. pullula* the occurrence of sex specific differences in the methylation pattern was observed (Negri et al., 2009a). Surprisingly, Random Amplification of Polymorphic DNA (RAPD) PCRs showed that *Wolbachia*-infected "intersex females" possess the same imprinting pattern of uninfected females (Negri et al., 2009a, 2009b). These data demonstrate that the infection disrupts the male imprinting thus influencing the expression of genes involved in sex differentiation and development. In addition, the alteration occurs only if the bacterium exceeds a density threshold, as "intersex males" maintain a male genome–methylation pattern (Negri et al., 2009a). Methylation-sensitive RAPD analyses were also carried out on gonads (testes and ovaries), confirming the occurrence of a sex-specific methylation of the genome, and strengthening the results obtained with somatic tissues in *Wolbachia*-infected specimens (Negri et al., 2009b). This suggests that *Wolbachia* is not only able to induce a feminization of genetic males, but may also cause the inheritance of female imprinting in gonads of feminized males. This is particularly intriguing since in gonads the parental imprinting is generally erased and re-established on the basis of the parent sex, and clearly indicates that feminized males act as true females establishing a female genomic imprinting in their genome. On the whole data demonstrate that Wolbachia may be considered an 'environmental' factor that promotes heritable epigenetic changes in the host gene expression: the epigenetic effects of Wolbachia symbiosis are manifested as a 'maternal effect', in which infection of the mother alters the offspring phenotype.

5. Possible interplay between steroid signalling and epigenetic pathways

5.1 Role of sex steroids in mammal sex differentiation

In humans the male-determining gene *Sry* on the male-specific Y chromosome is known to promote sexual development by inducing the bipotential gonads of the embryo to form testes. Then, the differentiated gonad produces the male sex steroid (i.e. testosterone) which activates gene transcription via androgen and estrogen receptors, thus driving the masculinisation processes of the whole body (Anway et al., 2005; Chang et al., 2006). In particular, sex hormone synthesis induces not only the sexual differentiation of the reproductive system, but also the sexual differentiation of the brain. This is known to occur in a carefully defined critical period, where a brief hormone exposure permanently organizes the brain sex differences (Dohier, 1998; Gabory et al., 2009; McCarthy et al., 2009). Indeed, gonadal hormones defeminize and masculinize the male brain, while a lack of gonadal steroids allows for feminization in the female. In rodents, for example, treatments with steroids during the critical period leads to a defeminized and masculinized neural phenotype, while blocking aromatization of testosterone to estradiol or antagonizing estrogen receptor binding inhibits a correct brain organization in males (Barraclough, 1961; Baum, 1979; Vreeburg et al., 1977).

The mechanisms exerted by sex hormones are strictly linked to the epigenetic machinery. For example, gonadal hormones are able to induce sex differences in DNA methylation, methyl-binding proteins and chromatin modifications necessary for a correct sexual differentiation of the brain (Nugent & McCarthy, 2011).

The role for steroids in modulating epigenetic changes is attracting the growing interest of many researchers. In particular, the field of endocrine disruption is shedding new light on the discipline of basic reproductive neuro-endocrinology, through studies on how early life exposures to endocrine-disrupting chemicals may alter gene expression via epigenetic mechanisms, including DNA methylation and histone acetylation/methylation. Importantly, these effects may be transmitted to future generations if the germ line is affected via trans-generational, epigenetic actions.

Recent evidence shows for example that androgen and estrogen receptors interact with histone modifying enzymes (Tsai et al., 2009). Measuring levels of acetylation and methylation of histones in neonatal mouse brains, Tsai and colleagues (2009) found that H3 histone modification is sexually dimorphic in some areas of the neonatal brain, and prenatal testosterone interacts with H3 acetylation to reverse this dimorphism.

In another study, tamoxifen - a selective estrogen receptor modulator - has been shown to interfere with imprinting at the specific locus Insulin-like growth factor 2/H19 in rat spermatozoa (Pathak et al., 2010). Since imprint at this locus is acquired during spermatogenesis in the male germ line, a role for estrogen signalling in the methylation dynamics of the testis is hypothesized. In particular it has been hypothesized that tamoxifen could exert an epigenetic action by directly affecting DNA methylation in the male germ cells. The observed reduction in sperm DNA methylation suggests imprinting error in the male germ-line mediated by defective estrogen signalling (Pathak et al., 2009; Pathak et al., 2010). Hence decipher interaction between estrogen signalling and DNA methylation pathways is of primary importance.

5.2 The *Wolbachia*-host interaction: A new perspective

The model proposed in Fig. 6 tries to explain a possible *Wolbachia*/host interaction involving host hormonal signalling and epigenetic regulation. In view of the absence of genes codifying for typical eukaryotic DNA methyltransferases in the sequenced genomes of *Wolbachia* strains isolated from *D. melanogaster* and the nematode *B. Malayi* (Foster et al., 2005; Wu et al., 2004), we cannot exclude that the bacterium encodes for some proteins interfering with ecdysteroids signalling pathway thus modulating the expression of the host DNMTs and/or histone modifying enzymes.

Hormone signalling orchestration is done by nuclear receptors, and over the past decade it has become increasingly clear that the recruitment of co-regulatory proteins to nuclear receptors is required for hormone-mediated transcriptional and biological activities. Many nuclear receptor co-regulators are key epigenetic regulators and utilize enzymatic activities to epigenetically modify the DNA and chromatin, through DNA methylation and histone acetylation/methylation (Hsia et al., 2010 Mahajan & Samuels, 2000; Rosenfeld et al., 2006).

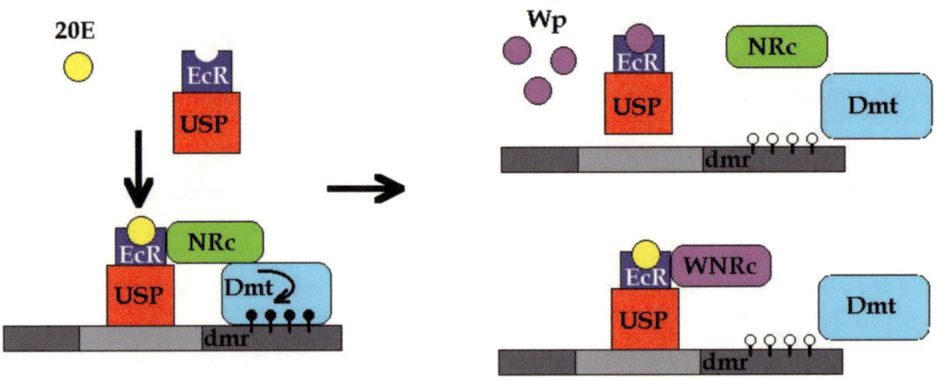

20E = 20-hydroxyecdysone; EcR = Ecdysone receptor; USP = Ultraspiracle; NRc = Nuclear Receptor co-regulator; Dmt = DNA-methyltransferase; dmr = Differentially metylated regions; Wp = *Wolbachia* product; WNRc = *Wolbachia* Nuclear Receptor co-regulator.
Filled lollypops and open lollypops indicate methylated and unmethylated CpGs, respectively.

Fig. 6. Model illustrating the possible interplay between ecdysone signaling and epigenetic regulation. For simplicity, among epigenetic mechanisms, only DNA methylation is considered.

In particular, as proposed in Fig. 6, once 20E is biosynthesized, it binds the nuclear receptor EcR which heterodimerizes with USP. Then, the EcR/USP complex binds DNA constitutively and complexes with nuclear receptors co-regulators, thus catalyzing DNA methyltransferases (and/or histone modifying enzymes) which results in a proper DNA methylation. In *Wolbachia*-infected insects, alterations of the methylation patterns may be due to hypothetical *Wolbachia* products (directly binding the nuclear-receptor or functioning as/or interfering with nuclear receptor co-regulators) that could inhibit EcR binding to DNA or DNA-methyltransferases (and/or histone modifying enzymes) recruitment, respectively.

Accordingly, studies on *Wolbachia*-host interactions should give great attention for example to selective nuclear receptor modulators; substances with an antagonist action on the ecdysone nuclear receptor; or co-regulators of nuclear receptors, in view of their emerging role in integrating transcriptional co-regulation with epigenetic regulation (Rosenfeld et al., 2006; Kato et al., 2011). This could eventually clarify the nature of this fascinating microbial symbiosis and the extraordinary effects on the host sexual development and reproduction.

6. Conclusion

An interaction between *Wolbachia* and host hormonal signalling pathways involving ecdysteroids may suggest the mechanistic way the bacterium uses for manipulating the host sexual behaviour and reproduction. Thus, the various phenotypic effects induced by the symbiont may be due to differences in the host physiology, considering that endocrine-related processes governing host development and reproduction display an enormous variability.

Recent data demonstrate a role of the symbiont in inducing epigenetic trans-generational changes in the host: by establishing intimate relationships with germ-line cells, epigenetic effects of *Wolbachia* symbiosis are manifested as a 'maternal effect', in which infection of the mother modulates the offspring phenotype. Indeed the *Wolbachia* infection is known to disrupt male imprinting, corresponding to changes in the genomic methylation pattern and in the host sexual phenotype towards females.

These observations raise a key question: what is the molecular basis of such an interaction? Some fascinating clues are provided by the recent demonstrations of interplay between hormone signalling and epigenetic pathways.

The mechanisms exerted by hormones are strictly linked to the epigenetic machinery, where steroids promote sex differences in DNA methylation, methyl-binding proteins and chromatin modifications, even if some epigenetic sex differences can also be directly attributed to the sex chromosomes. According to recent studies, selective nuclear receptor modulators and co-regulators of nuclear receptors are key factors in inducing epigenetic changes via DNA methylation and histone chemical modifications. These complex interactions influence the transcriptional output of many gene networks: the disruption of their normal function or expression by environmental factors can contribute to a vast spectrum of physiological abnormalities and disorders.

Hence, we propose a new perspective supporting a role of the symbiont *Wolbachia* as an "environmental factor" experienced by a mother that promotes heritable epigenetic changes by interaction with hormonal signalling pathways. Although further efforts are needed to fully clarify the genetic and molecular bases of such an interaction, new work hypotheses have been now offered for the study of the mechanisms (yet largely unknown) used by symbionts to dialogue with their hosts. Likewise, the *Wolbachia*-host interaction could become an emerging model system for the study of hormone signalling orchestration by nuclear receptors, and for shedding light on the role of nuclear receptor coregulators in integrating transcriptional coregulation with epigenetic regulation.

7. References

Anway, M.D., Cupp, A.S., Uzumcu, M. & Skinner, M.K. (2005). Epigenetic transgenerational actions of endocrine disruptors and male fertility, *Science* 308:1466- 1469.

Arakaki, N., Miyoshi, T. & Noda, H. (2001). *Wolbachia* mediated parthenogenesis in the predatory thrips *Franklinothrips vespiformis* (Thysanoptera: Insecta), *Proc. R. Soc. Lond. B* 268: 1011–1016.

Arumugam, S., Pfarr, K.M. & Hoerauf, A. (2008). Infection of the intermediate mite host with *Wolbachia*-depleted *Litomosoides sigmodontis* microfilariae: impaired L1 to L3 development and subsequent sex-ratio distortion in adult worms, *Int J Parasitol* 38: 981-7.

Barker, G.C., Mercer, J.G., Rees, H.H. & Howells, R.E. (1991). The effect of ecdysteroids on the microfilarial production of *Brugia pahangi* and the control of meiotic reinitiation in the oocytes of *Dirofilaria immitis, Parasitol Res* 77: 65–71.

Barraclough, C.A. (1961). Production of anovulatory, sterile rats by single injections of testosterone propionate, *Endocrinology* 1: 62–67.

Baum, M.J. (1979). Differentiation of coital behaviour in mammals: a comparative analysis, *Neurosci Biobehav Rev* 4: 265–284.

Beckstead, R.B., Lam, G. & Thummel, C.S. (2007). Specific transcriptional responses to juvenile hormone and ecdysone in *Drosophila, Insect Biochemistry and Molecular Biology* 37: 570–578.

Bender, J. (2004). DNA methylation and epigenetics, *Annu Rev Plant Biol* 55: 41-68.

Beukeboom, L.W., Kamping, A. & van de Zande, L. (2007). Sex determination in the haplodiploid wasp *Nasonia vitripennis* (Hymenoptera: Chalcidoidea): a critical consideration of models and evidence, *Sem Cell Dev Biol* 18: 371-8.

Biddinger, D., Hull, L., Huang, H., McPheron, B. & Loyer, M. (2006). Sublethal effects of chronic exposure to tebufenozide on the development, survival and reproduction of the tufted apple bud moth (Lepidoptera: Tortricidae), *J Econ Entomol* 99: 834-42.

Bouchon, D., Cordaux, R. & Grève, P. (2008). *Feminizing Wolbachia* and evolution of sex determination in isopods, In: *Insect symbiosis*, K. Bourtzis & T.A. Miller (Eds), 273-94, Boca Raton FL., Taylor and Francis Group.

Bownes, M., Blair, M., Kozma, R. & Dempster, M. (1983). 20E stimulates tissue-specific yolk-protein gene transcription in both male and female *Drosophila, J. Embryol. Exp. Morphol.* 78: 249–263.

Bownes, M., Ronaldson, E. & Mauchline, D. (1996). 20-Hydroxyecdysone, but not juvenile hormone, regulation of yolk protein gene Expression can be mapped to cis-acting DNA sequences, *Developmental Biology* 173: 475–489.

Burtis, K.C. & Baker, B.S. (1989). *Drosophila* doublesex gene controls somatic sexual differentiation by producing alternatively spliced mRNAs encoding related sex-specific polypeptides, *Cell* 56 (6): 997-1010.

Burtis, K.C. (2002). Doublesex in the Middle, *Science* 29 (5584): 1135-1136.

Carney, G.E. & Bender, M. (2000). The *Drosophila* ecdysone receptor (EcR) gene is required maternally for normal oogenesis, *Genetics* 154: 1203–1211.

Casiraghi, M., McCall, J.W., Simoncini, L., Kramer, L.H., Sacchi, L., Genchi, C., Werren, J.H. & Bandi, C. (2002). Tetracycline treatment and sex-ratio distortion: a role for *Wolbachia* in the moulting of filarial nematodes?, *Int J Parasitol* 32: 1457-68.
Casper, A.L. & Van Doren, M. (2009). The establishment of sexual identity in the *Drosophila* germline, *Development* 136 (22): 3821-30.
Chang, H.-S., Anway, M.D., Rekow, S.S. & Skinner M.K. (2006). Transgenerational epigenetic imprinting of the male germline by endocrine disruptor exposure during gonadal sex determination, *Endocrinology* 147(12): 5524–5541.
Charniaux-Cotton, H. (1954). Decouverte chez un Crustace Amphipode (*Orchestia gammarella*) d'une glande endocrine responsable de la differenciations des caracteres sexuels primaires et secondaires males, *C.R. Acad. Sci. Paris* 239 : 780–782.
Christiaens, O., Iga, M., Velarde, R. A., Rougé, P. &. Smagghe, G. (2010). Halloween genes and nuclear receptors in ecdysteroid biosynthesis and signalling in the pea aphid, *Insect Molecular Biology* 19 (2): 187–200.
Crossgrove, K., Maina, C.V., Robinson-Rechavi, M. & Lochner, M.C. (2008). Orthologues of the *Drosophila melanogaster* E75 molting control gene in the filarial parasites *Brugia malayi* and *Dirofilaria immitis, Mol Biochem Parasitol* 157: 92-7.
Crouse, H.V. (1960). The controlling element in sex chromosome behaviour in *Sciara, Genetics* 45: 1429-1443.
Cruz ,J., Mané Padròs, D., Belleés, X. & Martin, D. (2006). Functions of the ecdysone receptor isoform-A in the hemimetabolous insect *Blattella germanica* revealed by systemic RNAi in vivo, *Dev Biol* 297: 158-71.
Davis, M.B., Carney, G.E., Robertson, A.E. & Bender, M. (2005). Phenotypic analysis of EcR-A mutants suggests that EcR isoforms have unique functions during *Drosophila* development, *Dev Biol* 282: 385-96.
De Loof, A. & Huybrechts, R. (1998). '"Insects Do Not Have Sex Hormones": a myth?, *General and Comparative Endocrinology* 111: 245–60.
De Loof, A. (2006). Ecdysteroids: the overlooked sex steroids of insect? Males: the black box, *Insect Science* 13: 325-38.
De Loof, A. (2008). Ecdysteroids, juvenile hormone and insect neuropeptides: recent successes and remaining major challenges, *Gen Comp Endocrinol.* 155(1): 3-13.
DeFalco, T., Camara, N., Le Bras, S. & Van Doren, M. (2008). Non-autonomous sex determination controls sexually dimorphic development of the *Drosophila* gonad, *Dev Cell* 14: 275-86.
Dohier, K.D. (1998). Influence of hormones and hormone antagonists on sexual differentiation of the brain, *Arch Toxicol* 9: 131–141.
Dyer, K.A. & Jaenike, J. (2004). Evolutionarily stable infection by a male-killing endosymbiont in *Drosophila innubila*: molecular evidence from the host and parasite genomes, *Genetics* 168: 1443–1455.
Erdman, S.E. & Burtis, K.C. (1993). The *Drosophila* doublesex proteins share a novel zinc finger related DNA binding domain, *EMBO J* 12: 527–535.
Ewer, J. (2005a). How the ecdysozoan changed its coat, *PLoS Biology* 3: 1696-9.
Ewer, J. (2005b). Behavioral actions of neuropeptides in invertebrates: insights from *Drosophila, Hormones and Behavior* 48: 418 – 429.

Fialho, R.F. & Stevens, L. (2000). Male-killing *Wolbachia* in a flour beetle, *Proc. R. Soc. Lond. B* 267: 1469–1473.

Field, L.M., Lyko, F., Mandrioli, M. & Prantera, G. (2004). DNA methylation in insects, *Insect Mol Biol* 13: 109- 15.

Ford, A.T. (2008). Can you feminise a crustacean? *Aquatic Toxicology*, 88: 316–321.

Foster J., et al. (2005). The *Wolbachia* genome of *Brugia malayi*: endosymbiont evolution within a human pathogenic nematode, *PLoS Biol* 3: e121.

Frank, K., Frank, K. & Heald, R.D. (2010). The emerging role of *Wolbachia* species in heartworm disease, *Compend Contin Educ Vet.* 32(4): E1-5.

Frydman H. M., Li J.M., Robson D.N. & Wieschaus, E. (2006). Somatic stem cell niche tropism in *Wolbachia*, *Nature* 441: 509-512.

Gabory, A., Attig, L. & Junien, C. (2009). Sexual dimorphism in environmental epigenetic programming, *Molecular and Cellular Endocrinology* 304: 8–18.

Ganter, G.K., Walton, K.L., Merriman, J.O., Salmon, M.V., Brooks, K.M., Maddula, S. & Kravitz, E.A. (2007). Increased male male courtship in ecdysone receptor deficient adult flies, *Behav Genet* 37:507-12.

Gaziova, I., Bonnette, P.C., Henrich, V.C. & Jindra, M. (2004). Cell-autonomous roles of the ecdysoneless gene in *Drosophila* development and oogenesis, *Development* 131: 2715-25.

Ghedin, E., et al. (2007). Draft genome of the filarial nematode parasite *Brugia malayi*, *Science* 317: 1756- 60.

Gilbert L.I., Rybczynski, R. & Warren, J.T. (2002). Control and biochemical nature of the ecdysteroidogenic pathway, *Annu. Rev. Entomol.* 47: 883–916.

Gilbert, S.F. (2000). *Developmental Biology* (6th edition), Sinauer Associates, Sunderland (MA).

Giorgini, M., Monti, M.M., Caprio, E., Stouthamer, R. & Hunter, M.S. (2009). Feminization and the collapse of haplodiploidy in an asexual parasitoid wasp harboring the bacterial symbiont *Cardinium*, Heredity 102(4): 365-71.

Goll, M.G. & Bestor, T.H. (2005). Eukaryotic cytosine methyltransferases, *Annu. Rev. Biochem.* 74: 481–514.

Gonella, E., Negri, I., Marzorati, M., Mandrioli, M., Sacchi, L., Pajoro, M., Crotti, E., Rizzi, A., Clementi, E., Tedeschi, R., Bandi, C., Alma, A. & Daffonchio, D. (2011). Bacterial endosymbiont localization in *Hyalesthes obsoletus*, the insect vector of Bois Noir in *Vitis vinifera*, *Applied and Environmental Microbiology*, 77(4):1423-35.

Guiguen, Y., Fostier A., Piferrer, F. & Chang, C.F. (2010). Ovarian aromatase and estrogens: a pivotal role for gonadal sex differentiation and sex change in fish, *Gen Comp Endocrinol.* 165(3): 352-66.

Hahn, T., Liess, M. & Schulz, R. (2001). Effects of the hormone mimetic insecticide tebufenozide on *Chironomus riparius* larvae in two different exposure setups, *Ecotox Environ Safe* 49: 171-8.

Herpin, A. & Schartl, M. (2011). Dmrt1 genes at the crossroad: a widespread and central class of sexual development factors in fish, *FEBS J.* 278(7): 1010-9.

Hilgenboecker, K., Hammerstein, P., Schlattmann, P., Telschow, A. & Werren, J. H. (2008). How many species are infected with *Wolbachia*? — a statistical analysis of current data, *FEMS Microbiol. Lett.* 281: 215–220.

Hiroki, M., Kato, Y., Kamito, T. & Miura, K. (2002). Feminizationof genetic males by a simbiotic bacterium in a butterfly, *Eurema hecabe* (Lepidoptera: Pieridae), *Naturwissenschaften* 89: 67-70.

Höss, S. & Weltje, L. (2007). Endocrine disruption in nematodes: effects and mechanisms, *Ecotoxicology* 16: 15-28.

Hsia, E.Y., Goodson, M.L., Zou, J.X., Privalsky, M.L. & Chen, H.W. (2010). Nuclear receptor coregulators as a new paradigm for therapeutic targeting, *Adv Drug Deliv Rev.* 62 (13): 1227-37.

Huybrechts, R. & De Loof, A. (1977). Induction of vitellogenin synthesis in male *Sarcophaga bullata* by ecdysterone, *Journalof Insect Physiology* 23: 1359-1362.

Iturbe-Ormaetxe, I. & O'Neill, S. (2007). *Wolbachia*-host interactions: connecting phenotype to genotype, *CurrOpin Microbiol* 10:1-4.

Izumi, N., Yanagibori, R., Shigeno, S. & Sajiki, J. (2008). Effects of bisphenol A on the development, growth and sex ratio of the housefly *Musca domestica, Environ Toxicol Chem* 27: 1343-53.

Janer, G. & Porte, C. (2007). Sex steroids and potential mechanisms of non-genomic endocrine disruption in invertebrates, *Ecotoxicology* 16:145–160.

Jiggins, F.M., Hurst, G.D., Schulenburg, J. H. & Majerus, M. E. (2001). Two male-killing *Wolbachia* strains coexist within a population of the butterfly *Acraea encedon, Heredity* 86: 161–166.

Juchault, P. & Legrand, J.J. (1985). Mechanism of the refractory state of androgen hormone in *Armadillidium vulgare* Latr. (crustacean, isopod, oniscoid) harboring a feminizing bacteria, *Gen Comp Endocrinol* 60: 463-7.

Kageyama, D. & Traut, W. (2003). Opposite sex-specific effects of *Wolbachia* and interference with the sex determination of its host *Ostrinia scapulalis, Proc R Soc B* 271: 251-8.

Kamoda, S., Masui, S., Ishikawa, H. & Sasaki, T. (2000). *Wolbachia* infection and cytoplasmic incompatibility in the cricket *Teleogryllus taiwanemma, J Exp Biol* 203: 2503-9.

Kato, S., Yokoyama, A. & Fujiki, R. (2011). Nuclear receptor coregulators merge transcriptional coregulation with epigenetic regulation, *Trends in Biochemical Sciences* 36 (5): 272-281.

Kozlova, T. & Thummel, C.S. (2003). Essential roles for ecdysone signaling during *Drosophila* mid-embryonic development, *Science* 301:1911-4.

Laugé, G. (1985). Sex determination: Genetic and epigenetic factors, In: *Comprehensive Insect Physiology, Biochemistry and Pharmacology*, vol. 1, Embryogenesis and Reproduction, G. A. Kerkut & L. I. Gilbert (Eds), 295-318, Pergamon Press, Oxford.

Lee, S.-B. & Choi, J. (2007). Effects of bisphenol A and ethynyl estradiol exposure on enzyme activities, growth and development in the fourth instar larvae of *Chironomus riparius* (Diptera, Chironomidae), *Ecotoxicology and Environmental Safety* 68 (1): 84-90.

Legrand, J.J., Legrand-Hamelin, E. & Juchault, P. (1987). Sex determination in Crustacea, *Biol Rev* 62: 439-70.

Lobbia, S., Niitsu, S. & Fujiwara, H. (2003). Female-specific wing degeneration caused by ecdysteroid in the Tussock Moth, *Orgyia recens*: hormonal and developmental regulation of sexual dimorphism, *J Insect Sci* 3: 1-7.

Lyko, F. & Maleszka, R. (2011). Insects as innovative models for functional studies of DNA methylation, *Trends in Genetics* 27(4): 127-31.

Mahajan, M.A. & Samuels, H.H. (2000). A new family of nuclear receptor coregulators that integrate nuclear receptor signaling through CREB-binding protein, *Molecular and Cellular Biology* 20 (14): 5048-5063.

Martin, C.C. & McGowan, R. (1995). Genotype-specific modifiers of transgene methylation and expression in the zebrafish, *Danio rerio, Genet. Res.* 65: 21-28.

Martin, G., Juchault, P. & Legrand, J.J. (1973). Mise en évidence d'un micro-organisme intracytoplasmique symbiotede l'oniscoïde *Armadillidium vulgare* Latreille dont la présence accompagne l'intersexualité ou la féminisation totale des mâles génétiques de la lignée thélygène, *C R Acad Sc Paris* 276: 2313-6.

Martin, G., Sorokine, O., Moniatte, M., Bulet, P., Hetru, C. & Van Dorsselaer, A. (1999). The structure of a glycosylated protein hormone responsible for sex determination in the isopod, *Armadillidium vulgare, Eur J Biochem* 262: 727-36.

Matsuda M., Nagahama, Y., Shinomiya, A., Sato, T., Matsuda, C., Kobayashi, T., Morrey, C.E., Shibata, N., Asakawa, S., Shimizu, N., Hori, H., Hamaguchi, S. & Sakaizumi, M. (2002). DMY is a Y-specific DM-domain gene required for male development in the medaka fish, *Nature* 417: 559–563.

McCarthy, M.M., Auger, A.P., Bale, T.L., De Vries, G.J., Dunn, G.A., Forger, N.G., Murray, E.K., Nugent, B.M., Schwarz, J.M. & Wilson, M.E. (2009). The epigenetics of sex differences in the brain, *The Journal of Neuroscience* 29(41):12815–12823.

Motola, D.L., Cummins, C.L., Rottiers, V., Sharma, K.K., Li, T.T., Li, Y., Suino-Powell, K., Xu, H.E., Auchus, R.J., Antebi, A. & Mangelsdorf, D.J. (2006). Identification of ligands for DAF-12 that govern dauer formation and reproduction in *C. elegans, Cell* 124: 1209-23.

Mottier, V. , Siaussat, D., Bozzolan, F., Auzoux-Bordenave, S., Porcheron, P. & Debernard, S. (2004). The 20-hydroxyecdysone-induced cellular arrest in G2 phase is preceded by an inhibition of cyclin expression, *Insect Biochemistry and Molecular Biology* 34: 51–60.

Murphy, M.W., Sarver, A.L., Rice, D., Hatzi, K., Ye, K., Melnick, A., Heckert, Zarkower, D. & Bardwell, V.J. (2010). Genome-wide analysis of DNA binding and transcriptional regulation by the mammalian Doublesex homolog DMRT1 in the juvenile testis, *Proc Natl Acad Sci USA* 107 (30): 13360–13365.

Nakamura, M. J. (2010). The Mechanism of Sex Determination in Vertebrates—Are Sex Steroids the Key-Factor? *Exp. Zool.* 313: 381–398.

Nakamura, M.J. (2009). Sex determination in amphibians, *Semin Cell Dev Biol.* 20(3): 271-82.

Narita, S., Kageyama, D., Nomura, M. & Fukatsu, T. (2007). Unexpected mechanism of symbiont-induced reversal of insect sex: feminizing *Wolbachia* continuously acts on the butterfly *Eurema hecabe* during larval development, *Appl Environ Microbiol.* 73(13): 4332–4341.

Negri, I., Franchini, A., Gonella, E., Daffonchio, D., Mazzoglio, P.J., Mandrioli, M. & Alma, A. (2009a). Unravelling the *Wolbachia* evolutionary role: the reprogramming of the host genomic imprinting, *Proc R Soc B* 276: 2485-91.

Negri, I., Mazzoglio, P.J., Franchini, A., Mandrioli, M. & Alma, A. (2009b). Male or female? The epigenetic conflict between a feminizing bacterium and its insect host, *Communicative & Integrative Biology* 2 (6): 1-2.

Negri, I., Pellecchia, M., Grève, P., Daffonchio, D., Bandi, C. & and Alma, A. (2010). Sex and stripping: The key to the intimate relationship between *Wolbachia* and host? *Communicative & Integrative Biology* 3:2, 1-6.

Negri, I., Pellecchia, M., Mazzoglio, P.J., Patetta, A. & Alma, A. (2006). Feminizing *Wolbachia* in *Zyginidia pullula* (Insecta, Hemiptera), a leafhopper with an XX/X0 sex-determination system, *Proc R Soc B* 273: 2409-16.

Norris, D.O. & Carr, J.A. (2006). *Endocrine disruption: biological basis for health effects in wildlife and humans,* Oxford University Press, Oxford.

Nugent, B.M. & McCarthy, M.M. (2011). Epigenetic underpinnings of developmental sex differences in the brain, *Neuroendocrinology* 93(3): 150-8.

Oakes, M.B, Eyvazzadeh, A.D., Quint, E. & Smith, Y.R. (2008). Complete androgen insensitivity syndrome--a review, *J Pediatr Adolesc Gynecol.* 21(6): 305-10.

Oehlmann, J., Schulte-Oehlmann, U., Bachmann, J., Oetken, M., Lutz, I., Kloas, W. & Ternes, T.A. (2007). Bisphenol A induces superfeminization in the Ramshorn Snail *Marisa cornuarietis* (Gastropoda: Prosobranchia) at environmentally relevant concentrations, *Environmental Health Perspectives* 114 (1): 127-133.

Pathak, S., D'Souza, R., Ankolkar, M., Gaonkar, R. & Balasinor, N.H. (2010). Potential role of estrogen in regulation of the Insulin-like growth factor2–H19 locus in the rat testis, *Mol Cell Endocrinol.* 314(1): 110-7.

Pathak, S., Kedia-Mokashi, N., Saxena, M., D'Souza, R., Maitra, A., Parte, P., Gill-Sharma, M. & Balasinor, N.H. (2009). Effect of tamoxifen treatment on global and Insulin-like growth factor 2-H19 locus specific DNA methylation in rat spermatozoa and its association with embryo loss, *Fertil. Steril.* 91: 2253–2263.

Raikhel, A.S., Brown, M. & Belles, X. (2005). Hormonal control of reproductive processes, In: *Comprehensive Insect Physiology, Biochemistry, Pharmacology and Molecular Biology,* Vol. 3, Endocrinology, L. Gilbert, S. Gill & K. Iatrou (Eds), 433-491, Elsevier Press.

Raymond, C.S., Shamu, C.E., Shen, M.M., Seifert, K.J., Hirsch, B., Hodgkin, J. & Zarkower, D. (1998). Evidence for evolutionary conservation of sex-determining genes, *Nature* 391: 691–695.

Rewitz, K. F., O'Connor, M.B. & Gilbert, L. I. (2007). Molecular evolution of the insect Halloween family of cytochromeP450s: phylogeny, gene organization and functional conservation, *Insect Biochemistry and Molecular Biology,* 37: 741–753.

Riddiford, LM. (1993). Hormones and *Drosophila* development, In: *The Development of Drosophila melanogaster,* M. Bate & A.M. Arias (Eds), 899–939, Cold Spring Harbor Laboratory Press

Rideout, E.J., Dornan, A.J., Neville, M.C., Eadie S. & Goodwin, S.F. (2010). Control of sexual differentiation and behavior by the doublesex gene in *Drosophila melanogaster, Nature Neuroscience* 13: 458–466.

Rigaud, T. & Juchault, P. (1998). Sterile intersexuality in an isopod induced by the interaction between a bacterium (*Wolbachia*) and the environment, *Can J Zool* 76: 493-9.

Rigaud, T., Moreau, J. & Juchault, P. (1999). *Wolbachia* infection in the terrestrial isopod *Oniscus asellus*: sex ratio distortion and effect on fecundity, *Heredity* 83: 469-75.

Rosenfeld, M.G., Lunyak, V.V. & Glass, C.K. (2006). Sensors and signals: a coactivator/corepressor/epigenetic code for integrating signal-dependent programs of transcriptional response, *Genes & Development* 20: 1405–1428.

Sacchi, L., Genchi, M., Clementi, E., Negri, I., Alma, A., Ohler, S., Sassera, D., Bourtzis, K. & Bandi, C. (2010). Bacteriocyte-like cells harbour *Wolbachia* in the ovary of *Drosophila melanogaster* (Insecta, Diptera) and *Zyginidia pullula* (Insecta, Hemiptera), *Tissue Cell.* 42(5): 328-33.

Sagi, A. & Khalaila, I. (2001). The crustacean androgen: a hormone in an isopod and androgenic activity in decapods, *Amer. Zool.* 41: 477–484.

Sagi, A., Snir, E. & Khalaila, I. (1997). Sexual differentiation in decapod crustaceans: role of the androgenic gland, *Invertebr. Reprod. Dev.* 31: 55–61.

Sakamoto, H., Kageyama, D., Hoshizaki, S. & Yshikawa, Y. (2007). Sex specific death in the Asian corn borer moth (*Ostrinia furnacalis*) infected by *Wolbachia* occurs across larval development, *Genome* 50:645-52.

Schütt, C. & Nöthiger, R. (2000). Structure, function and evolution of sex-determining systems in Dipteran insects, *Development* 127: 667-77.

Sharman, G.B. (1971). Late DNA replication in the paternally derived X chromosome of female kangaroos, *Nature* 230: 231-232.

Smith, C.A., Roeszler, K.N., Ohnesorg, T., Cummins, D.M., Farlie, P.G., Doran, T.J. & Sinclair, A.H. (2009). The avian Z-linked gene DMRT1 is required for male sex determination in the chicken, *Nature* 461: 267–271.

Steinmann-Zwicky, M., Schmid, H. & Nöthiger, R. (1989). Cell-autonomous and inductive signals can determine the sex of the germ line of *Drosophila* by regulating the gene Sxl, *Cell* 57(1): 157-66.

Stouthamer, R., Breeuwer, J. A. & Hurst, G. D. (1999). *Wolbachia pipientis*: microbial manipulator of arthropod reproduction, *Annu. Rev. Microbiol.* 53: 71–102.

Stouthamer, R., Luck, R. F. & Hamilton, W. D. (1990). Antibiotics cause parthenogenetic *Trichogramma* (Hymenoptera/Trichogrammatidae) to revert to sex, *Proc. Natl Acad. Sci. USA* 87, 2424–2427.

Sugimoto, T.N., Fujii, T., Kayukawa, T., Sakamoto, H. & Ishikawa, Y. (2010). Expression of a *doublesex* homologue is altered in sexual mosaics of *Ostrinia scapulalis* moths infected with *Wolbachia, Insect Biochem Mol Biol.* 40(12): 847-54.

Surani, M.A. (1998). Imprinting and the initiation of gene silencing in the germ line, *Cell* 93: 309-312.

Suzuki, S. & Yamasaki, Y. (1998). Sex reversal by implantations of ethanol-treated androgenic glands of female isopods, *Armadillidium vulgare* (Malacostraca, Crustacea), *General and Comparative Endocrinology* 111: 367–375.

Swevers, L. & Iatrou, K. (2003). The ecdysone regulatory cascade and ovarian development in lepidopteran insects: insights from the silkmoth paradigm, *Insect Biochemistry and Molecular Biology* 33: 1285–1297.

Swevers, L., Raikhel, A.S., Sappington, T.W., Shirk, P. & Iatrou, K. (2005). Vitellogenesis and post-vitellogenic maturation of the insect ovarian follicle. In: *Comprehensive Molecular Insect Science,* vol.1, Reproduction and Development, L.I. Gilbert, K. Iatrou & S.S. Gill (Eds), 87-156, Elsevier Ltd., Oxford, UK.

Thummel , C.S. & Cory, J. (2002). Steroid signaling in plants and insects – common themes, different pathways, *Genes and Development* 16 (24): 3113–3129.

Tsai, H.-W., Grant, P.A. & and Rissman, E.F. (2009). Sex differences in histone modifications in the neonatal mouse brain, *Epigenetics* 4(1): 47–53.

Tsuzuki, S., Iwami, M. & Sakurai, S. (2001). Ecdysteroid-inducible genes in the programmed cell death during insect metamorphosis, *Insect Biochemistry and Molecular Biology* 31: 321–331.

Tzertzinis, G., Egaña, A.L., Palli, S.R., Robinson-Rechavi, M., Gissendanner, C.R., Liu, C., Unnasch, T.R. & Maina, C.V. (2010). Molecular evidence for a functional ecdysone signaling system in *Brugia malayi*, *PLoS Negl Trop Dis.* 4(3): e625.

Vreeburg, J., van der Vaart, P.D.M. & Van Der Schoot, P. (1977). Prevention of central defeminization but not masculinization in male rats by inhibition neonatally of oestrogen biosynthesis, *J Endocrinol* 74: 375-382.

Wang, C. & Croll, R.P. (2004). Effects of sex steroids on gonadal development and gender determination in the sea scallop, *Placopecten magellanicus*, *Aquaculture* 238: 483–498.

Warbrick, E.V., Barker, G.C., Rees, H.H. & Howells, R.E. (1993). The effect of invertebrate hormones and potential hormone inhibitors on the third larval moult of the filarial nematode, *Dirofilaria immitis*, in vitro, *Parasitology* 107: 459-63.

Waterbury, J. A., Horabin, J. I., Bopp, D. & Schedl, P. (2000). Sex determination in the *Drosophila* germline is dictated by the sexual identity of the surrounding soma, *Genetics* 155: 1741–1756.

Waterbury, J. A., Jackson, L. L. & Schedl, P. (1999). Analysis of the doublesex female protein in *Drosophila melanogaster*: role in sexual differentiation and behavior and dependence on intersex, *Genetics* 152: 1653–1667.

Weeks, A. R. & Breeuwer, J. A. (2001). *Wolbachia*-induced parthenogenesis in a genus of phytophagous mites, *Proc. R. Soc. Lond. B* 268, 2245–2251.

Werren, J.H., Baldo, L. & Clark, M.E. (2008). *Wolbachia*: master manipulators of invertebrate biology, *Nat RevMicrobiol* 6: 741-51.

White, M.J.D. (1973). *Animal cytology and Evolution* (Third Edition), Cambridge University Press, Cambridge.

Whiting, P.W., Greb, R.J. & Speicher, B.R. (1934). A new type of sex-intergrade, *Biol. Bull.* 66: 152-165.

Wu, M. et al. (2004). Phylogenomics of the reproductive parasite *Wolbachia pipientis* wMel: a streamlined genome overrun by mobile genetic elements, *PLoS Biol.* 2: 327–341.

Yoshimoto, S., Okada, E., Umemoto, H., Tamura, K., Uno, Y., Nishida-Umehara, C., Matsuda, Y., Takamatsu, N., Shiba, T. & Ito, M. (2008). A W-linked DM-domain gene, DM-W, participates in primary ovary development in *Xenopus laevis*, *Proc Natl Acad Sci USA* 105: 2469–2474.

Zeh, D. W., Zeh, J. A. & Bonilla, M. M. (2005). *Wolbachia*, sex ratio bias and apparent male killing in the harlequin beetle riding pseudoscorpion, *Heredity* 95: 41–49.

Zhu, J., Chen, L. & Raikhel, A.S. (2007). Distinct roles of Broad isoforms in regulation of the 20-hydroxyecdysone effector gene, Vitellogenin, in the mosquito *Aedes aegypti*, *Mol Cell Endocrinol.* 267(1-2): 97–105.

Zhu, L., Wilken, J., Phillips, N.B., Narendra, U., Chan, G., Stratton, S.M., Kent, S.B. & Weiss, M.A. (2000). Sexual dimorphism in diverse metazoans is regulated by a novel class of intertwined zinc fingers, *Genes Dev* 14: 1750–1764.

Zitnan, D., Kim, Y.-J., Zitnanova, I., Roller, L. & Adams, M.E. (2007). Complex steroid–peptide–receptor cascade controls insect ecdysis, *General and Comparative Endocrinology* 153: 88–96.

18

Tissue-Specific Regulation of Sex Hormone Biosynthesis and Metabolism: Novel Aspects on Hormonal Signalling and Maintenance of Cellular Steroid Levels

Maria Norlin and Kjell Wikvall
Department of Pharmaceutical Biosciences, Uppsala University, Uppsala, Sweden

1. Introduction

In this chapter, we intend to review our recent research in the context of contemporary research in the field of sex hormone biosynthesis and metabolism. Our findings have revealed novel aspects on the regulation of sex hormone metabolism and the metabolic control of cellular levels and effects of estrogens, androgens and neurosteroids. We will discuss our results in relation to current knowledge of metabolism and actions of estrogens and androgens. First, an introduction to this research field will be given.

2. Sex hormones: Biosynthesis, metabolism and actions

2.1 Biosynthesis and metabolism of sex hormones: An introduction

The sex hormones, estrogens and androgens, are present in almost all tissues and affect such diverse processes as bone formation, sexual function, brain development, cardiovascular and immune systems and growth of various organs (Arnal et al., 2007; Cheskis et al., 2007; Folkerd et al., 2010; Li & Al-Azzawi, 2009). One of the tissues, where hormonal control of growth is essential, is the prostate, where androgens as well as estrogens play a role (Prins & Korach, 2008; Weihua et al., 2002). Although the physiological levels are different, both androgens and estrogens are needed in both sexes.

The biosynthesis and metabolism of estrogens and androgens involve many different enzymes expressed in multiple organs (Miller et al., 2008; Norlin, 2008; Simard et al., 2005; Vihko et al., 2006). Large amounts of steroids, including sex hormone precursors are enzymatically formed in the adrenals, using cholesterol as starting material, and secreted to the circulation (Fig. 1). The formed sex hormone precursors may then be taken up by gonads and other organs for further metabolism to different androgenic and estrogenic compounds. The most important precursors for sex hormones are androstenedione and dehydroepiandrosterone (DHEA) and its sulphate, DHEA-S (Fig. 1). This large-scale production of precursors, available for transport to other tissues, is essential for reproductive functions and sexual development, including the formation of genitalia

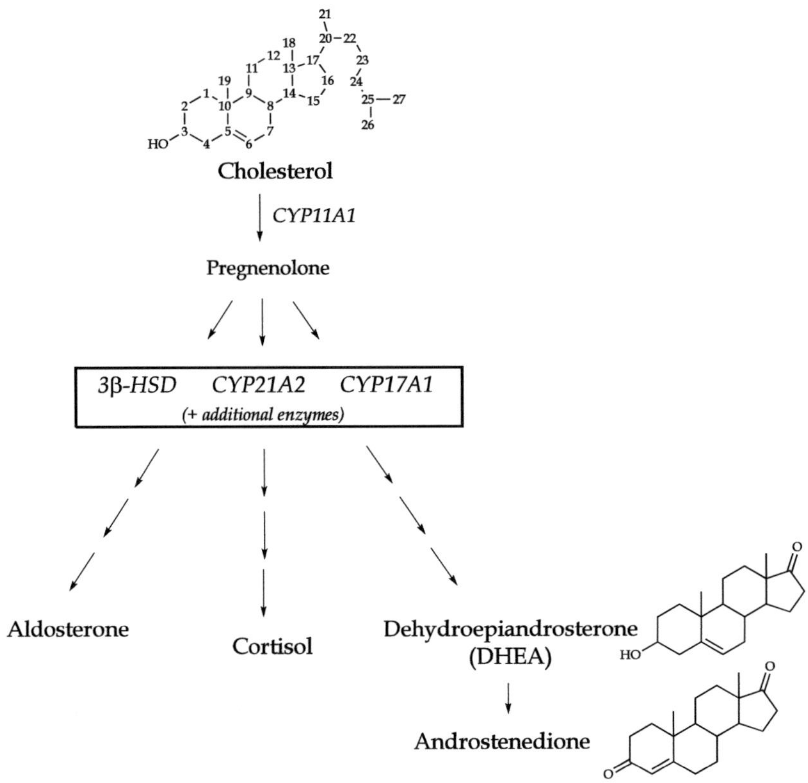

Fig. 1. A simplified overview on the biosynthesis of steroid hormones in the adrenal cortex.

(Rainey et al., 2004; Sultan et al., 2001). A sex hormone precursor may undergo different metabolic transformations in different cells, depending on which enzymes that are expressed in a certain tissue and how these enzymes are regulated. In addition to the uptake of precursors transported from the adrenals, many tissues have the ability to carry out all the steps in estrogen and androgen synthesis. Thus, cell-specific needs for these hormones may be controlled locally in each tissue (Hudak et al., 2006; Penning et al., 2000; Tsuchiya et al., 2005). Local metabolism, dependent on various tissue-specific enzymes, is essential to achieve hormonal effects and to eliminate excess hormone from the cells.

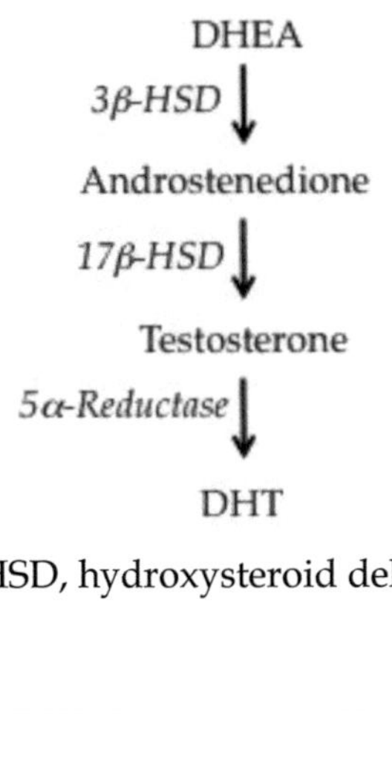

Fig. 2. Formation of androgens. HSD, hydroxysteroid dehydrogenases.

Several androgens are formed in humans (Bauman et al., 2006; Hudak et al., 2006; Weihua et al., 2002). A well-known androgen, testosterone, is formed in large amounts in several tissues, including the Leydig cells of the testes (Fig. 2). Testosterone levels are strongly influenced by the levels of its precursors, androstenedione and DHEA, in the blood circulation. Target tissues can convert testosterone into dihydrotestosterone (DHT), the most potent androgen, 10-fold more potent than testosterone (Fig. 2). Maintenance of adequate cellular levels of DHT is essential for a number of physiological processes, including sexual development and testicular function.

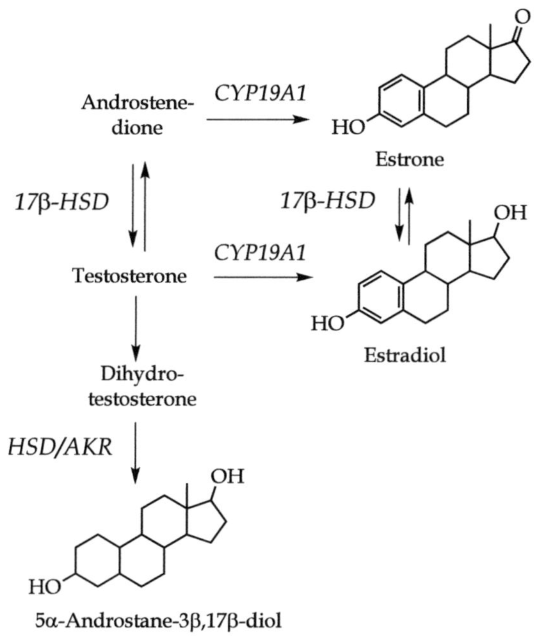

Fig. 3. Formation of some estrogens. HSD, hydroxysteroid dehydrogenases; AKR, aldo-keto reductases

The physiologically most potent estrogen is estradiol (17β-estradiol). The levels of estradiol are dependent on the enzymatic activity of aromatase (CYP19A1) which forms estradiol from testosterone (Bulun et al., 2009; Simpson et al., 2002) (Fig. 3). In addition, there are several other endogenous estrogens that affect various organs and cells (Norlin et al., 2008; Pettersson et al., 2008; Weihua et al., 2002; Zhu et al., 2005). Individual estrogens may be of different importance in different tissues. For instance, 5α-androstane-3β,17β-diol (3β-Adiol) has been described as particularly important for estrogenic function in the prostate (Weihua et al., 2002). An overview of enzymes in the formation of some estrogenic steroids is shown in Fig. 3.
The total body levels of sex hormones are regulated by signalling from the pituitary and by mechanisms for excretion by the kidneys or in the bile (Bourdeau & Stratakis, 2002; Hum et al., 1999; Waxman & Holloway, 2009). In addition, cell-specific factors and mechanisms are important for regulation of the local sex hormone synthesis and elimination (Jellinck et al., 2007; Norlin, 2008; Penning et al., 2000; Reddy, 2004). Estrogens and androgens are removed from the body via metabolism into inactive metabolites that are excreted in the urine and/or feces. Local metabolism of importance for tissue hormone levels vary for different steroids

and different tissues. Mechanisms believed to be of importance involve e. g. hydroxylation by cytochrome P450 (CYP) enzymes and conjugation with sulfate or glucuronic acid by the UDP-glucuronosyl transferases (UGT) and sulfotransferases (SULT) (Tang et al., 2006; Turgeon et al., 2001 Zhu et al., 2005) (Figs. 4 and 5).

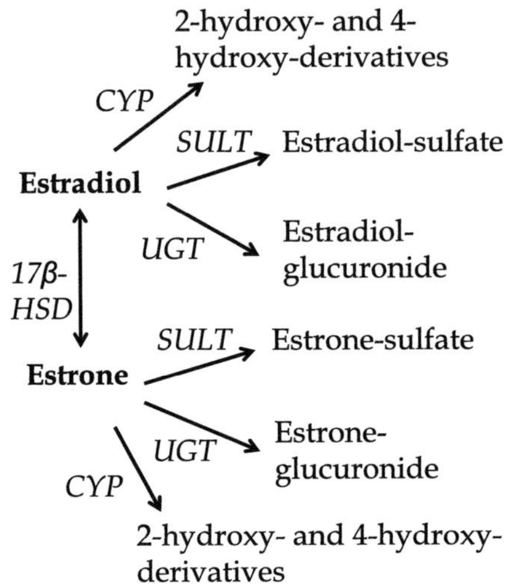

Fig. 4. Metabolic pathways that may affect the levels of estradiol and estrone. Please note that this figure is intended as an overview of potentially important pathways and does not necessarily describe the situation in any particular cell. AKR, aldo-keto reductases; CYP, cytochrome P450; HSD, hydroxysteroid dehydrogenases; SULT, sulfotransferases; UGT, UDP-glucuronosyl transferases.

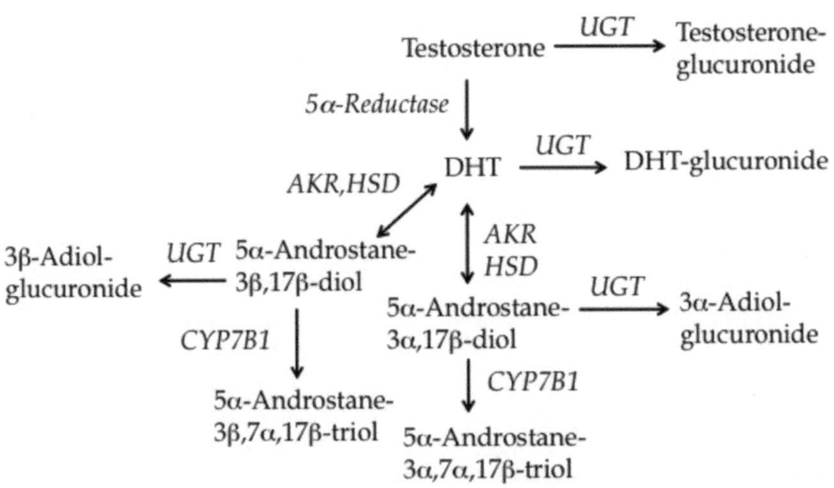

Fig. 5. Metabolic pathways that may affect the cellular levels of testosterone and its metabolites. Please note that this figure is intended as an overview of potentially important pathways and does not necessarily describe the situation in any particular cell. For abbreviations, see legend of Fig. 4.

2.2 Physiological and pharmacological actions of sex hormones and sex hormone-related compounds

Many of the cellular effects of estrogens and androgens are mediated via the classical sex hormone receptors, the androgen receptor, AR, and the two estrogen receptors, ERα and ERβ (Brinkmann et al., 1999; Cheskis et al., 2007; Li & Al-Azzawi, 2009; Prins & Korach, 2008). The actions of estrogens and androgens are often mediated via hormone-responsive sequences in target gene promoters, the "androgen response elements" (ARE) and "estrogen response elements" (ERE). Sex hormones are also able to act via mechanisms independent of the AR and ER (Bryant et al., 2006; Cheskis et al., 2007; Lorenzo & Saatcioglu 2008). Such mechanisms may involve signal transduction pathways, for instance MAPK (mitogen-activated protein kinase) or PI3K (phosphoinositide 3-kinase)/Akt signal pathways. Crosstalk between proteins of these signal pathways and estrogen receptors also have been reported for some hormonal targets. Additional pathways for hormonal action are believed to be mediated by different types of hormone receptors located at the cell membrane. Sex hormone-related compounds used in therapy include antagonists of ER and AR and selective hormone receptor modulators (SERMs and SARMs, respectively) (Bhasin & Jasuja, 2009; Cheskis et al., 2007; Jordan, 2007). Selective hormone receptor modulators function as agonists in some tissues and antagonists in others, resulting in different tissue-specific responses.

Despite the essential roles of sex hormones in a large number of physiological processes, excess amounts of these compounds can have a negative impact and even contribute to disease. Adverse effects of estrogens include e. g. intrahepatic cholestasis, which may occur in some women using oral contraceptives or during pregnancy, where this condition can result in premature delivery or fetal death (Yamamoto et al., 2006). Many breast tumours are dependent on estrogen for growth and are reported to exhibit increased estradiol biosynthesis. For this reason, inhibitors of the estradiol-forming aromatase (CYP19A1) are routinely used in treatment of breast cancer (Chen, 1998). Furthermore, although the growth-inducing effect of androgens are required for formation and normal function of the prostate, overproduction of androgens can contribute substantially to unwanted growth of this tissue e. g. in malignancy. Treatment to suppress androgen action and/or formation have therefore proven very useful in prostate cancer therapy as well as in treatment of benign prostate hyperplasia (Bauman et al., 2006; Hudak et al., 2006). In general, transformation into malignancy may elicit changes in both sex hormone concentrations and effects of sex hormones on growth (Bauman et al., 2006; Vihko et al., 2006). Marked changes in androgen and estrogen metabolism have been reported for many malignant cells. However, abnormalities in hormone synthesis and metabolism are not only found in malignancy. Although the functions of sex hormones formed in the CNS have been much less studied than those of the reproductive organs, disturbed synthesis and/or metabolism of several brain steroids have been described in neurodegenerative disease (Cossec et al., 2010; Schaeffer et al., 2006).

2.3 Cell- and tissue-specific steroid metabolism – role(s) for controlling cellular levels and effects of sex hormones

Steroid hormone metabolism is not the same everywhere in the body. Due to the different physiological demands that will arise in various tissues and during different conditions, the level of a certain hormone at a given time need to be carefully controlled. Also, not all cells need the same types of hormones. Often, a steroid hormone may potentially undergo several different metabolic pathways. However, one pathway may be particularly active in a certain tissue but absent in another tissue where a different pathway dominates. Metabolism of a steroid could also lead to a host of metabolites in the same tissue, via different enzymatic steps, all of which can be differentially affected by endogenous or exogenous regulators. Consequently, since the effect(s) of a hormone are dependent on its concentration, the metabolic pathways in a cell or tissue can have a considerable impact on which cellular actions that takes place.

An example of a steroid metabolized into many different compounds is dehydroepiandrosterone (DHEA) (Norlin, 2008; Rainey, 2004). This steroid is reported to have a number of effects of its own but, as described in the Introductory section, it is also essential as a precursor for a number of other hormones, with their own individual effects. The activity of the enzymes and genes involved in formation of these different products can all be differentially regulated.

Our knowledge on the cellular metabolic events that involve steroid hormones is far from sufficient. A proper understanding of these events would substantially increase the possibilities to intervene in physiological processes involving these hormones, such as cellular growth, dysfunctions of the reproductive and immune systems and a number of processes important for brain function. Even though there is a clear link between the serum levels of a hormone and its physiological effect(s), the levels of hormones present in a tissue often differs substantially from the levels measured in serum. Unfortunately, the steroid levels in tissue material are much more problematical to assay than the serum levels. Other complicating factors are the complex interplay of enzymes and regulatory molecules leading to formation of a certain compound and the existence of different cell-types with specific properties within the same tissue.

3. Sex hormones and vitamin D

In recent years, vitamin D has attracted increasing attention for its ability to regulate numerous genes in several physiological processes. In the following sections, a brief overview of the vitamin D hormone and discussion of data regarding the effects on sex hormone biosynthesis and metabolism will be given.

3.1 Vitamin D is activated to a multifunctional hormone with effects on gene expression

The prohormone vitamin D_3 (cholecalciferol) is synthesized in the skin on exposure to ultraviolet light and is also acquired from the diet (Holick, 1987). Vitamin D is needed for regulation of calcium levels in the body and vitamin D deficiency leads to skeletal diseases such as rickets in children and osteomalacia/osteoporosis in adults (Brown et al., 1999; DeLuca, 2004; Dusso et al., 2005; Jones et al., 1998). The role of vitamin D in human health and disease has received increased recognition in recent years. Although it was previously considered to be limited to regulation of calcium levels, recent data from epidemiological studies and basic sciences have expanded our understanding of its pivotal role in many biological processes. Vitamin D is important not only for endocrine functions, such as calcium homeostasis, but also for autocrine and/or paracrine functions, such as regulation of immune system, brain and fetal development, insulin secretion, apoptosis, cell proliferation and differentiation as well as involvement in cancer and the cardiovascular system. Most of these actions are mediated by transcriptional regulation of target genes through the vitamin D receptor (VDR), a member of the nuclear receptor superfamily of transcription factors (Armas & Heaney, 2011; Atkins et al., 2007; Norman, 2006, 2008; Verstuyf et al., 2010).

The active vitamin D_3 hormone, 1α,25-dihydroxy-vitamin D_3 (calcitriol), is formed through metabolic bioactivation by cytochrome P450 (CYP450) enzymes (Jones et al., 1998; Prosser & Jones, 2004; Wikvall, 2001). The activation of vitamin D requires two sequential hydroxylations (Fig. 6). The first step is a 25-hydroxylation of vitamin D_3 producing 25-hydroxyvitamin D_3 or calcidiol. A number of cytochrome P450-enzymes are capable of performing the 25-hydroxylation and in most organisms studied at least two 25-hydroxylases have been found - the mitochondrial CYP27A1 and the microsomal CYP2R1 (Cheng et al., 2003, 2004; Dahlbäck & Wikvall, 1988; Gascon-Barre et al., 2001). The second bioactivation step is a 1α-hydroxylation of calcidiol producing 1α,25-dihydroxyvitamin D_3 or calcitriol. The 1α-hydroxylation is carried out by CYP27B1 (Fu et al., 1997). Production of the circulating 1α,25-dihydroxyvitamin D_3 is initiated by hepatic 25-hydroxylation followed by renal 1α-hydroxylation. The circulating vitamin D hormone has mainly endocrine function e.g. in regulation of calcium homeostasis and maintenance of bone health. The normal serum levels of 25-hydroxyvitamin D_3 (20-250 nmol/L) are thousand times higher than the levels of 1α,25-dihydroxyvitamin D_3 (20-250 pmol/L). 1α,25-Dihydroxyvitamin D_3 is the most potent form of vitamin D_3 but 25-hydroxyvitamin D_3 can exert biological effects as well (Lou et al., 2004, 2010; Tuohimaa et al., 2005).

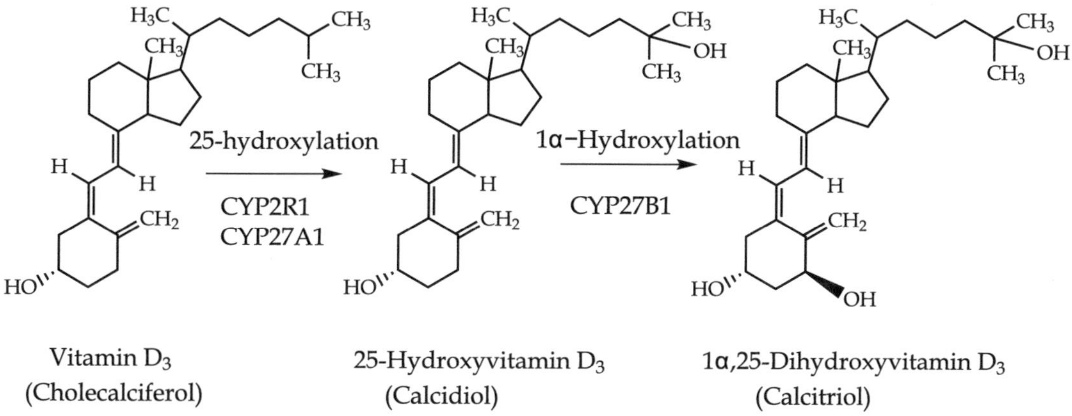

Fig. 6. Bioactivation of vitamin D_3.

Both calcidiol and calcitriol undergo further metabolism by the catabolizing enzyme CYP24A1 (Fig. 7). This enzyme 24-hydroxylates vitamin D metabolites and the 24-hydroxylation is a key point at which degradation of vitamin D begins. 24-Hydroxylated vitamin D metabolites are less biologically active and are then further metabolized by the multicatalytic CYP24A1 via side chain hydroxylation and oxidation to less active substances. Finally, after side chain cleavage, calcitroic acid is formed. Calcitroic acid is then excreted into the bile (Makin et al., 1989; Reddy and Tserng, 1989; Zimmerman et al., 2001).

The expression of both the activating (25- and 1α-hydroxylases) and the catabolizing (24-hydroxylase) enzymes by cells of certain tissues, indicates that the multifunctional hormone 1α,25-dihydroxyvitamin D_3 can be produced locally in some tissues, including cells in the skin, breast, colon, prostate, lung, and various cells of the immune system. The intracellular

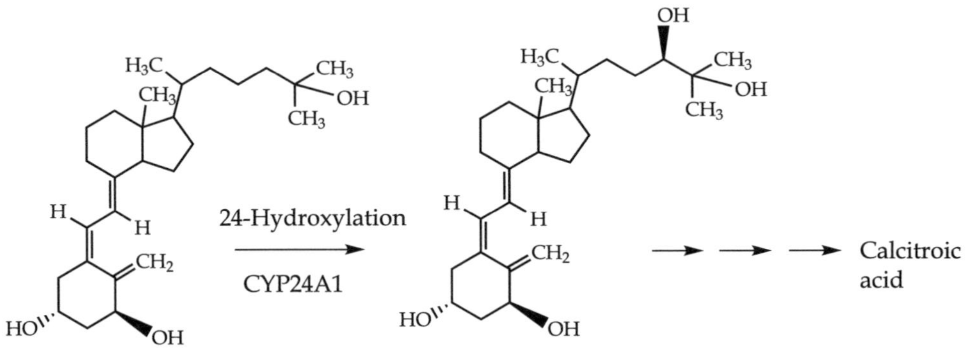

1α,25-Dihydroxyvitamin D_3 (Calcitriol)

1α,24,25-trihydroxyvitamin D_3 (1α,24,25-trihydroxycholecalciferol)

Fig. 7. Metabolism of 1α,25-dihydroxyvitamin D_3 (calcitriol) by CYP24A1 into less active metabolites. 25-Hydroxyvitamin D_3 is also catabolized by CYP24A1 in a similar way.

1α,25-dihydroxyvitamin D_3 is mainly used in an autocrine manner as a cofactor in the expression of many genes. This autocrine 1α,25-dihydroxyvitamin D_3 binds to VDR and modifies gene transcription. For example, genes involved in cell proliferation, differentiation and apoptosis are believed to be regulated by the internal 1α,25-dihydroxyvitamin D_3 of the cell. The activation, effects on gene expression and inactivation of 1α,25-dihydroxyvitamin D_3, is contained within the host cell. This active form of vitamin D is the major player in the internal autocrine action, but also 25-hydroxyvitamin D_3 can be formed within the cell and regulate gene expression (Lou et al., 2004; Tuohimaa et al., 2005; Verstuyf et al., 2010).
Recent data have revealed that vitamin D deficiency in the general population and even among young and healthy people is much more common than previously believed. Vitamin D deficiency not only causes rickets among children but also precipitates and exacerbates osteoporosis among adults and causes the painful bone disease osteomalacia. Interestingly, vitamin D deficiency is associated with increased risks of cardiovascular disease, multiple sclerosis, rheumatoid arthritis, type 1 diabetes mellitus and deadly cancers, such as prostate, breast and colon cancers (Adorini, 2002; Armas & Heaney, 2011; Giovannucci, 2007; Pérez-López, 2008; Schwartz, 2005; Zittermann, 2003).
The vitamin D receptor is widely expressed and it has been suggested that the active vitamin D_3 hormone may affect the expression of up to 200 genes in humans (Jones et al., 1998; Norman, 2008; Ramagopalan et al., 2010). It is probable that vitamin D_3 may have other roles yet undiscovered.

3.2 Vitamin D_3 exerts tissue-specific effects on estrogen and androgen metabolism

In recent reports from our laboratory, data are presented revealing vitamin D-mediated effects on the production of steroid hormones and expression of crucial steroidogenic enzymes in various cell lines (Lundqvist et al., 2010, 2011). As an example, the active vitamin D hormone 1α,25-dihydroxyvitamin D_3 decreases the production of dehydroepiandrosterone (DHEA) and DHEA-sulphate in adrenocortical NCI-H295R cells. DHEA is a precursor for both estrogen and androgen production. mRNA levels and enzyme activities for key enzymes in the steroidogenesis, such as CYP17A1 and CYP21A2 (cf. Fig. 1), were found to be altered by 1α,25-dihydroxyvitamin D_3 treatment (Lundqvist et al., 2010).

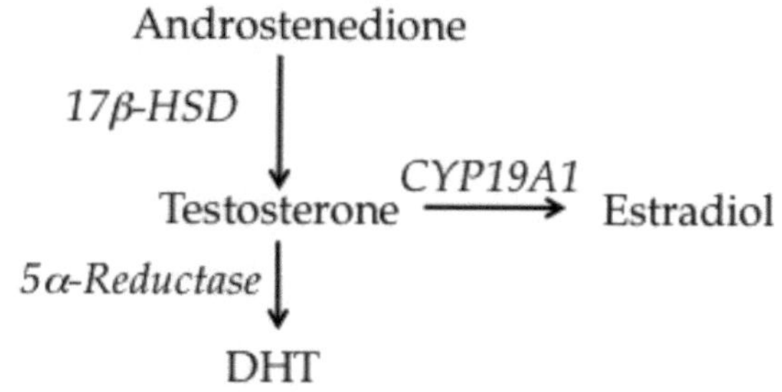

Fig. 8. Some important enzyme reactions in androgen and estrogen metabolism.

Accumulated data have revealed that sex hormone biosynthesis and metabolism may be regulated by vitamin D (Barrera et al., 2007; Krishnan et al., 2010; Lou et al., 2005; Lundqvist et al., 2011; Tanaka et al., 1996). Important reactions in the metabolism of androgens and estrogens are catalyzed by 5α-reductase and aromatase (CYP19A1) (Fig. 8). These two key enzymes determine the balance between androgen production and estrogen production. In addition to 5α-reductase and aromatase, the 17β-hydroxysteroid dehydrogenases are enzymes which regulate intracellular concentrations of active sex steroid hormones. Calcitriol has been found to up-regulate some types of 17β-hydroxysteroid dehydrogenase in human prostate cancer LNCaP and PC3 cells but not in stromal cells (Wang & Tuohimaa, 2007).

Estrogens are produced from androgenic precursors in a reaction catalyzed by aromatase (CYP19A1) (Figs. 3 and 8). Calcitriol increases aromatase activity in placental cells (Barrera et al., 2007), prostate cells (Lou et al., 2005) and osteoblasts (Tanaka et al., 1996) and vitamin D receptor null mutant mice have a decreased aromatase activity in the ovary, testis and epididymis (Kinuta et al., 2000). Interestingly, it was recently reported that 1α,25-dihydroxyvitamin D_3 regulates the expression of aromatase in a tissue-selective manner. Thus, calcitriol significantly decreased aromatase expression in human breast cancer cells and adipocytes but caused increased aromatase expression in human osteosarcoma cells and ovarian cancer cells (Krishnan et al., 2010). Calcitriol exerts cell line-specific effects on both estrogen and androgen metabolism, including the production of estrogens and androgens (Lundqvist et al., 2011). In breast cancer MCF-7 cells, aromatase gene expression and estradiol production were decreased, while production of androgens was markedly increased. In human adrenocortical NCI-H295R cells, 1α,25-dihydroxyvitamin D_3 stimulated aromatase expression and decreased dihydrotestosterone production. In prostate cancer LNCaP cells, aromatase expression increased after the same treatment, as did production of testosterone and dihydrotestosterone (Table 1). These findings are of interest for the research fields of breast cancer and prostate cancer. Vitamin D seems to be involved in the control also of prostate cancer cell growth (Flanagan et al., 2010; Tuohimaa et al., 2005). Analysis of effects of 1α,25-dihydroxyvitamin D_3 on aromatase promoter activities revealed differences between NCI-H295R cells and MCF-7 cells, where promoter I.3 and promoter I.4 were stimulated and promoter II were down regulated in NCI-H295R cells (Lundqvist et al., 2011) while all three promoters are down regulated in breast cancer MCF-7 cells (Krishnan et al., 2010).

The findings that 1α,25-dihydroxyvitamin D_3 specifically down regulates aromatase gene expression and activity and decreases production of estradiol in breast cancer cells are interesting in the context of 1α,25-dihydroxyvitamin D_3 as an anti cancer agent (Krishnan et al., 2010, Lundqvist et al., 2011)

	Cell line	Effect of treatment with 1α,25-dihydroxyvitamin D_3
Aromatase mRNA level	MCF-7	↓
	LNCaP	↑
	NCI-H295R	↑
Aromatase enzyme activity	MCF-7	↓
	LNCaP	-
	NCI-H295R	↑
Estradiol production	MCF-7	↓
	LNCaP	-
	NCI-H295R	↑/-
Dihydrotestosterone production	MCF-7	↑
	LNCaP	↑
	NCI-H295R	↓
Expression of promoter specific aromatase transcripts	MCF-7	↓ (p I.3, p I.4 and p II)
	LNCaP	No statistically significant alterations
	NCI-H295R	↑ (p I.3 and p I.4), ↓ (p II)

Table 1. Effects of calcitriol on estrogen and androgen metabolism. Please note that this table only summarizes the data obtained by our group (Lundqvist et al., 2011). Arrows indicate up- and down-regulation; -, unaltered.

Interestingly, 1α,25-dihydroxyvitamin D_3 increases androgen production in breast cancer MCF-7 cells (Lundqvist et al., 2011). The production of testosterone was increased by 60% and the production of dihydrotestosterone was increased 4-fold. The markedly increased production of dihydrotestosterone in MCF-7 cells after 1α,25-dihydroxyvitamin D_3 treatment appears not to be the result of increased 5α-reductase expression. An explanation for this effect could be that the decreased aromatase activity increases the concentration of testosterone, which is the precursor for dihydrotestosterone. The increased androgen production in breast cancer cells following vitamin D treatment needs to be studied further to elucidate its potential physiological roles.

The data showing that 1α,25-dihydroxyvitamin D_3 exerts tissue-specific effects on sex hormone production and metabolism provide important knowledge for further research in the fields of prostate and breast cancer. Prostate and breast are key tissues for estrogenic and androgenic pathways. Vitamin D deficiency is associated with increased risks of prostate and breast cancers (Holick, 2006; Thorne & Campbell, 2008; Bouillon et al., 2006). It is well-known that the active form of vitamin D, 1α,25-dihydroxyvitamin D_3, and analogs via binding to the vitamin D receptor exert anti-proliferative and pro-differentiative effects and have therefore been proposed to be of potential use as anti cancer agents (Deeb et al., 2007;

Masuda & Jones, 2006). Estrogens and androgens play a role in the pathogenesis of prostate cancer and a large group of all breast cancers involves estrogen-dependent mechanisms, i.e. they rely on estrogens to proliferate (Mathiasen et al., 2002; Sasano et al., 2009). The recent findings indicating regulation of intracellular levels of androgens and estrogens by vitamin D open new possibilities in prevention and treatment of prostate and breast cancer.

Aromatase (CYP19A1), the enzyme catalyzing the conversion of testosterone to estradiol, is critical for the progression of estrogen receptor-positive breast cancer in postmenopausal women. The aromatase expression is higher in breast cancer tissue than in normal breast tissue and the local estrogen levels in breast cancer tissue are higher than the circulating levels (Chen, 1998; Miller et al., 1990). Regulation of estradiol production and estrogenic signalling are key strategies in breast cancer treatment. Aromatase inhibitors and antiestrogens have therefore become important drugs in breast cancer treatment. Due to its effects on aromatase gene expression and enzyme activity, 1α,25-dihydroxyvitamin D_3 has been proposed as an interesting substance in breast cancer treatment and prevention. The vitamin D-mediated inhibition of aromatase seems to be tissue specific for breast cells, indicating that it is a potential drug target in treatment aiming to prevent estradiol production in breast but not in other tissues. This would reduce the risk of adverse effects due to effects on peripheral estrogen metabolism (e.g. osteoporosis). The vitamin D-induced tissue-selective regulation of aromatase expression and activity is an interesting strategy to affect estrogen levels in breast without effects on the peripheral estrogen metabolism.

High-dose vitamin D treatment will lead to adverse effects e.g. hypercalcemia. Therefore, synthetic vitamin D analogs with less pronounced hypercalcemic effect are potential drugs in treatment aiming to prevent estradiol production in breast but not in other tissues, a strategy that would lead to less adverse effects than the existing treatments. However, the mechanisms for these effects of vitamin D need to be clarified before vitamin D or analogs can be used in breast cancer treatment. It has been reported that the vitamin D analog EB1089 decreases the proliferation of breast cancer cells, especially anti-estrogen resistant breast cancer cells (Christensen et al., 2004; Larsen et al., 2001). EB1089 has undergone clinical trials phase I and II and was found to be a well tolerated substance (Dalhoff et al., 2003). However, it has not yet been tested in clinical trials against breast cancer. The new findings on vitamin D as a tissue-selective modulator of aromatase reinforce the interest for EB1089 as a potential drug in treatment of breast cancer, which may inhibit both estrogen-dependent and anti-estrogen resistant breast cancer.

Human adrenocortical NCI-H295R cells are widely used as a model for human adrenal cortex. It has been proposed that this adrenocortical carcinoma cell line could be suitable in a screening assay to study the effects of different chemicals on estradiol and testosterone production (Gracia et al., 2006; Hecker et al., 2006, 2007; Higley et al, 2010). We have examined whether adrenocortical NCI-H295R cells react in the same way as prostate cells and breast cells when they are treated with 1α,25-dihydroxyvitamin D_3. Interestingly, both estrogen and androgen metabolism were affected in a cell line-specific way (Table 1). The largest differences were observed between NCI-H295R cells and MCF-7 cells, where aromatase gene expression, estradiol production, aromatase promoter activity, testosterone production and dihydrotestosterone production were affected in opposite ways in the two cell lines. The discrepancies between NCI-H29R cells and LNCaP cells were smaller, but still noteworthy. Production of both testosterone and dihydrotestosterone was affected differentially in the two cell lines, as was the gene expression of 5α-reductase. Our data show that NCI-H295R cells respond in a different way than cells derived from important target tissues in estrogen and androgen production and metabolism (Lundqvist et al., 2011). These differences between NCI-H295R cells and cells derived from key endocrine target tissues need to be addressed and clarified if NCI-H295R cells should be used as a model for effects of different chemicals on estrogen and androgen metabolism.

4. Actions of CYP7B1 - potential role(s) for the levels and effects of estrogens, androgens and neurosteroids

In recent years we have carried out several studies on the effects and regulation of catalytic reactions mediated by CYP7B1, a widely expressed enzyme with a number of steroid substrates including DHEA. CYP7B1-mediated catalysis leads to formation of 6- or 7-hydroxymetabolites, mainly 7α-hydroxyderivatives (Pettersson et al, 2008; Rose et al., 1997; Tang et al., 2006; Stiles et al., 2009; Wu et al., 1999) (Fig. 9). This enzyme has been associated with several physiological processes, including brain function, immune system, cholesterol homeostasis and cellular viability and growth. Scientific publications in various areas have linked altered CYP7B1 levels and/or function to neurodegenerative processes, arthritis, and prostate cancer (Dulos et al., 2004; Olsson et al., 2007; Tsaousidou et al., 2008; Yau et al., 2003). However, the manner in which CYP7B1 affects these processes are in many cases unclear.

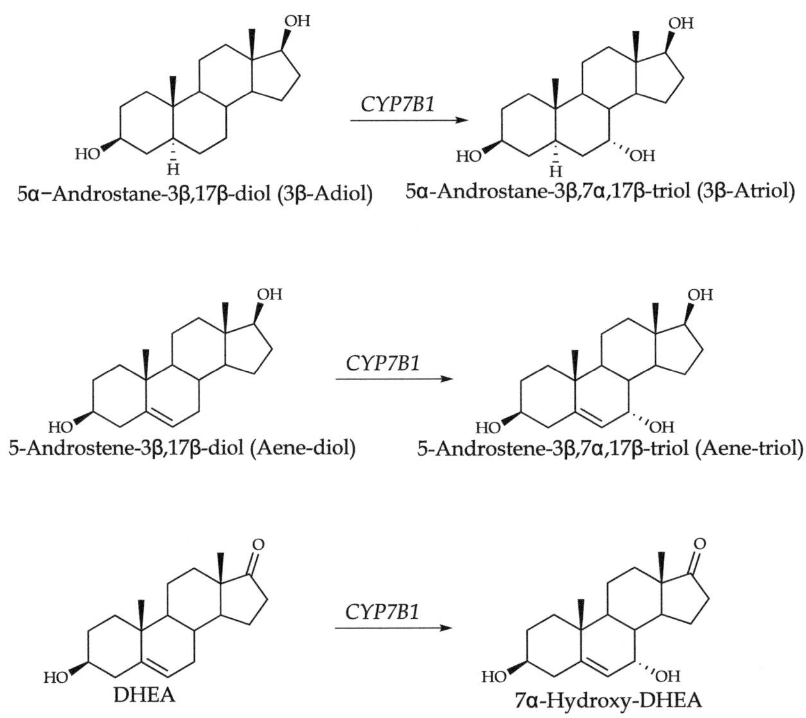

Fig. 9. CYP7B1-mediated catalytic reactions.

Substrates for CYP7B1 are neurosteroids, cholesterol derivatives and sex hormones, including some of the ligands for the estrogens receptors (ER). In recent studies we examined the role of CYP7B1-mediated catalysis for activation of the ER (Pettersson et al., 2008, 2010). Our studies, using ER-dependent luciferase reporter systems and ER-target genes, indicate significant stimulation of ER-response by the CYP7B1 substrates 5-androstene-3β,17β-diol (Aene-diol) and 5α-androstane-3β,17β-diol (3β-Adiol), for both ERα and β. In contrast, the CYP7B1-formed metabolites from these steroids have little or no estrogenic effects, indicating that CYP7B1-mediated metabolism abolishes the ER-stimulating effect of these compounds (Pettersson et al., 2010). In the course of our studies we have also found that DHEA induces both ER-dependent and AR-dependent responses in some cell types whereas 7α-hydroxy-DHEA has no or diminished effect (Norlin M. & Lundqvist J., unpublished results).

Our findings seem to indicate that actions by CYP7B1 might be a way to decrease estrogenic response, at least in some tissues. One of these may be the prostate, where signalling via ERβ has been reported to play a role in growth suppression. Gustafsson and collaborators proposed a pathway for hormonal control of proliferation where the role of CYP7B1 would be to counteract anti-proliferative action of ERβ by metabolizing its ligand 3β-Adiol (Weihua et al., 2002). This concept is supported by findings indicating that prostates of CYP7B1-/- mice are hypoproliferative. The roles of estrogens and estrogen receptors in prostate growth are however not well understood (Morani et al., 2008; Prins & Korach, 2008). Interestingly, Olsson et al. (2007) reported high expression of CYP7B1 protein in human high-grade prostatic intraepithelial neoplasia and adenocarcinomas. Enzymatic events of potential importance for intraprostatic hormone levels are of course not limited to actions by CYP7B1. Other enzymes of relevance include e. g. the conjugating enzymes, particularly some of the UDP-glucuronosyltransferases (UGT) expressed in prostate (Barbier & Bélanger, 2008). Also, the enzymes known to form important hormones in this tissue such as CYP17A1, 5α-reductase and the 3β- and 17β-hydroxysteroid dehydrogenases have attracted interest as potential or existing targets for therapy aimed at controlling cellular hormone levels (Hudak et al., 2006; Norlin; 2008; Sharifi, 2010; Vihko et al., 2006).

Considering its role in metabolism of ER ligands, CYP7B1 has been linked to estrogenic action by several studies and investigators (Petterson et al., 2010; Sugiyama et al., 2009; Weihua et al., 2002). However, the actions of CYP7B1 in sex hormone metabolism do not seem to be limited to estrogenic signalling. For instance, some of the steroids that are substrates for this enzyme may affect both estrogen and androgen receptors. This includes DHEA and Aenediol which are reported to be able to trigger both ER and AR signalling. It seems likely that the actual effects of these steroids in vivo may strongly depend on their local concentration. In addition, the presence or absence of other hormone ligands with higher affinitity for the receptor as well as the effects of tissue-specific comodulators should play important roles. These different possibilities open for enzymatic control of cell-specific actions, depending on e. g. comodulator expression, substrate availability, and substrate competition (Pettersson et al., 2008; Shapiro et al., 2011; Sugiyama et al., 2009).

The most potent androgenic hormone in the human body is dihydrotestosterone (DHT). Maintenance of normal DHT levels is essential for a number of physiological processes. On the other hand, excess levels of androgens, which strongly stimulate growth, may have a negative impact in disease. We recently identified a previously unknown androgenic substrate for CYP7B1 which is a metabolite of DHT (Pettersson et al., 2009) (Fig. 10). This steroid, 5α-androstane-3α,17β-diol (3α-Adiol), can itself induce androgenic responses, but since the effects of 3α-Adiol are weaker that those of DHT, conversion into 3α-Adiol is considered a means to reduce DHT-mediated effects on cell growth and other processes. 3α-Adiol can easily be converted back to DHT and is believed to serve as a source for this hormone (Auchus, 2004; Penning et al., 2000). 3α-Adiol is also believed to be of importance in the CNS, where it can modulate the action of gamma-amino butyric acid A ($GABA_A$) receptors and is reported to have anticonvulsant and analgesic properties (Reddy 2004; Frye, 2007).

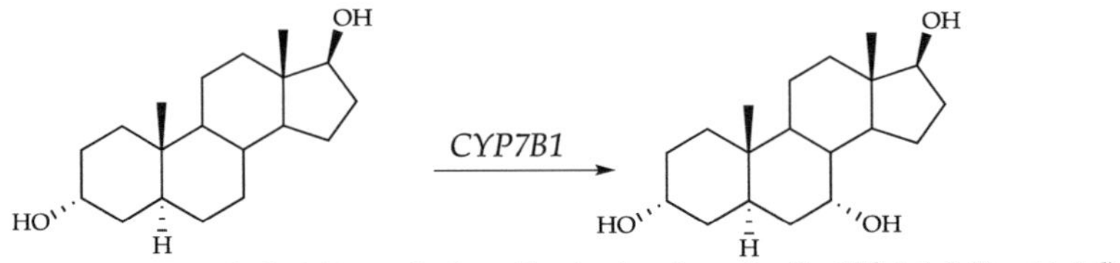

Fig. 10. CYP7B1-mediated metabolism of 5α-androstane-3α,17β-diol (3α-Adiol)

Local formation and functions in the CNS are features shared by other, previously characterized, substrates for CYP7B1, including DHEA, pregnenolone, Aenediol and 27-hydroxycholesterol, a cholesterol derivative believed to serve as a regulator of cholesterol homeostasis (Norlin & Wikvall 2007, Pikuleva; 2006). An important role for CYP7B1 in brain physiology is indicated by the recent studies revealing that disturbed function of this enzyme is linked to a human motor-neuron degenerative disease. Tsaousidou et al. (2008) first showed that hereditary spastic paraplegia (HSP) is associated with mutations in the CYP7B1 gene. Mutations in the coding region of this gene, which affects the functionality of the enzyme, is believed to be a frequent cause of this disease. The etiology and molecular mechanisms that underlies hereditary spastic paraplegia are however not known. It has been proposed that the mutated forms of CYP7B1 in patients suffering from HSP might lead to an abnormal brain cholesterol homeostasis due to an increase in 27-hydroxycholesterol levels (Tsaousidou et al., 2008). Despite the role of this steroid for maintenance of cholesterol homeostasis, 27-hydroxycholesterol negatively affects viability of some cells (Dasari et al., 2010). This steroid can also modulate estrogen receptor signalling in some tissues and has been described as an endogenous SERM (Du Sell et al. 2008; Umetani et al., 2008) However, it is also possible that the pathogenic basis for hereditary spastic paraplegia is connected to abnormal levels of other CYP7B1 substrates present in the brain, including DHEA. Although there is still much to be learned in this field, brain steroids are believed to influence several aspects of CNS function (Charalampopoulos et al., 2006; Maninger et al., 2009; Melcangi & Panzica, 2006). Various neurosteroids are considered to be involved in e. g. neuronal development, regulation of inflammatory responses, effects on cellular viability and modulation of the actions of various neurotransmitter receptors.

The concept of widely varying cell- and tissue-specific steroid metabolism is illustrated by the differences in metabolism of DHEA in different CNS cell types. Thus, whereas rat microglia, a cell type important for brain immune function, is reported to exclusively convert this steroid to Aenediol, the major route for DHEA metabolism in rat astrocytes seems to be 7α-hydroxylation, carried out by CYP7B1 (Fex Svenningsen et al., 2011; Jellinck et al., 2001; Jellinck et al, 2007). In contrast, the pathways using DHEA as an obligatory precursor for formation of testosterone and estradiol (see Introductory section), are much more dominant in cells outside the brain and are indeed essential for the development and functions of many endocrine organs. Very recently, we found that treatment with endogenous and synthetic estrogens strongly decreases CYP7B1-mediated DHEA hydroxylation in primary cultures of rat astrocytes (Fex Svenningsen et al., 2011). Since CYP7B1-mediated metabolism appears to be the main pathway for DHEA metabolism in these cells, we believe that estrogenic effects on this enzyme may lead to increase of the levels of DHEA via suppression of its metabolism. This could be one of the potential mechanisms whereby estrogens affect CNS, and may play a role for estrogen-dependent protection of CNS cells against injury (Brann et al., 2007; Melcangi & Panzica 2006).

5. Role of sex hormones in regulation of steroid-metabolizing enzymes

5.1 CYP7B1 is regulated by sex hormones

Our studies, carried out in several different cell types, indicate regulatory effects of both estrogen and androgens on CYP7B1 expression (Fex Svenningsen et al., 2011; Tang et al., 2006; Tang & Norlin, 2006) (Fig. 11). As described in the previous section, our results in primary rat CNS cultures showed decreased CYP7B1-mediated catalytic activity following estrogen treatment (Fex Svenningsen et al., 2011). In the studies on astrocytes we also found suppressive effects of estrogen on CYP7B1 mRNA levels. These findings, indicating suppression of the CYP7B1 gene, are different compared to some of our previous data concerning estrogen-dependent regulation of CYP7B1 in human kidney- and liver-derived cell lines (Tang et al., 2006, 2008). In kidney-derived HEK293 cells and liver-derived HepG2

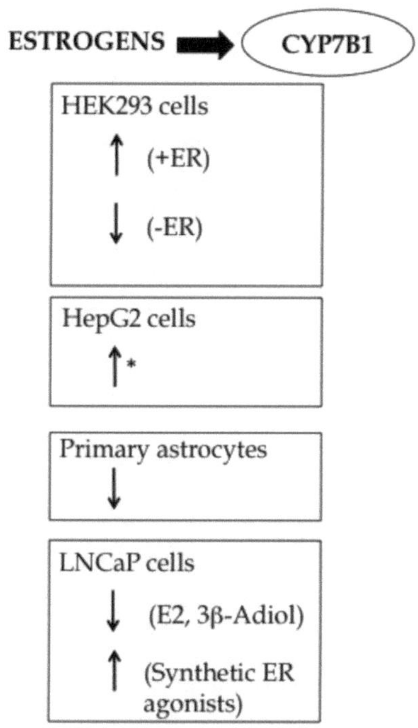

* Involvement of the PI3K/Akt pathway (Tang et al., 2008)

Fig. 11. Simplified overview of our findings on the effects of estrogens on the regulation of CYP7B1 in different cell types. For more information see text and references (Tang et al., 2006, 2008; Tang & Norlin, 2006; Fex Svenningsen et al., 2011)

cells, we have found that estradiol up-regulates CYP7B1 gene expression in the presence of estrogen receptors. Without overexpression of ER however, the kidney HEK293 cells, which have very low endogenous ER expression, react similarly as the astrocytes to estradiol treatment, suggesting that there might be both ER-dependent and ER-independent pathways for estrogen-mediated regulation of CYP7B1. Other possibilities are tissue- and/or species-specific differences in regulatory mechanisms. Species differences in enzymes may include enzyme localization. Data obtained by us and others show higher CYP7B1 levels in rat astrocytes than in rat neurons, whereas in humans CYP7B1 expression has been reported to be predominantly located in neurons (Fex Svenningsen et al., 2011; Trap et al., 2005; Zhang et al., 1997). However, in similarity with our results in human renal and hepatic cells, estrogen receptor-mediated upregulation of CYP7B1 has been shown also in mouse kidney and liver, indicating a similar effect in rodents as in humans and supporting an in vivo role for this regulatory mechanism (Jelinsky et al., 2003; Yamamoto et al., 2006).
Thus, from the results obtained by us and other investigators it seems that CYP7B1 not only affects hormonal actions but is itself regulated by hormones. Our studies have shown effects on CYP7B1 transcription and/or activity by both estrogens and androgens, although we observed differences depending on cell type (Fex Svenningsen et al., 2011; Tang et al., 2006, 2008; Tang & Norlin 2006). This may reflect different functions of CYP7B1 in different tissues or cells. In cell types where formation of estradiol is quantitatively important, the observed ER-mediated induction by estradiol on the CYP7B1-mediated pathway may be a means to divert DHEA from estradiol production, by increasing the amount of DHEA metabolized to 7α-hydroxyDHEA (Tang et al., 2006) (Fig. 12). In this way, estradiol-mediated regulation of CYP7B1 may decrease the levels of DHEA available for synthesis of estradiol in some tissues, functioning as a feed-back mechanism to balance the amount of estradiol formed. This could be of particular importance during fetal development as placental estrogen formation is dependent on C_{19}-steroid precursors such as DHEA which is secreted in large amounts by the fetal adrenal cortex. Although there are few data on the role(s) of CYP7B1 in fetal development, studies on tissues from both humans and rodents show markedly higher CYP7B1 mRNA levels in extrahepatic fetal tissues compared with the corresponding adult ones (Bean et al., 2001; Tang et al., 2006).

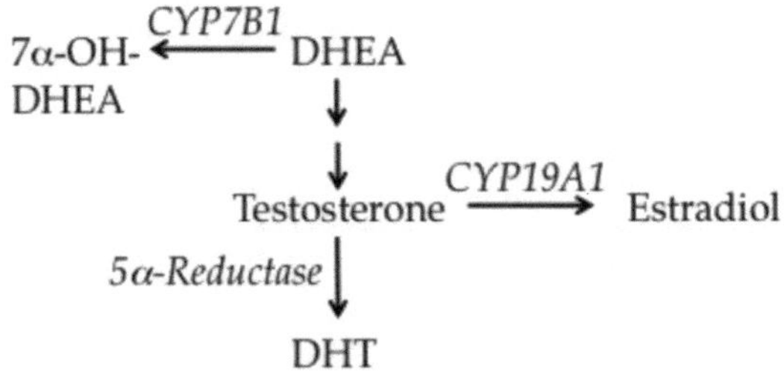

Fig. 12. Some of the alternate pathways for DHEA metabolism

Our data on estrogen-mediated upregulation of the CYP7B1 gene promoter in liver-derived human HepG2 cells showed involvement of the Akt/PI3K (phosphoinositide 3-kinase) cascade in the ER-mediated effects on CYP7B1 (Tang et al., 2008). The link between CYP7B1 and this signalling pathway, which is known to be of importance for cellular survival, suggests a possible connection between CYP7B1 action and viability. Also, as outlined

above, studies on this enzyme in the CNS point towards a potential role connected to neuroprotective events (Bean et al., 2001; Fex Svenningsen et al., 2011; Tsaousidou et al., 2008). Although CYP7B1 expression is abundant in tissues of humans and animals most immortalized cell lines lose their expression of CYP7B1. The reason for this is not known.
The estrogen-mediated regulation of CYP7B1 is of interest also because this enzyme catabolizes 27-hydroxycholesterol, recently identified as the first endogenous selective estrogen receptor modulator, SERM (Fig. 13). 27-Hydroxycholesterol is produced from cholesterol by the sterol 27-hydroxylase CYP27A1. Interestingly, CYP27A1 is also regulated by estrogens and androgens. The regulation of CYP27A1 by sex hormones is discussed below.

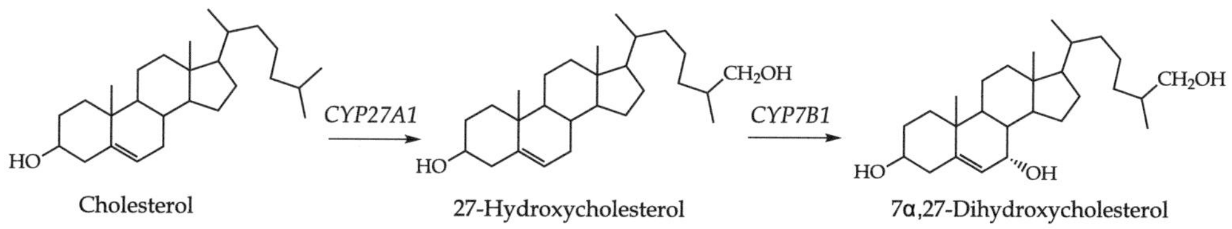

Fig. 13. Formation and metabolism of 27-hydroxycholesterol.

5.2 CYP27A1 is regulated by sex hormones

The sterol 27-hydroxylase CYP27A1 is an enzyme with several important roles (Norlin & Wikvall, 2007). CYP27A1 regulates cholesterol homeostasis including bile acid biosynthesis, cholesterol transport and cholesterol elimination. CYP27A1 is also a vitamin D 25-hydroxylase, catalyzing the first step in the bioactivation of vitamin D into the multifunctional hormone 1,25-dihydroxyvitamin D (Fig. 6). CYP27A1 is essential for the production of 27-hydroxycholesterol (Fig. 13), an oxysterol which has recently been identified as an endogenous selective estrogen receptor modulator, SERM (DuSell et al., 2008, 2010; Umetani et al., 2007, 2011). Considering these important functions, mechanisms for regulation of the human CYP27A1 gene are of great interest.
In studies carried out by our laboratory, we found that the cellular mRNA levels, enzyme activity and promoter activity of CYP27A1 are regulated by estrogens and androgens (Norlin et al., 2011; Tang et al., 2007) (Figs. 14 and 15). The responses to sex hormones are different in various cell lines and cells from different tissues. The hormonal action on the CYP27A1 promoter appears to be complex. In addition to cell-dependent effects, there are also differences between receptor subtypes and different promoter deletion constructs. For instance, whereas ERα suppressed the full-length promoter in HepG2 cells, deletion of a 3.4 kb long part of the promoter resulted in the opposite response. On the contrary, the response of different promoter constructs to ERβ was similar. The data available indicate that the CYP27A1 promoter contains sequences able to mediate both stimulation and suppression by ER (Tang et al., 2007). ER-mediated regulation of transcription is often associated with binding of ER homodimers to estrogen response elements (ERE) in target promotors. However, regulation by ER can also involve interaction with sequences containing Sp1 and activator protein (AP-1) sites (Safe, 2001; Schultz et al., 2005). Interestingly, it has been reported that ER-mediated regulation involving AP-1 sites may lead to opposite effects depending on ER subtype (Paech et al., 1997). As mentioned above, the CYP27A1 promoter contains several putative binding sites for ER, AP-1 and Sp1. It seems possible that cell-specific interactions with coactivators may be the reason for the different effects observed with different cell types and receptor subtypes.

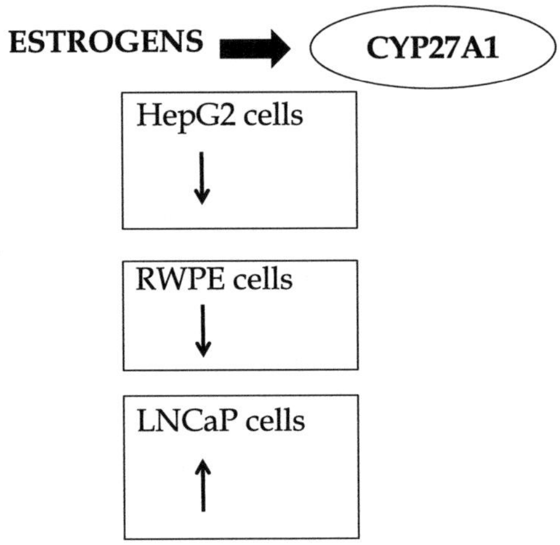

Fig. 14. Simplified overview of our findings on the effects of estrogens on the gene regulation of CYP27A1 in different cell types. For more information see text and references (Norlin et al., 2011; Tang et al., 2007).

Our studies on the mechanisms for the hormonal regulation of CYP27A1 have indicated the involvement of the JNK (c-jun N-terminal kinase)/c-jun pathway in androgen-mediated regulation of this enzyme (Norlin et al., 2011). It has been reported that the androgen receptor (AR) is phosphorylated by JNK and that stress kinase signaling regulates AR phosphorylation, transcription, and localization. Crosstalk between the JNK protein kinase and AR has been reported in several studies (Gioeli et al., 2006; Lazarevic et al, 2008; Lorenzo & Saatcioglu, 2008;). The link to JNK signaling is interesting since inflammatory processes, which can induce the JNK/c-jun pathway, may upregulate CYP27A1 to clear cholesterol from peripheral tissues.

The findings that estrogens downregulate and androgens upregulate CYP27A1 expression in liver-derived HepG2 cells are of interest for several reasons (Tang et al., 2007). The results are consistent with reports on an increased risk for cardiovascular disease in postmenopausal women treated with estrogen plus progestin. Also, increased testosterone levels in men have been associated with a favorable lipid profile (Alexandersen & Christiansen, 2004; Steinberg, 2006; Stoll & Bendszus, 2006; Tchernof et al., 1997; Zmuda et al., 1997). The difference in prevalence of atherosclerotic coronary disease between men and women can not be explained by effects of estrogens and androgens solely on CYP27A1 expression. However, the effects by sex hormones on the expression of CYP27A1 may have impact on several processes in cholesterol homeostasis. The findings that CYP27A1 is regulated by sex hormones imply that endogenous sex hormones as well as pharmacological compounds with estrogenic and androgenic effects may have an impact on several processes related to CYP27A1-mediated metabolism, such as cellular survival and growth, CNS function and cholesterol homeostasis. Because estrogens are used in oral contraceptives, in hormone therapy of postmenopausal women and in cancer treatment, the question arises how CYP27A1 is influenced by estrogens in different tissues. This question is of particular interest considering that anti-atherogenic properties have been ascribed to CYP27A1. The possibility of a tissue-specific regulation by sex hormones is supported by results with prostate cancer cells where estrogen increases the CYP27A1 transcriptional activity. The results also show that effects of sex hormones on CYP27A1 regulation are different in non-cancerous prostate RWPE-1 compared with prostate cancer LNCaP cells. Whether this difference in regulatory effects is due to different properties of different prostate cell lines or to altered properties of the CYP27A1 regulation in prostate cancer remain to be established.

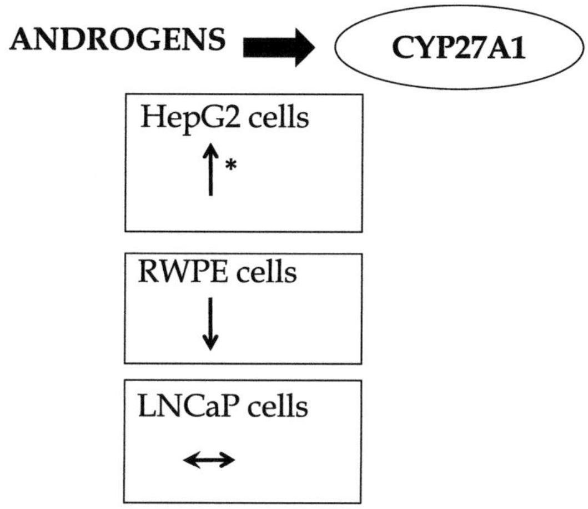

* Involvement of the JNK/c-jun kinase signalling pathway (Norlin et al., 2011).

Fig. 15. Simplified overview of our findings on the effects of androgens on the gene regulation of CYP27A1 in different cell types. For more information see text and references (Norlin et al., 2011; Tang et al., 2007).

5.3 Effects of sex hormones on vitamin D metabolism

Activated vitamin D metabolites, that can be formed by CYP27A1, are known to have beneficial effects on cell growth in extrahepatic tissues, such as in prostate cells and prostate cancer cells. As discussed above, novel data indicate that estrogens and androgens might regulate the intracellular levels of active hydroxyvitamin D_3 metabolites in prostate cells via regulation of CYP27A1 gene expression (Norlin et al., 2011; Tang et al., 2007). Another observation indicating that androgens can influence intracellular levels of active vitamin D metabolites was reported some years ago (Lou and Tuohimaa, 2006). These authors demonstrated that dihydrotestosterone (DHT) significantly suppressed the expression of the catabolizing enzyme CYP24A1 in androgen-sensitive prostate cancer LNCaP cells. Their data demonstrated that DHT enhances the antiproliferative activity of vitamin D_3 hormones by inhibiting their inactivating enzyme at physiological concentration of androgen. They suggested that the combined use of androgen and vitamin D_3 metabolites could be a promising treatment for prostate cancer.

6. Concluding remarks

Recent research using cell models has revealed novel and tissue-specific actions of sex hormones and vitamin D_3 in the regulation of enzymes in steroid metabolism. The active vitamin D hormone, calcitriol, has been found to affect genes in androgen and estrogen metabolism. Sex hormones regulate genes in neurosteroid metabolism and cholesterol homeostasis, including the CYP7B1 and CYP27A1 genes. The data available on the actions of the multifunctional and widely expressed CYP7B1 indicate potentially important roles of this enzyme for regulation of neurosteroid levels in the CNS as well as for control of the levels of sex hormones important in estrogenic and androgenic signalling in various cell types and tissues. Observed differences in effects and actions related to this enzyme reflect cell- and tissue-specificity of steroid-metabolizing enzymes of importance throughout the body. The new knowledge discussed in this review should be of importance for future research on brain function, endocrine signalling as well as treatment of estrogen- and androgen-dependent cancers, such as breast and prostate cancer.

7. Acknowledgments

The research in the authors` laboratory was supported by grants from the Swedish Research Council Medicine and the Åke Wiberg foundation (Sweden). We are grateful to Dr. Johan Lundqvist for assistance with some of the illustrations.

8. References

Adorini, L. (2002). Immunomodulatory effects of vitamin D receptor ligands in autoimmune diseases. *Int Immunopharmacol,* Vol. 2, pp. 1017-1028

Akwa, Y., Sananes, N., Gouezou, M., Robel, P., Baulieu, E.E. & Le Goascogne, C. (1993). Astrocytes and neurosteroids: metabolism of pregnenolone and dehydroepiandrosterone. Regulation by cell density. *J Cell Biol,* Vol. 121, pp. 135-143

Alexandersen, P. & Christiansen, C, (2004). The aging male: testosterone deficiency and testosterone replacement. An up-date. *Atherosclerosis.* Vol. 173, pp. 157-169

Armas, LAG. & Heaney, RP. (2011). Vitamin D: The iceberg nutrient. *J Renal Nutr,* Vol. 21, pp. 134-139

Arnal, JF., Scarabin, PY., Tremollieres, F., Laurell, H. & Gourdy, P. (2997). Estrogens in vascular biology and disease: where do we stand today? *Curr Opin Lipidol,* Vol. 18, pp. 554-560

Atkins GJ., Anderson, PH., Findlay, DM., Welldon, KJ., Vincent, C., Zannettino, ACW., O´Loughlin, PD. & Morris, HA. (2007). Metabolism of vitamin D_3 in human osteoblasts: evidence for autocrine and paracrine activities of 1a,25-dihydroxyvitamin D_3. *Bone,* Vol. 40, pp. 1517-1528

Auchus, RJ. (2004). The backdoor pathway to dihydrotestosterone. *Trends Endocrinol Metab,* Vol. 15, pp. 432-438

Barbier, O. & Bélanger, A. (2008). Inactivation of androgens by UDP-glucuronosyltransferases in the human prostate. *Best Pract Res Clin Endocrinol Metab,* Vol. 22, pp. 259-270

Barrera, D., Avila, E., Hernández, G., Halhali, A., Biruete, B., Larrea, F. & Díaz, L. (2007). Estradiol and progesterone synthesis in human placenta is stimulated by calcitriol. *J Steroid Biochem Mol Biol,* Vol. 103, pp. 529-532

Bauman, DR., Steckelbroeck, S., Peehl, DM. & Penning, TM. (2006). Transcript Profiling of the Androgen Signal in Normal Prostate, Benign Prostatic Hyperplasia, and Prostate Cancer. *Endocrinology,* Vol. 147, pp. 5806-5816

Bean, R., Seckl, JR., Lathe, R. & Martin, C. (2001). Ontogeny of the neurosteroid enzyme Cyp7b in the mouse. *Mol Cell Endocrinol,* Vol. 174, pp. 137-144

Bhasin, S. & Jasuja, R. (2009). Selective androgen receptor modulators as function promoting therapies.*Curr Opin Clin Nutr Metab Care,* Vol. 12, pp. 232-240

Bouillon, R., Eelen, G., Verlinden, L., Mathieu, C., Carmeliet, G. & Verstuyf, A. (2006). Vitamin D and cancer. *J Steroid Biochem Mol Biol,* Vol. 102, pp. 156-162

Bourdeau, I. & Stratakis, CA. (2002). Cyclic AMP-dependent signaling aberrations in macronodular adrenal disease. *Ann N Y Acad Sci,* Vol. 968, pp. 240-255

Brann, DW., Dhandapani, K., Wakade, C., Mahesh, VB. & Khan, MM. (2007). Neurotrophic and neuroprotective actions of estrogen: basic mechanisms and clinical implications. *Steroids,* Vol. 72, pp. 381-405

Brinkmann, AO., Blok, LJ., de Ruiter, PE., Doesburg, P., Steketee, K., Berrevoets, CA. & Trapman, J. (1999). Mechanisms of androgen receptor activation and function. *J Steroid Biochem Mol Biol,* Vol. 69, pp. 307-313

Brown, AJ., Dusso, A. & Slatopolsky, E. (1999). Vitamin D. *Am J Physiol,* Vol. 277, pp. F157-F175

Bryant, DN., Sheldahl, LC., Marriott, LK., Shapiro, RA. & Dorsa, DM. (2006). Multiple pathways transmit europrotective effects of gonadal steroids. *Endocrine* 29 (2006) 199-207

Bulun, SE., Lin, Z., Zhao, H., Lu, M., Amin, S., Reierstad, S. & Chen, D. (2009). Regulation of Aromatase Expression in Breast Cancer Tissue, *Ann N Y Acad Sci,* Vol. 1155, pp. 121-131

Charalampopoulos, I., Alexaki, VI., Tsatsanis, C., Minas, V., Dermitzaki, E., Lasaridis, I., Vardouli, L., Stournaras, C., Margioris, AN., Castanas, E. & Gravanis, A. (2006). Neurosteroids as endogenous inhibitors of neuronal cell apoptosis in aging. *Ann N Y Acad Sci,* Vol. 1088, pp. 139-152

Chen, S.(1998). Aromatase and breast cancer. *Frontiers in Bioscience,* Vol. 3, pp. d922-d933

Cheng, JB., Motola, DL., Mangelsdorf, DJ. & Russell, DW. (2003). De-orphanization of cytochrome P450 2R1: A microsomal vitamin D 25-hydroxylase. *J Biol Chem,* Vol. 278, pp. 38084-38093

Cheng, JB., Levine, MA., Bell, NH., Mangelsdorf, DJ. & Russell, DW. (2004). Genetic evidence that the human CYP2R1 enzyme is a key vitamin D 25-hydroxylase. Proc Natl Acad Sci U S A, Vol. 101, pp. 7711-7715

Cheskis, BJ., Greger, JG., Nagpal, S. & Freedman, LP. (2007). Signaling by estrogens. *J Cell Physiol,* Vol. 213, pp. 610-617

Christensen, GL., Jepsen, JS., Fog, CK., Christensen, IJ. & Lykkesfeldt, AE. (2004). Sequential Versus Combined Treatment of Human Breast Cancer Cells with Antiestrogens and the Vitamin D Analogue EB1089 and Evaluation of Predictive Markers for Vitamin D Treatment. *Breast Cancer Research and Treatment,* Vol. 85, pp. 53-63

Cossec, JC., Marquer, C., Panchal, M., Lazar, AN., Duyckaerts, C. & Potier, MC. (2010). Cholesterol changes in Alzheimer's disease: methods of analysis and impact on the formation of enlarged endosomes. *Biochim Biophys Acta,* Vol. 1801, pp. 839-845

Dahlbäck, H. & Wikvall, K. (1988). 25-Hydroxylation of vitamin D_3 by a cytochrome P-450 from rabbit liver mitochondria. *Biochem J,* Vol. 252, pp. 207-213

Dalhoff, K., Dancey, J., Astrup, L., Skovsgaard, T., Hamberg, KJ., Lofts, FJ., Rosmorduc, O., Erlinger, S., Bach Hansen, J., Steward, WP. Skov, T., Burcharth, F. & Evans, TRJ.

(2003). A phase II study of the vitamin D analogue Seocalcitol in patients with inoperable hepatocellular carcinoma. *Br J Cancer*, Vol. 89, pp. 252-257

Dasari, B., Prasanthi, JR., Marwarha, G., Singh, BB. & Ghribi, O. (2010). The oxysterol 27-hydroxycholesterol increases β-amyloid and oxidative stress in retinal pigment epithelial cells. *BMC Ophthalmol*, Vol. 10, p. 10-22

Deeb, KK., Trump, DL. & Johnson, CS. (2007). Vitamin D signaling pathways in cancer: potential for anticancer therapeutics. *Nature Reviews* Vol. 7, pp. 684-700

DeLuca, HF. (2004). Overview of general physiologic features and function of vitamin D. *American Journal of Clinical Nutrition*, Vol. 80, pp. 1689-1696

Dulos, J., Verbraak, E.. Bagchus, WM., Boots, AM. & Kaptein, A. (2004). Severity of murine collagen-induced arthritis correlates with increased CYP7B activity: enhancement of dehydroepiandrosterone metabolism by interleukin-1β, *Arthritis Rheum*, Vol. 50, pp. 3346-3353

DuSell, CD., Umetani, M., Shaul, PW., Mangelsdorf, DJ. & McDonnell, DP. (2008). 27-Hydroxycholesterol is an endogenous selective estrogen receptor modulator. *Mol Endocrinol*, Vol. 22, pp. 65-77

DuSell, CD., Nelson, ER., Wang, X., Abdo, J., Mödder, UI., Umetani, M., Gesty-Palmer, D., Javitt, NB., Khosla, S. & McDonnell, DP. (2010). The endogenous selective estrogen receptor modulator 27-hydroxycholesterol is a negative regulator of bone homeostasis. *Endocrinology*, Vol. 151, pp. 3675-3685

Dusso, AS., Brown, AJ. & Slatopolsky, E. (2005). Vitamin D. *American Journal of Physiology - Renal Physiology*, Vol.289, pp. 8-28

Fex Svenningsen, Å., Wicher, G., Lundqvist, J., Pettersson, H., Corell, M. & Norlin, M. (2011). Effects on DHEA levels by estrogen in rat astrocytes and CNS co-cultures via the regulation of CYP7B1-mediated metabolism. *Neurochem Int*, Vol. 58, pp. 620-624

Flanagan, JN., Zheng, S., Chiang, KC., Kittaka, A., Sakaki, T., Nakabayashi, S., Zhao, X., Spanjaard, RA., Persons, KS., Mathieu, JS., Holick, MF. & Chen TC. (2009). Evaluation of 19-nor-2a-(3-hydroxypropyl)-1α,25-dihydroxyvitamin D_3 as a therapeutic agent for androgen-dependent prostate cancer. *Anticancer Res*, Vol. 29, pp. 3547-3553

Folkerd, EJ. & Dowsett, M. (2010). Influence of Sex Hormones on Cancer Progression, *J Clin Oncol*, Vol. 28, pp. 4038-4044

Frye, CA. (2007). Some rewarding effects of androgens may be mediated by actions of its 5α-reduced metabolite 3α-androstanediol. *Pharmacol Biochem Behav*, Vol. 86, pp. 354-367

Fu, GK., Lin, D., Zhang, MYH., Bikle, DD., Shackleton, CHL., Miller, WL. & Portale, AA. (1997). Cloning of human 25-hydroxyvitamin D 1a-hydroxylase and mutations causing vitamin D-dependent rickets type 1. *Mol Endocrinol*, Vol. 11, pp. 1961-1970

Gascon-Barre, M., Demers, C., Ghrab, O., Theodoropoulos, C., Lapointe, R., Jones, G., Valiquette. L. & Ménard, D. (2001). Expression of CYP27A, a gene encoding a vitamin D-25 hydroxylase in human liver and kidney. *Clinical Endocrinology*, Vol. 54, pp. 107-115

Gioeli, D., Black, BE., Gordon, V., Spencer, A., Kesler, CT., Eblen, ST., Paschal, BM. & Weber, MJ. (2006). Stress kinase signaling regulates androgen receptor phosphorylation, transcription, and localization, *Mol Endocrinol*, Vol. 20, pp. 503-515

Giovannucci, E. (2007). Epidemiological evidence for vitamin D and colorectal cancer. *J Bone Miner Res*, Vol. 22, Suppl 2:V81-85

Gracia, T., Hilscherova, K., Jones, PD., Newsted, JL., Zhang, X., Hecker, M., Higley, EB., Sanderson, JT., Yu, RM., Wu, RS. & Giesy, JP. (2006). The H295R system for evaluation of endocrine-disrupting effects. *Ecotoxicology and Environmental Safety,* Vol. 65, pp. 293-305

Hecker, M., Newsted, JL., Murphy, MB., Higley, EB., Jones, PD., Wu, R. & Giesy, JP. (2006). Human adrenocarcinoma (H295R) cells for rapid in vitro determination of effects on steroidogenesis: Hormone production,*Toxicology and Applied Pharmacology,* Vol. 217, pp.114-124

Hecker, M., Hollert, H., Cooper, R., Vinggaard, AM., Akahori, Y., Murphy, M., Nellemann, C., Higley, E., Newsted, J., Laskey, J., Buckalew, A., Grund, S., Maletz, S., Giesy, J., Timm, G. (2011). The OECD validation program of the H295R steroidogenesis assay: Phase 3. Final inter-laboratory validation study. *Environ Sci Pollut Res Int,* Vol. 18, pp. 503-515

Higley, E., Newsted, J., Zhang, X., Giesy, J. & Hecker, M. (2010). Assessment of chemical effects on aromatase activity using the H295R cell line. *Environ Sci Pollut Res Int,* Vol. 17, pp. 1137-1148

Holick, MF. (1987). Photosynthesis of vitamin D in the skin: effect of environmental and life-style variables. *Fed Proc,* Vol. 46, pp. 1876-1882

Holick, MF. (2006) Vitamin D: Its role in cancer prevention and treatment. *Progr Biophys & Mol Biol,* Vol. 92, pp. 49-59

Jones, G, Strugnell, SA & DeLuca, HF (1998) Current understanding of the molecular actions of vitamin D. *Physiological Reviews,* Vol. 78, pp. 1193-231

Hudak, SJ., Hernandez, J. & Thompson, IM. (2006). Role of 5α-reductase inhibitors in the management of prostate cancer. *Clin Interv Aging,* Vol. 1, pp. 425-431

Hum, DW., Bélanger, A., Lévesque, E., Barbier, O., Beaulieu, M., Albert, C., Vallée, M., Guillemette, C., Tchernof, A., Turgeon, D. & Dubois, S. (1999). Characterization of UDP-glucuronosyltransferases active on steroid hormones. *J Steroid Biochem Mol Biol,* Vol. 69, pp. 413-423

Jelinsky, SA., Harris, HA., Brown, EL., Flanagan, K., Tunkey, C., Lai, K., Lane, MV., Simcoe, DK. & Evans, MJ. (2003). Global transcription profiling of estrogen activity: estrogen receptor a regulates gene expression in the kidney. *Endocrinology,* Vol. 144, pp. 701-710

Jellinck, PH., Lee, SJ. & McEwen, BS. (2001). Metabolism of dehydroepiandrosterone by rat hippocampal cells in culture: possible role of aromatization and 7-hydroxylation in neuroprotection. *J Steroid Biochem Mol Biol,* Vol. 78, pp. 313-317

Jellinck, PH., Kaufmann, M., Gottfried-Blackmore, A., McEwen, BS., Jones, G. & Bulloch, K. (2007). Selective conversion by microglia of dehydroepiandrosterone to 5-androstenediol- A steroid with inherent estrogenic properties. *J Steroid Biochem Mol Biol,* Vol. 107, pp. 156-162

Jordan, VC. (2007). SERMs: meeting the promise of multifunctional medicines. *J Natl Cancer Inst,* Vol. 99, pp. 350-356

Kinuta, K., Tanaka, H., Moriwake, T., Aya, K., Kato, S. & Seino, Y. (2000). Vitamin D Is an Important Factor in Estrogen Biosynthesis of Both Female and Male Gonads. *Endocrinology,* Vol. 141, pp. 1317-1324

Krishnan, AV., Swami, S., Peng, L., Wang, J., Moreno, J. & Feldman, D. (2010). Tissue-Selective Regulation of Aromatase Expression by Calcitriol: Implications for Breast Cancer Therapy. *Endocrinology,* Vol. 151, pp. 32-42

Larsen, SS., Heiberg, I. & Lykkesfeldt, AE. (2001). Anti-oestrogen resistant human breast cancer cell lines are more sensitive towards treatment with the vitamin D analogue EB1089 than parent MCF-7 cells. *Br J Cancer,* Vol. 84, pp. 686-690

Lazarevic, B., Karlsen, SJ. & Saatcioglu, F. (2008). Genistein differentially modulates androgen-responsive gene expression and activates JNK in LNCaP cells. *Oncol Rep,* Vol. 19, pp. 1231-1235

Li, J. & Al-Azzawi, F. (2009). Mechanism of androgen receptor action. *Maturitas,* Vol. 63, pp. 142-148

Lorenzo PJ. & Saatcioglu, F. (2008). Inhibition of apoptosis in prostate cancer cells by androgens is mediated through downregulation of c-Jun N-terminal kinase activation. *Neoplasia,* Vol. 10, 418-428

Lou, YR., Laaksi, I., Syvälä, H., Bläuer, M., Tammela, TLJ., Ylikomi, T., and Tuohimaa, P. (2004). 25-Hydroxyvitamin D_3 is an active hormone in human primary prostatic stromal cells. *FASEB J,* Vol. 18, pp. 332-334

Lou, YR., Murtola, T. & Tuohimaa, P. (2005). Regulation of aromatase and 5α-reductase by 25-hydroxyvitamin D_3, 1α,25-dihydroxyvitamin D_3, dexamethasone and progesterone in prostate cancer cells. *J Steroid Biochem Mol Biol,* Vol. 94, pp. 151-157

Lou, YR. & Tuohimaa, P. (2006). Androgen enhances the antiproliferative activity of vitamin D_3 by suppressing 24-hydroxylase expression in LNCaP cells. *J Steroid Biochem Mol Biol,* Vol. 99, pp. 44-49

Lou, YR., Molnár, F., Peräkylä, M., Qiao, S., Kalueff, AV., St-Arnaud, R., Carlberg, C. & Tuohimaa, P. (2010). 25-Hydroxyvitamin D_3 is an agonistic vitamin D receptor ligand. *J Steroid Biochem Mol Biol,* Vol. 118, pp. 162-170

Lundqvist, J., Norlin, M. & Wikvall, K. (2010). 1α,25-Dihydroxyvitamin D_3 affects hormone production and expression of steroidogenic enzymes in human adrenocortical NCI-H295R cells. *Biochim Biophys Acta - Mol Cell Biol Lipids,* Vol. 180, pp. 1056-1062

Lundqvist, J., Norlin, M. & Wikvall K. (2011). 1α,25-Dihydroxyvitamin D_3 exerts tissue-specific effects on estrogen and androgen metabolism. *Biochim Biophys Acta - Mol Cell Biol Lipids,* Vol. 1811, pp. 263-270

Makin, G., Lohnes, D., Byford, V., Ray, R. & Jones, G. (1989). Target cell metabolism of 1,25-dihydroxyvitamin D_3 to calcitroic acid. Evidence for a pathway in kidney and bone involving 24-oxidation. *Biochem J,* Vol. 262, pp. 173-180

Maninger, N., Wolkowitz, OM., Reus, VI., Epel, E.S. & Mellon, SH. (2009). Neurobiological and neuropsychiatric effects of dehydroepiandrosterone (DHEA) and DHEA sulfate (DHEAS). *Front Neuroendocrinol,* Vol. 30, pp. 65-91

Masuda, S. & Jones, G. (2006). Promise of vitamin D analogues in the treatment of hyperproliferative conditions. *Mol Cancer Ther,* Vol. 5, pp. 797-808

Mathiasen, IS., Sergeev, IN., Bastholm, L., Elling, F., Norman, AW. & Jäättelä, M. (2002). Calcium and Calpain as Key Mediators of Apoptosis-like Death Induced by Vitamin D Compounds in Breast Cancer Cells. *J Biol Chem,* Vol. 277, pp. 30738-30745

Melcangi, RC. & Panzica, GC. (2006). Neuroactive steroids: old players in a new game. *Neuroscience,* Vol. 138, 733-739

Miller, WR., Anderson, TJ. & Jack, WJL. (1990). Relationship between tumour aromatase activity, tumour characteristics and response to therapy, *J Steroid Biochem Mol Biol*, Vol. 37, pp. 1055-1059

Miller, W. (2008). Steroidogenic Enzymes. *Endocr Dev*, Vol. 13, 1-18

Morani, A., Warner, M. & Gustafsson, JA. (2008). Biological functions and clinical implications of oestrogen receptors α and β in epithelial tissues. *J Intern Med*, Vol. 264, pp. 128-142

Norlin, M & Wikvall, K. (2007). Enzymes in the conversion of cholesterol into bile acids. *Curr Mol Med*, Vol. 7, pp. 199-218

Norlin, M. (2008). Regulation of cellular steroid levels with special focus on oxysterol and estrogen metabolism. *Future Lipidol*, Vol. 3, pp. 337-346

Norlin, M., Pettersson, H., Tang, W. & Wikvall, K. (2011). Androgen receptor-mediated regulation of the anti-atherogenic enzyme CYP27A1 involves the JNK/c-jun pathway. *Arch Biochem Biophys*, Vol. 506, pp. 236-241

Norman, AW. (2006). Vitamin D Receptor: New Assignments for an Already Busy Receptor. *Endocrinology*, Vol. 147, pp. 5542-5548

Norman, AW. (2008). From vitamin D to hormone D: fundamentals of the vitamin D endocrine system essential for good health. *Am J Clin Nutr*. Vol. 88, pp. 491S-499

Olsson, M., Gustafsson, O., Skogastierna, C., Tolf, A., Rietz, BD., Morfin, R., Rane, A. & Ekström, L. (2007). Regulation and expression of human CYP7B1 in prostate: overexpression of CYP7B1 during progression of prostatic adenocarcinoma. *Prostate*, Vol. 67, pp. 1439-1446

Paech, K., Webb, P., Kuiper, GG., Nilsson, S., Gustafsson, J., Kushner, PJ. & Scanlan, TS. (1997). Differential ligand activation of estrogen receptors ERα and ERβ at AP1 sites. *Science*, Vol. 277, pp. 1508-1510

Penning, TM., Burczynski, ME., Jez, JM., Hung, CF., Lin, HK., Ma, H., Moore, M., Palackal, N. & Ratnam, K. (2000). Human 3α-hydroxysteroid dehydrogenase isoforms (AKR1C1-AKR1C4) of the aldo-keto reductase superfamily: functional plasticity and tissue distribution reveals roles in the inactivation and formation of male and female sex hormones. *Biochem J*, Vol. 351, pp. 67-77

Pérez-López, FR. (2008). Sunlight, the vitamin D endocrine system, and their relationships with gynaecologic cancer. *Maturitas*, Vol. 59, pp. 101-113

Pettersson, H., Holmberg, L., Axelson, M. & Norlin, M. (2008). CYP7B1-mediated metabolism of dehydroepiandrosterone and 5α-androstane-3β,17β-diol - potential role(s) for estrogen signaling. *Febs J*, Vol. 275, pp. 1778-1789

Pettersson, H., Lundqvist, J., Oliw, E. & Norlin, M. (2009). CYP7B1-mediated metabolism of 5α-androstane-3α,17β-diol (3α-Adiol): a novel pathway for potential regulation of the cellular levels of androgens and neurosteroids. *Biochim Biophys Acta*, Vol. 1791, pp.1206-1215

Pettersson, H., Lundqvist, J. & Norlin, M. (2010). Effects of CYP7B1-mediated catalysis on estrogen receptor activation. *Biochim Biophys Acta*, Vol. 1801, pp. 1090-1097

Pikuleva, IA. (2006). Cholesterol-metabolizing cytochromes P450. *Drug Metab Dispos*, Vol. 34, pp. 513-520

Prins, GS. & Korach, KS. (2008). The role of estrogens and estrogen receptors in normal prostate growth and disease. *Steroids*, Vol. 73, pp. 233-244

Prosser, DE. & Jones, G. (2004). Enzymes involved in the activation and inactivation of vitamin D. *Trends in Biochemical Sciences,* Vol. 29, pp. 664-673

Ramagopalan, SV., Heger, A., Berlanga, AJ., Maugeri, NJ., Lincoln. MR., Burrell, A., Handunnetthi, L., Handel, AE., Disanto ,G., Orton, SM., Watson, CT., Morahan, JM., Giovannoni, G., Ponting, CP., Ebers, GC. & Knight, JC. (2010). A ChiP-seq defined genome-wide map of vitamin D receptor binding: associations with disease and evolution. *Genome Res,* Vol. 20, pp. 1352-1360

Rainey, WE., Rehman, KS. & Carr, BR. (2004). The human fetal adrenal: making adrenal androgens for placental estrogens. *Semin Reprod Med,* Vol. 22, pp. 327-336

Reddy, DS. (2004). Testosterone modulation of seizure susceptibility is mediated by neurosteroids 3α-androstanediol and 17β-estradiol. *Neuroscience,* Vol. 129, pp. 195-207

Reddy, GS. & Tserng, KY. (1989). Calcitroic acid, end product of renal metabolism of 1,25-dihydroxyvitamin D_3 through the C-24 oxidation pathway. *Biochemistry,* Vol. 28, pp. 1763-1769

Rose, KA., Stapleton, G., Dott, K., Kieny, MP., Best, R,. Schwarz, M., Russell, DW., Björkhem, I., Seckl, J & Lathe, R (1997): Cyp7b, a novel brain cytochrome P450, catalyzes the synthesis of neurosteroids 7α-hydroxy dehydroepiandrosterone and 7α-hydroxy pregnenolone. *Proc Natl Acad Sci U S A,* Vol. 94, pp. 4925-4930

Safe, S. (2001). Transcriptional activation of genes by 17β-estradiol through estrogen receptor-Sp1 interactions. *Vitam Horm,* Vol. 62, pp. 231-252

Sasano, H., Miki, Y., Nagasaki, S. & Suzuki, T. (2009). In situ estrogen production and its regulation in human breast carcinoma: From endocrinology to intracrinology. *Pathol Int,* Vol. 59, pp. 777-789

Schaeffer, V., Patte-Mensah, C., Eckert, A. & Mensah-Nyagan, AG. (2006). Modulation of neurosteroid production in human neuroblastoma cells by Alzheimer's disease key proteins, *J Neurobiol,* Vol. 66, pp. 868-881

Schultz, JR., Petz, LN. & Nardulli, AM. (2005). Cell- and ligand-specific refulation of promoters containing activator protein-1 and Sp1 sites bt estrogen receptors a and b. *J Biol Chem,* Vol. 280, pp. 347-354

Schwartz, GG. (2005). Vitamin D and the epidemiology of prostate cancer. *Semin Dial,* Vol. 18, pp. 276-289

Shapiro, DJ., Mao, C. & Cherian, MT. (2011). Small molecule inhibitors as probes for estrogen and androgen receptor action. *J Biol Chem,* Vol. 286, pp. 4043-4048

Sharifi, N. (2010). New agents and strategies for the hormonal treatment of castration-resistant prostate cancer. *Expert Opin Investig Drugs,* Vol. 19, pp. 837-846

Simard, J., Ricketts, ML., Gingras, S., Soucy, P., Feltus, FA. & Melner, MH. (2005). Molecular biology of the 3β-hydroxysteroid dehydrogenase/Δ^5-Δ^4 isomerase gene family. *Endocr Rev,* Vol. 26, pp. 525-582

Simpson, ER., Clyne, C., Rubin, G., Boon, WC., Robertson, K., Britt, K., Speed, C. & Jones, M. (2002). Aromatase - a brief overview, *Ann Rev Physiol,* Vol. 64, pp. 93-127

Steinberg, D. (2006). Thematic review series: the pathogenesis of atherosclerosis. An interpretive history of the cholesterol controversy, part V: the discovery of the statins and the end of the controversy. *J Lipid Res,* Vol. 47, pp. 1339-1351

Stoll, G. & Bendszus, M. (2006). Inflammation and atherosclerosis: novel insights into plaque formation and destabilization. *Stroke,* Vol. 37, pp. 1923-1932

Stiles, AR., McDonald, JG., Bauman, DR. & Russell, DW. (2009). CYP7B1: one cytochrome P450, two human genetic diseases, and multiple physiological functions. *J Biol Chem,* Vol. 284, pp. 28485-28489

Sugiyama, N., Andersson, S., Lathe, R., Fan, X., Alonso-Magdalena, P., Schwend, T., Nalvarte, I., Warner, M. & Gustafsson, JA. (2009). Spatiotemporal dynamics of the expression of estrogen receptors in the postnatal mouse brain. *Mol Psychiatry,* Vol. 14, pp. 223-232

Sultan, C., Paris, F., Terouanne, B., Balaguer, P., Georget, V., Poujol, N., Jeandel, C., Lumbroso, S. & Nicolas, JC. (2001). Disorders linked to insufficient androgen action in male children, *Hum Reprod Update,* Vol. 7, pp. 314-322

Tanaka, S., Haji, M., Takayanagi, R., Tanaka, S., Sugioka, Y. & Nawata, H. (1996). 1,25-Dihydroxyvitamin D_3 enhances the enzymatic activity and expression of the messenger ribonucleic acid for aromatase cytochrome P450 synergistically with dexamethasone depending on the vitamin D receptor level in cultured human osteoblasts. *Endocrinology,* Vol. 137, pp. 1860-1869

Tang, W., Eggertsen, G., Chiang, JY. & Norlin, M. (2006). Estrogen-mediated regulation of CYP7B1: a possible role for controlling DHEA levels in human tissues. *J Steroid Biochem Mol Biol,* Vol. 100, pp. 42-51

Tang, W. & Norlin, M. (2006). Regulation of steroid hydroxylase CYP7B1 by androgens and estrogens in prostate cancer LNCaP cells. *Biochem Biophys Res Commun,* Vol. 344, pp. 540-546

Tang, W., Norlin, M. & Wikvall, K. (2007). Regulation of human CYP27A1 by estrogens and androgens in HepG2 and prostate cells. *Arch Biochem Biophys,* Vol. 462, pp. 13-20

Tang, W., Pettersson, H. & Norlin, M. (2008). Involvement of the PI3K/Akt pathway in estrogen-mediated regulation of human CYP7B1: identification of CYP7B1 as a novel target for PI3K/Akt and MAPK signalling. *J Steroid Biochem Mol Biol,* Vol. 112, pp. 63-73

Tchernof, AF., Labrie, F., Belanger, A., Prud´homme, D., Bouchard, C., Tremblay, A., Nadeau, A. & Despres, JP. (1997). Relationships between endogenous steroid hormone, sex hormone-binding globulin and lipoprotein levels in men: contribution of visceral obesity, insulin levels and other metabolic variables. *Atherosclerosis,* Vol. 133, pp. 235-244

Thorne, J. & Campbell, MJ. (2008). The vitamin D receptor in cancer. *Proc Nutr Soc,* Vol. 67, pp. 115-127

Trap, C., Nato, F., Chalbot, S., Kim, S.B., Lafaye, P. & Morfin, R. (2005). Immunohistochemical detection of the human cytochrome P4507B1: production of a monoclonal antibody after cDNA immunization. *J Neuroimmunol,* Vol. 159, pp. 41-47

Tsaousidou, MK., Ouahchi, K., Warner, TT., Yang, Y., Simpson, MA., Laing, NG., Wilkinson, PA., Madrid, RE., Patel, H., Hentati, F., Patton, MA., Hentati, A., Lamont, PJ., Siddique, T. & Crosby, AH. (2008). Sequence alterations within CYP7B1 implicate defective cholesterol homeostasis in motor-neuron degeneration. *Am J Hum Genet,* Vol. 82, pp. 510-515

Tsuchiya, Y., Nakajima, M. & Yokoi, T. (2005). Cytochrome P450-mediated metabolism of estrogens and its regulation in human. *Cancer Lett,* Vol. 227, pp. 115-124

Tuohimaa, P., Golovko, O., Kalueff, A., Nazarova, N., Qiao, S., Syvälä, H., Talonpoika, R. & Lou, YR. (2005). Calcidiol and prostate cancer. *J Steroid Biochem Mol Biol,* Vol. 93, pp. 183-190

Turgeon, D., Carrier, JS., Levesque, E., Hum, DW. & Belanger, A. (2001). Relative enzymatic activity, protein stability, and tissue distribution of human steroid-metabolizing UGT2B subfamily members. *Endocrinology,* Vol. 142, pp. 778-787

Umetani, M., Domoto, H., Gormley, AK., Yuhanna, IS., Cummins, CL., Javitt, NB., Korach, KS., Shaul, PW. (2007). Mangelsdorf DJ. 27-Hydroxycholesterol is an endogenous SERM that inhibits the cardiovascular effects of estrogen. *Nat Med,* Vol. 13, pp. 1185-1192

Umetani, M. & Shaul, PW. (2011). 27-Hydroxycholesterol: the first identified endogenous SERM. *Trends Endocrinol Metab,* Vol. 22, pp. 130-135

Verstuyf, A., Carmeliet, G., Bouillon, R. & Mathieu, C. (2010). Vitamin D: a pleiotropic hormone. *Kidney Int.* Vol. 78, pp. 140-145

Vihko, P., Herrala, A., Härkönen, P., Isomaa, V., Kaija, H., Kurkela, R. & Pulkka, A. (2006). Control of cell proliferation by steroids: the role of 17HSDs. *Mol Cell Endocrinol,* Vol. 248, pp. 141-148

Wang, JH. & Tuohimaa, P. (2007). Regulation of 17β-hydroxysteroid dehydrogenase type 2, type 4 and type 5 by calcitriol, LXR agonist and 5α-dihydrotestosterone in human prostate cancer cells. *J Steroid Biochem Mol Biol,* Vol. 107, pp. 100-105

Waxman, DJ. & Holloway, MG. (2009). Sex differences in the expression of hepatic drug metabolizing enzymes. Mol Pharmacol, Vol. 76, pp. 215-228

Weihua, Z., Lathe, R., Warner, M. & Gustafsson, JÅ. (2002). An endocrine pathway in the prostate, ERβ, AR, 5α-androstane-3β,17β-diol, and CYP7B1, regulates prostate growth. *Proc Natl Acad Sci U S A,* Vol. 99, pp. 13589-13594

Wikvall, K. (2001) Cytochrome P450 enzymes in the bioactivation of vitamin D to its hormonal form. *Int J Mol Med,* Vol. 7, pp. 201-209

Wu, Z., Martin, KO., Javitt, NB. & Chiang, JY. (1999). Structure and functions of human oxysterol 7α-hydroxylase cDNAs and gene CYP7B1. *J Lipid Res,* Vol. 40, pp. 2195-2203

Yamamoto, Y., Moore. R., Hess HA., Guo, GL., Gonzalez, FJ., Korach, KS., Maronpot, RR. & Negishi, M. (2006). Estrogen receptor a mediates 17α-ethynylestradiol causing hepatotoxicity. *J Biol Chem,* Vol. 281, pp. 16625-16631

Yau, JL., Rasmuson, S., Andrew, R., Graham, M, Noble, J., Olsson, T., Fuchs, E., Lathe, R. & Seckl, JR. (2003). Dehydroepiandrosterone 7-hydroxylase CYP7B: predominant expression in primate hippocampus and reduced expression in Alzheimer's disease. *Neuroscience,* Vol. 121, pp. 307-314

Zhang, J., Akwa, Y., el-Etr, M., Baulieu, EE. & Sjövall, J. (1997). Metabolism of 27-, 25- and 24-hydroxycholesterol in rat glial cells and neurons. *Biochem J,* Vol. 322, pp. 175-184

Zhu, BT. & Lee, AJ. (2005). NADPH-dependent metabolism of 17β-estradiol and estrone to polar and nonpolar metabolites by human tissues and cytochrome P450 isoforms. *Steroids,* Vol. 70, pp. 225-244

Zimmerman, DR., Reinhardt, TA., Kremer, R., Beitz, DC., Reddy, GS. & Horst, RL. (2001). Calcitroic acid is a major catabolic metabolite in the metabolism of 1α-dihydroxyvitamin D_2. *Arch Biochem Biophys,* Vol. 392, pp. 14-22

Zittermann, A. (2003). Vitamin D in preventive medicine: are we ignoring the evidence? *Br J Nutr,* Vol. 89, pp. 552-572

Zmuda JM, J.A. Cauley, A. Kriska, N.W. Glynn, J.P. Gutai, L.H. Kuller, *Am. J. Epidemiol.* 146 (1997) 609-617.

19

Solid State and Thermal Behavior of 17β-Estradiol in Ammonioethyl Methacrylate Ester Copolymer

Chutima Wiranidchapong
Faculty of Pharmacy, Srinakharinwirot University
Thailand

1. Introduction

17β-estradiol is the most potent form of naturally occurring estrogen secreted during the reproductive years (Andersson 2000; Paoletti 2001). It is an essential steroid hormone that regulates numerous endocrine functions through binding to two estrogen receptor (ER) isoforms, i.e., ERα and ERβ. The concentration of these receptor subtypes and the corresponding cofactors vary with tissue types, leading to tissue specific regulation of estrogen response and toxicity. However, the content of ER in tissues has been assumed to be time-invariant (Plowchalk 2002). This indicates that multiple or prolonged exposure to E_2 of ER in various tissues should not alter physiological and toxic responses.

Estradiol (E_2) is carried in the plasma in two forms, bound to plasma binding proteins (95-98 %) and unbound form or free estradiol (2-5 %) (Dunn 1983; Pardridge 1986; Plowchalk 2002). Both unbound and bound forms of E_2 manifest pharmacological actions. Bound form acts as a reservoir for E_2 in blood circulation (Plowchalk 2002). After menopause the primary circulating estrogen is estrone, which is less biologically active than E_2 (Kuhl 2005; Margolis 2010). Thus, E_2 is usually administered to control early menopausal symptoms such as hot flashes and night sweats. For long-term administration E_2 can prevent cardiovascular diseases and osteoporosis (Andersson 2000; Paoletti 2001). After administered E_2 reaches to blood circulation, it rapidly undergoes chemical conversions to estrone, driven in part by the body's need to maintain homeostasis. Other estrogens in conjugated forms either equine- or synthetic-derived also exist as a balance between the ingested form and estrone at steady state in the body. Margolis (Margolis 2010) indicated that the conversion of E_2 to estrone was reversible reaction. Therefore, estrone plays as a hormonally inert reservoir, capably converting to E_2. These conversions make the administered estrogen indistinguishable from naturally occurring E_2 in the body.

However, hormone therapy is not without risks. The FDA and several professional organizations currently recommend prescribing the lowest effective dose for the shortest duration of time in accordance with treatment goals for an individual woman (Mueck 2003; Utian 2008; Margolis 2010). Nowaday there are a wide variety of estrogen products, including oral tablets, transdermal patches, and topical sprays, gels, and lotions, as well as vaginal creams, tablets, and rings. Selection of an appropriate product is often based on patient's preference. Oral estrogen dosage form is preferred due to its convenient route of administration. To improve outcome of estrogen therapy, formulation properties and product pharmacokinetics should be considered for choosing an appropriate product.

2. Biopharmaceutics and pharmacokinetics of estrogen products

Oral administration of estrogen in tablet dosage form is the most favorable form for estrogen replacement therapy. The oral bioavailability of estrogen is dependent on its solubility in gastrointestinal (GI) fluid and permeability across membrane of endothelial cell lining in the gut wall. Unconjugated estrogens are hydrophobic molecules with low solubility in GI fluid. To improve the bioavailability their dissolution has to be increased. The methods normally used to enhance estrogen dissolution are chemical modification and reduction of the particle size.

Modification of chemical structure by conjugating with hydrophilic groups via esterification such as estradiol acetate and sulfonation such as sulfonated estrogens can improve drug dissolution. Conjugated estrogens exhibit better solubility than unconjugated form. However, most of conjugated estrogens have low affinity for ER. Thus, oral administration of conjugated form such as sulfonated estrogens may reduce undesired stimulation of ER within the GI tract. Since sulfonated estrogens are carried to target tissues, they are enzymatically hydrolyzed and then converted to bioactive estrogens (Margolis 2010). Similarly, estradiol acetate is also hydrolyzed in plasma and tissue and then transforms to active estrogen (Iwamori 2005; Margolis 2010).

Using micronized form of estrogen as an active ingredient in tablet formulation can improve estrogen dissolution by increasing surface area exposure to the dissolution medium. This phenomenon can be described by the Noyes-Whitney Equation (Shargel 1999);

$$\frac{dC}{dt} = \frac{DA}{h}(C_s - C) \tag{1}$$

where $\frac{dC}{dt}$ = rate of drug dissolution at time t, D = diffusion rate constant, A = surface area of the drug particles, C_s = concentration of drug in the stagnant layer (equal to solubility of the drug), C = concentration of drug in bulk solution, h = thickness of the stagnant layer.

From Noyes-Whitney equation, rate of drug dissolution at time t $\left(\frac{dc}{dt}\right)$ is directly increased as the surface area of the drug particles (A) is increased. Using micronized estrogen in tablet formulation results in the increase of surface area of the drug particles and consequently increases estrogen dissolution. Furthermore, design of tablet disintegration by using specific disintegrants in the formulation affects the duration to allow estrogen to dissolve in the GI fluid and then absorb into the blood stream. Product design potentially affects the bioavailability of estrogen.

During hormone therapy estrogens are orally administered once a day according to prolonged terminal elimination half-life (Plowchalk 2002). Oral dosage form of estrogens is often formulated in immediate-release tablet. This kind of product rapidly releases estrogen after administered. Due to rapid absorption of estrogens into the blood circulation (Margolis 2010), plasma estrogen concentration versus time profile reveals peaks and troughs pattern. Therefore, oral administration of immediate-release estrogen tablets has the potential to produce high spikes in blood levels, which possibly lead to estrogen-excess symptoms such as breast tenderness, headaches, nausea, vomiting, mood swings, bleeding, or spotting.

Boyd et al. (Boyd 2003; Margolis 2010) reported the decrease in maximum concentration ranging from 3% to 36% in a fed state as compared to a fasting state in subjects, taking estrogen tablet with a high-fat meal. This report met an agreement with the reason of some patients undergone breakthrough hot flashes when taking their estrogen products with food (Margolis 2010). In addition, the variation of estrogen concentration in blood level probably comes from intestinal and hepatic first-pass metabolism of orally administered estrogen (Meli 1968; Longcope 1985; Plowchalk 2002). This characteristic results in low oral bioavailability of estrogen, which is only 2-5 % (Bawaarshi-Hassar 1989; Kuhnz 1993; Plowchalk 2002). Thus, trend of estrogen product development has been tempted to abandon oral administration and shifted to non-oral administrations.

Non-oral estrogen administration avoids hepatic first-pass effect, allowing smaller dose to be used and preventing undesirable changes from liver stimulation (Pentikis 1998; Munoz 1999; Rohr 1999; Andersson 2000; Paoletti 2001; Anderson 2002). However, desirable estrogen product is not only containing the lowest effective dose but also maintaining estrogen in blood level within a therapeutic range over a conveniently long dosing interval. These characteristics ensure adequate concentration of estrogen in blood for preventing both daytime hot flashes and night sweats, while not reaching overly high or peaky blood levels that may cause adverse events, such as breast tenderness, headache, nausea, vomiting, mood swings, bleeding, or spotting.

In the past, the only way to eliminate the peak and trough plasma levels of drug therapy was to deliver continuous intravenous (IV) infusion to a patient at a constant rate based on pharmacokinetics of the drug. However, this kind of drug administration requires health care professionals to monitor drug concentration in the plasma, thus usually cannot be performed at home. To alleviate this problem, various types of controlled-release drug delivery system have been developed to release the drug at a constant rate, replacing the administration via continuous IV infusion. In 1937, Parks and Dansby had formulated compressed pure crystalline estrogen pellets and administered them by subcutaneous injection to livestock. The results showed a continuous release of hormone over 3 months in several animals. Their work was presented at the Royal Society of Medicine in London. This led to a widespread idea of hormonal implantation in animals, which became the standard practice in the 1950s (Dash 1998). This discovery sparked an interest area of implantable drug delivery systems, leading to extended studies and continuous discoveries until the present time.

Implantable drug delivery systems have basically been classified into two major classes, i.e., drug implants and implantable pumps containing the drug. The first class utilizes various types of polymer matrices and polymeric membranes to control the kinetics of drug release from the delivery systems (Danckwerts 1991; Dash 1998). The second class consists of mechanical pump-type implants, which utilize an infusion pump-type action to control release of the drug. For estrogen therapy, the goal of the delivery system is to release estrogens at a constant rate throughout an intended period of time. Controlled release of estrogen products either transdermal patches or vaginal rings utilize polymer matrices and/or polymeric membranes as rate-controlling element similar to drug implants. To clearly understand how polymer matrices and polymer membranes can facilitate the release of estrogen, the fundamentals of rate-controlling drug delivery should be addressed.

3. Basic concepts of rate-controlled estrogen delivery

The majority of recent literatures have been focused on sustained-release and controlled-release drug delivery systems. Sustained-release drug product is referred to a dosage form formulated to retard the release of a therapeutic agent. Thus, the drug in the systemic

circulation is delayed the onset, prolonged its plasma concentration and provided longer duration of action (Chien 1992). On the other hand, controlled-release drug product is pointed to the delivery system giving a release profile not only predictable kinetically but also reproducible from one unit to another (Chien 1982; Chien 1989; Chien 1992).
Basic principles in the rate-controlled drug released from both polymer matrix and polymeric membrane is governed by Fick's laws of diffusion (Grant 1968; Chien 1992), which define the flux of diffusion (J_D) across a plane surface of unit area as shown;

$$J_D = -D\frac{dc}{dx} \tag{2}$$

where D is the diffusivity of drug molecule in a medium of solid, solution, or gas, $\left(\frac{dc}{dx}\right)$ is the concentration gradient of the drug molecule across a diffusional path with thickness dx, and a negative sign is used to define the direction of diffusion from a region with high concentration to a region with low concentration. The drug concentration gradient acts as the energy element for the diffusion of drug molecules.
In order to identify the mechanism of drug release, governed by Fick's laws of diffusion, the following assumptions need to be established (Chien 1992);

1. Dissolution of drug crystals into their surrounding medium is the first step of the drug release process.
2. A pseudo-steady state exists in the process of controlled drug release.
3. The diffusion coefficient of a drug molecule in a given medium is invariable with time and distance.
4. The interfacial partitioning of a drug molecule from polymer toward solution is related to its solubility in polymer (C_p) and in solution (C_s) as defined by

$$K = \frac{C_s}{C_p} \tag{3}$$

where K is defined as the partition coefficient.
Kinetically released of drug molecules from these types of rate-controlled drug delivery should be illustrated at each mechanism of drug release.

3.1 Polymer membrane permeation-controlled drug release

Polymer membrane permeation-controlled drug release has been appeared in a pharmaceutical dosage form in which a drug is totally or partially encapsulated within a drug reservoir compartment. The drug reservoir may exist in solid, suspension, or solution forms. The encapsulation of drug formulation inside the reservoir compartment is performed by spray coating, injection molding, hot-melt extrusion, microencapsulation, or other techniques.
The examples of this kind of rate-controlled drug delivery system are Progestasert IUD, an intrauterine device and Norplant, subdermal implant. Progestasert IUD contains a suspension of progesterone crystals in silicone medical fluid, encapsulated in a nonporous membrane of ethylene vinyl acetate copolymer in a T-shaped device. This product can continuously release progesterone in the uterine cavity at rate of at least 65 μg/day for a year (Chien 1992). For Norplant, the active drug is levonorgestrel, encapsulated in nonporous silicone medical-grade tubing with both ends sealed with medical-grade adhesive silicone. The development of this product has been found in 2 generations. The first is composed of 6 units of levonorgestrel crystals encapsulated in silicone tubes and the second is composed of 2 units of silicone tubes

containing levonorgestrel dispersing in silicone elastomer matrix inside. Both are designed to continuously liberate the active drug at a daily dosage rate of 30 μg for up to 7 years (Croxatto 1981; Weiner 1981; Diaz 1982; Segal 1983; Chien 1992).

The release process begins on the outermost layer of drug particles dissociating themselves from the crystal state and then dissolving in the surrounding medium, partitioning and diffusing through the polymer structure, and finally partitioning into the elution medium surrounding the device. During the device is sink in the surrounding medium, the hydrodynamic diffusion layer occurs on the immediate surface of the device. Therefore, the diffusion path length in which drug molecules diffuse across under a concentration gradient is the addition of the thickness of polymeric membrane and the hydrodynamic diffusion layer.

The cumulative amount of drug (Q) released from a unit surface area of a polymer membrane permeation-controlled drug delivery system is expressed as shown (Chien 1992);

$$Q = \frac{C_p K D_d D_p}{K D_d h_p + D_p h_d} t - \frac{D_p D_d}{K D_d h_p + D_p h_d} \int_0^t C_{b(t)}\, dt \quad (4)$$

where C_p is the drug solubility in the polymer, K is the partition coefficient as defined by Equation (3), D_p and D_d are the drug diffusivities in the polymer membrane with thickness h_p and in the hydrodynamic diffusion layer with thickness h_d, respectively. $C_{b(t)}$ is the concentration of drug in the interface of diffusion layer/ bulk solution, t is time, and dt is a differential length of time.

In the case of sink condition throughout the course of controlled drug release, the saturated concentration of drug in the solution (C_s) is much higher than the concentration of the drug in the bulk solution ($C_{b(t)}$); $C_s >> C_{b(t)}$ or $C_{b(t)} \approx 0$. Thus, Equation (4) can be reduced to

$$Q = \frac{C_p K D_d D_p}{K D_d h_p + D_p h_d} t \quad (5)$$

The rate of drug released from this system can be defined by rearrangement of Equation (5) into

$$\frac{Q}{t} = \frac{C_p K D_d D_p}{K D_d h_p + D_p h_d} \quad (6)$$

Equation (6) indicates that the rate of drug release per unit time is equal to a constant value, i.e., the solubility of drug in the polymer, the partition coefficient, the diffusivity of drug molecule, and the thickness of the rate-controlling membrane. This implies that the polymer membrane permeation-controlled drug delivery gives a constant drug release profile. Equation (6) has considerably described the release of progesterone from Progestasert IUD (Chien 1992).

In case of a thick polymer membrane (h_p) and/or extremely low diffusivity of drug molecules in a polymer (D_p), which is dependent on the type of polymer material, the term of KD_dh_p is much higher than the term of D_ph_d. Thus, Equation (6) can be simplified to

$$\frac{Q}{t} = \frac{C_p D_p}{h_p} \quad (7)$$

Under this condition the rate of drug release is a function of the solubility and diffusivity of drug in the polymer and is inversely proportional to the thickness of the polymer membrane. So the release of drug molecules is governed by the membrane-modulated permeation process.

In case of a very low interfacial partition coefficient (K) or a thick hydrodynamic diffusion layer (h_d), in which a condition is little movement of the surrounding medium, the KD_dh_p term is significantly smaller than the D_ph_d term. Equation (6) can be reduced to

$$\frac{Q}{t} = \frac{C_pKD_d}{h_d} \quad (8)$$

From Equation (2), since $C_pK = C_s$, Equation (8) can be rewritten as;

$$\frac{Q}{t} = \frac{C_sD_d}{h_d} \quad (9)$$

Under this condition the rate of drug release is a function of drug solubility in the surrounding medium and drug diffusivity in the hydrodynamic diffusion layer and is inversely proportional to the thickness of the hydrodynamic diffusion layer. Thus, the release of drug molecules is governed by the diffusion layer-limiting partition-controlled process.

From the principle of controlled release of drug from a dosage form in which the drug is encapsulated inside the polymer membrane, solubility of the drug strongly affects the rate of drug release. Under the condition in which the polymeric membrane plays the leading role in modulation of drug release, drug solubility in that polymer is a significant factor influencing the rate of drug release. On the other hand, under the condition of the hydrodynamic diffusion layer-limiting partition-controlled process, drug solubility in the surrounding medium affects the rate of drug release. Thus, an alteration in drug solubility either in polymer membrane or in the surrounding medium can also affect the rate of drug released from this kind of drug delivery system.

3.2 Polymer matrix diffusion-controlled drug release

Delivery system, controlling drug release by polymer matrix diffusion-controlled drug release, is prepared by homogeneously dispersing drug particles in a rate-controlling polymer matrix. The drug dispersion in the polymer matrix can be produced by dissolving the drug and the polymer in an appropriate solvent, followed by solvent evaporation at an elevated temperature and/or under a vacuum, or mixing finely ground drug particles with a rubbery polymer at an elevated temperature. The drug-polymer dispersion is then compressed, molded, or extruded to form a drug delivery device of various shapes and sizes designed for specific application.

An example of this type of drug delivery system is Compudose subdermal implant, fabricated by dispersing micronized estradiol (E_2) crystals in a viscous silicone elastomer and then coating the E_2-dispersing polymer around a rigid (drug-free) silicone rod by extrusion to form a rod-shaped implant. This product has been used for growth promotion in steers. It can release E_2 at controlled dose for 200 to 400 days (Hsieh 1987; Chien 1992).

The release of drug dispersing in a matrix environment is based on the hypothesis that the drug particles cannot move from their individual positions in the polymer matrix. The drug solids in the layer closer to the surface of the device are first diffused, so that this layer becomes a drug depletion zone. Then, the drug particles in the next layer begin to dissolve and diffuse, resulting in the growing thickness of drug depletion layer. This thickness becomes greater and greater as more drug solids are eluted out of the device, leading to inward advancement of the interface of drug dispersion zone/ drug depletion zone into the core of the device for another thickness(dh_p). Therefore, the rate of drug release from the polymer matrix diffusion-controlled drug delivery system is time-dependent and progressively decreases in response to increase in the thickness of the diffusional path as time goes by. At steady state the rate of drug release $\left(\frac{dQ}{dt}\right)$ is defined as followed (Chien 1992);

$$\frac{dQ}{dt} = \left(\frac{AC_pD_p}{2t}\right)^{\frac{1}{2}} \tag{10}$$

where A is the initial drug loading dose in the polymer matrix, C_p is the drug solubility in the polymer, which is also the drug reservoir concentration in the system, and D_p is the diffusivity of the drug molecules in the polymer matrix.

Integration of Equation (10) gives the relationship of the cumulative amount of drug release (Q) directly varied with the square root of time as the following equation;

$$Q = \left(2AC_pD_p\right)^{\frac{1}{2}}(t)^{\frac{1}{2}} \tag{11}$$

From Equation (11), the cumulative amount of drug released from the polymer matrix diffusion-controlled drug delivery system is controlled by the loading dose, solubility and diffusivity of the drug in the polymer matrix. This confirms that the drug solubility in the polymer is also one of significant factors affecting the amount of drug released from this delivery system.

One major drawback of the polymer matrix diffusion-controlled drug delivery system is its inability to achieve a constant release due to the variable thickness of the drug depletion zone. The thickness of the drug depletion zone increases as the release of drug proceeds. Therefore, the rate of drug release decreases with the reciprocal of the square root of time. Rippe and Johnso (Rippie 1969), Cobby et al. (Cobby 1974), and Hsieh et al. (Hsieh 1983) revealed that the shape of a matrix could be a factor affecting drug release, so that several researches since last 2 decades have been done in development of new designs of matrix system in order to achieve the zero-order or near zero-order release kinetics.

3.2.1 Hemipheric polymer matrix diffusion-controlled drug release

Drug released from hemispheric polymer matrix device has been designed to achieve a constant release (Hsieh 1983). The device is composed of the drug dispersing in a hemispheric polymer matrix, coated with an impermeable material except for a small cavity cut into the center of the flat surface as shown in Figure 1. Only a cavity in the center where

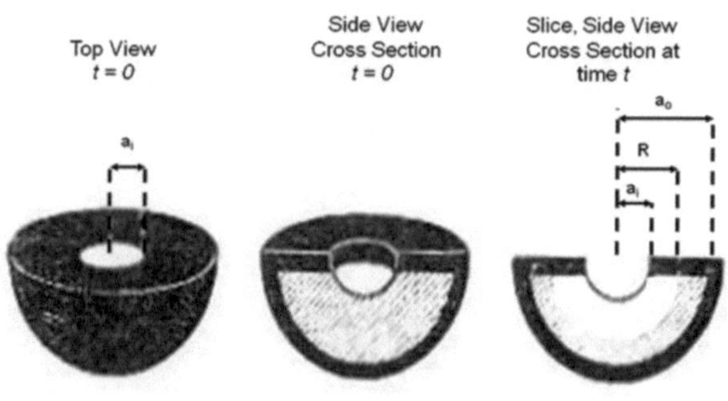

Fig. 1. Diagram of a hemispheric polymer matrix device: a_i was the inner radius; a_o was the outer radius; R was the distance to the interface between the drug depletion zone (white area) and the drug dispersing zone (diagonal lines); and black represented coated regions through which the drug release could not occur (From Hsieh, et. al., 1983).

the drug can be released the interface between drug depletion zone and drug dispersing zone moves into the interior as a front. The inwardly-releasing hemisphere increases the available area, where the drug can be released, so as to compensate the increase in diffusion distance of drug transport.

The rate of drug release $\left(\frac{dQ}{dt}\right)$ from the hemispheric polymer matrix device can be expressed as (Hsieh 1983);

$$\frac{dQ}{dt} = 2\pi C_s D_p a_i \left(\frac{R}{R-a_i}\right) \tag{12}$$

where π is a constant value, C_s is drug solubility in the surrounding medium, D_p is the diffusivity of drug molecules in the polymer matrix, a_i is radius of the cavity, and R is radial distance to interface between drug depletion zone and drug dispersing zone within the matrix.

Since R-a_i becomes equal to R when $R \gg a_i$. Equation (12), then, can be simplified to;

$$\frac{dQ}{dt} = 2\pi C_s D_p a_i \tag{13}$$

Each of the terms in Equation (13) is a constant. Thus, the rate of drug released from the hemispheric polymeric matrix device with small a_i is essentially constant. The theoretical analysis has been agreed with the experimental data obtained from Hsieh et al. (Hsieh 1983). Their study addressed that hemispheric matrices acted as constant release systems for both sodium salicylate and bovine serum albumin, which were represented as small molecule and macromolecule, respectively.

3.2.2 A hollow cylindrical polymer matrix diffusion-controlled drug release

Drug released from a hollow cylindrical matrix device demonstrates a constant release profile because mechanism of drug released from this device is almost similar to that of the hemispheric polymer matrix device. This device has been fabricated by Vandelli and Cameroni since 1993 (Vandelli 1993a; Vandelli 1993b). It is a cylindrical polymer-drug matrix with a hole bored in the center of the flat surface through both sides of the matrix as displayed in Figure 2. All surfaces of the device are coated with an impermeable polymer except a central hole where the drug can be released, similar to the hemispheric polymer matrix device.

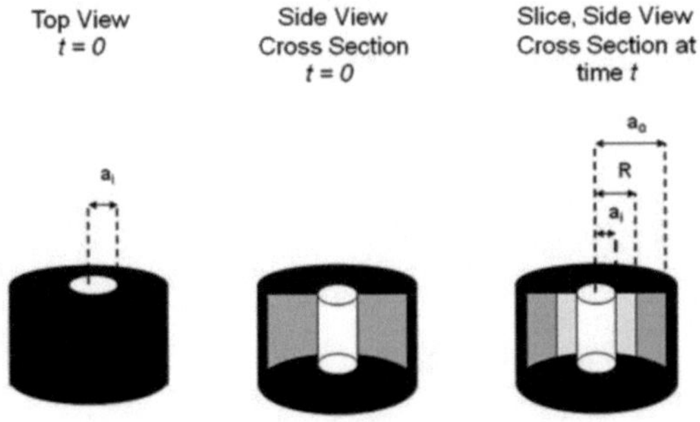

Fig. 2. Diagram of a hollow cylindrical matrix device: a_i was the inner radius; a_o was the outer radius; R is the distance to the interface between the drug depletion zone (light gray area) and the drug dispersing zone (dark gray area); and black representing coated regions through which the drug release could not take place (Reproduced from Wiranidchapong, 2006).

In addition, the swelling polymer used in the matrix can modulate the drug release following pseudo-zero order kinetics regardless of the loaded drug. This device regulates the drug release by swelling process and the effect of matrix geometry (Vandelli 1993b).

3.2.3 The three-layer polymer matrix diffusion-controlled drug release

The three-layer polymer matrix device has been designed to achieve zero-order kinetics of the drug release under the trade name of Geometrix® Technology since 1992 (Conte 1993; Conte 1996; Conte 2000; Abdul 2004). In fact, this device is a multi-layer tablet, which comprises of a matrix core containing an active drug and one or more barriers applied to the core directly during the tableting process. The barriers reduce the burst release of the drug in the core by limiting the available surface for the drug release and controlling the solvent penetration rate at the same time. During the subsequent portions of the barriers dissolve, the erosion of these swollen barriers is dominated and the surface available for the drug release slowly increases. In this way the decrease of delivery rate due to the increase of diffusion path-length, corresponding to the increase of drug depletion zone, is counterbalanced by the simultaneous increase of the available area for drug release. Thus, the drug release can be maintained at a relatively constant level during the swelling and erosion of the barriers.

Maggi et al. (Maggi 2000) declared that release profiles of the three-layer matrices with the same cores and different barriers were different. The barriers containing polymers of higher viscosity were stronger reduction in the rate of drug release than those containing polymers of lower viscosity. In the same way, the cores containing the polymers of higher viscosity released the drug at a lower rate than those containing the polymers of lower viscosity. However, the dissolution profiles of the three-layer systems with the same barriers but different polymers used in the cores were similar. Their work was focused on the modulation of highly water-soluble drug released such as diltiazem hydrochloride. Therefore, the core had less effect on the modulation of drug release while the barriers played the leading role in controlling drug release from the three-layer matrix system used a highly water-soluble drug as a model drug.

The three-layer polymer matrix containing 17β-estradiol (E_2) as a model drug was produced by Wiranidchapong (Wiranidchapong 2006). E_2 dispersing in poly(ethyl acrylate-methyl methacrylate-trimethylammonioethyl methacrylate chloride) 1:2:0.1 or Eudragit® RS (ERS) at weight percent of 10, 20, and 30 was used in the core component while ERS free drug was used as polymeric barriers on both sides of the core. In vitro release of E_2 from the three-layer matrices exhibited 80 % of cumulative amount of E_2 released within 7 days in all cases as shown in Figure 3(a). E_2 daily release rate from these matrices is shown in Figure 3(b). The increase in weight percent of E_2 in the core did not significantly increase E_2 daily release rate.

To compare E_2 release profiles obtained from the three-layer matrices containing different weight percents of E_2 used in the cores, the similarity factor (f_2) was used in the assessment. The f_2 test adopted by the Center for Drug Evaluation and Research (FDA) and by Human Medicines Evaluation Unit of the European Agency for the Evaluation of Medicine Products (EMEA) can be defined as the following equation (Costa 2001).

$$f_2 = 50 \times log\left[\left\{1 + \left(\frac{1}{n}\right)\sum_{j=1}^{n}\left|R_j - T_j\right|^2\right\}^{-0.5} \times 100\right] \quad (14)$$

where n is the sampling number, R_j and T_j are the percent dissolved of two comparative formulations at each time point j. FDA and EMEA have suggested that two dissolution profiles are declared similar if f_2 is between 50 and 100. The higher f_2 value, the more similar dissolution profiles are obtained (Costa 2001).

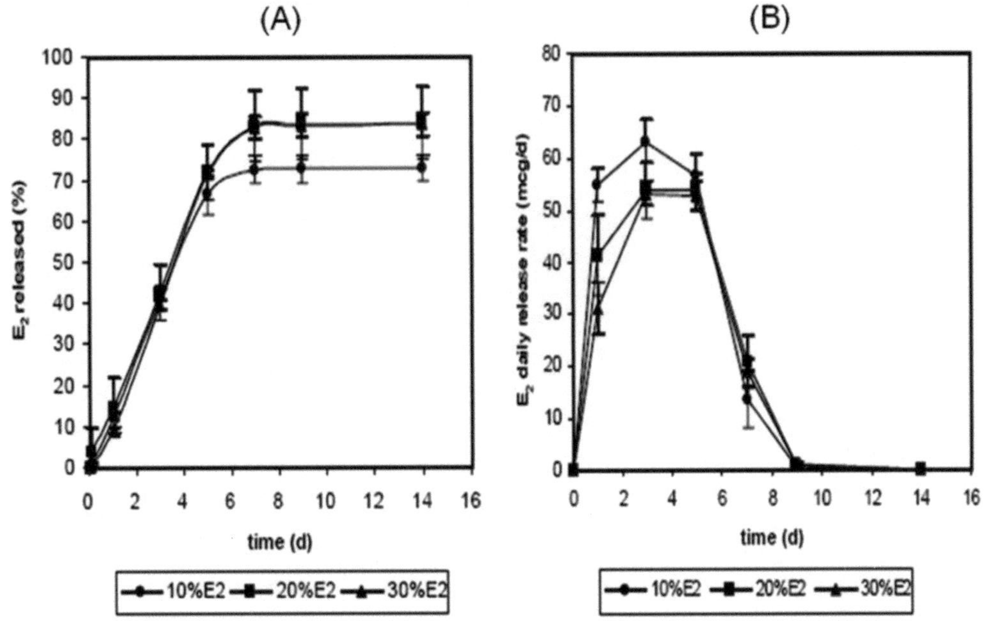

Fig. 3. In vitro release (A) and the daily rate (B) of E_2 released from the three-layer matrices containing 10, 20, and 30 % w/w E_2 in ERS used in the cores (Reproduced from Wiranidchapong, 2006).

f_2 values of E_2 release profiles of the core containing 10 % w/w E_2 compared with those containing 20 and 30 % w/w E_2 were 57.18 and 58.16, respectively. In addition, f_2 values obtained from the comparison of E_2 release profiles of the core containing 20 % w/w E_2 with those containing 30 % w/w E_2 was 77.77 (Wiranidchapong 2006). Thus, E_2 release profiles of the three-later polymer matrices containing 10, 20, and 30 % w/w E_2 in ERS used in the cores were similar.

In the case of the increase in weight percent of drug in the matrix, the porosity upon drug depletion is increased and the tortuosity is reduced, so that rate of drug release should increase. However, the rate of E_2 release did not increase as weight percent of E_2 in the cores increased. This suggested that the increase in porosity and the decrease in tortuosity in the core of the three-layer matrix could not elevate the E_2 release rate. The porosity and the tortuosity might not be the important factors in controlling E_2 release from this system.

Similar study was investigated with norethindrone (NET), the other poorly water-soluble drug, used in the core and ERS employed as barriers of the three-layer matrix (Wiranidchapong 2006). The cumulative release and the daily release rate of NET from the three-layer matrices containing 30, 40, and 50 % w/w NET in ERS used in the cores are shown in Figure 4. NET release profiles showed 80 % of NET released within 14 days in all cases. NET daily release rate exhibited relatively constant within 9 days.

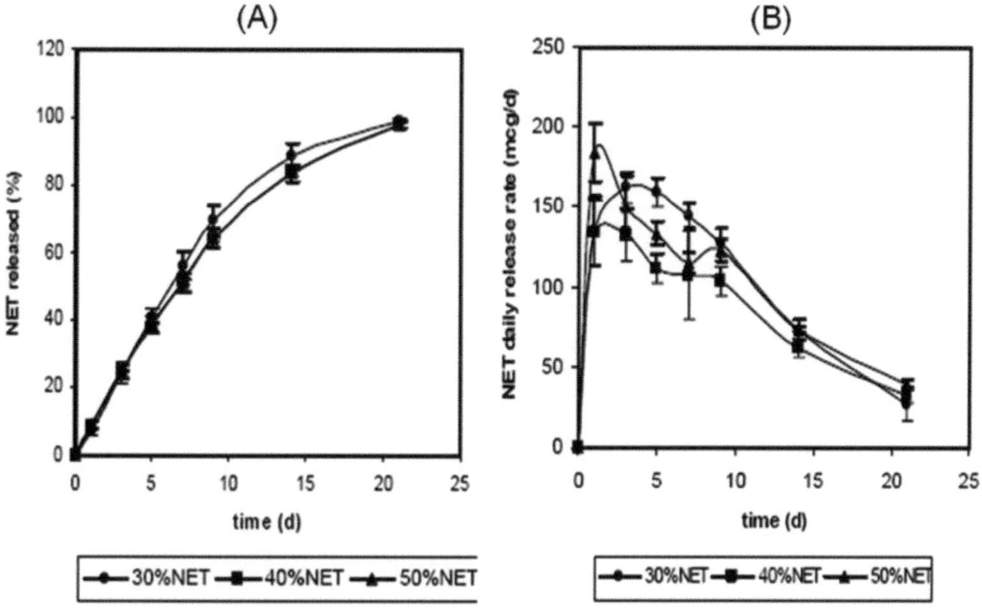

Fig. 4. In vitro release (A) and the daily rate (B) of NET released from the three-layer matrices containing 30, 40, and 50 % w/w NET in ERS used in the cores (Reproduced from Wiranidchapong, 2006).

From preliminary study conducted at 37°C, 120 rpm, the solubility of E_2 and NET in 3.5 % w/v benzalkonium chloride in phosphate buffer pH 7.4 used as release medium were 891.29 µg/ml and 460.16 µg/ml, respectively. The solubility of NET in the release medium is around two times lower than that of E_2 corresponding to two times longer extended release of NET than that of E_2.

The f_2 values obtained from the comparison of NET release profile of the three-layer matrix in which core containing 30 % w/w NET with those containing 40 and 50 % w/w NET were 73.23 and 72.55, respectively. Furthermore, f_2 values obtained from NET release profile of the core containing 40 % w/w NET compared with that of 50 % w/w NET was 96.69. This indicated the similarity among NET release profiles obtained from the three-layer polymer matrices containing 30, 40, and 50 % w/w NET in the polymeric cores.

This study represented that the intrinsic solubility of E_2 and NET affected the duration of drug released from the three-layer matrix. The increase in weight percent of E_2 and NET used in the core corresponding to the increase of the porosity and decrease of the tortuosity did not increase the daily release rate. The solubility of E_2 and NET in the release medium predominated in controlling the E_2 and NET release when compared with the porosity and the tortuosity upon drug depletion.

Further study was to investigate the effect of the barrier and the type of polymer used in the core and barrier on NET released from the three-layer matrix (Wiranidchapong 2006). Poly(ethyl acrylate-methyl methacrylate-trimethylammonioethyl methacrylate chloride) 1:2:0.1 and 1:2:0.2 or Eudragit® RS (ERS) and Eudragit® RL (ERL), respectively have been used as rate controlling polymers. ERL is more permeable than ERS because of higher content of quaternary ammonium groups in the structure. The NET released profile obtained from the three-layer matrix using ERL in the core was compared with that of ERS.

In addition, the NET released profiles obtained from the three-layer matrices having the same cores but different kinds of polymer used in the barriers and without the barriers were also investigated. The percentage of drug loading was set at 30.

The cumulative release of NET from the three-layer matrices using ERL in the cores with barrier layers of either ERL or ERS exhibited 80 % of NET released within 2 days whereas those of ERS in the cores with either ERS or ERL in the barriers and without the barriers exhibited 80 % of NET release within 14 days as illustrated in Figure 5. The difference of polymer used in the core significantly changed NET release profile but the difference of polymer used in the barriers, including without the barriers did not significantly change NET release profile. Therefore, the core exerted more influence on the modulation of a poorly water-soluble drug release than the barrier did.

NET release profiles of the devices containing ERS in the cores were compared with each other. The f_2 values of NET release profiles obtained from the device using ERS in the barriers compared with those of ERL and without the barriers were 75.36 and 77.76, respectively. In addition, f_2 value of NET release profile obtained from the device using ERL in the barriers compared with that of without barriers was 86.00. The NET release profiles obtained from the devices using ERS in the cores with the barriers using either ERS or ERL and without the barriers were similar. Thus, the three-layer design did not affect the NET release.

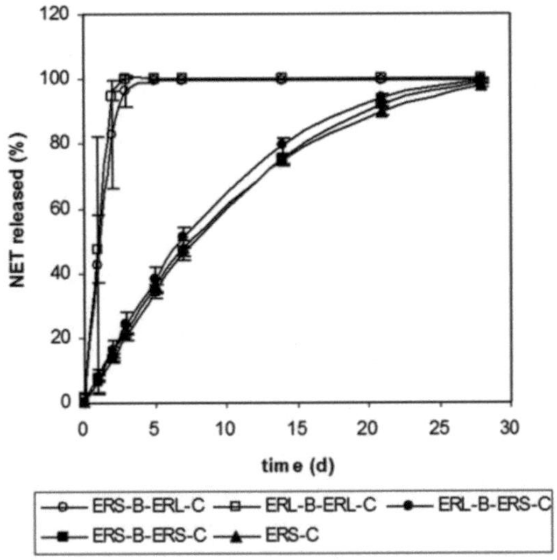

Fig. 5. In vitro release of NET from the three-layer matrices containing ERS or ERL used in the cores and ERS or ERL used in the barriers, including without the barriers (Reproduced from Wiranidchapong, 2006).

Approximately 60 % of either E_2 or NET released from the three-layer matrices investigated in this study were well fitted with the zero-order released model by linear regression analysis. The coefficient of determination (R^2) obtained from each fit was in the range of 0.9946 - 0.9999 (Wiranidchapong 2006). The zero-order model was apparently appropriate to describe either E_2 or NET released from the matrices using ERS as the rate-controlling polymer. As previously mentioned, the zero-order kinetic of drug released is accomplished in the polymer membrane permeation-controlled drug delivery system in both conditions governed by the polymeric membrane-modulated permeation process and the diffusion layer-limiting partition-controlled process. In case of incompletely coated membrane such as the three-layer polymeric matrix, the hydrodynamic diffusion layer (h_d) predominates in controlling the drug release. As seen in Equation (9), the rate of drug release is a result of drug solubility in the surrounding medium.

Chandrasekaran and Paul (Chandrasekaran 1982) announced that the solubility of poorly water-soluble drug predominated and offered as the limiting resistance to drug release. This resulted in the saturated concentration of dissolved drug at the inside of matrix pores when drug loading exceeded the drug solubility under the given condition. Non-dissolved drug was not available for diffusion but it acted as a drug reservoir for keeping constant the absolute amount of drug release within a certain period of time. The zero-order release kinetic could be achieved under this condition (Siepmann 2001). Furthermore, Kim (Kim 2000) indicated that the geometry was not an important factor for a drug dissolution controlled release system and the increase in the porosity and the reduction in the tortuosity did not influence the kinetics of drug release. Therefore, the zero-order kinetic of either E_2 or NET released from the matrices was a result of the inherent solubility of E_2 and NET providing the drug dissolution controlled release system (Wiranidchapong 2006).

The E_2 released from the polymeric matrix is controlled by the dissolution of E_2 in the surrounding medium. Therefore, an alteration in the solid state of E_2 dispersing in the polymer matrix can modify the characteristic of E_2 release. Solid state of E_2 should be revealed in both cases of pure drug and the drug dispersing in the polymer under various conditions, which might be appeared in the manufacturing process.

4. Solid state properties of estradiol

The most common form of E_2 is the hemihydrates (Variankaval 2000; Wiranidchapong 2008). However, E_2 can exist in various kinds of pseudopolymorphs as hemisolvates, dependent on the type of solvent used in the crystallization. For an example, E_2-hemisolvate of methanol was produced by crystallization in saturated solution of E_2 in methanol (Variankaval 2000). In addition, either polymorphs or pseudopolymorphs exhibit the definite arrangement of molecules inside the crystal lattice. This directly affects on a crystal habit, which is an external shape of the crystal. Thus, crystal morphology is a specific characteristic for each polymorphic form. An alteration in polymorphic state possibly changes the crystal habit and/or even crystal morphology, leading to significant variation in raw-material characteristics such as particle orientation, flowability, packing, compaction, suspension stability and dissolution. This can lead to serious implications of physical stability in dosage forms (Niazi 2007).

E_2 can exist in the amorphous form and at least three crystalline forms, including E_2-hemihydrate (Variankaval 2000; Wiranidchapong 2006; Wiranidchapong 2008). Differential scanning calorimetry (DSC) curve reveals that the three crystal forms and amorphous form of E_2 are inter-convertible under various thermal conditions as displayed in Figure 6(A) (Wiranidchapong 2006; Wiranidchapong 2008). This indicates that the polymorphic transformation of E_2 possibly occurs during manufacturing process in which optimal thermal energy has been utilized. Thus, inconsistency of E_2 polymorphs have probably been found in pharmaceutical products obtained from inadequate quality control of manufacturing procedures. Different polymorphs exhibit dramatic change in physical and chemical properties. This leads to inconsistency in dissolution rate, rate of drug release from controlled-release product, and bioavailability. To control the product quality, physicochemical properties of E_2 polymorphs should be verified.

4.1 Characterization by DSC and TGA

From DSC analysis, E_2-hemihydrate exhibited the melting point onset at 179.2 °C corresponding to the third endotherm observed in the first heating run (DSC; 0-182 °C at 10 K/min). The first endotherm (onset at 110 °C) and second endotherm (onset at 174 °C) in the first heating run corresponded to the partial release of hydrogen bonded water and the complete loss of water lattice, respectively. The water loss observed in the first scan was agreed with a weight loss of 3.2 % of E_2 measured by thermogravimetric analysis (TGA) as illustrated in Figure 6(B) (Wiranidchapong 2006; Wiranidchapong 2008). This result indicated that the stoichiometry of E_2 should be $C_{18}H_{24}O_2.\frac{1}{2}H_2O$.

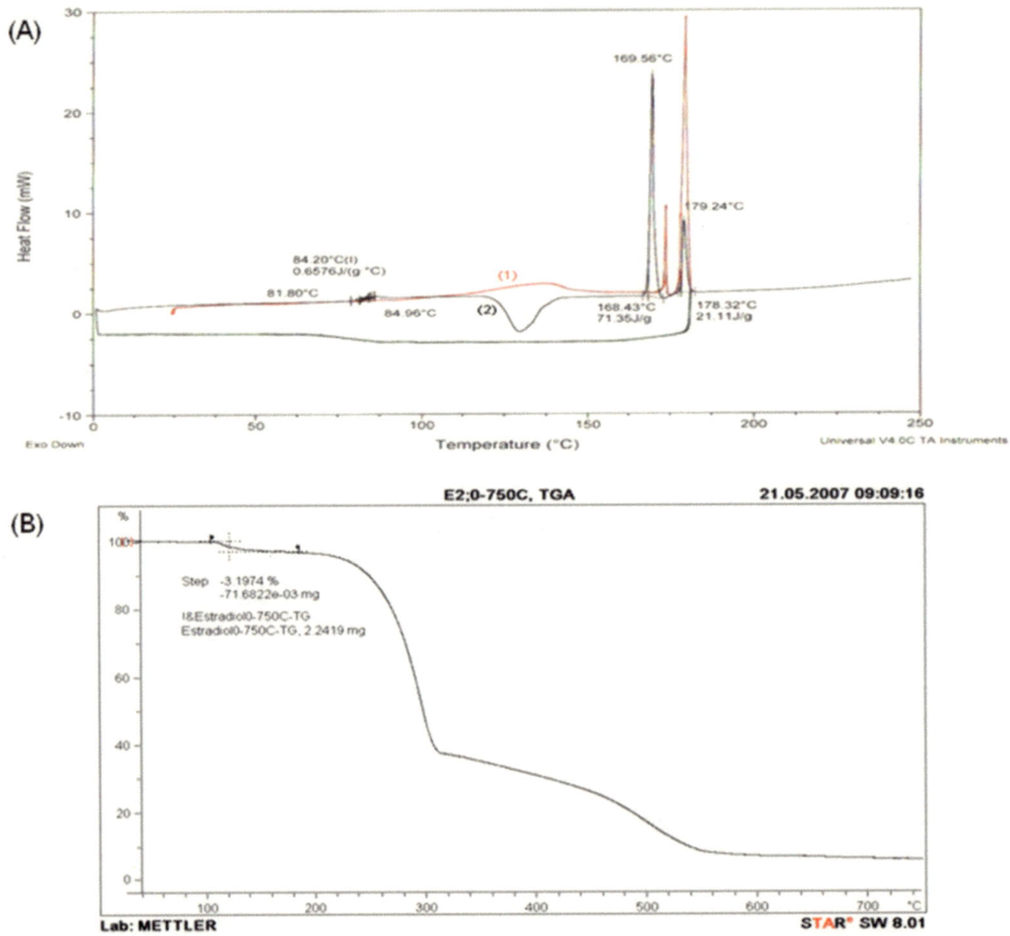

Fig. 6. (A) DSC curve of E_2 scanned with the program: (1) heating to 182 °C, 10 K/min, cooling to 0 °C, 20 K/min, and then (2) heating to 250 °C, 10 K/min; (B) TGA of E_2 (Reproduced from Wiranidchapong, 2008).

On cooling (DSC; 182-0 °C at 20 K/min) the glass transition temperature (T_g) was observed around 84.2 °C, correlating to that observed in the second heating (DSC; 0-250 °C at 10 K/min). This aspect revealed an appearance of amorphous E_2 after E_2-hemihydrate had been melted and then rapidly cooled. In the second heating the amorphous E_2 in glassy state was changed to that in rubbery state when the temperature reached the T_g, followed by recrystallization into ED form as stated by Variankaval et al. (Variankaval 2000) and anhydrous E_2 exhibiting their melting points at 169.6 °C and 179.2 °C, respectively (Variankaval 2000; Wiranidchapong 2006; Wiranidchapong 2008).

4.2 Characterization by X-ray powder diffraction

Each polymorph of E_2 exhibits the definite X-ray powder diffraction (XRPD) patterns as illustrated in Figure 7. E_2-hemihydrate demonstrates characteristic peaks at 13.14, 15.74, 18.26, 22.62, and 26.58° (Latsch 2003; Park 2005; Wiranidchapong 2006; Wiranidchapong 2008). Anhydrous E_2 prepared by heating E_2-hemihydrate from 0-175 °C and 0-180.5 °C at heating rate of 5 K/min exhibited the characteristic peaks at 13.60, 16.78, 21.00, and 24.72°, which were not observed in the diffraction pattern of E_2-hemihydrate.

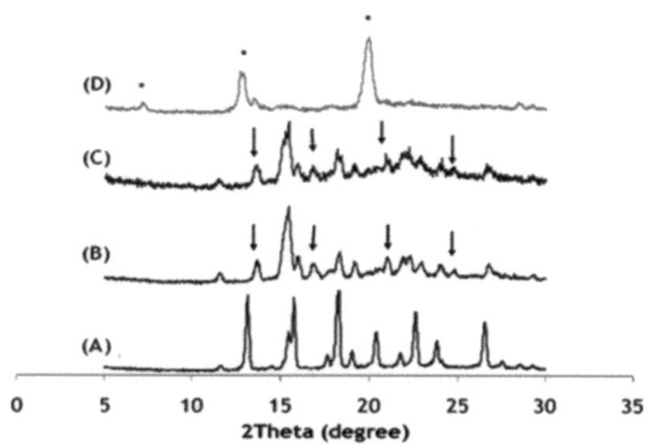

Fig. 7. XRPD of E_2-hemihydrate (A); anhydrous E_2 produced from either heating to 175 °C, 5 K/min (B); or heating to 180.5 °C, 5 K/min (C); and ED form of E_2 (D) (Reproduced from Wiranidchapong, 2008).

The relative peak intensity of anhydrous E_2 obtained from heating to 180.5 °C was less than that of anhydrous E_2 obtained from heating to 175 °C. In addition, the diffraction peaks of anhydrous E_2 obtained from heating to 180.5 °C did not significantly separate from baseline, indicating a mixture of crystalline form and amorphous form. This represents the inconsistency in the appearance of E_2 polymorph when the process slightly changes. ED form of E_2 prepared by heating E_2-hemihydrate to 180.5 °C at 5 K/min and cooling to 0 °C at 20 K/min and finally heating to 140 °C at 5 K/min manifested the definite diffraction pattern, which exhibited the characteristic peaks at 12.64 and 19.94°. This feature indicates that XRPD analysis can be used to investigate polymorphic forms of E_2, which are inter-convertible under various thermal conditions.

4.3 Characterization by FTIR

FTIR spectra of E_2-hemihydrate, anhydrous E_2, and the mixture of anhydrous E_2 with amorphous E_2 are displayed in Figure 8. E_2-hemihydrate exhibited very broad bands centered at 3435.95 and 3232.06 cm^{-1} attributed to O-H stretching of hydroxyl group adjacent to C-17 and C-3 positions in E_2 chemical structure, respectively (Barnett 1995; Wiranidchapong 2006; Wiranidchapong 2008; Wiranidchapong 2009). The broad band characteristic indicates the hydrogen-bonded hydroxyl group with water entrapped in the crystal structure.

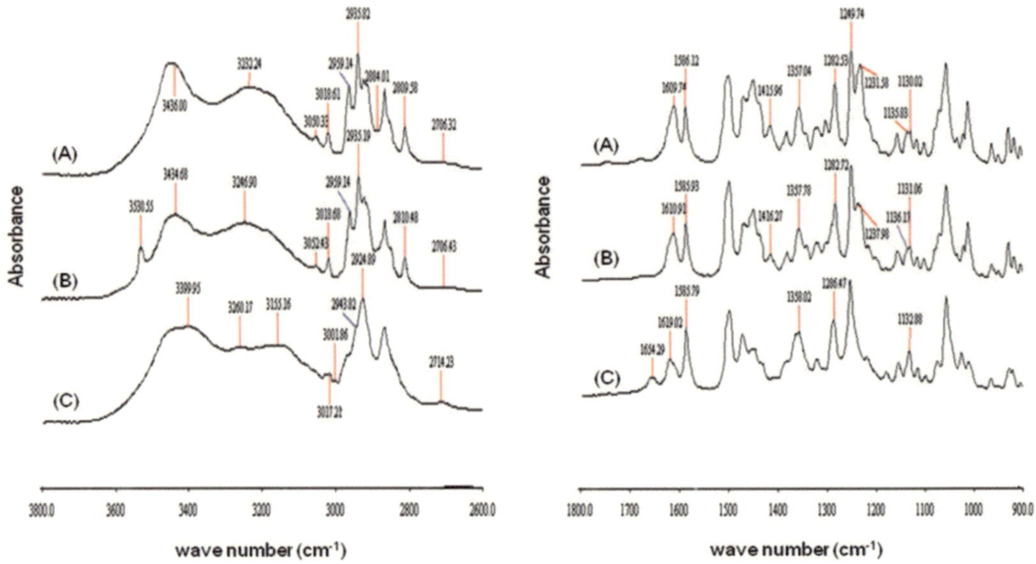

Fig. 8. FTIR spectra of E_2-hemihydrate (A); anhydrous E_2 (B); and the mixture of anhydrous E_2 with amorphous E_2 (C), recorded at room temperature in the range of 3800-2600 cm^{-1} (left) and 1800-900 cm^{-1} (right).

Anhydrous E_2 prepared by heating E_2-hemihydrate to 175 °C at 5 K/min displayed the peak around 3530 cm^{-1} in the FTIR spectrum. This peak corresponded to free hydroxyl group absorption (Kuo 2001a; Kuo 2001b; Wiranidchapong 2006; Wiranidchapong 2008; Wiranidchapong 2009). The appearance of this peak was agreed with the water loss during heating. However, broad bands centered at 3434.27 and 3245.29 cm^{-1} attributed to O-H stretching of hydroxyl group adjacent to C-17 and C-3 positions respectively in the E_2 chemical structure, were still observed.

For FTIR spectrum of E_2 heated to 220 °C at 5 K/min, which was presumably the mixture of anhydrous E_2 with amorphous E_2, the O-H stretching bands of hydroxyl groups adjacent to the C-17 and C-3 positions and C-H stretching vibration of aromatic ring in the regions of 3100-3000 cm^{-1} (Silverstein 1991) shifted to lower wavenumber when compared with those of E_2-hemihydrate and anhydrous E_2. Furthermore, three consecutive peaks in the range of 1655-1580 cm^{-1} attributed to absorption of the mixtures of tautomeric keto and enol forms (Silverstein 1991) were noticed in FTIR spectrum of E_2 heated to 220 °C whereas only two consecutive peaks in this region were observed in FTIR spectra of E_2-hemihydrate and anhydrous E_2. Due to the absorption peak in this region affected by physical state, electronic and mass effects of neighboring substitutes, conjugation, hydrogen bonding, and ring strain (Silverstein 1991), this might be the characteristics of amorphous E_2 blended with anhydrous

E_2. In addition, the peaks in the regions of 1300-900 cm^{-1} illustrated different shapes from those of E_2-hemihydrate, and anhydrous E_2.

According to drug dissolution and drug solubility in the polymer affecting the rate of drug released from either polymer membrane permeation- or polymer matrix diffusion-controlled release systems, solid state of E_2 dispersing in the polymer should also influence on the rate of E_2 release. Solid dispersion prepared by solvent evaporation is generally used to distribute drug into the polymeric matrix (Serajuddin 1999). Solid dispersions containing E_2 in ERS at 1 and 2 % w/w exhibited amorphous state of E_2 in the dispersion while those containing E_2 at 10, 20, and 30 % w/w illustrated crystalline state of E_2 in the dispersion (Wiranidchapong 2006). This interpretation was supported by photomicrographs of ERS, solid dispersion containing 1, 2, 10, 20, and 30 % w/w of E_2 in ERS and E_2 under polarized light microscope as shown in Figure 9. The absence of birefringence was observed in ERS and solid dispersions containing 1 and 2 % w/w of E_2. This is a characteristic of amorphous substance, which cannot turn plane polarized light and cannot reflect purple light to other wavelengths of visible lights. On the other hand, the birefringence was observed in solid dispersions containing 10, 20, and 30 % w/w of E_2 and E_2 crystal powder. This is a characteristic of crystalline substance, which is able to turn plane polarized light and reflect purple light to other visible wavelengths.

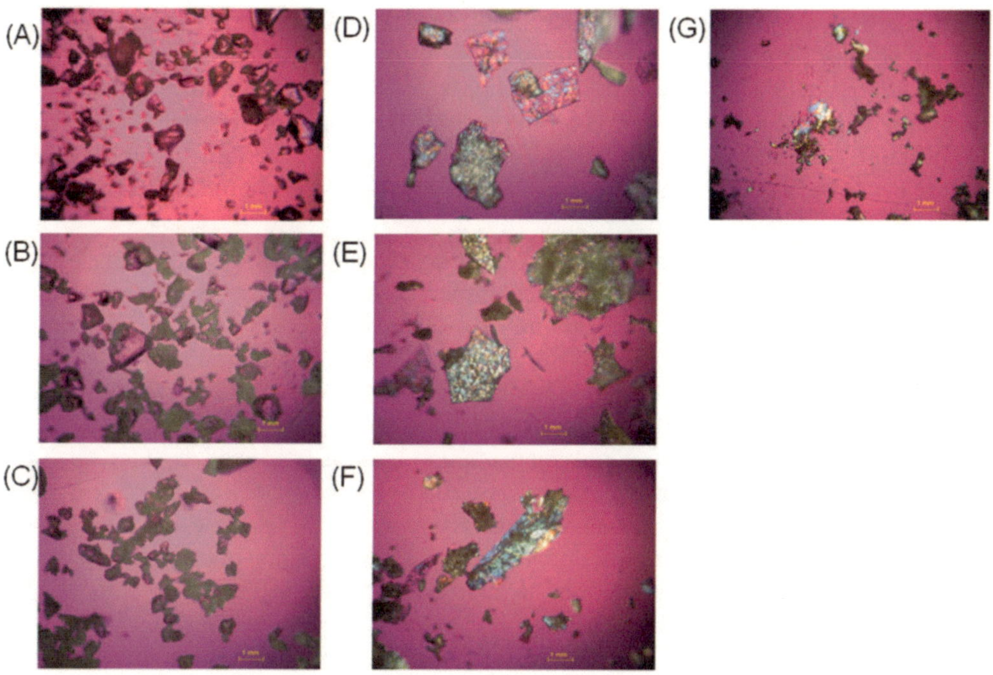

Fig. 9. Photomicrographs obtained from polarized light microscope: (A) ERS; solid dispersions containing E_2 in ERS at weight percent of (B) 1; (C) 2; (D) 10; (E) 20; (F) 30; and (G) E_2-hemihydrate (Reproduced from Wiranidchapong, 2006).

To compare with approximately 80 % of the E_2 released from the matrices containing E_2 at 10, 20, and 30 % w/w in the dispersion within 7 days, the matrices, which were composed of E_2 at 1 and 2 % w/w in the dispersions released approximately 60-80 % of the E_2 within 3 days (Wiranidchapong 2006). This study was in accordance with the finding of amorphous E_2 in the dispersion containing E_2 at 1 and 2 % w/w. Amorphous state is thermodynamically unstable. The molecular interactions of amorphous substance are weakened and usually gone into breaking. Therefore, amorphous E_2 exhibited higher dissolution rate than crystalline E_2, so that the rate of E_2 release from matrix containing amorphous E_2 is higher than that of the matrix containing crystalline E_2.

The polymorphic state of E_2 in the polymer matrix can be observed not only by polarized light microscope but also by DSC and/or MTDSC (modulated temperature differential scanning calorimetry) (Wiranidchapong 2006; Wiranidchapong 2008; Wiranidchapong 2009). To understand how DSC and/or MTDSC can differentiate between amorphous state and crystalline state of E_2 dispersing in the polymer matrix. Thermal behavior of solid dispersion containing E_2 in ERS should be explored.

5. Thermal behavior of E_2 in ERS solid dispersion

In general, T_g is one of thermal properties of an amorphous material observed by thermal analysis. Likewise, the melting point is a thermal property of a crystalline material. In the case of the amorphous E_2 existing in the polymer matrix, either E_2 or polymer in the matrix are amorphous materials. Thus, both amorphous E_2 and the polymer can manifest their T_g. A question is how the T_g behavior of this solid dispersion is. Which one between a single T_g or both T_g of amorphous E_2 and the polymer should be observed? For a solid dispersion composed of crystalline E_2 in the polymer matrix, what the temperature should be the melting point of E_2 in the dispersion? Does the polymer influence on the melting point of E_2? To understand the thermal behaviors of E_2 in ERS solid dispersion, the theory of the miscibility between the binary mixtures in which a polymer blend should be addressed.

5.1 T_g behavior described by the Gordon Taylor equation

In polymer sciences, the miscibility of a polymer blend composed of two amorphous polymers can be determined by thermal analysis. A single T_g point is an indication of full miscibility of a polymer blend (Kuo 2001a; Kuo 2001b; Maldonado-Santoyo 2004). On the contrary, an immiscible polymer blend exhibits more than one T_g representing T_g of amorphous pure polymers used as components (Kuo 2001a). In general, T_g of a miscible blend lies between T_g of the pure polymers, which can be predicted by Gordon-Taylor equation or its modified version equation (Maldonado-Santoyo 2004). Either T_g or weight fraction of binary polymer components are major factors in predicting the T_g of a miscible polymer blend by Gordon-Taylor equation and its modified version equation.

Gordon-Taylor equation has been proposed for the composition dependence on the T_g of miscible polymer blends derived under these assumptions (Schneider 1988);

1. The contacts due to the interaction between the components of the blend are responsible for conformational arrangement, free volume distribution, and conformational energy barriers.
2. The probabilities of binary contact are related to the volume fractions of the components, so that the composition dependence on the T_g has been related to the volume fractions (Ø) of the components.

The Gordon-Taylor equation with respect to the volume fraction ($Ø_2$) of the stiffer polymer component (with T_{g2}) has been defined as the following relationship (Schneider 1988);

$$\frac{T_g - T_{g1}}{T_{g2} - T_{g1}} = (1 + K_1)\emptyset_2 - (K_1 + K_2)\emptyset_2^2 + K_2\emptyset_2^3 \quad (15)$$

The parameters K_1 and K_2 are related to the difference of the T_g of the polymer components $(T_{g2} - T_{g1})$, so that

$$K_1 = \frac{K_1^*}{(T_{g2} - T_{g1})} \quad (16)$$

and

$$K_2 = \frac{K_2^*}{(T_{g2} - T_{g1})} \quad (17)$$

The system-specific constant K_1^* is related to the interaction energy differences between hetero- and homo-contacts, whereas K_2^* considers the energetic effects on the binary contacts of the molecular surrounding.

The ideal behavior of the polymer blend exhibits the equality of the different energetic effects. This means the identical energetic effects of both hetero- and homo-contacts and the equality of the contact energy of the molecular neighborhood. So both K_1^* and K_2^* are equal to zero in the idealized condition of the T_g behavior of miscible polymer blend. The Gordon-Taylor equation resulted from the idealized condition can be expressed;

$$\frac{T_g - T_{g1}}{T_{g2} - T_{g1}} = \emptyset_2 \quad (18)$$

$$T_g = \emptyset_2 T_{g2} + (1 - \emptyset_2)T_{g1} \quad (19)$$

Because of $\emptyset_1 + \emptyset_2 = 1$, and then

$$T_g = \emptyset_2 T_{g2} + \emptyset_1 T_{g1} \quad (20)$$

To express in term of the temperature-dependent weight fraction (w_i), the volume fractions $(\emptyset_i)$ are given by the expression;

$$\emptyset_i = \frac{(\Delta\alpha_i \times w_i)/\rho_i}{\sum_i\{(\Delta\alpha_i \times w_i)/\rho_i\}} \quad (21)$$

where ρ_i is the density of the components and $\Delta\alpha_i$ is the difference between the expansion coefficients of the melt (L) and the glass (gl) at T_{gi} $(\Delta\alpha_i = \alpha_{L,i} - \alpha_{gl,i})$.

Introducing Equation (21) into Equation (20), yielding the Gordon-Taylor equation expressed in term of the temperature-dependent weight fraction as displayed;

$$T_g = \frac{\rho_2\Delta\alpha_1 w_1 T_{g1} + \rho_1\Delta\alpha_2 w_2 T_{g2}}{(\rho_2\Delta\alpha_1 w_1 + \rho_1\Delta\alpha_2 w_2)} \quad (22)$$

Due to $K = \frac{\rho_1\Delta\alpha_2}{\rho_2\Delta\alpha_1}$, so that Equation (22) can be rearranged as;

$$T_g = \frac{w_1 T_{g1} + K w_2 T_{g2}}{w_1 + K w_2} \quad (23)$$

In the case of polymer blends exhibiting the behavior deviating from the ideal behavior, the fit of Gordon-Taylor equation to experimental data fails. This suggests an interaction contribution to the Gordon-Taylor parameters (K). The Kwei equation is recommended in this case. The Kwei relation is identical to a second-order equation of the proposed model expressed in Equation (15). It considers different energetic effects of the binary contact ($K_1 \neq 0$), but neglects the effects of the immediate neighborhood of contacts ($K_2 = 0$). Therefore, Equation (15) can be written under this assumption as shown;

$$\frac{T_g - T_{g1}}{T_{g2} - T_{g1}} = (1 + K_1)\emptyset_2 - K_1\emptyset_2^2 \tag{24}$$

Equation (24) can be illustrated in term of the corrected weight fraction (w_{ic}) as the following equations;

$$\frac{T_g - T_{g1}}{T_{g2} - T_{g1}} = (1 + K_1)w_{2c} - K_1 w_{2c}^2 \tag{25}$$

$$T_g = w_{1c}T_{g1} + w_{2c}T_{g2} + \left(T_{g2} - T_{g1}\right)(K_1 w_{2c} w_{1c}) \tag{26}$$

Due to $w_{1c} = w_1/(w_1 + Kw_2)$ and $w_{2c} = Kw_2/(w_1 + Kw_2)$, so that Equation (26) can be rewritten as displayed;

$$T_g = \frac{w_1 T_{g1} + K w_2 T_{g2}}{w_1 + K w_2} + \left(T_{g2} - T_{g1}\right)\frac{K_1 K w_2 w_1}{(w_1 + K w_2)^2} \tag{27}$$

Because of $q = \left(T_{g2} - T_{g1}\right)\frac{K_1 K}{(w_1 + K w_2)^2}$, then Equation (27) can be illustrated as;

$$T_g = \frac{w_1 T_{g1} + K w_2 T_{g2}}{w_1 + K w_2} + q w_2 w_1 \tag{28}$$

Equation (28) is the Kwei equation, which is the second order equation of the proposed model. The q parameter reflects the balance between breaking the intra bonding and forming the inter bonding. Normally the q parameter corresponds to the strength of hydrogen bonding. The q value of the polymer blend should depend on an entropy change corresponding to the change in the number of hydrogen bonding interactions. In the case of negative q value, it indicates that the self-associated hydrogen bonding is stronger than the inter-associated hydrogen bonding. In reciprocal way, the positive q value indicates that the self-associated hydrogen bonding is weaker than the inter-associated hydrogen bonding. The higher q value, the stronger hydrogen bonding (Kuo 2001a; Kuo 2001b).

The third order equation of the proposed model considers the contact interaction energies ($K_1 \neq 0$) and the influence of the molecular neighborhood on the contact energy ($K_2 \neq 0$), so that Equation (15) can be written in the term of the corrected weight fraction of the stiffer polymer (w_{2c}) as displayed below;

$$\frac{T_g - T_{g1}}{T_{g2} - T_{g1}} = (1 + K_1)w_{2c} - (K_1 + K_2)w_{2c}^2 + K_2 w_{2c}^3 \tag{29}$$

The Equation (29) can be resolved for the T_g of the blend as the following expression;

$$T_g = \frac{(1 - w_2)T_{g1} + K w_2 T_{g2}}{1 + (K-1)w_2} + \frac{K_1^* K}{\{1 + (K-1)w_2\}^2} \times (1 - w_2)w_2 - \frac{-K_2^* K_2}{\{1 + (K-1)w_2\}^3} \times (1 - w_2)w_2^2 \tag{30}$$

Equation (30) is an extended Gordon-Taylor equation, which is written in term of the weight fraction of the stiffer polymer (w_2). Due to Equations (16) and (17), K_1^* and K_2^* are related to K_1 and K_2, respectively, so that the influence of the weight fraction of the components on the T_g is included both K_1 and K_2.

The application of Gordon-Taylor equation and its modified version equation has been extended to describe the T_g behavior of E_2 in ERS solid dispersion (Wiranidchapong 2006; Wiranidchapong 2008; Wiranidchapong 2009). The study revealed that solid dispersions containing E_2 in ERS at weight percent of 1-90 manifested a single T_g lying between the T_g of ERS (66.21 °C) and E_2 (83.77 °C) as displayed in Figure 10.

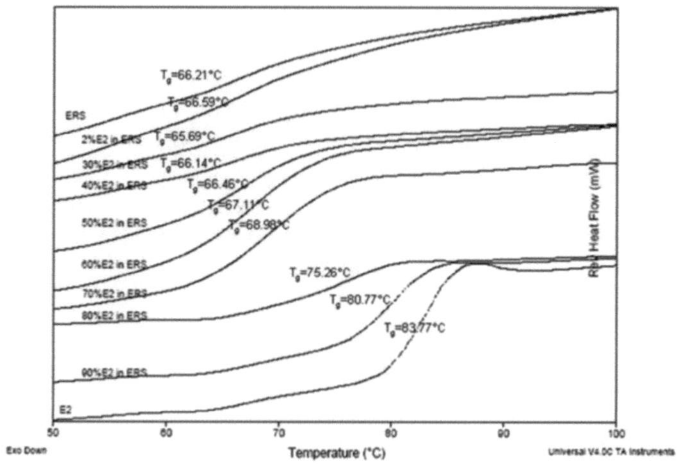

Fig. 10. T_g of E_2 in ERS solid dispersions at concentration range of 0-100 % w/w investigated by MTDSC with the program: heating to 182 °C, 10 K/min, cooling to 25 °C, 20 K/min, an isothermal period for 5 min at 25 °C, and finally heating to 250 °C, 5 K/min (Reproduced from Wiranidchapong, 2008).

In addition, the T_g shifted toward the T_g of E_2 when weight fractions of E_2 in the dispersions increased. This behavior was observed in E_2 in ERS solid dispersions investigated by MTDSC with the program of heating from 25 to 182 °C at 10 °C/min, cooling to 25 °C at 20 °C/min, an isothermal period for 5 min at 25 °C, and finally heating to 250°C at 5 °C/min. This heating program provided the transformation of E_2-hemihydrate into amorphous E_2 blended with ERS as the same as a blend of amorphous polymers. Thus, the T_g behavior of these blends could be described by the principle of Gordon-Taylor equation. However, the experimental T_g values were better fitted to Kwei equation than the Gordon-Taylor equation. The q value, the Kwei equation parameters, obtained from the curve-fitting was not equal to zero, which implied an interaction between E_2 and ERS in the blend.

5.2 The melting point behavior described by the flory-huggins theory

In the case of a crystalline polymer blended with an amorphous polymer, the melting point depression of a crystalline polymer in blend indicates the miscibility and interaction between the polymer components. Partially miscible or immiscible blends do not typically show the depression of melting point whereas a miscible blend displays the melting point depression when the content of amorphous polymer increases. The temperature reduction was a result of morphological effects and thermodynamic reasons (Kuo 2001a; Kuo 2001b). In a thermodynamically miscible blend, an amorphous polymer resides inside the interlamellar regions of a semi-crystalline polymer. It expands the interlamellar regions. The spherulite radial growth rate, time to half volume crystallization and melting temperature of semi-crystalline component generally decrease as the concentration of the amorphous polymer increases. The mean field self-consistent theory used to a model of a blend containing di-block copolymers composing of crystallisable and amorphous copolymer blocks has been proposed. The free energy based on this theory can be expressed as a sum of free energy of free crystalline and amorphous blocks, entropy and enthalpy of interactions between these two blocks. For long chain polymers, the effect of the end groups can be ignored. The change in partial free energy of the crystals in a miscible blend (Δg_{2b}) can be expressed (Rostami 2000);

$$\Delta g_{2b} = \Delta g_2 + \Delta g_m \tag{31}$$

where Δg_2 is the change in partial free energy of crystalline unit of a homopolymer and Δg_m is the change in partial free energy of the mixture.
The equilibrium melting temperature is defined as the last temperature that infinitely long crystal melts. By definition, at the equilibrium melting temperature of the blends, where the last crystal melts, Δg_{2b} becomes zero, so that Equation (31) can be expressed as following equations;

$$\Delta g_2 = -\Delta g_m \tag{32}$$

$$\Delta h_2 - T_{mb}\Delta S_2 = -\Delta g_m \tag{33}$$

$$1 - \frac{T_{mb}\Delta S_2}{\Delta h_2} = \frac{-\Delta g_m}{\Delta h_2} \tag{34}$$

where Δh_2 is the heat of fusion of a crystalline polymer, T_{mb} is the equilibrium melting point of a blend, and ΔS_2 is the entropy of crystalline unit in a blend.
In condition of a narrow temperature range between T_{mb} and T_m, which is the equilibrium melting point of a crystalline polymer, it is reasonable to assume that Δh_2 and ΔS_2 are temperature independent hence;

$$T_m = \frac{\Delta h_2}{\Delta S_2} \tag{35}$$

Introducing Equation (35) into Equation (34), so that Equation (34) can be expressed as the following equation;

$$1 - \frac{T_{mb}}{T_m} = \frac{-\Delta g_m}{\Delta h_2} \tag{36}$$

A popular equation for Δg_m is given by the classic Flory-Huggins mean field model. When a crystalline polymer is designated as the second component in the mixture, the lattice model gives;

$$\Delta g_m = \frac{RT_{mb}V_2}{V_1}\left\{\ln\left(\frac{\phi_2}{r_2}\right) + \left(\frac{1}{r_2} - \frac{1}{r_1}\right)\phi_1\right\} + \frac{RT_{mb}V_2}{V_1}\lambda_{21}\phi_1^2 \tag{37}$$

where Ø is the volume fraction and r is the chain length of each component denoted by the subscript used. V_1 and V_2 are the molar volume of the amorphous unit and the crystalline unit, respectively. λ_{21} is the polymer-polymer interaction parameter. R is the universal gas constant. T_{mb} is the temperature of the blends. The term in the square bracket represents contribution from the combinatorial entropy to the chemical potential changes per mole of crystalline unit in the mixture. As a major contribution to the molar free energy changes of the mixture is provided by the enthalpy term, which is the second term of Equation (37). The entropy contribution is neglected, so that Δg_m can be written in term of an approximate chemical potential form as displayed;

$$\Delta g_m = \frac{-RT_{mb}V_2}{V_1}\lambda_{21}\phi_1^2 \tag{38}$$

Substituting this approximated term into Equation (36) and rearranging, so that the resulting relationship is given as the following equation (Rostami 2000; Pimbert 2002);

$$\frac{1}{T_{mb}} - \frac{1}{T_m} = \frac{-RV_2\lambda_{21}\phi_1^2}{\Delta h_2 V_1} \tag{39}$$

According to $\lambda_{21} = \frac{BV_1}{RT_{mb}}$, Equation (39) can be written as the following expression (Nishi 1975; Kuo 2001a);

$$T_m - T_{mb} = \frac{-T_m B V_2 \emptyset_1^2}{\Delta h_2} \tag{40}$$

where B is the interaction energy density characteristic of the polymer pair. The resulting equation, Equation (40), is the Nishi-Wang equation (Nishi 1975; Kuo 2001a; Kuo 2001b).
From the investigation of the E_2 melting point in solid dispersions containing E_2 in ERS at the concentration range of 0-100 % w/w (Wiranidchapong 2006; Wiranidchapong 2008), the melting point depression as a function of composition was revealed as displayed in Figure 11. The behavior of the E_2 melting point in ERS solid dispersion was in accordance with that of a crystalline polymer blended with an amorphous polymer. Fitting experimental melting point of E_2 in the dispersion to the Nishi-Wang equation exhibited good agreement between experimental values and predicted values, with randomly distributed residuals and the coefficient of determination (R^2) of 0.9804. In addition, B value obtained from curve-fitting was -0.281 J/(g*cm^3) (Wiranidchapong 2006; Wiranidchapong 2008). This indicated validity of the Nishi-Wang equation to predict the melting point of E_2 in ERS solid dispersions, miscibility and interaction between E_2 and ERS in the molten state.

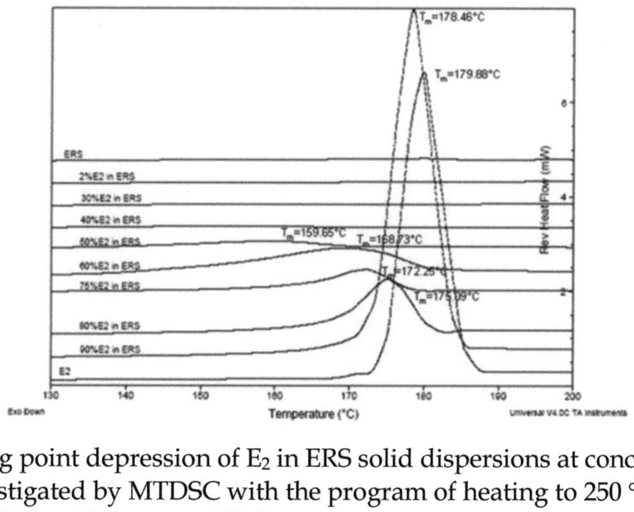

Fig. 11. The melting point depression of E_2 in ERS solid dispersions at concentration range of 0-100 % w/w investigated by MTDSC with the program of heating to 250 °C, 5 K/min (Reproduced from Wiranidchapong, 2006).

5.3 The interaction between E_2 and ERS in solid dispersion

Both Kwei equation and Nishi-Wang equation predicted an existence of a specific interaction between E_2 and ERS in the molten state. FTIR analysis was used to investigate the interaction between E_2 and ERS in solid dispersions. FTIR spectra of E_2 in ERS solid dispersions heated from 25-175 °C at 5 K/min were compared with those of anhydrous E_2 and ERS as illustrated in Figure 12. The peak around 3530 cm^{-1}, corresponding to free hydroxyl group absorption (Kuo 2001a; Kuo 2001b; Wiranidchapong 2006; Wiranidchapong 2008; Wiranidchapong 2009), in FTIR spectrum of anhydrous E_2 was also observed in that of 75 % w/w E_2 in ERS solid dispersion heated from 25-175 °C. This indicated the water loss during the heating process, so that the free hydroxyl group of E_2 was observed. Additionally, the band at 1732 cm^{-1} corresponding to the ester C=O stretching vibration of free carbonyl group (Pignatello 2002; Wiranidchapong 2006; Wiranidchapong 2008; Wiranidchapong 2009) was displayed in FTIR spectrum of ERS.

The interaction between E_2 and ERS was affirmed by the shift of broad band centered at 3434 cm^{-1}, attributed to O-H stretching of hydroxyl groups adjacent to C-17 positions in E_2, to 3411 cm^{-1} with a shoulder of the ester C=O stretching band in 75 %w/w E_2 in ERS solid dispersion heated from 25-175 °C. The shoulder around 1710 cm^{-1} corresponding to the hydrogen-bonded carbonyl group (Kuo 2001a; Kuo 2001b; Wiranidchapong 2006; Wiranidchapong 2008; Wiranidchapong 2009) suggested the inter-associated hydroxyl-carbonyl bond. The shoulder around 1710 cm^{-1} was also observed in FTIR spectra of 50 and 20 %w/w E_2 in ERS solid dispersions heated from 25-175 °C. Thus, the inter-associated hydrogen bonding between the free hydroxyl group of E_2 and the ester C=O group of ERS was occurred in solid dispersion of E_2 in ERS in the molten state in which water was removed from the E_2 crystal. This occurrence was in accordance with the prediction by Kwei equation and Nishi-Wang equation.

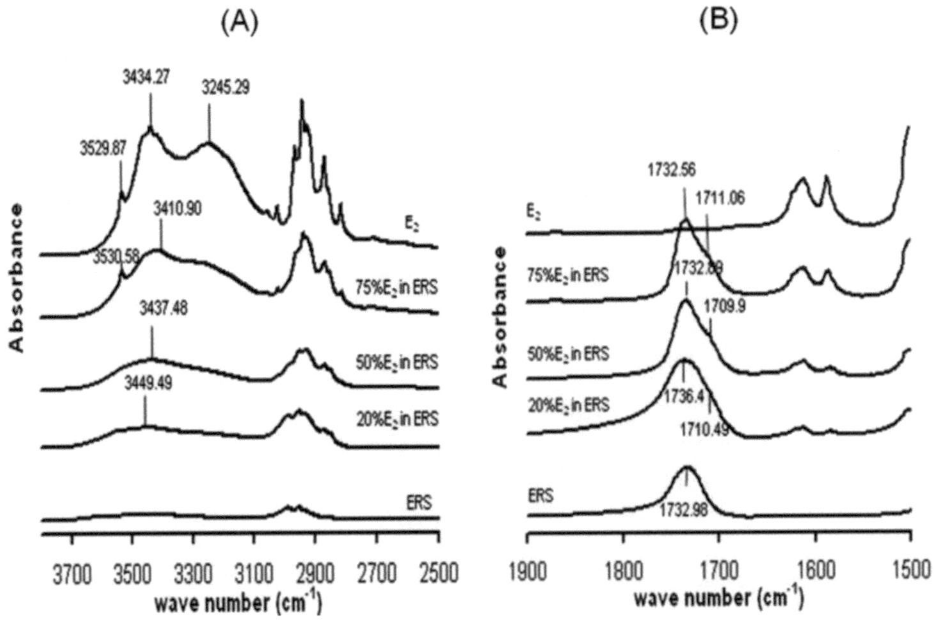

Fig. 12. FTIR spectra of E_2 in ERS solid dispersions at concentration range of 0-100 % w/w heated from 25-175 °C, 5 K/min, recorded at room temperature in the range of 3800-2600 cm^{-1} (A) and 1800-900 cm^{-1} (B) (Reproduced from Wiranidchapong, 2008).

6. Conclusions

E_2 is an essential steroid hormone that regulates numerous endocrine functions secreted during the reproductive years. Early phase in menopause symptoms can be relieved by administration of E_2 mimic the menstrual cycle. The treatment goal requires the lowest effective dose delivered into the blood circulation at a constant rate. This manner can prevent estrogen-insufficient symptoms and/or estrogen-excess symptoms according to peak and trough pattern of plasma estrogen concentration versus time profile. Polymer matrix diffusion controlled-release drug delivery system can provide a relatively constant rate of E_2 release. The accomplishment of a constant release is a result of the inherent solubility of E_2 providing the drug dissolution controlled-release system.
Polymorphic state of E_2 dispersing in the polymer matrix directly affects the solubility of E_2 in the surrounding medium and consequently the rate of E_2 released. Thermal analysis can be used to verify the polymorphic state of E_2 dispersing in the polymer matrix. In the case of amorphous E_2 dispersing in the polymer matrix, the T_g behavior can be described by the principle of Gordon-Taylor equation. On the other hand, the melting point depression of crystalline E_2 dispersing in the polymer matrix can be described by the Flory-Huggins theory. Additionally the interaction between E_2 and ERS used as a polymer matrix can be predicted by both theories.

7. Acknowledgment

This work is performed to celebrate Associate Professor Poj Kulvanich's sixty birthday. I wish to express my gratitude to my Ph.D. supervisor, Associate Professor Poj Kulvanich for providing me an opportunity to do the research at School of Pharmacy, University of Otago, New Zealand in 2005. The virtue of this work is given to Professor Ian Tucker, who makes me know how valuable the fitting model is. My acknowledgment is extended to Professor Thomas Rades, who firstly introduces me the principle of Gordon-Taylor equation. My special thanks are given to Boonta Chutvirasakul, lecturer in Pharmaceutical Chemistry, Faculty of Pharmacy, Srinakharinwirot University for her assistance to proof the language of this work. Finally, I would like to express my gratitude to my mother and older brother for their support and encouragement.

8. References

Abdul, S., and Poddar, S. S. (2004). "A flexible technology for modified release of drugs: Multi layered tablets." J Control Release 97: 393-405.

Anderson, P. O., Knoben, J. E., and Troutman, W. G. (2002). Handbook of clinical drug data, McGraw-Hill.

Andersson, T. L. G., Stehle, B., Davidsson, B., and Höglund, P. (2000). "Drug concentration effect relationship of estradiol from two matrix transdermal delivery systems: Menorest^Ò^ and Climara^Ò^." Maturitas 35: 245-252.

Barnett, S. M., Butler, I. S., Top, S., and Jaouen, G. (1995). "Pressure-tuning infrared and solution Raman spectroscopic studies of 17β-estradiol and several A-ring and 17α-ethynylestradiol derivatives." Vib Spectros 8: 263-277.

Bawaarshi-Hassar, R. N., Hussain, A. A., and Crooks, P. A. (1989). "Nasal absorption and metabolism of progesterone and 17beta-estradiol in the rat." Drug Matab Dispos 17: 248.

Boyd, R. A., Zegarac, E. A., Eldon, M. A. (2003). "The effect of food on the bioavailability of norethindrone and ethinyl estradiol from norethindrone acetate/ethinyl estradiol tablets intended for continuous hormone replacement therapy." J Clin Pharmacol 43(1): 52-58.
Chandrasekaran, S. K., and Paul, D. R. (1982). "Dissolution-controlled transport from dispersed matrixes." J Pharm Sci 71: 1399-1402.
Chien, Y. W. (1982). Novel drug delivery systems: Fundamentals, developmental concepts and biomedical assessments. New York, Marcel Dekker.
Chien, Y. W. (1989). "Rate-control drug delivery systems: Controlled release vs. sustained release." Medical Progress Through Technology 15: 21-46.
Chien, Y. W. (1992). Novel drug delivery system. New York, Marcel Dekker.
Cobby, J., Mayershon, M., and Walker, G. C. (1974). "Influence of shape factors on kinetics of drug release from matrix tablets: I. Theoretical." J Pharm Sci 63: 725-733.
Conte, U., and Maggi, L. (1996). "Modulation of the dissolution profiles from Geomatrix® multi-layer matrix tablets containing drugs of different solubility." Biomaterials 17: 889-896.
Conte, U., and Maggi, L. (2000). "A flexible technology for the linear, pulsatile and delayed release of drugs, allowing for easy accommodation of difficult in vitro targets." J Control Release 64: 263-268.
Conte, U., Maggi, L., Colombo, P., and La Manna, A. (1993). "Multi-layered hydrophilic matrices as constant release devices (Geomatrix™ system)." J Control Release 26: 39-47.
Costa, P., and Lobo, J. M. S. (2001). "Modeling and comparison of dissolution profiles." Eur J Pharm Sci 13: 123-133.
Croxatto, H. B., et. al. (1981). "Plasma levels of levonorgestrel in women during long-term use of Norplant." Contraception 23(197).
Danckwerts, M., and Fassihi, A. (1991). "Implantable controlled release drug delivery systems: A review." Drug Dev Ind Pharm 17: 1465-1502.
Dash, A. K., and Cudworth II, G. C. (1998). "Therapeutic applications of implantable drug delivery systems." Journal of Pharmacological and Toxicological Methods 40(1): 1-12.
Diaz, S., et. al. (1982). "A five-year clinical trial of levonorgestrel silastic implants (Norplant)." Contraception 25: 447.
Dunn, J. F. (1983). Transport of estrogens in human plasma. Catechol Estrogens. G. R. Merriam. New York, Raven: 167-176.
Grant, J., and Park, G. S. (1968). Diffusion in polymers. New York, Academic Press.
Hsieh, D. S. T., Rhine, W. D., and Langer, R. (1983). "Zero-order controlled-release polymer matrices for micro- and macro-molecules." J Pharm Sci 72: 17-22.
Hsieh, D. S. T., Smith, N., and Chien, Y. W. (1987). "Subcutaneous controlled delivery of estradiol by Compudose implants: In vitro and in vivo evaluations." Drug Dev Ind Pharm 13: 2651-2666.
Iwamori, M. (2005). "Estrogen sulfatase." Methods Enzymol 400: 293-302.
Kim, C.-J. (2000). Drug dissolution/diffusion controlled systems. Controlled release dosage form design. C.-J. Kim. Pennsylvania, Technomic Publishing: 75-82.
Kuhl, H. (2005). "Pharmacology of estrogens and progestogens: Influence of different routes of administration." Climacteric 8(Suppl 1): 3-63.
Kuhnz, W., Gansau, C., and Mahler, M. (1993). "Pharmacokinetics of estradiol, free and total estrone, in young women following single intraveneous and oral administration of 17β-estradiol." Arzneim-Forsch/Drug Res 43: 966-973.

Kuo, S. W., and Chang, F. C. (2001a). "Miscibility and hydrogen bonding in blends of poly (vinylphenol-co-methyl methacrylate) with poly (ethylene oxide)." Macomolecules 34: 4089-4097.

Kuo, S. W., Huang, C. F., and Chang, F. C. (2001b). "Study of hydrogen-bonding strength in poly (ε-caprolactone) blends by DSC and FTIR." J Polym Sci Part B: Polym Phys 39: 1348-1359.

Latsch, S., Selzer, T., Fink, L., and Kreuter, J. (2003). "Crystallization of estradiol containing TDDS determined by isothermal microcalorimetry, x-ray diffraction, and optical microscopy." Eur J Pharm Biopharm 56: 43-52.

Longcope, C., Gorbach, S., Goldin, B., Woods, M., Dwyer, J., and Warram, J. (1985). "The metabolism of estradiol; oral compared to intraveneous administration." J Steroid Biochem 23: 1065-1070.

Maggi, L., Bruni, R., and Conte, U. (2000). "High molecular weight polyethylene oxides (PEOs) as an alternative to HPMC in controlled release dosage forms." Int J Pharm 195: 229-238.

Maldonado-Santoyo, M., et al. (2004). "Miscibility behavior and hydrogen bonding in blends of poly (vinyl phenyl ketone hydrogenated) and poly (2-ethyl-2-oxazoline)." J Polym Sci Part B: Polym Phys 42: 636-645.

Margolis, M. B. (2010). "How drug delivery and pharmacokinetics impact estrogen therapy." The Female Patient(Suppl 5): 1-8.

Meli, A., Cargill, D. I., Giannina, T., and Steinetz, B. G. (1968). "Studies on the transport of estrogens by the rat small intestine in vivo." Proc Soc Exp Biol Med 129: 937-944.

Mueck, A. O., and Seeger, H. (2003). "Smoking, estradiol metabolism and hormone replacement therapy." Arzneimittelforschung 53(1): 1-11.

Munoz, A. (1999). "Oesclim©: An advanced delivery system for HRT." Maturitas 33(s39-s47).

Niazi, S. K. (2007). Handbook of Preformulation: Chemical, Biological, and Botanical Drugs. New York, Informa Healthcare USA.

Nishi, T., and Wang, T. T. (1975). "Melting point depression and kinetic effects of cooling on crystallization in poly(vinylidine fluoride)-poly(methyl methacrylate) mixtures." Macromolecules 8: 909-915.

Paoletti, A. M., Pilia, I., Nannipieri, F., Bigini, C., and Melis, G. B. (2001). "Comparison of pharmacokinetic profiles of a 17β-estradiol gel 0.6 mg/g (Gelestra) with a transdermal delivery system (Estraderm TTS 50) in postmenopausal women at steady state." Maturitas 40: 203-209.

Pardridge, W. M. (1986). "Serum bioavailability of sex steroid hormones." Clin Endocrinol Metab 15: 259-278.

Park, J.-S., Kang, H. W., Park, S. J., and Kim, C-K. (2005). "Use of CP/MAS solid-state NMR for the characterization of solvate molecules within estradiol crystal forms." Eur J Pharm Biopharm 60: 407-412.

Pentikis, H. S., Mullin, M. E., Howard, M., Boutouyrie, B., and Rhodes, G. (1998). "Evaluation of the bioavailability and dose proportionality of three formulations of a combination estrogen and progestin adhesive-based matrix transdermal delivery system." Curr Ther Res 59: 681-691.

Pignatello, F., M., and Puglisi, G. (2002). "Preparation of solid dispersions of nonsteroidal anti-inflammatory drugs with acrylic polymers and studies on mechanisms of drug-polymer interactions." AAPS Pharm Sci Tech 3: 1-11.

Pimbert, S., Avignon-Poquillon, L., and Levesque, G. (2002). "Calorimetric study of fluorinated methacrylic and vinyl polymer blends: Part 2: Correlation between

miscibility, chemical structure and c_{12} interaction parameter in binary systems." Polymer 43: 3295-3302.
Plowchalk, D. R., and Teeguarden, J. (2002). "Development of a physiologically based pharmacokinetic model for estradiol in rats and humans: A biologically motivated quantitative framework for evaluating responses to estradiol and other endocrine-active compounds." Toxicological Sciences 69: 60-78.
Rippie, E. G., and Johnson, J. R. (1969). "Regulation of dissolution rate by pellet geometry." J Pharm Sci 58: 428-431.
Rohr, U. D., Nauert. C., and Stehle, B. (1999). "17β-estradiol delivered by three different matrix patches 50 mg/day: A three way cross-over study in 21 postmenopausal women." Maturitas 33: 45-48.
Rostami, S. D. (2000). "Advances in theory of equilibrium melting point depression in miscible polymer blends." Eur Polym J 36: 2285-2290.
Schneider, H. A. (1988). "The Gordon-Taylor equation. Additivity and interaction in compatible polymer blends." Makromol Chem 189: 1941-1955.
Segal, S. J. (1983). "The development of Norplant implants." Studies in Family Planning 14: 161.
Serajuddin, A. T. M. (1999). "Solid dispersion of poorly water-soluble drugs: Early promises, subsequent problems, and recent breakthroughs." J Pharm Sci 88: 1058-1066.
Shargel, L., and Yu, A. (1999). Applied biopharmaceutics and pharmacokinetics. New Jersey, Prentice-Hall International.
Siepmann, J., and Peppas, N. (2001). "Modeling of drug release from delivery systems based on hydroxypropyl methylcellulose (HPMC)." Adv Drug Deliv Rev 48: 139-157.
Silverstein, R. M., Bessler, G. C., and Morrill, T. C. (1991). Infrared spectrometry. Spectrometric identification of organic compounds. J. Stiefel. Singapore, John Wiley and Sons: 91-164.
Utian, W. H., Archer, D. F., Bachmann, G. A., et al; North American Menopause Society (2008). "Estrogen and progestogen use in postmenopausal women: July 2008 position statement of the North American Menopause Society." Menopause 15(4(pt 1)): 584-602.
Vandelli, M. A., and Cameroni, R. (1993a). "Selective coating of cylindrical matrices with a central hole. I. An interpretation of the swelling process." Int J Pharm 100: 107-114.
Vandelli, M. A., Coppi, G., and Cameroni, R. (1993b). "Selective coating of cylindrical matrices with a central hole. II. An interpretation of the release process." Int J Pharm 100: 115-121.
Variankaval, N. E., Jacob, K. I., and Dinh, S. M. (2000). "Characterization of crystal forms of β-estradiol-thermal analysis, Raman microscopy, X-ray analysis and solid-state NMR." J Cryst Growth 217: 320-331.
Weiner, E., et. al. (1981). "Plasma levels of d-norgestrel after oral administration." Contraception 23: 197.
Wiranidchapong, C. (2006). Development of 17b-estradiol and norethindrone implants using acrylate polymers as release controlling agent Pharmaceutics. Bangkok, Chulalongkorn University. Doctor of Philosophy in Pharmaceutics: 107.
Wiranidchapong, C., Rades, T., Tucker, I. G., Kulvanich, P. (2009). "Method of preparation does not affect the miscibility between steroid hormone and polymethacrylate." Thermochimica Acta 485: 57-64.
Wiranidchapong, C., Tucker, I. G., Rades, T., Kulvanich, P. (2008). "Miscibility and interactions between 17b-estradiol and Eudragit® RS in solid dispersion." J Pharm Sci 97(11): 4879-4888.